Sarcoma: Diagnosis and Treatment

Sarcoma: Diagnosis and Treatment

Edited by Serenity Hodges

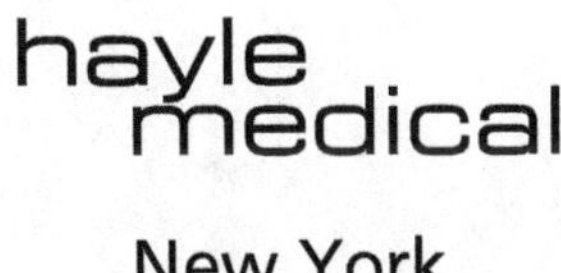

New York

Hayle Medical,
750 Third Avenue, 9th Floor,
New York, NY 10017, USA

Visit us on the World Wide Web at:
www.haylemedical.com

ISBN: 978-1-63241-901-9

Cataloging-in-Publication Data

Sarcoma : diagnosis and treatment / edited by Serenity Hodges.
p. cm.
Includes bibliographical references and index.
ISBN 978-1-63241-901-9
1. Sarcoma. 2. Sarcoma--Diagnosis. 3. Sarcoma--Treatment. 4. Cancer. 5. Tumors. I. Hodges, Serenity.
RC270 .S27 2020
616.994--dc23

Table of Contents

Preface

A sarcoma is the cancer of the transformed cells of mesenchymal origin. All malignant tumors of cancellous bone, fat, cartilage, muscle, vascular or hematopoietic tissues are considered sarcomas. These are named based on the tissue of origin and are assigned a grade depending on the presence of cellular and subcellular characteristics that are associated with malignant biological behavior as well as their frequency. High-grade tumors can undergo metastasis and therefore need aggressive treatment. Surgery is important in the treatment of sarcomas. Other treatments such as chemotherapy and radiation therapy may also be administered, whether before or after surgery. These can improve prognosis and increase chances of survival. This book unravels the recent studies in sarcoma. It unfolds the innovative aspects in the management of sarcoma which will be crucial for the progress of oncology in the future. It will help new researchers by foregrounding their knowledge in this medical condition.

This book is a comprehensive compilation of works of different researchers from varied parts of the world. It includes valuable experiences of the researchers with the sole objective of providing the readers (learners) with a proper knowledge of the concerned field. This book will be beneficial in evoking inspiration and enhancing the knowledge of the interested readers.

In the end, I would like to extend my heartiest thanks to the authors who worked with great determination on their chapters. I also appreciate the publisher's support in the course of the book. I would also like to deeply acknowledge my family who stood by me as a source of inspiration during the project.

Editor

1

The use of Radiation Therapy in Well-Differentiated Soft Tissue Sarcoma of the Extremities

Alexander L. Lazarides,[1] William C. Eward,[2] Paul J. Speicher,[3] Chun-Han Hou,[4] Daniel P. Nussbaum,[3] Cindy Green,[2] Dan G. Blazer III,[3] David G. Kirsch,[5] and Brian E. Brigman[2]

[1]*School of Medicine, Duke University, Durham, NC 27710, USA*
[2]*Department of Surgery, Division of Orthopedic Surgery, Duke University Medical Center, Durham, NC 27710, USA*
[3]*Department of Surgery, Duke University Medical Center, Durham, NC 27710, USA*
[4]*Department of Orthopedic Surgery, National Taiwan University Hospital, Taipei 10617, Taiwan*
[5]*Department of Radiation Oncology, Duke University Medical Center, Durham, NC 27710, USA*

Correspondence should be addressed to William C. Eward; william.eward@dm.duke.edu

Academic Editor: Peter C. Ferguson

Objective. This study investigated patterns of utilization of radiation therapy (RT) and correlated this with overall survival by assessing patients with well-differentiated soft tissue sarcoma of the extremity (STS-E) in the National Cancer Database (NCDB). *Methods*. All patients diagnosed with well-differentiated STS-E between 1998 and 2006 were identified in the NCDB. Patients were stratified by use of surgery alone versus use of adjuvant RT after surgery and analyzed using multivariate analysis, Kaplan-Meier analysis, and propensity matching. *Results*. 2113 patients with well-differentiated STS-E were identified in the NCDB for inclusion with a mean follow-up time of 74 months. 69% of patients were treated with surgery alone, while 26% were treated with surgery followed by adjuvant RT. Patients undergoing amputation were less likely to receive adjuvant RT. There was no difference in overall survival between patients with well-differentiated STS treated with surgery alone and those patients who received adjuvant RT. *Conclusions*. In the United States, adjuvant RT is being utilized in a quarter of patients being treated for well-differentiated STS-E. While the use of adjuvant RT may be viewed as a means to facilitate limb salvage, this large national database review confirms no survival benefit, regardless of tumor size or margin status.

1. Introduction

Soft tissue sarcomas (STS) are a heterogeneous group of rare tumors that share a mesenchymal origin. Despite a low incidence of less than 1% of new cases per year [1, 2], sarcoma is disproportionately lethal, which is mostly attributable to the development of pulmonary metastasis [3]. Established prognostic factors for poor outcomes in patients with STS of the extremities (STS-E) include grade, size, depth, and patient age [4, 5]. Of these, tumor grade is probably the most sensitive indicator of a tumor's biological behavior and the strongest predictor of metastasis and death from disease [6, 7]. Well-differentiated tumors have dramatically different biological behavior from their intermediate- and high-grade counterparts. Patients with well-differentiated STS-E have a much lower likelihood of developing metastasis and dying from disease. For such patients, the role of adjuvant radiation therapy (RT) has been to limit local recurrence rather than have an impact upon survival [8, 9].

When adjuvant RT should be utilized in the treatment of well-differentiated STS-E, or if it should be utilized at all, it remains a matter of controversy. The goals of treatment are achieving local control, preserving function of the involved limb, and reducing the risk of death from disease. Radiation therapy is regarded as unlikely to reduce the already low risk for death from disease and it has the potential to worsen function of the involved limb. For these reasons, some physicians believe that the risks of RT outweigh its potential benefits with regard to well-differentiated STS-E [10]. In a recent review of the SEER database, Koshy et al. reported that adjuvant radiation utilization was associated with a survival benefit for high grade, but not low grade STS [11].

At present, the National Comprehensive Cancer Network NCCN guidelines state that, regardless of depth, low grade tumors less than 5 cm should be treated with surgery alone; consideration may be given for RT if margins are inadequate, which is defined by the NCCN as a goal of margins >1 cm [12]. Low grade tumors greater than 5 cm should be treated with surgery and RT for all patients whose margins are inadequate. Given that an exact amount of margin that is sufficient has never been determined, it is probably impractical to make blanket recommendations for RT utilization, especially for low-grade tumors where survival is not likely to be affected. Using the large patient cohort with well-differentiated STS captured by the National Cancer Database (NCDB), the goals of our project were to investigate patterns of utilization of RT with regard to several known prognostic factors and to correlate the use of RT on survival in this subset of patients.

2. Methods

The Duke University Institutional Review Board approved this retrospective analysis of the American College of Surgeons/American Cancer Society National Cancer Data Base (NCDB). More than 1500 Commission on Cancer- (CoC-) accredited facilities contributed to this registry, accounting for a large majority of new cases of cancer every year in the USA. To identify patients who underwent resection of an extremity soft tissue sarcoma, the NCDB Participant User File for 1998 through 2011 was utilized first queried for all patients treated at a NCDB participating institution for tumors in the arms or legs with International Classification of Diseases for Oncology, 3rd Edition (ICD-O-3) topography codes C47.1, C47.2, C49.1, and C49.2. Relevant histologic subtypes were selected based on a series of ICD-O-3 histology codes, all of which represented soft-tissue sarcomas. Other inclusion criteria included malignant behavior, primary cancer diagnosis, no distant metastasis, and known status for preoperative radiation therapy.

National trends in the rate of adjuvant RT, defined by the NCDB as "radiation therapy given after surgery to the primary site," were examined with the Cochran-Armitage trend test in patients with well-differentiated soft tissue sarcomas of the extremities. The use of adjuvant RT was then used to classify subjects into two groups. Baseline characteristics and outcomes between groups were compared using Pearson's chi-square test for categorical variables and analysis of variance (ANOVA) for continuous variables. Multivariable logistic regression was used to predict factors that were associated with the administration of adjuvant RT. Patients who received neoadjuvant RT, defined by the NCDB as "radiation therapy given before surgery to the primary site," were excluded to avoid potential biases in a comparison of sarcomas graded from a biopsy prior to preoperative radiation therapy with sarcomas graded from the entire resected tumor. Furthermore, grading sarcomas after preoperative radiation therapy and resection could be altered by radiation effects. To control for confounding in the use of adjuvant RT, we used propensity matching, which is defined as "conditional probability of assignment to a particular treatment given a vector of observed covariates" [13]. Using this system, we developed propensity scores, which were defined as the a priori conditional probability of being treated with RT prior to surgery. Patients were then matched on these propensity scores, using a 1 : 1 nearest neighbor algorithm, which included the following variables: age, sex, race, Charlson/Deyo comorbidity score, patient census tract education and income levels, tumor size, histologic subtype, histologic grade, tumor location (upper versus lower extremity), treatment facility type (academic or community hospital), and extent of resection. Adjusted medians and proportions between the propensity-matched groups were then compared. With propensity-matched analyses, we hoped to employ a method that corrects, at least partially, for confounding factors.

To ensure the accuracy of survival data, the NCDB only provides vital status for patients five years following the date of surgery. Therefore, survival from the time of diagnosis was assessed for all patients who underwent resection prior to 2007. Prior to analysis, subjects who underwent resection from 1998 to 2006 were rematched using the aforementioned variables. Then, long-term survival among groups was evaluated using the Kaplan-Meier method with comparisons based on the log-rank test.

A more specific analysis was carried out for patients with margin negative tumors and margin positive tumors. Within these groups, an analysis was carried out for size smaller than 5 cm and size greater than 5 cm. The above analyses were again repeated with patients with well-differentiated liposarcoma of the extremities only. It is not possible to determine rates of local recurrence for patients with STS-E enrolled in this database.

Results are reported as median (IQR), proportions (%), and odds ratios (OR, 95% CI) as applicable. p values < 0.05 indicate statistical significance, and we controlled for type I error at the level of the comparison. All statistical analyses were performed using R (the R Foundation for Statistical Computing, version 3.0.2, Vienna, Austria).

3. Results

3.1. Demographics and Patient Characteristics. A total of 2340 patients were identified in the NCDB who had undergone resection of an STS-E with a well-differentiated histologic grade. Five hundred seventy-three patients (27%) received adjuvant RT; 1540 patients (73%) were treated with surgery alone. A small number of patients ($n = 98$) who received neoadjuvant RT or combined neoadjuvant and adjuvant ($n = 12$) were excluded due to the potential challenge in grading the sarcoma following definitive resection because of radiation effect. Furthermore, 98 patients had missing RT treatment data and were therefore excluded from the study, leaving a remaining 2113 patients to be evaluated.

Baseline characteristics are shown in Table 1. There were no statistically significant differences between groups with regard to age, sex, distance to cancer center, preoperative

TABLE 1: Baseline characteristics for all patients with well-differentiated tumors.

Variable	Overall (n = 2113)	Surgery alone (n = 1540)	Adjuvant RT (n = 573)	p value
Patient characteristics				
Age, yrs. (IQR)	55 (43, 68)	55 (43, 69)	54 (43, 67)	0.419
Female	1,035 (48%)	752 (48.1%)	283 (47.8%)	0.957
Race				0.792
White	1,774 (84%)	1,290 (84%)	484 (84%)	
Black	255 (12.1%)	188 (12.2%)	67 (11.6%)	
Other	83 (3.9%)	58 (3.8%)	25 (4.3%)	
Charlson Comorbidity Score				0.777
0	1,265 (88.6%)	908 (88.3%)	357 (89.5%)	
1	140 (9.8%)	103 (10%)	37 (9.3%)	
≥2	22 (1.5%)	17 (1.7%)	5 (1.3%)	
Education above median	1,239 (60.9%)	878 (59.7%)	361 (63.9%)	0.091
Income above median	1,406 (69.1%)	1,005 (68.3%)	401 (71%)	0.269
Distance to cancer center (IQR)	13.4 (5.6, 36.4)	14.7 (5.7, 41.3)	10.9 (5.1, 24.6)	0.611
Treatment facility				0.288
Community Cancer Program	117 (5.5%)	82 (5.4%)	35 (6%)	
Comprehensive Community Cancer Program	827 (39.2%)	585 (38.3%)	242 (41.5%)	
Academic/Research Program	1,165 (55.2%)	859 (56.3%)	306 (52.5%)	
Uninsured	76 (3.7%)	53 (3.5%)	23 (4%)	0.697
Tumor characteristics				
Limb location				0.61
Upper limb and shoulder	499 (23.1%)	367 (23.5%)	132 (22.3%)	
Lower limb and hip	1,658 (76.9%)	1,198 (76.5%)	460 (77.7%)	
Tumor size (mm)	90 (40, 170)	84 (35, 170)	97 (50, 159.2)	0.504
Tumor size				**<0.001**
<5 cm	582 (31.3%)	449 (33.9%)	133 (24.7%)	
5–9.9 cm	406 (21.8%)	268 (20.2%)	138 (25.7%)	
10–19.9 cm	527 (28.3%)	344 (26%)	183 (34%)	
>20.0 cm	347 (18.6%)	263 (19.9%)	84 (15.6%)	
Histology				**0.001**
Clear cell sarcoma	4 (0.2%)	4 (0.3%)	0 (0%)	
Epithelioid sarcoma	8 (0.4%)	5 (0.3%)	3 (0.5%)	
Fibrosarcoma	91 (4.2%)	73 (4.7%)	18 (3%)	
Leiomyosarcoma	231 (10.7%)	185 (11.8%)	46 (7.8%)	
Liposarcoma	1,418 (65.7%)	1,014 (64.8%)	404 (68.2%)	
Malignant fibrous histiocytoma	103 (4.8%)	70 (4.5%)	33 (5.6%)	
Mixed mesenchymal sarcoma	3 (0.1%)	3 (0.2%)	0 (0%)	
MPNST	64 (3%)	44 (2.8%)	20 (3.4%)	
Myxosarcoma	19 (0.9%)	9 (0.6%)	10 (1.7%)	
Rhabdomyosarcoma	2 (0.1%)	1 (0.1%)	1 (0.2%)	
Sarcoma NOS	122 (5.7%)	98 (6.3%)	24 (4.1%)	
Small cell sarcoma	2 (0.1%)	0 (0%)	2 (0.3%)	
Spindle cell sarcoma	45 (2.1%)	33 (2.1%)	12 (2%)	
Synovial sarcoma	44 (2%)	25 (1.6%)	19 (3.2%)	
Undifferentiated sarcoma	1 (0%)	1 (0.1%)	0 (0%)	

TABLE 1: Continued.

Variable	Overall (n = 2113)	Surgery alone (n = 1540)	Adjuvant RT (n = 573)	p value
Treatment specifics				
Surgery type				**0.002**
Local excision	723 (33.5%)	525 (33.5%)	198 (33.4%)	
Radication resection	1,365 (63.3%)	976 (62.4%)	389 (65.7%)	
Limb amputation	65 (3%)	60 (3.8%)	5 (0.8%)	
Major amputation	4 (0.2%)	4 (0.3%)	0 (0%)	
Amputation (versus no amputation)	69 (3.2%)	64 (4.1%)	5 (0.8%)	**<0.001**
Days to definitive surgery (IQR)	0 (0, 34)	0 (0, 33)	10 (0, 35.2)	0.598
Neoadjuvant chemo	1 (0.3%)	0 (0%)	1 (1.2%)	0.256
Adjuvant chemo	6 (1.8%)	1 (0.4%)	5 (6%)	**0.005**
Endpoints and outcomes				
Surgical margins				**0.001**
Negative	1,534 (78.5%)	1,133 (80.5%)	401 (73.3%)	
Microscopic	234 (12%)	146 (10.4%)	88 (16.1%)	
Macroscopic	186 (9.5%)	128 (9.1%)	58 (10.6%)	
30-day readmission	35 (2.6%)	27 (2.7%)	8 (2.1%)	0.626
Hospital LOS (IQR)	1 (0, 3)	1 (0, 3)	1 (0, 3)	0.427

comorbidities, income, or education. Additionally, there were no statistically significant differences in Charlson Comorbidity Scores between the two groups.

3.2. Tumor Characteristics and Treatment Choices. With regard to tumor characteristics, patients who received adjuvant RT were more likely to have tumors larger than 5 cm ($p <$ 0.001, Table 1). When categorized by histologic subtype, adjuvant RT was more commonly utilized in patients with liposarcoma (68.2% receiving adjuvant RT versus 64.8% receiving surgery alone), malignant fibrous histiocytoma (5.6% versus 4.5%), MPNST (3.4% versus 2.8%), and myxosarcoma (1.7% versus 0.6%) when compared to other histologic subtypes. Patients who underwent adjuvant RT were also more likely to have received adjuvant chemotherapy than those who did not receive adjuvant RT (6% versus 0.4%, p = 0.005). They were also more likely to undergo radical resections (65.7% versus 62.4%, p = 0.002) than local excisions. Of the 69 patients treated with an amputation, 64 of those were treated with surgery alone. Only 5 patients (0.8% of the RT group) were managed with a combination of amputation and adjuvant RT. Patients with microscopically or macroscopically positive margins were more likely to receive adjuvant RT (26.7% versus 19.5%, p = 0.001) (Table 1). A multivariable logistic regression analysis found no independent predictors of adjuvant RT use (Table 1). There were no differences in surgery type, surgical margins, 30-day mortality, readmission rates, or hospital length of stay.

3.3. Survival Outcomes. Five-year survival from the time of diagnosis for all patients (n = 2113; Figure 1(a)) was not statistically different between patients treated with surgery alone and patients receiving adjuvant RT (89.5% versus 92.1%, p = 0.614). These patients were rematched on the propensity to receive adjuvant RT, adjusting for confounding variables (Table 3). Again, the analysis showed no statistically significant differences in survival (89.5% versus 92.2%, p = 0.984).

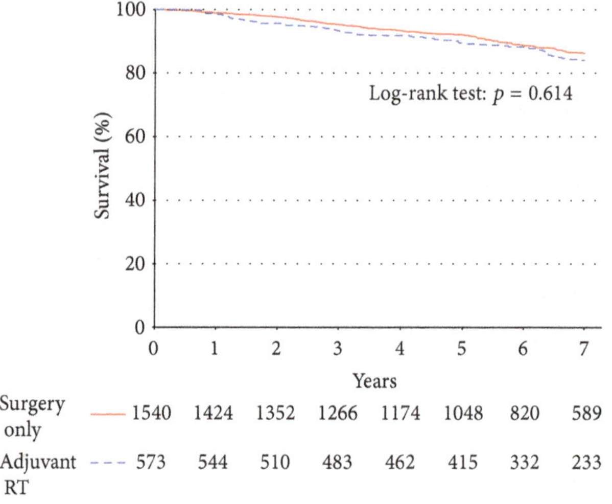

FIGURE 1: There is no difference in unadjusted survival for patients with well-differentiated tumors when stratified by adjuvant RT versus surgery alone.

For patients who had a negative surgical margin (n = 1496; Figure 2(a)), there was no statistically significant difference in 5-year survival rates based on the addition of adjuvant RT (91.6% versus 94.5%, p = 0.887). These patients were rematched on the propensity to receive adjuvant RT, adjusting for confounding variables (Table 3). This showed no statistically significant survival difference for patients treated with adjuvant RT (91.6% versus 94.5%, p = 0.85).

TABLE 2: Baseline characteristics for patients with well-differentiated liposarcoma only.

Variable	Overall (n = 1418)	No RT (n = 1014)	Adjuvant only (n = 404)	p value
Patient characteristics				
Age, yrs. (IQR)	57 (45, 70)	57 (46, 70)	54 (44, 68)	**0.006**
Female	676 (47.7%)	484 (47.7%)	192 (47.5%)	0.991
Race				0.875
White	1,171 (84.2%)	837 (84%)	334 (84.6%)	
Black	160 (11.5%)	117 (11.7%)	43 (10.9%)	
Other	60 (4.3%)	42 (4.2%)	18 (4.6%)	
Charlson Comorbidity Score				0.791
0—none	836 (88.2%)	600 (88%)	236 (88.7%)	
1—one point	97 (10.2%)	72 (10.6%)	25 (9.4%)	
2—two or more points	15 (1.6%)	10 (1.5%)	5 (1.9%)	
Education above median	820 (61.2%)	576 (60.4%)	244 (63.2%)	0.367
Income above median	922 (68.8%)	647 (67.8%)	275 (71.2%)	0.246
Distance to cancer center (IQR)	14.2 (5.8, 39.5)	15.5 (6.2, 44.5)	11 (5.3, 26.8)	0.867
Treatment facility				**0.021**
Community Cancer Program	74 (5.3%)	47 (4.8%)	27 (6.8%)	
Comprehensive Community Cancer Program	534 (38.5%)	364 (36.8%)	170 (42.6%)	
Academic/Research Program	780 (56.2%)	578 (58.4%)	202 (50.6%)	
Uninsured	43 (3.1%)	30 (3.1%)	13 (3.3%)	0.956
Tumor characteristics				
Limb location				0.856
Upper limb and shoulder	212 (15%)	150 (14.8%)	62 (15.3%)	
Lower limb and hip	1,206 (85%)	864 (85.2%)	342 (84.7%)	
Tumor size (mm)	130 (70, 200)	133 (70, 200)	121 (71.5, 185)	**0.009**
Tumor size				**0.002**
5 cm	197 (15.7%)	149 (16.9%)	48 (12.8%)	
5–9.9 cm	262 (20.9%)	173 (19.7%)	89 (23.7%)	
10.0–19.9 cm	457 (36.4%)	300 (34.1%)	157 (41.9%)	
>20.0 cm	339 (27%)	258 (29.3%)	81 (21.6%)	
Histology				0.999
Liposarcoma	1,418 (100%)	1,014 (100%)	404 (100%)	
Treatment specifics				
Surgery type				0.439
Local excision	461 (32.5%)	337 (33.2%)	124 (30.7%)	
Radical resection	938 (66.1%)	661 (65.2%)	277 (68.6%)	
Limb amputation	18 (1.3%)	15 (1.5%)	3 (0.7%)	0.31
Major amputation	1 (0.1%)	1 (0.1%)	0 (0%)	
Days to definitive surgery (IQR)	0 (0, 27)	0 (0, 24)	9 (0, 34.5)	0.393
Selection of adjuvant RT by surgical margin				
Surgical margins				**0.014**
Negative	946 (74.9%)	684 (76.7%)	262 (70.6%)	
Positive margin, microscopic	182 (14.4%)	112 (12.6%)	70 (18.9%)	
Positive margin, macroscopic	135 (10.7%)	96 (10.8%)	39 (10.5%)	
30-day readmission	25 (2.7%)	21 (3.2%)	4 (1.6%)	0.257
Hospital LOS (IQR)	1 (0, 3)	1 (0, 3)	1 (0, 3)	0.452

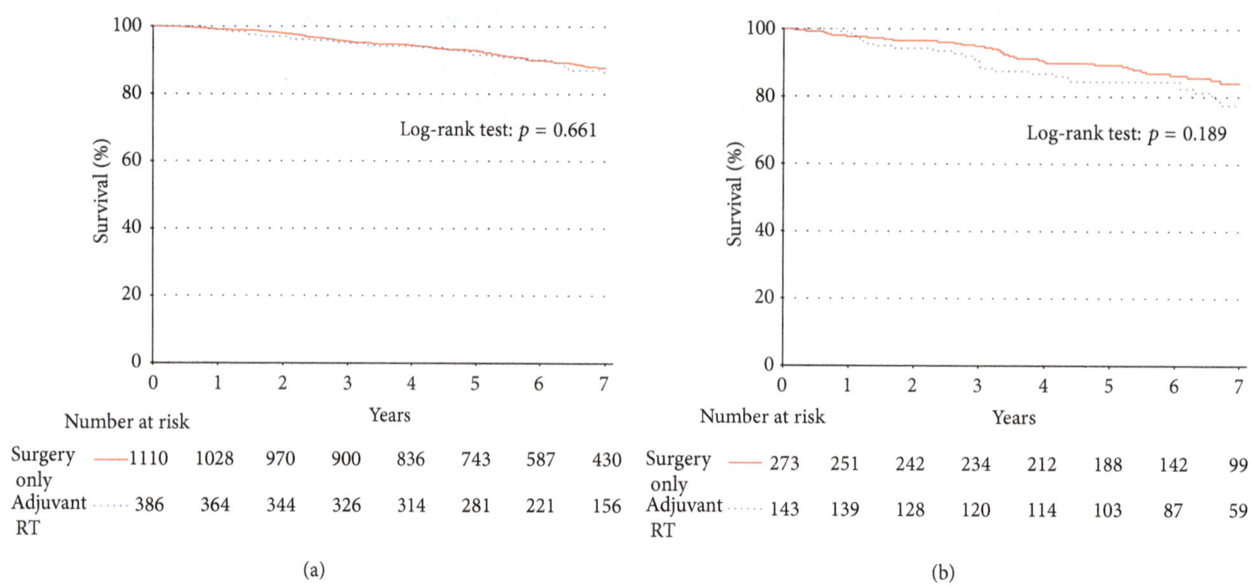

FIGURE 2: There is no difference in unadjusted survival for (a) patients with well-differentiated tumors when stratified by adjuvant RT versus surgery on the basis of negative margins. There was also no difference when stratified on the basis of positive margins (b).

TABLE 3: Five year propensity matched survival.

Grouping	Number of patients	Surgery only	Adjuvant RT	p value
Well-differentiated tumors when stratified by adjuvant RT versus surgery alone	1146	92.2% (89.9–94.6%)	89.5% (86.9–92.2%)	0.984
Well-differentiated tumors when stratified by adjuvant RT versus surgery on the basis of negative margins	772	94.5% (92–97%)	91.6% (88.7–94.6%)	0.85
Well-differentiated tumors when stratified by adjuvant RT versus surgery on the basis of positive margins	286	92.4% (88–97.1%)	84.4% (78.5–90.8%)	0.096
Well-differentiated liposarcoma when stratified by adjuvant RT versus surgery alone	808	91.7% (88.8–94.7%)	90% (87–93.1%)	0.84
Well-differentiated liposarcoma when stratified by adjuvant RT versus surgery on the basis of negative margins	524	93.7% (90.6–97%)	91.3% (87.7–95%)	0.891
Well-differentiated liposarcoma when stratified by adjuvant RT versus surgery on the basis of positive margins	218	90.8% (85.3–96.7%)	87.5% (81.4–94.1%)	0.735

For patients who had a positive surgical margin (n = 416; Figure 2(b)), there were also no statistically significant differences in survival rates for patients treated with adjuvant RT (84.4% versus 89.4%, p = 0.189). These patients were rematched on the propensity to receive adjuvant RT, adjusting for confounding variables (Table 3). No statistically significant survival difference was shown for patients treated with adjuvant RT (84.4% versus 92.4%, $p = 0.096$).

For patients with large (greater than 5 cm) tumors, use of adjuvant RT had no influence on survival. Survival was plotted among all patients who had margin-negative, well-differentiated tumors less than 5 cm (n = 464; Figure 3(a)) and greater than 5 cm ($n = 862$; Figure 3(b)). This revealed no statistically significant difference in survival rates for patients receiving the adjuvant RT (90.7% versus 95.1%, $p = 0.648$ and 91.9% versus 91.8%, $p = 0.296$), respectively, for these groups.

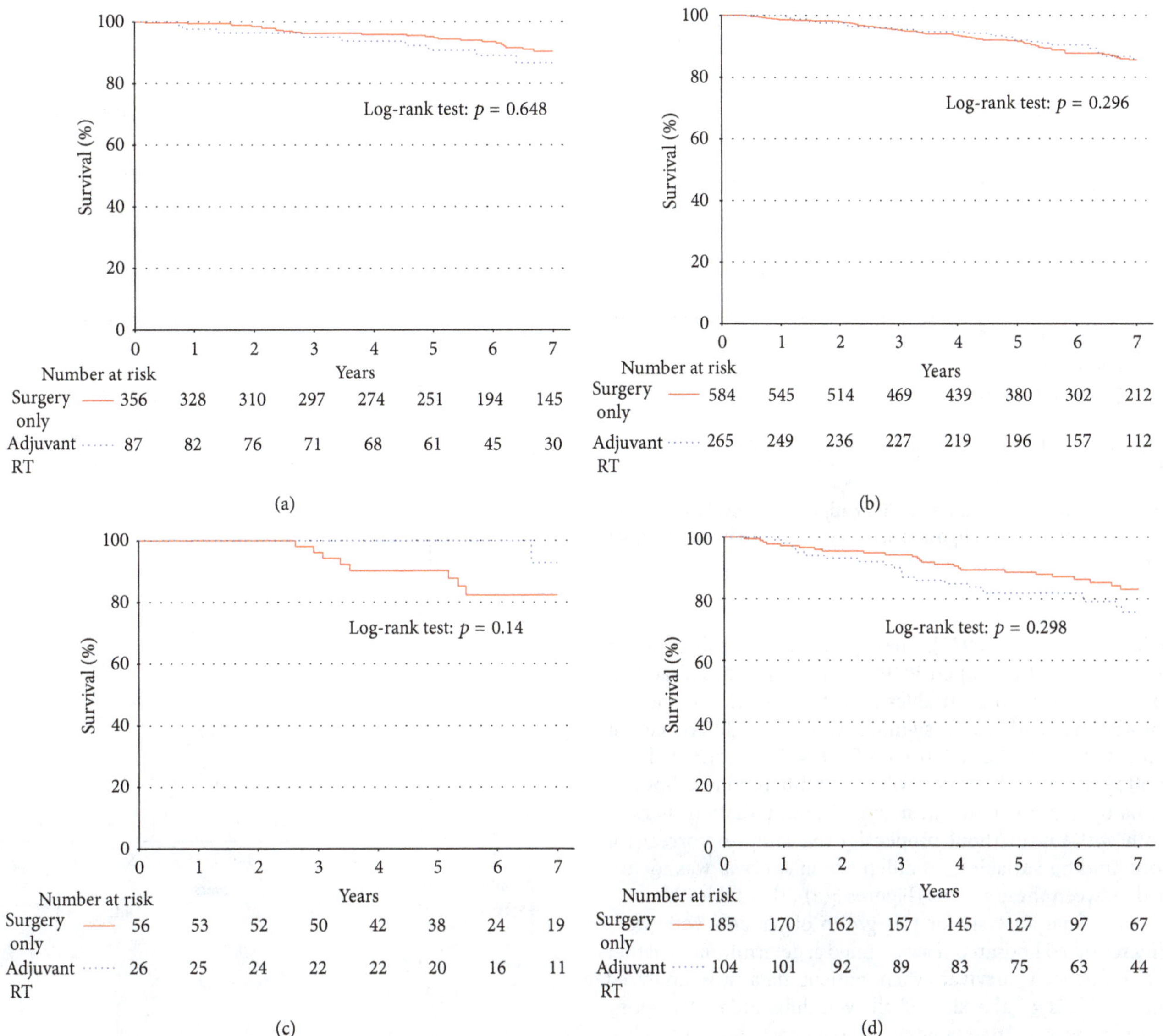

FIGURE 3: There is no difference in unadjusted survival for patients with well-differentiated tumors when stratified by adjuvant RT versus surgery on the basis of size <5 cm (a) and >5 cm (b) for patients with negative margin status. There was also no difference when stratified on the basis of size in patients with positive margin status ((c) and (d), resp.).

A similar analysis was carried out for patients who underwent surgery who had margin-positive well-differentiated tumors less than 5 cm ($n = 84$; Figure 3(c)) and greater than 5 cm ($n = 291$; Figure 3(d)). There were no statistically significant differences in survival rates for patients receiving adjuvant RT compared to those who did not (100% versus 90.2%, $p = 0.14$ and 81.8% versus 88.6%, $p = 0.298$) in each of these two groups.

3.4. Well-Differentiated Liposarcoma. Because the well-differentiated liposarcoma is its own unique and common subtype [14], we repeated our analysis to evaluate the large group of patients with this tumor. Out of the initial 2157 patient cohort, a total of 1418 patients were identified who had undergone resection of a well-differentiated liposarcoma of an extremity. Subjects were again grouped by surgery with adjuvant RT (404 patients, 28%) versus surgery alone (1014 patients, 72%). Baseline characteristics are shown in Table 2. Patients who underwent adjuvant RT were more likely to be older (57 versus 54 years old, $p = 0.006$). There were no statistically significant differences in sex, distance to cancer center, tumor characteristics, preoperative comorbidities, income, education, or Charlson Comorbidity Scores. After surgery, there were no statistically significant differences between groups with regard to margin status, 30-day hospital readmission or hospital LOS (Table 2).

Survival from the time of diagnosis was evaluated for all patients who underwent resection of a well-differentiated liposarcoma. First, survival was plotted among all patients who underwent surgery during this period ($n = 1418$; Figure 4), which revealed no statistically significant difference in survival rates for patients receiving the addition

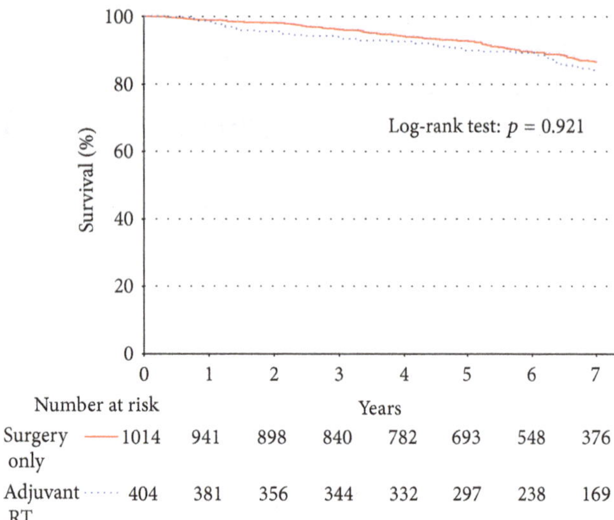

FIGURE 4: There is no difference in unadjusted survival for patients with well-differentiated liposarcoma when stratified by adjuvant RT versus surgery alone.

adjuvant RT (p = 0.921). These patients were subsequently rematched on the propensity to receive adjuvant RT, adjusting for confounding variables (Table 3). Again, the analysis showed no statistically significant survival difference for patients treated with adjuvant RT (p = 0.84). Survival was plotted among all patients with well-differentiated liposarcoma by margin status, with and without radiation therapy. Both with and without propensity matching to correct for confounding variables, no difference in survival was identified between these groups (Figures 5(a)-5(b), Table 3).

Our final analysis for this group of patients with well-differentiated liposarcoma was aimed at determining whether RT influenced survival when patient data was analyzed on the basis of the size of all well-differentiated tumors. Survival was plotted among all patients who underwent surgery during this period who had margin-negative well-differentiated tumors less than 5 cm (n = 148; Figure 6(a)) and greater than 5 cm (n = 697; Figure 6(b)). These analyses revealed no statistically significant differences in the survival rates for patients receiving the adjuvant RT for either of these groups (less than 5 cm: 90.9% versus 95.4%, p = 0.862 and greater than 5 cm: 89.2% versus 92%, p = 0.789). A similar analysis was carried out for patients who underwent surgery who had margin-positive well-differentiated tumors less than 5 cm (n = 35; Figure 6(c)) and greater than 5 cm (n = 251; Figure 6(d)). Again no statistically significant differences in 5-year survival rates were observed for patients receiving the adjuvant RT in either group (less than 5 cm: 100% versus 90.2%, p = 0.159 and greater than 5 cm: 85.4% versus 89.2%, p = 0.948).

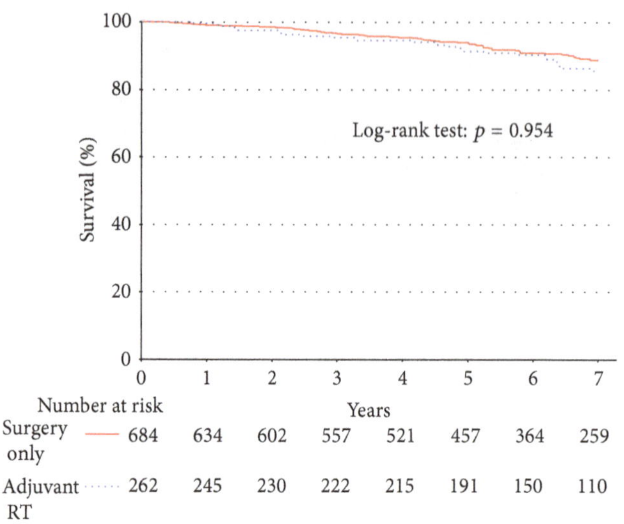

(a)

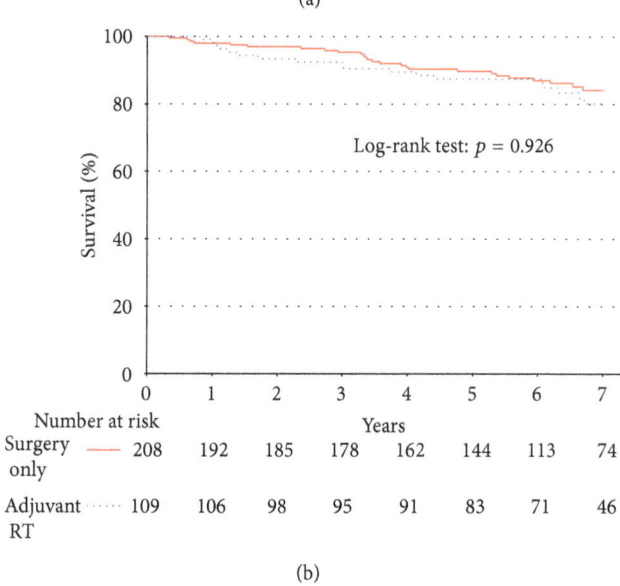

(b)

FIGURE 5: There is no difference in unadjusted survival for (a) patients with well-differentiated liposarcoma when stratified by adjuvant RT versus surgery on the basis of negative margins. There was also no difference when stratified on the basis of positive margins (b).

4. Discussion

Soft tissue sarcomas of the extremities (STS-E) represent a heterogeneous group of tumors with a wide variation in biologic behavior. Much of the data that influences treatment decisions is limited by small numbers and by a failure to investigate tumors of a specific grade. Grade is arguably the single most important independent predictor of behavior and well-differentiated STS-E have a limited capacity for metastasis and causing death from disease [15]. With access to the NCDB, this study represents the largest patient cohort to date focusing specifically on patterns of radiation therapy usage and outcomes of patients with well-differentiated STS-E. The primary objective of this retrospective cohort study was to examine the usage patterns of adjuvant radiation therapy in well-differentiated STS-E patients.

The goal of surgery for soft tissue sarcomas of the extremities is en bloc resection of the tumor with a negative margin [16, 17]. However, with surgery alone the rate of

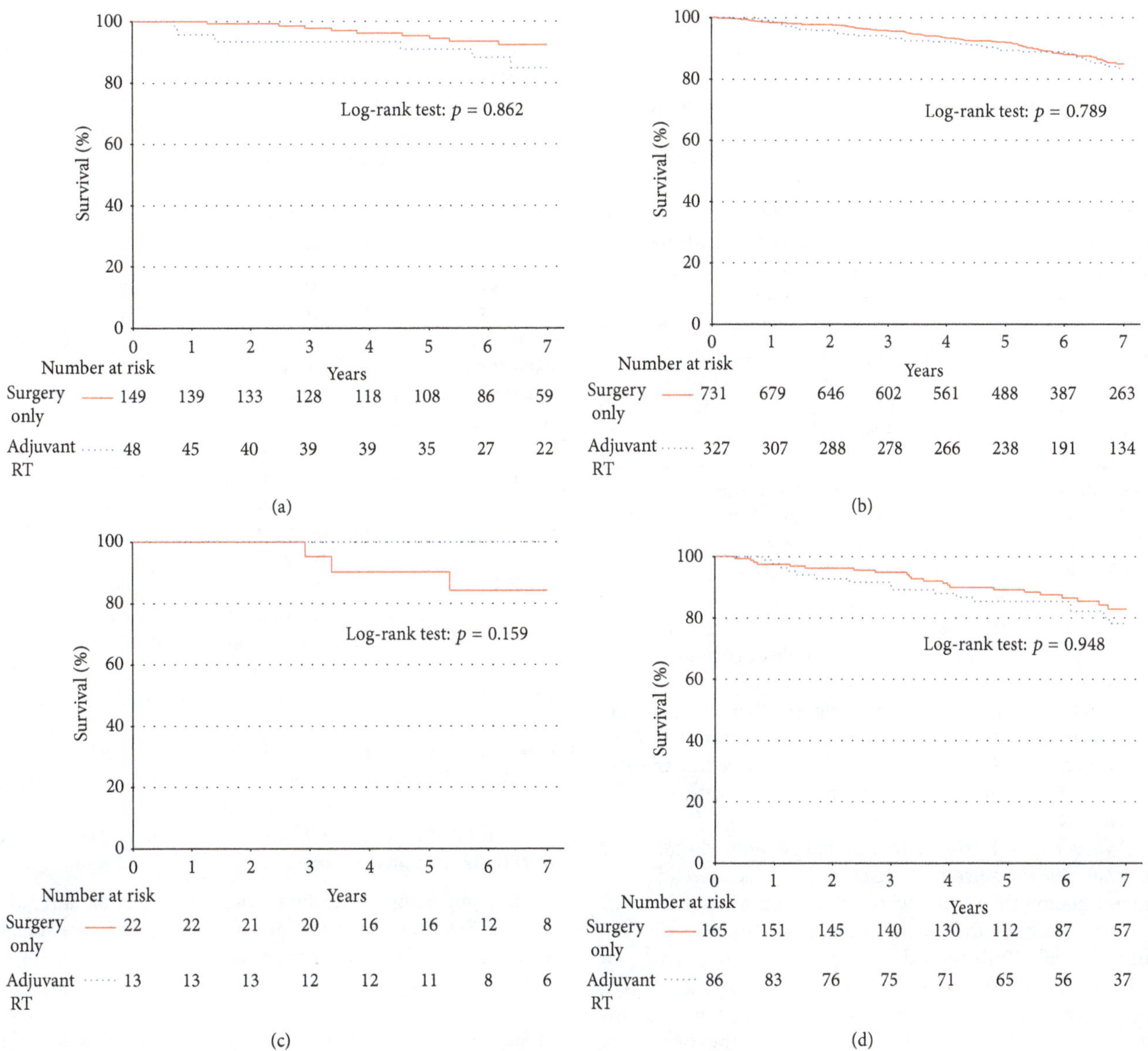

FIGURE 6: There is no difference in unadjusted survival for patients with well-differentiated liposarcoma tumors when stratified by adjuvant RT versus surgery on the basis of size <5 cm (a) and >5 cm (b) for patients with negative margin status. There was also no difference when stratified on the basis of size in patients with positive margin status ((c) and (d), resp.).

local recurrence approaches 40 percent for all sarcomas [18, 19]. The addition of radiation therapy improves the rate of local control to over 90% [20]. While the impact of local recurrence on metastasis and survival remains a subject of debate, local control is an important aspect of sarcoma management, as local recurrences can have major morbidity that may compromise limb function as a consequence of tumor progression or from the need for subsequent surgery and/or adjuvant therapies [21]. One limitation of this study is the ability to determine rates of local recurrence from the NCDB.

A large study conducted of 8249 patients with soft tissue sarcoma of any anatomic location from the Florida Cancer Data System confirmed that low-grade tumors demonstrated a significant survival advantage compared to other sarcomas [22]; they also found that there was no survival benefit with the addition of radiation therapy, though they did not specifically examine by location. A study by Pisters et al. included a cohort of 46 patients with well-differentiated soft tissue sarcomas receiving brachytherapy [9]. Their findings indicated that well-differentiated soft tissue sarcomas exhibited no improvement in local tumor control with the addition of brachytherapy. In contrast, a study by Yang et al. ($n = 55$) found that external beam RT improved the rates of local control in well-differentiated STS of the extremities [8]. Regardless of the impact on local control, neither study showed a survival benefit with the addition of radiation therapy following surgery. Additionally, the studies that demonstrate LR to be an independent risk factor for metastasis and death have not looked specifically at well-differentiated tumors. Some authors have questioned whether or not well-differentiated tumors are even likely to respond to RT, given their latent biology.

With these points in mind, one might wonder why adjuvant RT would be considered at all for patients with well-differentiated tumors. At our institution, adjuvant RT is reserved for those patients with well-differentiated STS-E in whom the morbidity of a subsequent resection would be unacceptable. Therefore, we were surprised to find that 27% of all patients with well-differentiated STS-E in the NCDB were treated with adjuvant radiation therapy. One might expect that this would result from patients with challenging or high-risk disease being disproportionately treated with adjuvant RT. Yet this was not the case. Patients with positive margins received RT 36% of the time and patients with tumors >5 cm received RT 32% of the time. In a separate analysis of the NCDB focusing exclusively on patients with high grade STS-E, we found that RT was utilized only 62% of the time (Hou et al., in press). These data suggest that adjuvant RT is underutilized in patients with high grade STS-E while being overutilized in patients with low grade STS-E. We did find that the use of adjuvant RT for well-differentiated sarcomas was associated with a significantly lower rate of limb amputation as the index procedure (0.8% in the RT group versus, 4.1% in the surgery alone group, $p < 0.001$). This pattern may suggest that surgeons are considering adjuvant RT as a means of limiting the need for amputation. Alternatively, it may simply reflect the fact that patients requiring a limb amputation have little need for adjuvant RT.

We were also intrigued to find that patients who received adjuvant RT were also more likely to have received adjuvant chemotherapy than those who did not receive adjuvant RT. The role of chemotherapy in treating soft tissue sarcoma is controversial. While some data supports a survival benefit for utilizing chemotherapy to treat large, deep, high grade STS [23], there is no evidence supporting the use of chemotherapy to treat low grade STS [24]. In general, the benefit of systemic therapy for soft tissue sarcoma is improved survival, rather than improved local control. A large analysis from the Sarcoma Meta-Analysis Collaboration found that the use of doxorubicin and ifosfamide improved survival by 11% but provided no benefit with regard to local disease control. For low-grade tumors, the risk of death from disease is already low so there would seem to be little role for utilizing chemotherapy for most tumors. One possibility we consider is that the patients in our series receiving systemic therapy may have had erroneous pathologic diagnoses entered into the database. The NCCN guidelines recommend that all patients with STS be evaluated by a multidisciplinary team with experience managing STS. In this setting, experienced surgeons and radiation oncologists can work together to optimize therapy to achieve local control and preserve limb function whenever possible.

Our analysis of patients in the NCDB indicates that radiotherapy does not improve or decrease overall survival in low-grade lesions. This is consistent with the large cohort of study of the SEER database by Koshy et al. examining 2317 patients with "low grade" histology. Of note, tumor grade in this study was categorized into low or high even though sarcomas are typically graded using a three-tier system consisting of low, intermediate, and high grades [25, 26]. A study by Mollabashy et al. looked at a smaller cohort of 108 patients with low grade STS and found that the addition of RT to surgical excision had no effect on either local control or overall survival [27]. The addition of RT had a higher rate of complications as compared to surgery, specifically postoperative lymphedema.

Factors that carry a poor prognostic outcome for soft tissue sarcoma of the extremities include size greater than 5 cm and positive margin status following resection [28]. We examined the effect of these prognostic factors on overall survival in patients with well-differentiated STS-E and found no significant effect on overall survival. Therefore, these results are consistent with tumor grade being the most important prognostic factor for patients with soft tissue sarcoma. There was no overall survival benefit associated with adjuvant radiation therapy when compared to surgery alone in these groups. These findings are in contrast to a small study by Choong et al. They reviewed 132 patients with low-grade STS-E and found that patients with tumors larger than 5 cm and positive margins benefited from the addition of RT with decreased local recurrence and increased metastasis-free survival. Overall survival was not directly addressed [6]. As expected, patients with small lesions (<5 cm) and negative margins showed no benefit in overall survival with the addition of RT. But, in contrast with what has been previously suggested, our data indicates that RT also conferred no survival benefit on patients with large tumors (>5 cm) and resections with positive margins.

In comparing our findings with Choong et al. and Yang et al., important limitation of our study becomes evident: it is not possible to determine rates of local recurrence or metastasis using the NCDB. Local recurrence is thought to be a significant predictor of poor prognosis; particularly in high-grade sarcomas, studies show that patients with local recurrences have higher rates of metastasis and shorter overall survival rates [29, 30]. While RT may not impact overall survival, in combination with limb-sparing surgery moderate doses of RT can eliminate microscopic disease beyond the area of gross resection and reduce rates of local recurrence [20]. The addition of LR and metastasis data to the NCDB would offer two specific utilities. First, it would help to elucidate the role of RT in reducing rates of local recurrence. Second, it would allow investigation of the impact of local recurrence on distant recurrence, disease specific survival, and overall survival in this population of patients with WD tumors.

Another limitation of our study is that it was limited to survival data acquisition prior to 2006. It is possible that trends in RT usage and management have changed in the past 8 years and therefore the outcomes with contemporary RT technology may be different. Indeed, recent reports of IMRT for STS-E suggest increased local control with decreased morbidity [31, 32]. Another limitation of the present study relates to how specimens were obtained for grading. Histology can be evaluated from a core needle biopsy specimen or from the entire tumor specimen following resection. Evaluations from a biopsy could be a source of sampling error, which may affect our results. It is also unclear if tumor grading changed after resection; it is possible that the information entered into the database represents the original biopsy and not the final pathology. We kept this possibility in consideration in our analysis. A small number of patients (125) who received neoadjuvant RT were excluded due to the challenge of grading the tumor following definitive resection as a consequence of radiation effect.

Atypical fatty tumors such as well-differentiated liposarcoma of the extremities remain a unique subset of STS-E with a particularly favorable biological behavior [33, 34]. Though they can be locally aggressive, well-differentiated liposarcomas exhibit lower rates of metastasis [35] and higher rates of overall survival [36, 37]. Radiation therapy is still frequently used in the management of these well-differentiated tumors; this practice remains routine at some institutions [38, 39]. Our study found no significant effect on overall survival with the addition of radiation therapy when compared to surgery alone; this extended to patients with positive margins and patients with tumors greater than 5 cm. Therefore, limb-sparing surgery alone is a reasonable option for well-differentiated liposarcoma of the extremity arising in a location where additional surgical treatment of a local recurrence would not be anticipated to cause significant functional impairment.

Soft tissue sarcomas of the extremities are a diverse and heterogenous group of tumors, which can be challenging to manage. The subset of these tumors that are histologically well-differentiated represents a group of tumors with a more indolent biological behavior. Using a large database, we describe patterns of usage of adjuvant radiation therapy in the United States. In examining this aim, we demonstrate that adjuvant radiation therapy, as expected, does not improve or decrease survival. While radiation therapy will continue to have an important role in reducing the risk of local recurrence for certain well-differentiated STS of the extremities, our results suggest that RT will not impact survival, regardless of tumor size or margin status. Because RT to the extremity can cause short-term toxicity and late effects [40, 41], adjuvant RT should be utilized to treat well-differentiated STS-E when improving local control outweighs these side effects and not to try to improve overall survival [8]. The decision about whether or not to utilize adjuvant RT should be made in the setting of a multidisciplinary discussion with consideration given to each patient's unique situation.

Disclosure

The data in the PUF have been deidentified to the extent that they are no longer a limited data set as defined by Health Insurance Portability and Accountability Act (HIPAA). William C. Eward is co-first author.

References

[1] A. Jemal, R. Siegel, J. Xu, and E. Ward, "Cancer statistics, 2010," *CA Cancer Journal for Clinicians*, vol. 60, no. 5, pp. 277–300, 2010.

[2] R. W. Miller, J. L. Young Jr., and B. Novakovic, "Childhood cancer," *Cancer*, vol. 75, supplement 1, pp. 395–405, 1995.

[3] G. B. Mann, J. J. Lewis, and M. F. Brennan, "Adult soft tissue sarcoma," *Australian and New Zealand Journal of Surgery*, vol. 69, no. 5, pp. 336–343, 1999.

[4] S. Sinha and A. H. S. Peach, "Diagnosis and management of soft tissue sarcoma," *British Medical Journal*, vol. 341, Article ID c7170, 2010.

[5] R. Hussein and M. A. Smith, "Soft tissue sarcomas: are current referral guidelines sufficient?" *Annals of the Royal College of Surgeons of England*, vol. 87, no. 3, pp. 171–173, 2005.

[6] P. F. M. Choong, I. A. Petersen, A. G. Nascimento, and F. H. Sim, "Is radiotherapy important for low-grade soft tissue sarcoma of the extremity?" *Clinical Orthopaedics and Related Research*, no. 387, pp. 191–199, 2001.

[7] G. K. Zagars, M. T. Ballo, P. W. T. Pisters et al., "Prognostic factors for patients with localized soft-tissue sarcoma treated with conservation surgery and radiation therapy: an analysis of 1225 patients," *Cancer*, vol. 97, no. 10, pp. 2530–2543, 2003.

[8] J. C. Yang, A. E. Chang, A. R. Baker et al., "Randomized prospective study of the benefit of adjuvant radiation therapy in the treatment of soft tissue sarcomas of the extremity," *Journal of Clinical Oncology*, vol. 16, no. 1, pp. 197–203, 1998.

[9] P. W. Pisters, L. B. Harrison, D. H. Leung, J. M. Woodruff, E. S. Casper, and M. F. Brennan, "Long-term results of a prospective randomized trial of adjuvant brachytherapy in soft tissue sarcoma," *Journal of Clinical Oncology*, vol. 14, no. 3, pp. 859–868, 1996.

[10] S. M. M. Sommerville, J. T. Patton, J. C. Luscombe, D. C. Mangham, and R. J. Grimer, "Clinical outcomes of deep atypical lipomas (well-differentiated lipoma-like liposarcomas) of the extremities," *ANZ Journal of Surgery*, vol. 75, no. 9, pp. 803–806, 2005.

[11] M. Koshy, S. E. Rich, and M. M. Mohiuddin, "Improved survival with radiation therapy in high-grade soft tissue sarcomas of the extremities: a SEER analysis," *International Journal of Radiation Oncology Biology Physics*, vol. 77, no. 1, pp. 203–209, 2010.

[12] National-Comprehensive-Cancer-Network, *Soft Tissue Sarcoma Version 2.2014*, 2014, http://www.nccn.org/professionals/physician_gls/PDF/sarcoma.pdf.

[13] P. R. Rosenbaum and D. B. Rubin, "The central role of the propensity score in observational studies for causal effects," *Biometrika*, vol. 70, no. 1, pp. 41–55, 1983.

[14] S. Singer, C. R. Antonescu, E. Riedel, M. F. Brennan, and R. E. Pollock, "Histologic subtype and margin of resection predict pattern of recurrence and survival for retroperitoneal liposarcoma," *Annals of Surgery*, vol. 238, no. 3, pp. 358–371, 2003.

[15] M. F. Brennan, C. R. Antonescu, N. Moraco, and S. Singer, "Lessons learned from the study of 10,000 patients with soft tissue sarcoma," *Annals of Surgery*, vol. 260, no. 3, pp. 416–422, 2014.

[16] R. Kandel, N. Coakley, J. Werier, J. Engel, M. Ghert, and S. Verma, "Surgical margins and handling of soft-tissue sarcoma in extremities: a clinical practice guideline," *Current Oncology*, vol. 20, no. 3, pp. e247–e254, 2013.

[17] K. K. Tanabe, R. E. Pollock, L. M. Ellis, A. Murphy, N. Sherman, and M. M. Romsdahl, "Influence of surgical margins on outcome in patients with preoperatively irradiated extremity soft tissue sarcomas," *Cancer*, vol. 73, no. 6, pp. 1652–1659, 1994.

[18] A. Alho, T. A. Alvegard, O. Berlin et al., "Surgical margin in soft tissue sarcoma. The Scandinavian Sarcoma Group experience," *Acta Orthopaedica Scandinavica*, vol. 60, no. 6, pp. 687–692, 1989.

[19] A. Azzarelli, "Surgery in soft tissue sarcomas," *European Journal of Cancer Part A: General Topics*, vol. 29, no. 4, pp. 618–623, 1993.

[20] S. A. Rosenberg, J. Tepper, E. Glatstein et al., "The treatment of soft-tissue sarcomas of the extremities: prospective randomized evaluations of (1) limb-sparing surgery plus radiation therapy compared with amputation and (2) the role of adjuvant chemotherapy," *Annals of Surgery*, vol. 196, no. 3, pp. 305–315, 1982.

[21] C. S. Trovik, "Local recurrence of soft tissue sarcoma: a Scandinavian sarcoma group project," *Acta Orthopaedica Scandinavica—Supplement*, vol. 72, no. 300, pp. 1–31, 2001.

[22] J. C. Gutierrez, E. A. Perez, D. Franceschi, F. L. Moffat Jr., A. S. Livingstone, and L. G. Koniaris, "Outcomes for soft-tissue sarcoma in 8249 cases from a large state cancer registry," *Journal of Surgical Research*, vol. 141, no. 1, pp. 105–114, 2007.

[23] A. le Cesne, S. Cresta, R. G. Maki et al., "A retrospective analysis of antitumour activity with trabectedin in translocation-related sarcomas," *European Journal of Cancer*, vol. 48, no. 16, pp. 3036–3044, 2012.

[24] N. Pervaiz, N. Colterjohn, F. Farrokhyar, R. Tozer, A. Figueredo, and M. Ghert, "A systematic meta-analysis of randomized controlled trials of adjuvant chemotherapy for localized resectable soft-tissue sarcoma," *Cancer*, vol. 113, no. 3, pp. 573–581, 2008.

[25] A. T. Deyrup and S. W. Weiss, "Grading of soft tissue sarcomas: the challenge of providing precise information in an imprecise world," *Histopathology*, vol. 48, no. 1, pp. 42–50, 2006.

[26] C. D. Fletcher, "WHO classification of tumours of soft tissue and bone," in *World Health Organization Classification of Tumours*, IARC Press, Lyon, France, 4th edition, 2013.

[27] A. Mollabashy, W. W. Virkus, R. A. Zlotecki, B. H. Berrey, and M. T. Scarborough, "Radiation therapy for low-grade soft tissue sarcoma," *Clinical Orthopaedics and Related Research*, no. 397, pp. 190–195, 2002.

[28] H. D. Suit, H. J. Mankin, W. C. Wood et al., "Treatment of the patient with stage M0 soft tissue sarcoma," *Journal of Clinical Oncology*, vol. 6, no. 5, pp. 854–862, 1988.

[29] A. Gronchi, R. Miceli, M. Fiore et al., "Extremity soft tissue sarcoma: adding to the prognostic meaning of local failure," *Annals of Surgical Oncology*, vol. 14, no. 5, pp. 1583–1590, 2007.

[30] J. J. Lewis, D. Leung, M. Heslin, J. M. Woodruff, and M. F. Brennan, "Association of local recurrence with subsequent survival in extremity soft tissue sarcoma," *Journal of Clinical Oncology*, vol. 15, no. 2, pp. 646–652, 1997.

[31] B. O'Sullivan, A. M. Griffin, C. I. Dickie et al., "Phase 2 study of preoperative image-guided intensity-modulated radiation therapy to reduce wound and combined modality morbidities in lower extremity soft tissue sarcoma," *Cancer*, vol. 119, no. 10, pp. 1878–1884, 2013.

[32] F. Roeder, B. Lehner, T. Schmitt et al., "Excellent local control with IOERT and postoperative EBRT in high grade extremity sarcoma: results from a subgroup analysis of a prospective trial," *BMC Cancer*, vol. 14, no. 1, article 350, 2014.

[33] R. J. Canter, S. Beal, D. Borys, S. R. Martinez, R. J. Bold, and A. S. Robbins, "Interaction of histologic subtype and histologic grade in predicting survival for soft-tissue sarcomas," *Journal of the American College of Surgeons*, vol. 210, no. 2, pp. 191–198.e2, 2010.

[34] J. B. Koea, D. Leung, J. J. Lewis, and M. F. Brennan, "Histopathologic type: an independent prognostic factor in primary soft tissue sarcoma of the extremity?" *Annals of Surgical Oncology*, vol. 10, no. 4, pp. 432–440, 2003.

[35] J.-M. Coindre, P. Terrier, L. Guillou et al., "Predictive value of grade for metastasis development in the main histologic types of adult soft tissue sarcomas: a study of 1240 patients from the French Federation of Cancer Centers sarcoma group," *Cancer*, vol. 91, no. 10, pp. 1914–1926, 2001.

[36] D. R. Lucas, A. G. Nascimento, B. K. S. Sanjay, and M. G. Rock, "Well-differentiated liposarcoma: the Mayo Clinic experience with 58 cases," *The American Journal of Clinical Pathology*, vol. 102, no. 5, pp. 677–683, 1994.

[37] C. A. Smith, S. R. Martinez, W. H. Tseng et al., "Predicting survival for well-differentiated liposarcoma: the importance of tumor location," *Journal of Surgical Research*, vol. 175, no. 1, pp. 12–17, 2012.

[38] K. M. Dalal, C. R. Antonescu, and S. Singer, "Diagnosis and management of lipomatous tumors," *Journal of Surgical Oncology*, vol. 97, no. 4, pp. 298–313, 2008.

[39] G. K. Zagars, M. S. Goswitz, and A. Pollack, "Liposarcoma: outcome and prognostic factors following conservation surgery and radiation therapy," *International Journal of Radiation Oncology, Biology, Physics*, vol. 36, no. 2, pp. 311–319, 1996.

[40] A. M. Davis, B. O'Sullivan, R. Turcotte et al., "Late radiation morbidity following randomization to preoperative versus postoperative radiotherapy in extremity soft tissue sarcoma," *Radiotherapy and Oncology*, vol. 75, no. 1, pp. 48–53, 2005.

[41] B. O'Sullivan, A. M. Davis, R. Turcotte et al., "Preoperative versus postoperative radiotherapy in soft-tissue sarcoma of the limbs: a randomised trial," *The Lancet*, vol. 359, no. 9325, pp. 2235–2241, 2002.

2

Intraoperative Radiotherapy in the Management of Locally Recurrent Extremity Soft Tissue Sarcoma

Christopher L. Tinkle,[1] Vivian Weinberg,[1] Steve E. Braunstein,[1] Rosanna Wustrack,[2] Andrew Horvai,[3] Thierry Jahan,[4] Richard J. O'Donnell,[2] and Alexander R. Gottschalk[1]

[1] *Department of Radiation Oncology, University of California, San Francisco, 1600 Divisadero Street, MZ Building R H1031, San Francisco, CA 94143, USA*
[2] *Department of Orthopaedic Surgery, University of California, San Francisco, San Francisco, CA, USA*
[3] *Department of Pathology, University of California, San Francisco, San Francisco, CA, USA*
[4] *Department of Medicine, University of California, San Francisco, San Francisco, CA, USA*

Correspondence should be addressed to Alexander R. Gottschalk; alexander.gottschalk@ucsf.edu

Academic Editor: Peter C. Ferguson

Purpose. To investigate the efficacy and morbidity of limb-sparing surgery with intraoperative radiotherapy (IORT) for patients with locally recurrent extremity soft tissue sarcoma (ESTS). *Methods and Materials.* Twenty-six consecutively treated patients were identified in a single institution retrospective analysis of patients with locally recurrent ESTS treated with IORT following salvage limb-sparing resection from May 2000 to July 2011. Fifteen (58%) patients received external beam radiotherapy (EBRT) prior to recurrence (median dose 63 Gy), while 11 (42%) patients received EBRT following IORT (median dose 52 Gy). The Kaplan-Meier product limit method was used to estimate disease control and survival and subsets were compared using a log rank statistic, Cox's regression model was used to determine independent predictors of disease outcome, and toxicity was reported according to CTCAE v4.0 guidelines. *Results.* With a median duration of follow-up from surgery and IORT of 34.9 months (range: 4 to 139 mos.), 10 patients developed a local recurrence with 4 subsequently undergoing amputation. The 5-year estimate for local control (LC) was 58% (95% CI: 36–75%), for amputation-free was 81% (95% CI: 57–93%), for metastasis-free control (MFC) was 56% (95% CI: 31–75%), for disease-free survival (DFS) was 35% (95% CI: 17–54%), and for overall survival (OS) was 50% (95% CI: 24–71%). Prior EBRT did not appear to influence disease control (LC, $p = 0.74$; MFC, $p = 0.66$) or survival (DFS, $p = 0.16$; OS, $p = 0.58$). Grade 3 or higher acute and late toxicities were reported for 6 (23%) and 8 (31%) patients, respectively. The frequency of both acute and late grade 3 or higher toxicities occurred equally between patients who received EBRT prior to or after IORT. *Conclusions.* IORT in combination with oncologic resection of recurrent ESTS yields good rates of local control and limb-salvage with acceptable morbidity. Within the limitations of small subsets, these data suggest that prior EBRT does not significantly influence disease control or toxicity.

1. Introduction

With the demonstration of comparable overall and disease-free survival rates with oncologic resection coupled with adjuvant radiotherapy compared to amputation, limb-sparing surgery and radiation have become the standard curative therapy for extremity soft tissue sarcoma (ESTS) [1]. This multimodality approach yields long-term overall local failure rates of approximately 20% [1–3]. However, subsets of patient defined by clinicopathologic features, including surgical margins status and tumor grade, size, depth, and location, have varying risk of recurrence. For example, in carefully selected patients with small tumors resected and widely clear margins, a 10-year local recurrence rate of ~10% has been observed following surgery alone [4], while series of patients with positive surgical margins treated with adjuvant radiotherapy suggest ~30% local recurrence rate [5, 6]. For patients who experience an isolated local recurrence after definitive limb-sparing therapy, outcomes of both subsequent local control and overall survival are generally inferior to that observed with primary, localized disease, and yet it has long been recognized that a significant fraction of these patients can be salvaged [7–9].

The treatment algorithm of locally recurrent ESTS has been proposed to follow a similar workflow of that of primary ESTS, with long-term salvage local control rates ranging widely from 42 to 67% [10–12]. Data are conflicting regarding the role of adjuvant reirradiation in those patients treated initially with conservative surgery and radiation, however, with reports of superior local control through the use of combined surgery and reirradiation compared to surgery alone [13], while others have observed no significant improvement in local control with the addition of reirradiation [11]. Furthermore, significant postsalvage toxicity has been reported in patients treated with reirradiation [11, 13, 14]. While brachytherapy and external beam radiotherapy (EBRT) have historically been employed in the recurrent setting, more recently an alternative technique through the use of intraoperative external beam radiotherapy (IORT) has also been reported [15–18]. IORT may be used to rapidly deliver highly localized, high dose treatment with the added advantages of direct visualization of the tumor bed at the time of surgery, the ability to displace or shield nearby critical structures, and the possibility to administer lower dose adjuvant EBRT. With the exception of the recent large Spanish cooperative study [19], however, many of these reports have included analysis of patients with both primary and locally recurrent disease, making it more difficult to assess the role of IORT in the management of recurrent disease.

Since 1998 our institution has employed single fraction electron-based IORT through the use of a mobile linear accelerator for patients at risk for close or microscopically positive margins, in both the primary and recurrent setting, as well as for those patients with recurrent tumors within a previously irradiated field. In this study, we report mature treatment outcomes and toxicities for patients treated with limb-sparing surgery and IORT for locally recurrent ESTS at high risk for subsequent local recurrence.

2. Methods and Materials

2.1. Patients. The committee on human research approved this retrospective study of patients with extremity STS treated with IORT between May, 2000, and July, 2011, at the University of California, San Francisco (UCSF). Twenty-six consecutively treated patients were identified with a diagnosis of locally recurrent ESTS, with or without distant metastasis, who underwent limb-sparing reresection and IORT. STS were restricted to tumors within the "Soft Tissue Sarcoma" section of the 7th edition American Joint Committee on Cancer (AJCC) Staging Manual [20]. Workup included a history and physical exam, routine laboratory studies, and, depending on the individual case, exam under anesthesia, chest radiograph, computed tomography (CT) of chest, abdomen, and pelvis, magnetic resonance imaging (MRI) of the extremity of interest, or positron emission tomography (PET). Fine needle aspirate (FNA) or incisional biopsy was done prior to planned oncologic resections. Final tumor size was determined from pathologic data and AJCC staging using the retreatment classification was done at the time of reresection and IORT. The time to development of any initial relapse (local or distant) was defined from end of initial prerelapse treatment to first recurrence. Patients were presented and multimodality management recommendations made at the multidisciplinary UCSF sarcoma tumor board.

2.2. Surgery. A single senior orthopaedic oncologist (RJO) performed all definitive reresections. Pathology for all cases was reviewed at UCSF and assigned a grade according to the FNCLCC grading system (Coindre system) [21], with grade 1 tumors considered as low grade and grades 2 and 3 tumors considered as high grade. Surgical margins were considered positive when tumor cells were found at the margin of the resected specimen and close when margins were ≤2 mm. For patients where intraoperative margin status based on frozen section was reported ($n = 20$), there were no discrepancies on final permanent pathology.

2.3. Radiation. The indications for IORT and the target fields were determined jointly by the surgeon and radiation oncologist. The most common indications were the expectation of a close or positive margin adjacent to a critical structure and recurrence after prior irradiation. Additional indications included high grade pathology, bulky recurrence (>5 cm), and multiply recurrent disease. The Mobetron linear accelerator (IntraOp Medical Corporation, Nevada) was used at the time of definitive resection to deliver 4 to 12 MeV electrons through flat or beveled cones ranging from 2.5 to 10 cm in internal diameter. Dose was typically prescribed to the 85–90% isodose line. Total delivered dose was determined based on surgical bed volumes and intraoperative frozen pathologic margin status. Critical structures, particularly uninvolved nerves or vessels, were either mobilized away from the treatment field or protected with lead shielding. Tissue bolus was used in select cases to spare sensitive structures located deep to the tumor bed. Recommendations for adjuvant EBRT were based on the absence of prior in-field EBRT, final pathologic margins, and high risk disease (positive margins outside direct IORT field and bulky, deep, high grade disease). EBRT consisted of 3D conformal technique with a clinical target volume (CTV) encompassing the surgical bed, drain sites, and scar plus a 3 cm radial margin and a 5 cm longitudinal margin based on the preoperative gross tumor volume (GTV) extent defined on preoperative CT and/or MRI and was employed 4–8 weeks postoperatively.

2.4. Chemotherapy. Initiation of chemotherapy was based on high risk disease features (high grade disease, advanced group stage, and multiply recurrent tumors), symptomatology (pain and/or neuropathy), tumor proximity to critical structures, and desired presurgical shrinkage, as well as patient age, comorbidities, and performance status. The most commonly employed chemotherapy regimen consisted of a combination of anthracycline and ifosfamide.

2.5. Follow-Up. Patients were evaluated 3 to 6 weeks after reresection and IORT, then at 3- to 6-month intervals for disease status and toxicity assessments for 2 to 3 years, and then at annual intervals. Surveillance imaging of the site of interest and chest was obtained at 6- to 12-month intervals. Postreresection and IORT failure was defined at the time of biopsy or resection proven recurrence, except in cases of patient or physician deferred biopsy which were diagnosed clinically. Local recurrence was defined as a recurrence within the IORT and/or EBRT treatment field, while distant metastasis was defined as spread of the primary disease outside the irradiated field.

Local and distant metastasis-free disease control were each measured from the date of reresection and IORT to the date of recurrence, while the amputation-free duration was from the date of surgery and IORT to the date of amputation. The durations for patients without documented disease recurrence or amputation were censored at the date of last disease follow-up. Overall survival (OS) was defined as the period of time from the date of reresection and IORT to death from any cause. The durations for patients without documented death were censored at the date the patients were last known to be alive. Disease-free survival (DFS) was defined as the period of time from reresection and IORT to the date of first documented evidence of disease recurrence or death from any cause, whichever occurred first. The durations for surviving patients remaining disease-free were censored at the last date of follow-up. The time to initial recurrence was defined as the interval from end of initial definitive therapy to date of first recurrence.

Physician reported morbidity was assessed according to the Common Toxicity Criteria for Adverse Events, version 4.0 (CTCAE V4.0) [22], with acute and late events defined as those arising within 90 days or beyond 90 days of reresection and IORT, respectively. Recorded events were of those considered to be medically significant to severe (grade 3 or higher). To assess limb function, the worst individual toxicity was reported for joint function, weakness, or gait. Moderate wound complications included seromas requiring multiple aspirations and infections managed with operative debridement.

2.6. Statistical Analysis. Descriptive statistics (e.g., medians with minimum and maximum values and percentages) were calculated to summarize patient and disease features and treatment toxicities. Baseline and treatment subsets were compared using either Fisher's exact test for categorical features or t-test for continuous variables. The Kaplan-Meier product limit method was used to estimate the 5-year probabilities and presented with 95% confidence intervals (CIs) of overall survival and disease-free survival and of remaining free of local recurrence, metastatic recurrence, and amputation. Patient subsets were compared using a log rank statistic. Cox's regression model was used univariately to determine whether the duration to first recurrence was a predictor of each disease outcome following reresection and IORT. Significance was determined by the likelihood ratio (LLR) test with results summarized with a hazard ratio (HR) and 95% CIs. The same method was applied to identify independent predictors of each disease outcome. Due to the total sample size, following convention at most 2 predictors were included in a model. For all analyses a probability value less than 0.05 was considered to be statistically significant. Analyses were performed using Statistica (StatSoft v6).

3. Results

3.1. Patient Characteristics. The median age at the time of definitive reresection and IORT was 51 years with a range of 12 to 76 years. Upper extremity tumors were somewhat more common, occurring in 15 (58%) patients. Tumors were deep to the superficial fascia in 22 (85%) patients and 14 (54%) patients had tumors >5 cm in largest diameter. High grade (FNCLCC grade 2 or 3) tumors comprised the majority of cases (77%), with undifferentiated pleomorphic sarcoma (27%) and synovial sarcoma (19%) representing the most common histologies. AJCC group stage II or higher was found in 20 (77%) patients. Of the 6 patients with low grade tumors, 4 had positive margins, 5 were deep in location, and 4 were larger than 5 cm. A single local recurrence prior to reresection and IORT was observed in 20 (77%) patients, while 6 (23%) patients experienced more than one recurrence (range: 2–5). The median time to first local recurrence from the end of initial treatment was 17 months, with a range of 3 to 199 months. Close to half of first recurrences were detected beyond two years from initial treatment (46%). Distant metastasis prior to reresection and IORT was detected in 4 (15%) patients, all with spread to lung. The baseline patient characteristics are summarized in Table 1.

3.2. Treatment Characteristics. All patients achieved a gross total resection, yet margins were found to be microscopically positive in 12 (46%) specimens and close (≤2 mm) in 7 (27%). Median cone size used for IORT was 7 cm (range: 3–10 cm) and 5 (19%) patients were treated with >1 IORT field. Median IORT prescription dose was 15 Gy (range: 10–18 Gy). With the exception of one patient who received both EBRT prior to recurrence (60 Gy) and following reresection and IORT (40 Gy) and one patient who received only IORT, each patient who received EBRT prior to recurrence underwent IORT alone and each patient without a history of prior EBRT underwent both IORT and adjuvant EBRT. Median EBRT prescription dose prior to recurrence was 63 Gy with a range of 25 to 72 Gy. Median adjuvant EBRT following IORT was 52 Gy with a range of 22 to 60 Gy. Chemotherapy as part of initial definitive treatment prior to recurrence was given to 6 (25%) patients, while peri-IORT chemotherapy was given to 13 (54%) patients. A combination of anthracycline and ifosfamide containing regimen was the most commonly employed, and peri-IORT chemotherapy was restricted to high grade tumors in all cases. The treatment characteristics are summarized in Table 2.

3.3. Disease Control Outcomes. From the date of reresection and IORT, the median follow-up was 34.9 months (range: 4–139 months) for all patients and 45.1 months (range: 26–139 months) for living patients. Ten patients developed

TABLE 1: Baseline patient characteristics at time of reresection and IORT ($n = 26$).

Patient characteristic	Number of patients (%)
Age	
Median	51 years
Range	12–76 years
≤18	1 (4%)
19–50	12 (46%)
>50	13 (50%)
Gender	
Female	15 (58%)
Male	11 (42%)
Site	
Lower extremity	11 (42%)
Upper extremity	15 (58%)
Histology	
Undifferentiated pleomorphic sarcoma	7 (27%)
Synovial sarcoma	5 (19%)
Liposarcoma	4 (15%)
Fibrosarcoma	3 (11.5%)
Spindle cell sarcoma	3 (11.5%)
Leiomyosarcoma	1 (4%)
Malignant peripheral nerve sheath tumor	1 (4%)
Rhabdomyosarcoma	1 (4%)
Soft tissue sarcoma, NOS	1 (4%)
T stage	
T1	12 (46%)
T2	14 (54%)
Depth	
Superficial	4 (15%)
Deep	22 (85%)
Grade (FNCLCC)	
1	6 (23%)
2	6 (23%)
3	14 (54%)
AJCC group stage	
I	6 (23%)
II	11 (42%)
III	5 (19%)
IV	4 (15%)
Initial local recurrence type	
Single	20 (77%)
Multiple	6 (23%)
Time to initial recurrence	
Median	17 mo.
Range	3–199 mo.

TABLE 2: Treatment characteristics.

Treatment characteristic	Number of patients (%)
Surgical margins	
Positive	12 (46%)
Close (≤2 mm)	7 (27%)
Negative	7 (27%)
Radiation therapy	
EBRT prior to recurrence	15 (58%)
Median dose (range)	63 Gy (25–72)
EBRT following IORT	11 (42%)
Median dose (range)	52 Gy (22–60)
IORT cone size	
Median	7 cm
Range	3–10 cm
IORT dose	
Median	15 Gy
Range	10–18 Gy
Chemotherapy ($n = 24$)	
As part of initial therapy	6 (25%)
Peri-IORT	13 (54%)
Peri-IORT chemotherapy schedule	
Pre-IORT alone	6 (25%)
Post-IORT alone	6 (25%)
Pre- & Post-IORT	1 (4%)

a local recurrence following reresection and IORT with a median duration of 10 months (2–30 months), and 10 patients developed new or progressive distant metastasis with a median duration of 8 months (2–50 months). Four patients with local recurrence subsequently underwent amputation. Of the 8 patients who experienced a local recurrence and were without metastasis at the time of reresection and IORT, 3 patients also developed distant metastasis, 2 at the time of local recurrence and 1 following local recurrence. Of the 4 patients with metastasis at the time of reresection and IORT, 2 developed a subsequent local recurrence and all four developed new or progressive distant metastasis. Of the 10 patients who have died, 9 expired with metastatic disease after disease recurrence, while one patient died without disease recurrence. The 5-year Kaplan-Meier estimate for local control was 58% (95% CI: 36–75%), for amputation-free was 81% (95% CI: 57–93%), for metastasis-free control was 56% (95% CI: 31–75%), for disease-free survival was 35% (95% CI: 17–54%), and for overall survival was 50% (95% CI: 24–71%) (Figures 1 and 2).

In comparing patients with or without a history of prior EBRT for initial management, there was no significant difference in any of the clinicopathologic variables analyzed (Fisher's exact test, $p > 0.05$). Analysis of disease outcomes by course of EBRT revealed no difference between those patients who received EBRT as part of their initial management followed by reresection and IORT alone compared to those who underwent adjuvant EBRT following salvage surgery and IORT (Log rank, $p > 0.05$). The Kaplan-Meier 5-year estimate of local control of those patients who received prior EBRT and those patients who did not receive prior EBRT was 55% and 61%, respectively. Using Cox's regression model the longer the duration of the time to first recurrence was found to be a significant predictor of prolonging metastasis-free control, disease-free survival, and overall survival but not local control (LLR test, $p = 0.002$, 0.009, 0.001, and

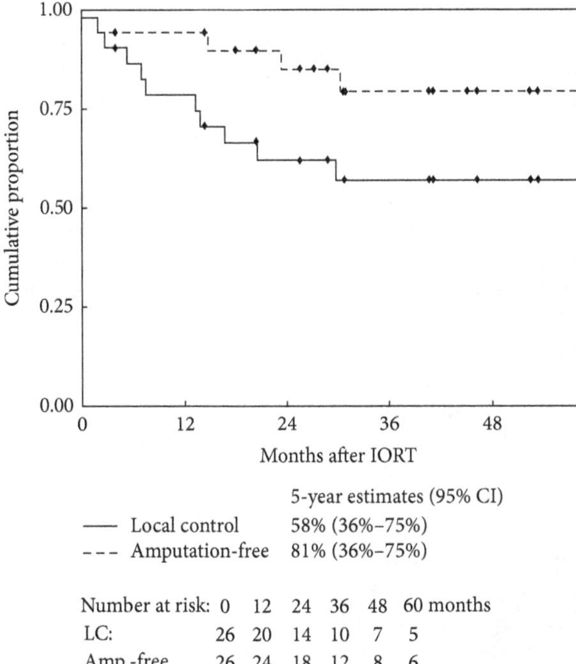

FIGURE 1: Kaplan-Meier probability distributions of local disease control and free of amputation after oncologic reresection and intraoperative radiotherapy (IORT) with 5-year estimates. CI = confidence interval.

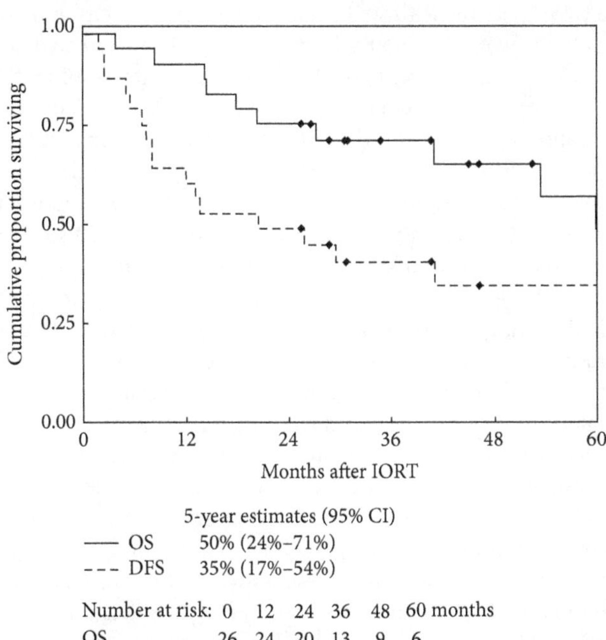

FIGURE 2: Kaplan-Meier probability distributions of disease-free survival (DFS) and overall survival (OS) after oncologic reresection and IORT with 5-year estimates. CI = confidence interval.

TABLE 3: Incidence of grade 3 acute and late toxicity.

Toxicity	Acute* Number of patients (%)	Late* Number of patients (%)
Wound complications		
EBRT prior to recurrence	2 (8%)	3 (15%)
EBRT following IORT	1 (4%)	1 (4%)
Limb/joint dysfunction		
EBRT prior to recurrence	1 (4%)	3 (12%)
EBRT following IORT	2 (8%)	3 (12%)
Total	6 (23%)	8 (31%)

*Five of the 6 patients with grade 3 acute toxicity also had late toxicity of the same type, and 7 patients had multiple grade 3 toxicities.

0.09, resp.). The interval to first recurrence was also a significant predictor of metastasis-free control, disease-free survival, and overall survival when limited to those patients without metastases at the time of reresection and IORT (p = 0.03, 0.04, and 0.02, resp.). T stage was the only independent predictor of local control for the overall patient cohort (p = 0.02, HR = 5.35, 95% CI: 1.13–25.4), while no significant predictor was found when limited to patients without metastasis at recurrence. The presence of metastasis at the time of reresection and IORT was a significant predictor of inferior overall survival (p = 0.04, HR = 5.70, 95% CI: 1.12–29.15).

3.4. Toxicity. Acute medically significant toxicity (grade 3) developed in 6 (23%) patients and late grade 3 toxicity developed in 8 (31%) patients, while no patient developed grade 4 or higher acute toxicity (Table 3). A total of 8 patients experienced any grade 3 toxicity with 7 developing multiple severe events. Gait disturbance and functional impairment of the limb due to joint stiffness or weakness were the most common events and occurred acutely in 3 (12%) patients and in the late phase in 6 (23%) patients, including the 3 patients with acute events. However, eventual improvement or resolution was noted in 5 of these patients. Significant toxicity related to limb/joint function occurred in 3 patients who received EBRT prior to recurrence and in 3 patients who received adjuvant EBRT following reresection and IORT. Acute grade 3 wound complications, both infectious and noninfectious, occurred in 3 (12%) patients, with 2 patients treated with EBRT prior to recurrence and 1 patient treated with EBRT after recurrence. Late grade 3 wound complications occurred in 4 (15%) patients including 2 who had acute events, with 3 patients treated with EBRT prior to recurrence and 1 patient treated with EBRT following recurrence. Each wound complication resolved with intravenous antibiotics and/or surgical intervention. Three patients experienced both wound and joint/limb function-related grade 3 toxicity.

4. Discussion

The value of adjuvant radiotherapy (RT) for improved local control following oncologic limb-preserving surgery of ESTS has been well established [1, 2, 23, 24]. In addition to several patient- and tumor-related predictive factors related to local control following this treatment paradigm, locally recurrent disease course has been associated with inferior local control [5, 7, 25]. When feasible salvage limb-sparing surgery remains the primary treatment modality for these patients [12], however, the role of radiation, particularly in the reirradiation setting, is less well defined [13, 14]. Given the potential for compounded toxicity in the recurrent setting, varied advanced radiation techniques including brachytherapy and IORT have been employed to deliver conformal high dose irradiation while minimizing normal tissue toxicity. The direct visualization provided by intraoperative external beam may have further advantages for targeting and critical structure protection and may allow for relatively reduced doses of large field adjuvant EBRT [26]. In this study, disease control and treatment toxicity outcomes were analyzed for patients treated at our institution for locally recurrent high risk ESTS treated with salvage limb-sparing resection and IORT.

Using an approach of salvage oncologic resection combined with IORT where adjuvant EBRT is largely restricted to those without prior radiation, we find encouraging long-term disease outcomes in this high risk population with 5-year local control, limb salvage, and overall survival estimates of 58%, 81%, and 50%, respectively. A limited number of groups have reported disease outcomes in cohorts of patients with locally recurrent ESTS treated with salvage limb-sparing surgery and IORT [15–19, 26–28]. While the majority of these studies have included patients with both primary and locally recurrent disease, with inclusion of patients with STS of various sites in some series, our results do appear to compare favorably with these reports. In the report from the group at the University of Heidelberg of 153 patients with ESTS, 58 patients with recurrent disease were included, the majority of whom (49 patients) received prior EBRT and underwent reresection and IORT alone for recurrence [26]. Interestingly, there did not appear to be a significant difference in outcomes between patients with recurrent and primary disease in this study, with 5-year estimates of local recurrence-free survival and OS of 69% versus 73% and 64% versus 78%, respectively. However, significant differences in patient and tumor characteristics or follow-up duration, if any, were not reported. A report from Stanford University of 50 patients with either locally advanced or recurrent STS of various sites (4 patients with ESTS) included 35 patients with recurrent disease, approximately half of whom (16 patients) received prior EBRT. Additional therapy, RT and/or systemic therapy, was given to 16 patients, and while the use of adjuvant EBRT appeared to significantly improve disease specific survival, the use of and outcomes with adjuvant EBRT in previously irradiated patients were not described. Overall 5-year patient outcomes were 55%, 24%, and 30% for in-field control (within the IORT field), locoregional control (within anatomic site), and disease-specific survival, respectively.

In a more recent report focusing on an extensive patient cohort with nonmetastatic recurrent STS, Calvo et al. [19] conducted a pooled analysis of 103 patients following reresection and IORT with or without adjuvant EBRT from three Spanish institutions with a median follow-up of 57 months. Approximately one-third of patients ($n = 31$) received EBRT prior to recurrence, 17 of whom underwent reirradiation. Two-thirds of the patients had extremity or trunk wall STS and one-third had retroperitoneal STS. Overall 5-year local control and disease-free survival estimates were 60% and 52%, respectively. Importantly, the use of adjuvant EBRT was a significant predictor of local control on multivariable analysis. While there did not appear to be a significant difference in local control (or other outcomes) between those patients with a history of prior EBRT and those who received reirradiation compared to all others, outcomes between those treated with reresection and IORT alone after failing EBRT and those treated without prior EBRT with reresection, IORT, and adjuvant EBRT were not separately reported. Collectively, disease control and survival outcome results from our cohort as well as those from the series described above are in line with those observed in patients with locally recurrent STS treated with reresection and either EBRT [11] or brachytherapy [29, 30].

With regard to toxicity, we found a moderate occurrence of both acute and late toxicities within this group of heavily treated patients, the majority of whom completed several rounds of multimodality treatment. Acute and late grade 3 toxicity developed in 23% and 31% of patients, respectively, and were predominantly related to gait disturbance or functional impairment of the limb due to joint stiffness or weakness. No grade 4 or 5 toxicity was observed, and no patient required amputation secondary to treatment associated toxicity. Toxicity reported from the Spanish cooperative study by Calvo et al. [19], assessed through the Radiation Therapy Oncology Group/European Organization for Research and Treatment of Cancer (RTOG/EORTC) criteria [31], included 16 (16%) patients with acute grade 3 or higher toxicity, mostly related to wound complications, while significant late toxicity developed in 13 (13%) patients and consisted predominantly of neuropathy and edema. While acute or late toxicity did not appear to differ significantly between those who received adjuvant EBRT and those that did not, toxicity related to reirradiation was not reported. Tran et al. [17] reported grades 3/4 toxicity in 4 (8%) patients, and this consisted of wound breakdown, fistula, neuropathy, and hydronephrosis. Acute grades 2–4 toxicity reported from the University of Heidelberg group developed in 35 (23%) patients, while late grades 2–4 toxicity, per RTOG/EORTC criteria, was reported in 26 (17%) of patients. Acute toxicity consisted predominately of wound-healing disturbances, while late toxicity was most commonly related to joint contracture/fibrosis and neuropathy. Evaluation of toxicity by disease course or prior EBRT was not specified in the above two studies. Overall, review of these data suggests that the moderate toxicity observed in this study is representative of those observed in patients with recurrent STS managed with salvage surgery and IORT. Furthermore, evaluation of toxicity from studies employing EBRT [11, 13, 14] or brachytherapy [29, 30] in the recurrent setting indicates that complications reported from our study are comparable, with significant complications ranging from 18 to 80%.

An interesting report, in abstract form, from members of the Spanish cooperative IORT group in which a similar treatment paradigm to that of ours for recurrent ESTS was employed, has suggested inferior local control and increased toxicity in patients who received prior EBRT [32]. Fifty patients with an isolated local recurrence of ESTS underwent reresection with either IORT or high dose-rate (HDR) brachytherapy. Adjuvant EBRT was given only to patients without prior local radiation (24 patients), while previously irradiated patients underwent reresection and IORT alone (26 patients). The five-year locoregional control estimate in patients with prior EBRT was significantly lower compared to those without prior EBRT (26% versus 81%, $p = 0.001$), and of the 13 (26%) patients with grade 3 or 4 toxicity, 9 patients required reintervention and all were within the prior EBRT group. In our series we did not find statistically significant differences in either disease control outcomes or toxicity between previously irradiated patients and those without prior EBRT. Reasons for these discrepancies are unclear, yet may reflect differences in our highly selected study populations, IORT application (electron beam versus brachytherapy), or other unforeseen variables. It must also be acknowledged that limitations to our study, as well as many of the described studies above, including the retrospective study design and accompanying small sample size limit definitive conclusions are at best hypothesis generating. An additional possible limitation to this study is the inclusion of patients with known distant metastatic disease at the time of recurrence. Indeed, each of the four patients with metastatic disease at the time of initial recurrence progressed distantly and succumbed to their disease.

In conclusion, this study demonstrates that incorporation of IORT as a component of multimodality management of patients with locally recurrent ESTS achieves high rates of local control and limb salvage with acceptable treatment morbidity and suggests that prior EBRT does not significantly influence disease control or toxicity. This technique offers a method of delivering focal therapy to achieve local control for the majority of patients who otherwise may require more radical surgical procedures. Larger, prospective trials are necessary to more fully evaluate the role of IORT in disease control and toxicity outcomes in patients with ESTS.

References

[1] S. A. Rosenberg, J. Tepper, E. Glatstein et al., "The treatment of soft-tissue sarcomas of the extremities: prospective randomized evaluations of (1) limb-sparing surgery plus radiation therapy compared with amputation and (2) the role of adjuvant chemotherapy," *Annals of Surgery*, vol. 196, no. 3, pp. 305–315, 1982.

[2] P. W. Pisters, L. B. Harrison, D. H. Leung, J. M. Woodruff, E. S. Casper, and M. F. Brennan, "Long-term results of a prospective randomized trial of adjuvant brachytherapy in soft tissue sarcoma," *Journal of Clinical Oncology*, vol. 14, no. 3, pp. 859–868, 1996.

[3] M. F. Brennan, C. R. Antonescu, N. Moraco, and S. Singer, "Lessons learned from the study of 10,000 patients with soft tissue sarcoma," *Annals of Surgery*, vol. 260, no. 3, pp. 416–422, 2014.

[4] P. W. T. Pisters, R. E. Pollock, V. O. Lewis et al., "Long-term results of prospective trial of surgery alone with selective use of radiation for patients with T1 extremity and trunk soft tissue sarcomas," *Annals of Surgery*, vol. 246, no. 4, pp. 675–681, 2007.

[5] G. K. Zagars and M. T. Ballo, "Significance of dose in postoperative radiotherapy for soft tissue sarcoma," *International Journal of Radiation Oncology Biology Physics*, vol. 56, no. 2, pp. 473–481, 2003.

[6] K. M. Alektiar, J. Velasco, M. J. Zelefsky, J. M. Woodruff, J. J. Lewis, and M. F. Brennan, "Adjuvant radiotherapy for margin-positive high-grade soft tissue sarcoma of the extremity," *International Journal of Radiation Oncology Biology Physics*, vol. 48, no. 4, pp. 1051–1058, 2000.

[7] D. J. Biau, P. C. Ferguson, P. Chung et al., "Local recurrence of localized soft tissue sarcoma: a new look at old predictors," *Cancer*, vol. 118, no. 23, pp. 5867–5877, 2012.

[8] G. K. Zagars, M. T. Ballo, P. W. T. Pisters, R. E. Pollock, S. R. Patel, and R. S. Benjamin, "Prognostic factors for disease-specific survival after first relapse of soft-tissue sarcoma: analysis of 402 patients with disease relapse after initial conservative surgery and radiotherapy," *International Journal of Radiation Oncology Biology Physics*, vol. 57, no. 3, pp. 739–747, 2003.

[9] J. J. Lewis, D. Leung, M. Heslin, J. M. Woodruff, and M. F. Brennan, "Association of local recurrence with subsequent survival in extremity soft tissue sarcoma," *Journal of Clinical Oncology*, vol. 15, no. 2, pp. 646–652, 1997.

[10] L. Moureau-Zabotto, L. Thomas, B. N. Bui et al., "Management of soft tissue sarcomas (STS) in first isolated local recurrence: a retrospective study of 83 cases," *Radiotherapy and Oncology*, vol. 73, no. 3, pp. 313–319, 2004.

[11] M. A. Torres, M. T. Ballo, C. E. Butler et al., "Management of locally recurrent soft-tissue sarcoma after prior surgery and radiation therapy," *International Journal of Radiation Oncology Biology Physics*, vol. 67, no. 4, pp. 1124–1129, 2007.

[12] S. Singer, K. Antman, J. M. Corson, and T. J. Eberlein, "Long-term salvageability for patients with locally recurrent soft-tissue sarcomas," *Archives of Surgery*, vol. 127, no. 5, pp. 548–554, 1992.

[13] C. Catton, A. Davis, R. Bell et al., "Soft tissue sarcoma of the extremity. Limb salvage after failure of combined conservative therapy," *Radiotherapy and Oncology*, vol. 41, no. 3, pp. 209–214, 1996.

[14] D. J. Indelicato, K. Meadows, C. P. Gibbs Jr., C. G. Morris, M. T. Scarborough, and R. A. Zlotecki, "Effectiveness and morbidity associated with reirradiation in conservative salvage management of recurrent soft-tissue sarcoma," *International Journal of Radiation Oncology Biology Physics*, vol. 73, no. 1, pp. 267–272, 2009.

[15] A. Kretzler, M. Molls, R. Gradinger, P. Lukas, H.-U. Steinau, and F. Würschmidt, "Intraoperative radiotherapy of soft tissue sarcoma of the extremity," *Strahlentherapie und Onkologie*, vol. 180, no. 6, pp. 365–370, 2004.

[16] T. Lehnert, M. Schwarzbach, F. Willeke et al., "Intraoperative radiotherapy for primary and locally recurrent soft tissue sarcoma: morbidity and long-term prognosis," *European Journal of Surgical Oncology*, vol. 26, supplement, pp. S21–S24, 2000.

[17] P. T. Tran, W. Hara, Z. Su et al., "Intraoperative radiation therapy for locally advanced and recurrent soft-tissue sarcomas

in adults," *International Journal of Radiation Oncology Biology Physics*, vol. 72, no. 4, pp. 1146–1153, 2008.

[18] I. Azinovic, R. M. Monge, J. J. Aristu et al., "Intraoperative radiotherapy electron boost followed by moderate doses of external beam radiotherapy in resected soft-tissue sarcoma of the extremities," *Radiotherapy and Oncology*, vol. 67, no. 3, pp. 331–337, 2003.

[19] F. A. Calvo, C. V. Sole, M. Cambeiro et al., "Prognostic value of external beam radiation therapy in patients treated with surgical resection and intraoperative electron beam radiation therapy for locally recurrent soft tissue sarcoma: a multicentric long-term outcome analysis," *International Journal of Radiation Oncology Biology Physics*, vol. 88, no. 1, pp. 143–150, 2014.

[20] S. B. Edge and C. C. Compton, "The american joint committee on cancer: the 7th edition of the AJCC cancer staging manual and the future of TNM," *Annals of Surgical Oncology*, vol. 17, no. 6, pp. 1471–1474, 2010.

[21] J.-M. Coindre, "Grading of soft tissue sarcomas: review and update," *Archives of Pathology & Laboratory Medicine*, vol. 130, no. 10, pp. 1448–1453, 2006.

[22] W. F. Sindelar, T. J. Kinsella, P. W. Chen et al., "Intraoperative radiotherapy in retroperitoneal sarcomas: final results of a prospective, randomized, clinical trial," *Archives of Surgery*, vol. 128, no. 4, pp. 402–410, 1993.

[23] J. C. Yang, A. E. Chang, A. R. Baker et al., "Randomized prospective study of the benefit of adjuvant radiation therapy in the treatment of soft tissue sarcomas of the extremity," *Journal of Clinical Oncology*, vol. 16, no. 1, pp. 197–203, 1998.

[24] B. O'Sullivan, A. M. Davis, R. Turcotte et al., "Preoperative versus postoperative radiotherapy in soft-tissue sarcoma of the limbs: a randomised trial," *The Lancet*, vol. 359, no. 9325, pp. 2235–2241, 2002.

[25] P. W. Pisters, D. H. Leung, J. Woodruff, W. Shi, and M. F. Brennan, "Analysis of prognostic factors in 1,041 patients with localized soft tissue sarcomas of the extremities," *Journal of Clinical Oncology*, vol. 14, no. 5, pp. 1679–1689, 1996.

[26] S. Oertel, M. Treiber, A. Zahlten-Hinguranage et al., "Intraoperative electron boost radiation followed by moderate doses of external beam radiotherapy in limb-sparing treatment of patients with extremity soft-tissue sarcoma," *International Journal of Radiation Oncology, Biology, Physics*, vol. 64, no. 5, pp. 1416–1423, 2006.

[27] M. G. Haddock, I. A. Petersen, D. Pritchard, and L. L. Gunderson, "IORT in the management of extremity and limb girdle soft tissue sarcomas," *Frontiers of Radiation Therapy and Oncology*, vol. 31, pp. 151–152, 1997.

[28] J. A. Call, S. L. Stafford, I. A. Petersen, and M. G. Haddock, "Use of intraoperative radiotherapy for upper-extremity soft-tissue sarcomas: analysis of disease outcomes and toxicity," *American Journal of Clinical Oncology*, vol. 37, no. 1, pp. 81–85, 2014.

[29] D. B. Pearlstone, N. A. Janjan, B. W. Feig et al., "Re-resection with brachytherapy for locally recurrent soft tissue sarcoma arising in a previously radiated field," *Cancer Journal from Scientific American*, vol. 5, no. 1, pp. 26–33, 1999.

[30] K. M. Alektiar, K. Hu, L. Anderson, M. F. Brennan, and L. B. Harrison, "High-dose-rate intraoperative radiation therapy (HDR-IORT) for retroperitoneal sarcomas," *International Journal of Radiation Oncology Biology Physics*, vol. 47, no. 1, pp. 157–163, 2000.

[31] J. D. Cox, J. Stetz, and T. F. Pajak, "Toxicity criteria of the Radiation Therapy Oncology Group (RTOG) and the European organization for research and treatment of cancer (EORTC)," *International Journal of Radiation Oncology, Biology, Physics*, vol. 31, no. 5, pp. 1341–1346, 1995.

[32] M. Cambeiro, J. Aristu, M. Moreno, L. Arbea, and R. M. Monge, "Conservative surgery and intraoperative radiation therapy for locally recurrent soft-tissue sarcomas of the extremities and the superficial trunk," *International Journal of Radiation Oncology*Biology*Physics*, vol. 84, no. 3, pp. S170–S171, 2012.

3

Preoperative Diagnosis of usual Leiomyoma, Atypical Leiomyoma, and Leiomyosarcoma

M. Matsuda,[1] T. Ichimura,[1] M. Kasai,[1] M. Murakami,[1] N. Kawamura,[2] T. Hayashi,[3] and T. Sumi[1]

[1] *Department of Obstetrics and Gynecology, Osaka City University Graduate School of Medicine, 1-5-7 Asahimachi, Abeno-ku, Osaka 545-8585, Japan*

[2] *Department of Obstetrics and Gynecology, Osaka City General Hospital, Osaka 534-0021, Japan*

[3] *Department of Immunology and Infectious Disease, Shinshu University Graduate School of Medicine, Nagano 390-8621, Japan*

Correspondence should be addressed to M. Matsuda; m1163079@med.osaka-cu.ac.jp

Academic Editor: Akio Sakamoto

Uterine smooth muscle tumors (SMTs) are common pelvic tumors in women, and most of them are diagnosed as usual leiomyoma (UL). Exclusion of malignant disease is important in the management of SMTs. However, differentiation of SMTs remains difficult. In this study, we aimed to improve the preoperative diagnosis of SMTs. We examined 21 ULs, 7 atypical leiomyomas (ALs), and 6 leiomyosarcomas (LMSs), all of which were diagnosed by uterine tumor biopsy. Immunohistochemical findings (low-molecular-mass polypeptide 2 (LMP2) and Ki-67) and clinical features (serum lactate dehydrogenase level and menopause) were evaluated. Statistically significant differences in the expression of LMP2 and Ki-67 were observed between UL and AL and between UL and LMS. The combined LMP2 and Ki-67 score was significantly different between UL and AL, between UL and LMS, and between AL and LMS. The combined immunohistochemistry and clinical findings score (total score) was also significantly different between pathological types. The findings of this study suggest that the accuracy of the preoperative diagnosis of SMTs may be improved by using a combination of immunohistochemical and clinical findings.

1. Introduction

Uterine smooth muscle tumors (SMTs) are common pelvic tumors in women, and most of them are usual leiomyomas (ULs). Leiomyosarcoma (LMS) is rare, constituting only about 1% of uterine cancers; however, it has a poor prognosis [1]. Diagnosis of LMS depends on the presence of cytologic atypia, a high mitotic index (MI), and coagulative tumor cell necrosis (CTCN). Some cases partially have these features, which helps to distinguish between UL and other SMTs. Atypical leiomyoma (AL) is one such SMT, and its pathological features lie between those of LMS and UL; however, its degree of malignancy is uncertain [2]. Although most LMSs arise in postmenopausal women, several cases have been reported in women of reproductive age [1, 3]. Patients with AL are younger than those with LMS and often desire to have children [4].

Various treatments are available for the management of symptomatic UL. Uterus-preserving treatments such as myomectomy, administration of gonadotropin-releasing hormone analog, uterine arterial embolization, and focused ultrasound surgery are widely performed. With the exception of myomectomy, surgical specimens are not obtained using these techniques, and a pathological diagnosis is impossible. Therefore, pretreatment differentiation of SMTs is important. Imaging modalities, especially magnetic resonance imaging (MRI) and fluorodeoxyglucose- (FDG-) positron emission tomography, are useful for the diagnosis of SMTs. However, distinguishing among the different types of SMT remains difficult in many cases [5, 6].

Since 1994, we have performed transcervical needle biopsy to improve the preoperative differential diagnosis of SMTs [7]. Although this procedure enables us to directly evaluate the tumor tissues, the biopsy specimens are very small and the diagnosis may be underestimated. We have attempted to improve the preoperative diagnosis using immunohistochemistry (IHC). We previously reported that the expression of Ki-67 in LMS was higher than that in UL using biopsy specimens [8].

A recent study reported that defective expression of low-molecular-mass polypeptide 2 (LMP2) may initiate the development of spontaneous human uterine LMS [9]. LMP2 is encoded in the major histocompatibility complex class region of the 20S proteasome, which is part of the 26s complex that degrades ubiquitin-conjugated proteins [10]. LMP knockout mice were shown to develop uterine LMS [9].

To improve the quality of preoperative diagnosis of SMTs, we performed a retrospective evaluation of the clinical and IHC features of SMTs by anti-LMP2 and Ki-67 examination of specimens obtained by transcervical needle biopsy.

2. Materials and Methods

2.1. Case Selection. We performed a search of all inpatient files from the Department of Gynecology at Osaka City University Hospital for all patients with uterine SMTs with available needle biopsy specimens in the years 2000 and 2013. All patients underwent transcervical needle biopsy because of unusual MRI findings (high intensity on T1- and/or T2-weighted images) or a rapidly enlarging tumor. Thirty-four cases of SMT were found: 6 cases of LMS, 7 of AL, and 21 of UL. AL was defined as an SMT with moderate to severe atypia, an MI of <10 per 10 high-power fields, and no CTCN.

All tissues were used with the approval of the Ethics Committee of Osaka City University after written informed consent had been obtained from the patients.

2.2. Transcervical Needle Biopsy of Uterine SMTs. Transcervical needle biopsy of uterine SMTs was performed under transabdominal guidance using a Pro-Mag 2.2 biopsy system (Manan Medical Products, Northbrook, IL) with an automatic cutting needle (25 cm long, 16-gauge, and 17 mm notch) and a 20 cm long straight stainless steel guide pipe (4 mm maximum external dimension, 3 mm maximum internal dimension, Honest Medical, Tokyo, Japan). To prevent sampling error, three or more biopsy specimens per patient were obtained [7].

2.3. IHC Staining Procedures. Expression of LMP2 and Ki-67 was investigated in paraffin-embedded sections using the avidin-biotin peroxidase complex method. The 4 μm thick paraffin sections were deparaffinized and immersed in 3% hydrogen peroxidase to block endogenous peroxidase activity. Next, an antigen retrieval procedure was performed only for the sections undergoing examination of Ki-67 expression by immersing the slides in 10 mM citrate buffer (pH 6.0) and heating in an autoclave at 120°C for 20 min. The protocol for the DAKO LSAB 2 peroxidase kit (DAKO, Kyoto, Japan) was followed. The sections undergoing examination of Ki-67 expression were incubated overnight with the primary antibody in a humidified chamber at 4°C, and the sections undergoing examination of LMP2 expression were incubated for 1 hour with primary antibody in a humidified chamber at room temperature. The primary antibodies used for this study were monoclonal mouse anti-human Ki-67 and polyclonal rabbit antiproteasome 20s LMP2. The working dilutions for each primary antibody were 1 : 20 for anti-Ki-67 and 1 : 100 for anti-LMP2. Sections were rinsed with PBS three times and incubated for 10 min with the secondary antibody (biotinylated goat anti-mouse and rabbit immunoglobulin G secondary antibody). The sections were then incubated with streptavidin-peroxidase complex, and 3,3′-diaminobenzidine was used as a chromogen. The sections were counterstained with Mayer's hematoxylin. The specificity of the IHC reactions was checked by omitting the primary antibody [8].

Table 1: (a) LMP2 score. (b) Ki-67 score.

(a)

Score	0	1	2
Intensity	Negative	Weakly positive	Positive
Range	Negative	Focal	Diffuse

(b)

Score	0	1	2
LI	≥15	>5, <15	≤5

2.4. IHC Scoring. LMP2 expression positivity was indicated by brown-staining cytoplasm. The staining intensity was scored as positive = 2 points, weakly positive = 1 point, and negative = 0 points. The stained area was classified as negative = 0 points, focal = 1 point, and diffuse = 2 points (Table 1(a)).

Expression of Ki-67 was evaluated using the labeling index (LI). We counted the positive cells with a brown-stained nucleus at high magnification (×40 objective and ×10 ocular); an LI of ≤5% was assigned 2 points, an LI of >5 to <15% was assigned 1 point, and an LI of ≥15% was assigned 0 points (Table 1(b)). We observed all the areas of all cores and then chose the most active area and calculated LI for each case.

Finally, we calculated the product of each score as the IHC score. The product of the IHC and clinical scores was defined as the total score.

2.5. Clinical Features. We also evaluated each patient's serum lactate dehydrogenase (LD) level and menstrual situation. For the serum LD level, we calculated the LD ratio as the maximum serum LD value/the upper limit of the normal range. When the LD ratio was >1.2, we determined that the patient had a high serum LD level and assigned a score of 0 points (Table 2(a)). We assigned a score of 1 point for premenopausal patients (Table 2(b)).

2.6. Statistical Analysis. The Mann-Whitney U test was used to compare the scores among the analyzed groups (UL, AL, and LMS). P values of <0.05 were considered statistically significant. SPSS version 21 (IBM) was used for all calculations.

TABLE 2: (a) LD score. (b) Menopause score.

(a)

Score	0	1
LD ratio	>1.2	≤1.2

(b)

Score	0	1
Menopause	After	Before

TABLE 3: Clinical features in SMTs.

	UL ($n = 21$)	AL ($n = 7$)	LMS ($n = 6$)
Age (median)	43	46	55
Menopause	1 (5%)	1 (14%)	5 (83%)
High level LD	0	0	3 (50%)

3. Results

3.1. Clinical Features. The patients' clinical features are summarized in Table 3. The patients' ages ranged from 31 to 69 years with a median age of 43 years in patients with UL, 46 years in patients with AL, and 56 years in patients with LMS. No patients took medication, hormones, and supplements. One, one, and three patients with UL, AL, and LMS were postmenopausal, respectively. A high LD level was recorded in only three patients with LMS. Three patients with UL and one with AL underwent myomectomy; the remaining patients underwent total hysterectomy. No patients with AL developed recurrence.

3.2. IHC Findings. Figure 1 shows the immunochemical staining results for LMP2 and Ki-67. The results of the IHC studies are shown in Figures 2–4.

The LMP2 score for UL was 2 to 4 points (median, 3 points), that for AL was 0 to 4 points (median, 3 points), and that for LMS was 0 to 2 points (median, 0 points). A significant difference was found in the product score of UL and LMS ($P < 0.01$) and of UL and AL ($P < 0.05$) (Figure 2).

The Ki-67 score for UL was 1 to 2 points (median, 2 points), that for AL was 0 to 2 points (median, 2 points), and that for LMS was 0 to 2 points (median, 0.5 points). A significant difference was found in the product score of UL and LMS ($P < 0.01$) and of UL and AL ($P < 0.05$) (Figure 3).

The IHC score for UL was 4 to 6 points (median, 5 points), that for AL was 2 to 5 points (median, 4 points), and that for LMS was 0 to 3 points (median, 1.5 points). A significant difference was found in the product score of UL and LMS, of UL and AL, and of AL and LMS ($P < 0.01$) (Figure 4). All cases of UL scored >4 points, and all cases of LMS scored <5 points. With respect to differentiation between AL and UL, the accuracy of inspection was the best when the cut-off score was set at 4 points: the sensitivity was 71.4% (95% CI, 41.8–88.5%) and the specificity was 90.5% (95% CI, 80.6–96.2%). With respect to differentiation between LMS and AL, the accuracy of inspection was the best when the cut-off score was set at 2 points: the sensitivity was 83.3% (95% CI, 54.4–95.3%) and the specificity was 71% (95% CI, 46.3–82.8%).

The total scores are shown in Figure 5. The total score for UL was 5 to 8 points (median, 7 points), that for AL was 3 to 7 points (median, 6 points), and that for LMS was 0 to 4 points (median, 2 points). A significant difference was found in the product score of UL and LMS, of UL and AL, and of AL and LMS ($P < 0.01$). With respect to differentiation between AL and UL, the accuracy of inspection was the best when the cut-off score was set at 6 points: the sensitivity was 71.4% (95% CI, 41.8–88.5%) and the specificity was 90.5% (95% CI, 80.6–96.2%). These results were the same as the IHC scores. With respect to differentiation between LMS and AL, the accuracy of inspection was the best when the cut-off score was set at 3 points: the sensitivity was 83.3% (95% CI, 54.4–95.3%) and the specificity was 85.7% (95% CI, 60.9–96.0%). The total score was more accurate than the IHC score.

4. Discussion

Statistically significant differences were found between UL and LMS and between UL and AL using one measure of IHC in the present study. However, there was no significant difference between AL and LMS. The combination of IHC findings and clinical features enabled detection of significant differences between AL and LMS.

The most important modality for preoperative diagnosis of SMTs is MRI. MRI findings suggestive of LMS include large heterogeneous masses and hemorrhage or cystic necrosis [11]. However, these findings are often present in cases of cellular leiomyoma, degenerated leiomyoma, and atypical leiomyoma. Recent reports have shown that the signal intensity on diffusion-weighted images may be useful for the differential diagnosis of SMTs [12]. Goto et al. reported that the combined use of dynamic MRI and serum LD measurement was useful for the diagnosis of LMS and degenerated leiomyoma [13]. FDG positron emission tomography findings of LMS feature moderate to intense FDG uptake. However, UL rarely shows high FDG uptake and LMS rarely shows mild FDG uptake [6], making it difficult to distinguish SMTs.

We aimed to improve the preoperative diagnosis of SMTs using transcervical uterine tumor biopsy [7]. We performed this technique, transcervical needle biopsy, on over 600 patients from 1994. No major complications, such as infection, intraperitoneal hemorrhage, or an injury of adjacent structures that required surgery, were reported to have occurred. For prevention of infection, we injected antibiotics during transcervical needle biopsy. To avoid injury of adjacent structures and major vessels, we perform transcervical biopsy carefully under transabdominal ultrasonography guidance [14]. Biopsy enables direct evaluation of tumor tissues. However, the diagnosis may be underestimated because the biopsy specimens are very small. Diagnosis of LMS requires two of the three following pathological features: cytologic atypia, a high MI, and CTCN. Small specimens sometimes cannot contain all features. CTCN is often confused with ischemic-type necrosis, and diagnosis of CTCN

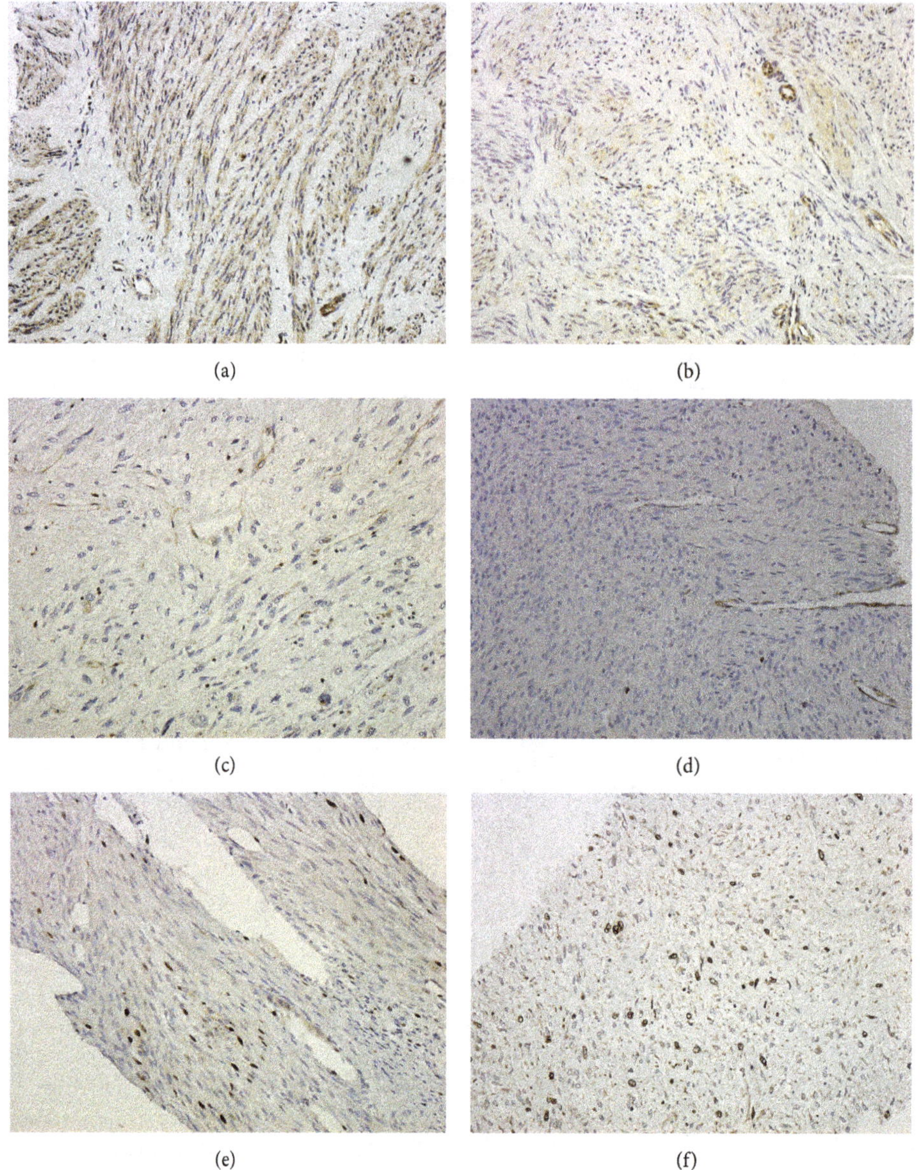

(a) (b) (c) (d) (e) (f)

Figure 1: LMP2 and Ki-67 expression. (a) Positive expression of LMP2 in UL. (b) Weakly positive expression of LMP2 in UL. (c) Negative expression of LMP2 in LMS. (d) Ki-67 expression in UL (LI ≤ 5). (e) Ki-67 expression in UL (5 < LI < 15). (f) Ki-67 expression in LMS (LI ≥ 15).

is difficult. Lim et al. reported that when six pathologists reviewed the occurrence of CTCN in 34 cases of LMS, full agreement regarding the presence or absence of CTCN was reached in only 12 cases (7 were thought to show CTCN) [15]. To prevent sampling error, three and over pieces of biopsy core were sampled. Considering the malignancy of LMS, we checked pathological findings of biopsy specimens in all the areas of all the cores strictly. If we suspected malignancy a little, we recommended the operation to the patients. In more detail, we think of the possibility of the malignancy, when there are some mild atypical nuclei (moderate to severe atypia which is one feature of LMS), less than 10 mitotic figures in all areas, or necrosis which cannot be clearly diagnosed as hyaline necrosis. On the other hand, because of that reason, we cannot exclude some patients of false positive.

Several studies have reported the IHC findings in SMTs. In LMS, the proliferative index of cells (Ki-67, PHH3) is often high and cell cycle regulatory proteins (p16, p53, p27, p21, and cyclins A and E) are often highly expressed. The expression of these markers is sometimes increased in cases of AL [16–19]. We herein reported the IHC staining results of Ki-67 in SMTs. For differentiation between LMS and UL, the best cut-off LI for Ki-67 with biopsy specimens was 5%. In the IHC evaluation of Ki-67 using surgical specimens, all LMS specimens showed an LI of ≥15%. Therefore, we classified the Ki-67 LI as 5% and 15% [8]. In the present study,

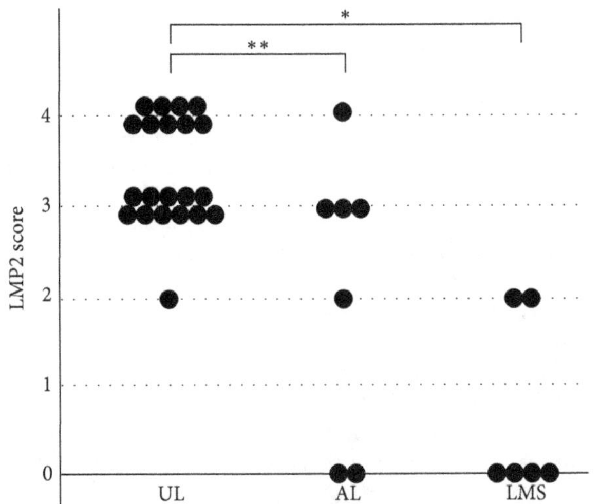

FIGURE 2: LMP score in SMTs. A significant difference was found in the LMP2 score for UL and AL and for UL and LMS ($^*P < 0.01$, $^{**}P < 0.05$).

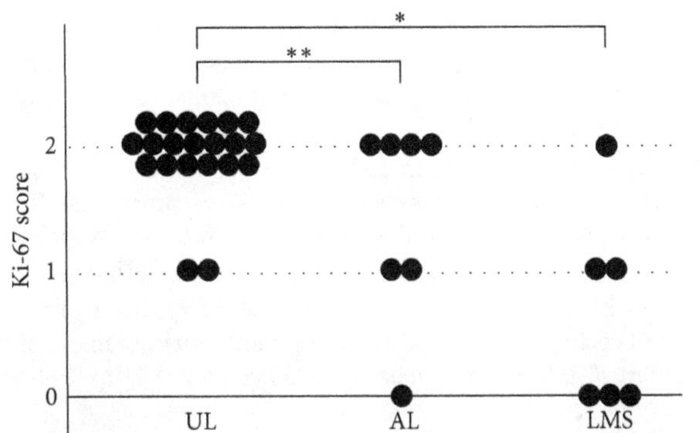

FIGURE 3: Ki-67 score in SMTs. A significant difference was found in the LMP2 score for UL and AL and for UL and LMS ($^*P < 0.01$, $^{**}P < 0.05$).

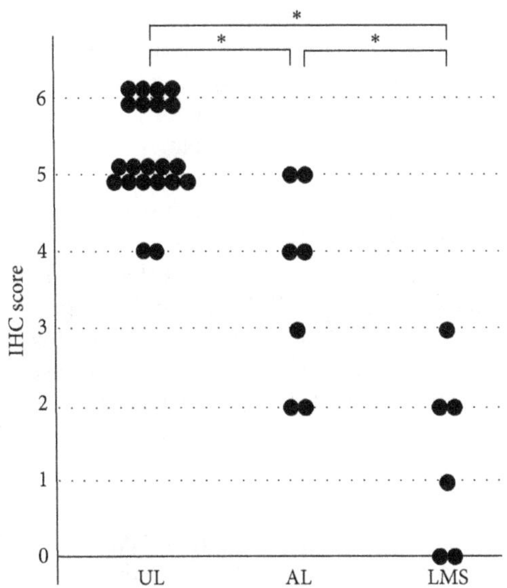

FIGURE 4: IHC score in SMTs. A significant difference was found in the LMP2 score for UL and AL, for UL and LMS, and for AL and LMS ($^*P < 0.01$).

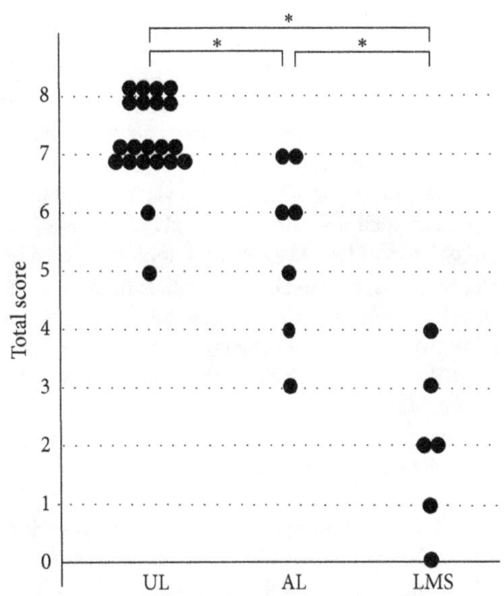

FIGURE 5: Total score in SMTs. A significant difference was found in the LMP2 score for UL and AL, for UL and LMS, and for AL and LMS ($^*P < 0.01$).

the expression of Ki-67 was high in LMS, but there was no difference between AL and LMS.

Hayashi et al. reported the occurrence of LMP2 deficiency associated with the development of LMS. In IHC examination of LMP2 in resected specimens, 46 of 55 cases of LMS were negative, while all 48 cases of UL were positive [20]. The correlation between defective LMP2 function and uterine LMS tumorigenesis is not clearly understood. However, LMP2 has been suggested to play the role of a tumor suppressor by inducing reduced expression of interferon regulatory factor 1 and calponin 1 [21]. Likewise, the present study revealed differences in the staining pattern between UL and LMS in biopsy specimens (Figure 2). The combination of IHC analyses of Ki-67 and LMP2 was helpful for discrimination between LMS and AL.

SMTs have similar presenting symptoms including dysmenorrhea, menorrhagia, anemia, and pelvic masses. Serum levels of total LD in patients with LMS are often abnormally high, but those in patients with degenerated myoma and certain types of leiomyoma are also often elevated [13]. We examined which clinical indicators (chief complaint, MRI findings, serum LD levels, and menopause) are the most useful for the diagnosis of SMTs. Seven patients with AL and eight with LMS were analyzed, and significant differences in the serum LD level and menopause status were noted between patients with AL and those with LMS. The best cut-off LD ratio was 1.2; thus, we defined a high level of LD as >1.2 in this study. Most patients with LMS were postmenopausal; premenopausal patients were assigned 1 point.

The degree of malignancy associated with AL is unknown; most patients undergo hysterectomy to exclude LMS. Ly et al. found that the risk of recurrence in patients with AL is low and that treatment for atypical leiomyoma by myomectomy is therefore a viable option for women of childbearing age; confirmation of pregnancy is also possible after this procedure [4]. Thus, discrimination between AL and LMS is important.

In conclusion, this study suggests that the accuracy of a preoperative diagnosis of SMTs may be improved using a combination of IHC and clinical findings. However, the sample size of this study was small, and more cases need to be examined to reach a definitive conclusion.

References

[1] R. L. Giuntoli II, D. S. Metzinger, C. S. DiMarco et al., "Retrospective review of 208 patients with leiomyosarcoma of the uterus: prognostic indicators, surgical management, and adjuvant therapy," *Gynecologic Oncology*, vol. 89, no. 3, pp. 460–469, 2003.

[2] S. W. Bell, R. L. Kempson, and M. R. Hendrickson, "Problematic uterine smooth muscle neoplasms: a clinicopathologic study of 213 cases," *The American Journal of Surgical Pathology*, vol. 18, no. 6, pp. 535–558, 1994.

[3] D. Milman, Y. Zalel, H. Biran et al., "Unsuspected uterine leiomyosarcoma discovered during treatment with a gonadotropin-releasing hormone analogue: a case report and literature review," *European Journal of Obstetrics Gynecology and Reproductive Biology*, vol. 76, no. 2, pp. 237–240, 1998.

[4] A. Ly, A. M. Mills, J. K. McKenney et al., "Atypical leiomyomas of the uterus: a clinicopathologic study of 51 cases," *American Journal of Surgical Pathology*, vol. 37, no. 5, pp. 643–649, 2013.

[5] K. Sato, N. Yuasa, M. Fujita, and Y. Fukushima, "Clinical application of diffusion-weighted imaging for preoperative differentiation between uterine leiomyoma and leiomyosarcoma," *The American Journal of Obstetrics and Gynecology*, vol. 210, no. 4, pp. 368.e1–368.e8, 2014.

[6] K. Kitajima, K. Murakami, Y. Kaji, and K. Sugimura, "Spectrum of FDG PET/CT findings of uterine tumors," *The American Journal of Roentgenology*, vol. 195, no. 3, pp. 737–743, 2010.

[7] N. Kawamura, T. Ichimura, F. Ito et al., "Transcervical needle biopsy for the differential diagnosis between uterine sarcoma and leiomyoma," *Cancer*, vol. 94, no. 6, pp. 1713–1720, 2002.

[8] C. Yoshida, T. Ichimura, N. Kawamura et al., "A scoring system for histopathologic and immunohistochemical evaluations of uterine leiomyosarcomas," *Oncology Reports*, vol. 22, no. 4, pp. 725–731, 2009.

[9] T. Hayashi and D. L. Faustman, "Development of spontaneous uterine tumors in low molecular mass polypeptide-2 knockout mice," *Cancer Research*, vol. 62, no. 1, pp. 24–27, 2002.

[10] M. Gaczynska, K. L. Rock, T. Spies, and A. L. Goldberg, "Peptidase activities of proteasomes are differentially regulated by the major histocompatibility complex-encoded genes for LMP2 and LMP7," *Proceedings of the National Academy of Sciences of the United States of America*, vol. 91, no. 20, pp. 9213–9217, 1994.

[11] Y. O. Tanaka, M. Nishida, H. Tsunoda, Y. Okamoto, and H. Yoshikawa, "Smooth muscle tumors of uncertain malignant potential and leiomyosarcomas of the uterus: MR findings," *Journal of Magnetic Resonance Imaging*, vol. 20, no. 6, pp. 998–1007, 2004.

[12] T. Namimoto, Y. Yamashita, K. Awai et al., "Combined use of T2-weighted and diffusion-weighted 3-T MR imaging for differentiating uterine sarcomas from benign leiomyomas," *European Radiology*, vol. 19, no. 11, pp. 2756–2764, 2009.

[13] A. Goto, S. Takeuchi, K. Sugimura, and T. Maruo, "Usefulness of Gd-DTPA contrast-enhanced dynamic MRI and serum determination of LDH and its isozymes in the differential diagnosis of leiomyosarcoma from degenerated leiomyoma of the uterus," *International Journal of Gynecological Cancer*, vol. 12, no. 4, pp. 354–361, 2002.

[14] N. Kawamura, T. Ichimura, K. Takahashi, A. Tsujimura, O. Ishiko, and S. Ogita, "Transcervical needle biopsy of uterine myoma-like tumors using an automatic biopsy gun," *Fertility and Sterility*, vol. 77, no. 5, pp. 1060–1064, 2002.

[15] D. Lim, T. Alvarez, M. R. Nucci et al., "Interobserver variability in the interpretation of tumor cell necrosis in uterine leiomyosarcoma," *American Journal of Surgical Pathology*, vol. 37, no. 5, pp. 650–658, 2013.

[16] A. M. Mills, A. Ly, B. L. Balzer et al., "Cell cycle regulatory markers in uterine atypical leiomyoma and leiomyosarcoma: immunohistochemical study of 68 cases with clinical follow-up," *The American Journal of Surgical Pathology*, vol. 37, no. 5, pp. 634–642, 2013.

[17] L. Chen and B. Yang, "Immunohistochemical analysis of p16, p53, and Ki-67 expression in uterine smooth muscle tumors," *International Journal of Gynecological Pathology*, vol. 27, no. 3, pp. 326–332, 2008.

[18] M. Sanci, C. Dikis, S. Inan, E. Turkoz, N. Dicle, and C. Ispahi, "Immunolocalization of VEGF, VEGF receptors, EGF-R and Ki-67 in leiomyoma, cellular leiomyoma and leiomyosarcoma," *Acta Histochemica*, vol. 113, no. 3, pp. 317–325, 2011.

[19] Y. L. Zhai, T. Nikaido, T. Shiozawa et al., "Expression of cyclins and cyclin-dependent kinases in smooth muscle tumors of the uterus," *International Journal of Cancer*, vol. 84, pp. 244–250, 1999.

[20] T. Hayashi, A. Horiuchi, K. Sano et al., "Potential role of LMP2 as tumor-suppressor defines new targets for uterine leiomyosarcoma therapy," *Scientific Reports*, vol. 1, article 180, 2011.

[21] T. Hayashi, A. Horiuchi, K. Sano et al., "Molecular approach to uterine leiomyosarcoma: LMP2-deficient mice as an animal model of spontaneous uterine leiomyosarcoma," *Sarcoma*, vol. 2011, Article ID 476498, 6 pages, 2011.

4

A Clinicopathological Analysis of Soft Tissue Sarcoma with Telangiectatic Changes

Hiroshi Kobayashi,[1,2] Keisuke Ae,[1] Taisuke Tanizawa,[1] Tabu Gokita,[1] Noriko Motoi,[3] and Seiichi Matsumoto[1]

[1]*Department of Orthopedic Surgery, Cancer Institute Hospital, Ariake 3-8-31, Koutou-ku, Tokyo 135-8550, Japan*
[2]*Department of Orthopedic Surgery, The University of Tokyo Hospital, Hongo 7-3-1, Bunkyo-ku, Tokyo 113-8655, Japan*
[3]*Department of Pathology, Cancer Institute Hospital, Ariake 3-8-31, Koutou-ku, Tokyo 135-8550, Japan*

Correspondence should be addressed to Hiroshi Kobayashi; hkobayashi-tky@umin.ac.jp

Academic Editor: Sophie Taieb

Background. Soft tissue sarcoma with a hemorrhagic component that cannot be easily diagnosed by needle biopsy is defined here as soft tissue sarcoma with telangiectatic changes (STST). *Methods.* We retrospectively reviewed clinicopathological data of STST from 14 out of 784 patients (prevalence: 1.8%) with soft tissue sarcoma. *Results.* Tumors were found mostly in the lower leg. Histological diagnoses were undifferentiated pleomorphic sarcoma ($n = 5$), synovial sarcoma ($n = 5$), epithelioid sarcoma ($n = 2$), and malignant peripheral nerve sheath tumor and fibrosarcoma ($n = 1$). No history of trauma to the tumor site was recorded in any patient. Needle aspiration transiently reduced the tumor volume, but subsequent recovery of tumor size was observed in all cases. Out of 14 patients, 9 presented with a painful mass. MRI characteristics included intratumoral nodules (64.3%). The local recurrence rate was 14.3%, and the 2-year event-free survival rate was poorer (50%) than that of most sarcomas. *Conclusions.* STST is unique in its clinicopathological presentation. Painful hematomas without a trauma history, intratumoral nodules within a large hemorrhagic component, and subsequent recovery of tumor size after aspiration are indicative of the presence of STST.

1. Introduction

Needle biopsies are useful for histological diagnosis, since most soft tissue sarcomas are solid. However, small segments of soft tissue sarcoma cannot be diagnosed by needle biopsy because the tumor contains a large, fluid-filled hemorrhagic component. This phenomenon is generally not well appreciated, resulting in delayed diagnosis and poor prognosis [1]. We defined this tumor as a soft tissue sarcoma with telangiectatic changes (STST). Fourteen patients were examined for their unique clinicopathological features, imaging characteristics, diagnostic procedures, and long-term outcomes. The aims of this study are to raise awareness of a rare but distinct clinical form of STST and to assist clinicians in distinguishing between STST and other similar pathologies (hematomas, benign tumors, etc.).

2. Patients and Methods

We retrospectively reviewed 764 cases of soft tissue sarcoma treated in our hospital between 1984 and 2006. Among these patients, 14 (1.8%) developed soft tissue sarcoma of the extremities, which presented with a significant hemorrhagic mass on MRI prior to the initiation of chemotherapy.

The mean age of these patients was 35.9 years (range: 18–66 years). The male to female ratio was 1.8 : 1. The mean follow-up period was 6 years (range: 1–19 years) after the diagnosis of STST.

Of these 14 patients, 7 developed lung metastases, 2 developed lymph node metastases, and 1 developed subcutaneous metastases. Seven patients had died of exacerbation of lung metastases. Information was reviewed from medical records detailing demographic characteristics, clinical presentation of the primary tumor, imaging characteristics, local

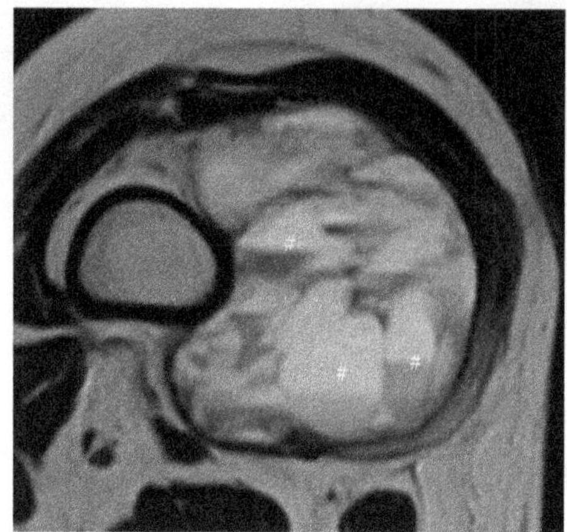
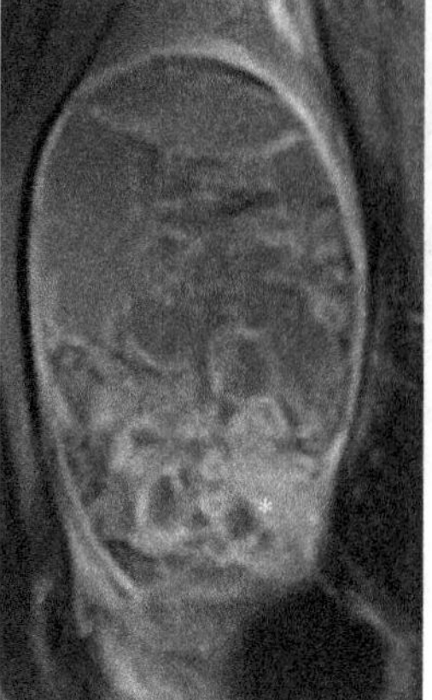

Figure 1: MRI characteristics of soft tissue sarcoma with telangiectatic changes (STST) images showed typical MRI features of STST: (#) fluid-fluid levels, (∗) tumor nodules.

recurrence of the primary tumor site, treatment procedure of the primary site and any lung metastasis, the diagnostic procedure, and oncological outcome. The clinical features of STST were subsequently analyzed.

3. Results

3.1. Clinical and Pathologic Characteristics. No history of trauma to the tumor site was recorded in any patient. The primary complaints were swelling (14 cases), pain (9 cases), and local inflammation (7 cases). Most tumors were located in the thigh (7 cases), followed by the lower thigh (3 cases), buttocks (2 cases), and knee and neck (1 case each).

All cases were categorized as high-grade sarcomas, with histological diagnoses of undifferentiated pleomorphic sarcoma (UPS; 5 cases), synovial sarcoma (5 cases), epithelioid sarcoma (2 cases), and malignant peripheral nerve sheath tumor (MPNST) and fibrosarcoma (1 case each) (Table 1). Tumor size was >5 cm in 12 cases and <5 cm in 2 cases.

3.2. Imaging Characteristics. MRI was performed in 10 out of 14 patients (71%). All tumors were observed to contain blood in over 70% of the tumor area. Tumor nodules on the side of the blood-filled mass were observed in all cases (Figure 1, ∗), although the size of tumor nodules varied in each case. Four out of 10 cases contained fluid-fluid levels (Figure 1, #).

3.3. Diagnostic Procedure. Fine-needle aspiration was performed in 5 patients, resulting in a diagnosis of malignancy in only 1 patient. Needle aspiration temporarily reduces tumor volume, but subsequent recovery of the tumor size was observed in all cases. Core needle biopsies were performed in 6 patients; cytological diagnosis is a sensitivity of 57.1%, but histological diagnosis is a sensitivity of 28.6%. Open biopsies were performed in 10 patients because an accurate diagnosis could not be determined by needle biopsy in 8 cases, and small size precluded needle biopsy in the remaining 2 cases. Incisional and excisional biopsies were performed in 6 and 4 patients, respectively, with a sensitivity of 100% (Table 2). The mean interval between the first visit and pathologic diagnosis was 4 months (Table 3). Repeated aspiration of the tumor after recovery of the tumor size resulted in delayed diagnosis of STST of up to 36 months, because the tumors present as fluctuating masses that may be confused with a hematoma.

Table 1: Clinicopathological characteristics of 14 patients with soft tissue sarcoma with telangiectatic changes (STST).

Sex	
Male	9
Female	5
Trauma	
+	0
−	14
Clinical presentation	
Swell	14
Pain	9
Local inflammation	7
Anatomical location	
Thigh	7
Lower thigh	3
Buttock	2
Knee	1
Neck	1
Histological diagnosis	
UPS	5
Synovial sarcoma	5
Epithelioid sarcoma	2
MPNST	1
Fibrosarcoma	1

UPS: undifferentiated pleomorphic sarcoma.
MPNST: malignant peripheral nerve sheath tumor.

3.4. Treatment and Prognosis. Wide resection of tumors with limb-sparing surgery was performed in 11 cases, and amputation was performed in 3 cases, resulting in wide-margin tumor resection in all cases. Local recurrence was observed

TABLE 2: Relationship among biopsy strategy, surgery, and local recurrence in 14 patients.

Case number	Needle biopsy			Open biopsy		Surgery	Local recurrence
	FNA	CNB		Incisional biopsy	Excisional biopsy		
		Cytology	Histology				
1	Negative	—	—	+	−	Amputation	−
2	Negative	—	—	+	−	Amputation	−
3	Negative	—	—	−	+	Limb-sparing surgery	−
4	—	—	—	+	−	Limb-sparing surgery	−
5	—	Negative	Neurogenic tumor	−	+	Limb-sparing surgery	−
6	—	—	—	−	−	Limb-sparing surgery	−
7	—	Positive	Spindle cell tumor	+	−	Amputation	+
8	Positive	—	—	−	−	Limb-sparing surgery	−
9	Negative	Negative	Fat tissue	−	+	Limb-sparing surgery	−
10	—	Positive	Spindle cell tumor	+	−	Limb-sparing surgery	−
11	—	Negative	Hemangioma	−	+	Limb-sparing surgery	−
12	—	Positive	UPS	−	−	Limb-sparing surgery	−
13	—	—	—	+	−	Limb-sparing surgery	−
14	—	Positive	UPS	−	−	Limb-sparing surgery	+

FNA: fine-needle aspiration.
CNB: core needle biopsy.
UPS: undifferentiated pleomorphic sarcoma.

TABLE 3: Interval between first visit and diagnosis in 14 patients.

Interval (month)	
0	3
1	7
3	1
6	1
36	1
Unknown	1

in 2 cases (14%) and was not related to biopsy procedures and surgery (Table 2). The rate of metastasis was 50%, involving lungs (7 cases), lymph nodes (2 cases), and subcutaneous tissue (1 case). Out of the 7 cases of lung metastasis, an acute increase of lung nodules was observed because of telangiectatic changes in 3 cases (Figure 2). Chemotherapy was performed in all 7 cases of lung metastases postoperatively, but all 7 patients died of complications resulting from lung metastases. The 2-year event-free survival (EFS) rate was 50%.

4. Discussion

Weiss and Enzinger reported on this rare subset of tumors in their 1978 review of 200 cases of MFH [2]. The authors maintained that 5% of MFHs undergo such extreme hemorrhaging that they present clinically as fluctuating masses, which may be confused with hematoma. This study revealed a rare but distinct clinical form of STST. The prevalence of STST was reported to be in the range of 2.9–3.2% [3, 4]. In our study, the rate was relatively low, at 1.8%, as we analyzed only a subset of soft tissue sarcomas (i.e., those that had been difficult to diagnose by needle biopsies because of a hemorrhagic component). Telangiectatic changes occur in a variety of high-grade soft tissue sarcomas, such as MFH, primitive neuroectodermal tumors (PNET) synovial sarcoma, leiomyosarcoma, myxofibrosarcoma, and epithelioid sarcoma. However, intermediate grade sarcoma (e.g., angiomatoid fibrous histiocytoma) and benign tumors (e.g., hemangiomas and schwannomas) could present with a hemorrhagic change [5]. The anatomic distribution defining the presentation of STST correlates well with the sites for soft tissue sarcomas observed in our study, as reported previously [3].

Most high-grade STSTs often present as a painless, gradually enlarging mass [6]. In our study, 9 out of 14 patients (64%) complained of a painful mass but had no prior trauma history. Sternheim et al. reported a higher rate of 80% [3]. The reason of pain from the mass may be caused by intratumoral bleeding and the resulting rapid stretching of surrounding tissues. The lesion is often initially misdiagnosed as a deep intramuscular hematoma for the following reasons: (i) swelling is rapid; (ii) imaging displays a fluid-filled mass; and (iii) hematomas are more common than sarcomas [3].

In our study, repeated puncture of the masses misdiagnosed as hematomas led to a delay of STST diagnosis and treatment. Therefore, subsequent recovery of tumor size after aspiration is an important clue to the presence of STST [1, 7, 8].

In imaging, chronically expanding hematomas have been shown to have large central collections of heterogeneous signal material in both T1- and T2-weighted MRI series [9]. Unlike STSTs, hematomas are usually surrounded by a thick pseudocapsule of material (with a very low intensity T2 signal) composed of fibrous tissue, hemosiderin deposits, and iron-laden macrophages [10]. Therefore, the presence of

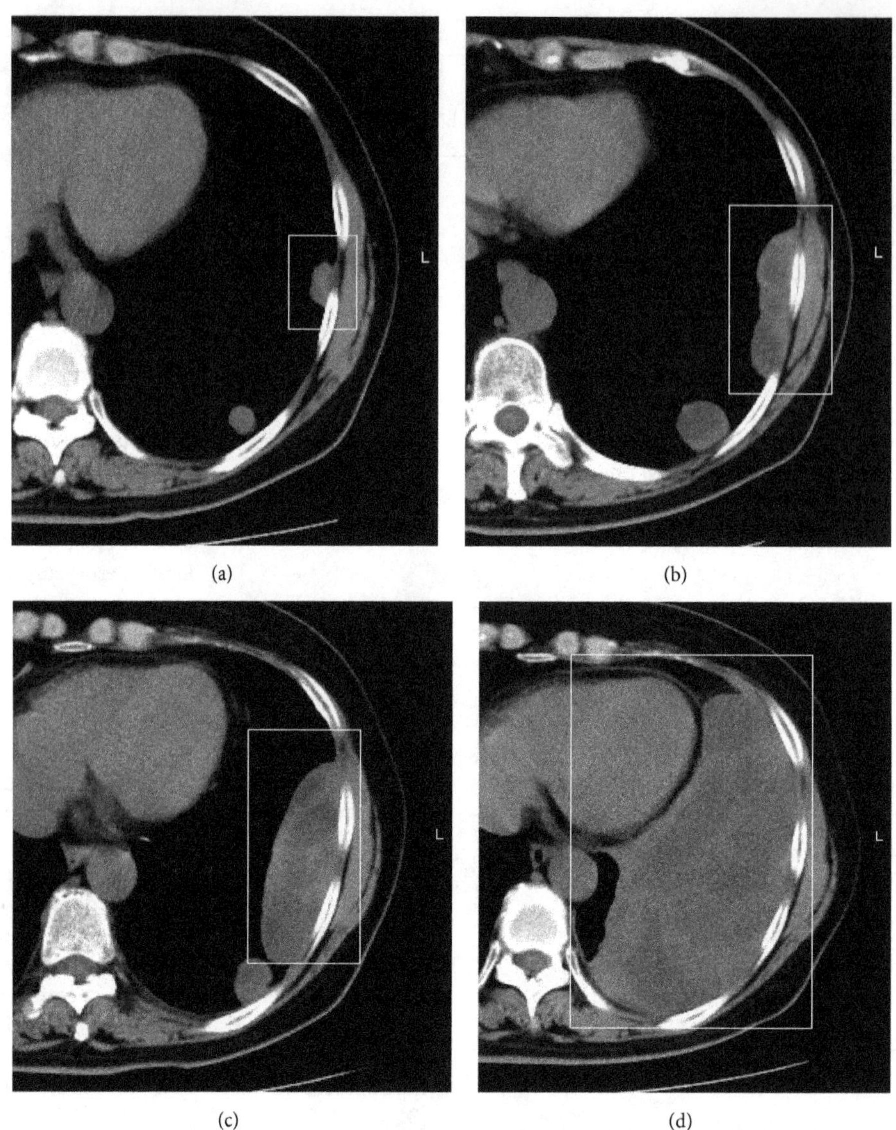

(a) (b) (c) (d)

FIGURE 2: Lung metastases also presented telangiectatic change and resulted in rapid deterioration. (a) First detection of lung metastases. (b) Two months after first detection. (c) Three months after first detection. (d) Four months after first detection.

the nodule enhanced in the tumor is often used to distinguish between hematomas and hemorrhagic neoplasms on MRI and CT scans. In our study, tumor nodules were observed in all cases. However, chronically expanding hematomas with intratumoral nodules have been reported in some instances [10]; therefore, the presence of a nodule does not definitively indicate the existence of a malignancy. On the other hand, a hemorrhagic mass without a nodule could be observed in a hematoma or a benign tumor but not in STST. The presence of fluid-fluid levels was observed in 40% of cases (4 out of 10). However, fluid-fluid levels can be observed in several types of benign tumor, such as hemangiomas and schwannomas; thus, this result did not help in differentiating benign from malignant neoplasms [5].

It is clinically and radiologically impossible to differentiate chronic hematomas from sarcomas; therefore, biopsies must be performed. Since STSTs tend to be misdiagnosed as hematomas as a result of imaging results, tumor aspiration is initially performed in most cases. In this study, fine-needle aspiration resulted in a diagnosis of malignancy in only 1 out of 5 patients. Another study reported a similar diagnostic rate of aspiration-biopsy cytology, that is, 1 out of 6 patients [1]. Fluid analysis showed the presence of numerous erythrocytes, a moderate presence of inflammatory cells (including lymphocytes, macrophages cells, and unaltered neutrophils) like those observed in hematomas. Even when no tumor or atypical cells are observed, reductions in mass size after aspiration followed by rapid mass recovery should be considered a clue to the possible presence of STST. In our study, repetitive aspiration-biopsy cytology alone would have led to the correct diagnosis of STST at the outset. Core needle biopsies were performed in 6 patients, demonstrating that cytological diagnosis was 57.1% sensitivity and histological diagnosis was 28.6% sensitivity. A past study reported a sensitivity of 100% in their subject population [3]. The low rate of diagnosis by core needle biopsy observed in our study was caused by an inability to target the small intratumoral nodule. By contrast, open biopsies were performed with 100% diagnostic sensitivity in our study. We performed excisional biopsies of tumors whose nodules were very small and thus not easily accessible. If internal patchy gadolinium enhancement is observed in the mass, a chronically expanding hematoma remains a possible diagnosis, but immediate aspiration, targeted biopsy, or surgical excision would be necessary to exclude the diagnosis of a hemorrhagic sarcoma because of overlapping imaging characteristics [10].

Sternheim et al. reported a relatively high local recurrence rate of 30% [3], substantially higher than the 14% rate (2 out of 14 cases) observed in our study (which is the same rate as overall soft tissue sarcomas); this is because a wide surgical margin was achieved in our cases. This evidence indicates that STST is not the manifestation of local aggressive behavior. In this study, the overall survival rate was 50%—a poor prognosis—confirming previous reports [3]. In our study, metastatic lung lesions caused intratumoral hemorrhaging and acute increases in tumor size, which, in addition to delayed diagnoses, resulted in a poorer patient prognosis and a relatively more rapid deterioration than those observed in prior reports.

5. Conclusion

STST is a rare and unique clinicopathological entity. STSTs present with characteristic MR imaging patterns, but precise differentiation from benign neoplasms is challenging. However, reduction in size after aspiration and subsequent rapid recovery of tumor size are suggestive to the clinician of the possible presence of STST, and cytological and pathological analyses should be performed through repeated aspiration and needle biopsies. In the instance that no malignancy is observed by needle biopsy, incisional and excisional biopsy should be performed to precisely diagnose STST. STSTs present with aggressive biological behavior and hemorrhagic changes, even at the metastatic lesions; therefore, prompt excision of the metastatic lesions could improve overall outcomes.

References

[1] S. Imaizumi, T. Morita, A. Ogose et al., "Soft tissue sarcoma mimicking chronic hematoma: value of magnetic resonance imaging in differential diagnosis," *Journal of Orthopaedic Science*, vol. 7, no. 1, pp. 33–37, 2002.

[2] S. W. Weiss and F. M. Enzinger, "Malignant fibrous histiocytoma: an analysis of 200 cases," *Cancer*, vol. 41, no. 6, pp. 2250–2266, 1978.

[3] A. Sternheim, X. Jin, B. Shmookler, J. Jelinek, and M. M. Malawer, "'Telangiectatic' transformation in soft tissue sarcomas. A clinicopathology analysis of an aggressive feature of high-grade sarcomas," *Annals of Surgical Oncology*, vol. 15, no. 1, pp. 345–354, 2008.

[4] P. V. Dyck, F. M. Vanhoenacker, J. Vogel et al., "Prevalence, extension and characteristics of fluid-fluid levels in bone and soft tissue tumors," *European Radiology*, vol. 16, no. 12, pp. 2644–2651, 2006.

[5] F. Alyas, J. Lee, M. Ahmed, D. Connell, and A. Saifuddin, "Prevalence and diagnostic significance of fluid-fluid levels in soft-tissue neoplasms," *Clinical Radiology*, vol. 62, no. 8, pp. 769–774, 2007.

[6] J. B. Koea, D. Leung, J. J. Lewis, and M. F. Brennan, "Histopathologic type: an independent prognostic factor in primary soft tissue sarcoma of the extremity?" *Annals of Surgical Oncology*, vol. 10, no. 4, pp. 432–440, 2003.

[7] K. Okada, T. Augiyama, H. Kato et al., "Chronic expanding hematoma mimicking soft tissue neoplasm," *American Society of Clinical Oncology*, vol. 19, pp. 2971–2972, 2001.

[8] H. A. Mann, A. Hilton, N. J. Goddard et al., "Synovial sarcoma mimicking haemophilic pseudotumour," *Sarcoma*, vol. 2006, Article ID 27212, 3 pages, 2006.

[9] O. Cebesoy, E. Tutar, and O. Arpacioglu, "Spontaneous giant expanding thigh hematoma mimicking soft tissue neoplasm," *Joint Bone Spine*, vol. 75, no. 1, pp. 64–66, 2008.

[10] P. T. Liu, K. O. Leslie, C. P. Beauchamp, and S. F. Cherian, "Chronic expanding hematoma of the thigh simulating neoplasm on gadolinium-enhanced MRI," *Skeletal Radiology*, vol. 35, no. 4, pp. 254–257, 2006.

5

Computer-Assisted Planning and Patient-Specific Instruments for Bone Tumor Resection within the Pelvis: A Series of 11 Patients

François Gouin,[1,2] Laurent Paul,[3] Guillaume Anthony Odri,[1,2] and Olivier Cartiaux[3]

[1] *Clinique Chirurgicale Orthopédique et Traumatologique, CHU Hôtel-Dieu, Place Alexis-Ricordeau 1, 44093 Nantes Cedex 1, France*
[2] *Laboratoire Physiopathologie de la Résorption Osseuse, Inserm UI957, Faculté de Medecine, Université de Nantes, rue Gaston Veil, 44000 Nantes, France*
[3] *Computer Assisted and Robotic Surgery (CARS), Institut de Recherche Expérimentale et Clinique, Université Catholique de Louvain, Avenue Mounier 53, 1200 Brussels, Belgium*

Correspondence should be addressed to Laurent Paul; laurent.paul@uclouvain.be

Academic Editor: Charles Catton

Pelvic bone tumor resection is challenging due to complex geometry, limited visibility, and restricted workspace. Accurate resection including a safe margin is required to decrease the risk of local recurrence. This clinical study reports 11 cases of pelvic bone tumor resected by using patient-specific instruments. Magnetic resonance imaging was used to delineate the tumor and computerized tomography to localize it in 3D. Resection planning consisted in desired cutting planes around the tumor including a safe margin. The instruments were designed to fit into unique position on the bony structure and to indicate the desired resection planes. Intraoperatively, instruments were positioned freehand by the surgeon and bone cutting was performed with an oscillating saw. Histopathological analysis of resected specimens showed tumor-free bone resection margins for all cases. Available postoperative computed tomography was registered to preoperative computed tomography to measure location accuracy (minimal distance between an achieved and desired cut planes) and errors on safe margin (minimal distance between the achieved cut planes and the tumor boundary). The location accuracy averaged 2.5 mm. Errors in safe margin averaged −0.8 mm. Instruments described in this study may improve bone tumor surgery within the pelvis by providing good cutting accuracy and clinically acceptable margins.

1. Introduction

Limb salvage surgery is now the preferred procedure for most patients with bone tumors of pelvis and the lower limb. However, resection of bone tumors within the pelvis remains highly challenging because of the complex three-dimensional (3D) geometry of the pelvic bone and the proximity of important organs and neurovascular structures. This complex and restricted working space can explain the high complication rate usually observed in pelvic bone tumor surgery, particularly the local recurrence rate ranging from 28 to 35% [1]. Accurate resections with wide margins are required since it is highly associated with a low local recurrence rate [2–7].

A previous study investigated the ability of experienced surgeons to perform wide margins during simulated tumor cutting of the pelvis [8]. This in vitro study, while performed under optimal conditions, clearly demonstrated that freehand cutting of bone tumors of the pelvis is not accurate enough to ensure wide margins: the errors on the desired safe margin averaged 5.3 mm with a standard deviation ranging from 2.7 to 5.3 mm among the experienced surgeons, and two resections (out of twelve) were intralesional.

Intraoperative navigation systems have been developed for bone tumor surgery, specifically within the pelvis [9–12]. Several authors have reported their experience in using navigation technology to resect bone tumors [13–21]. Their results are highly encouraging since significant improvements in surgical margins can be observed. A significantly decreased local recurrence rate has been shown by Jeys et al. [18] but should be confirmed with a long-term follow-up (13 months

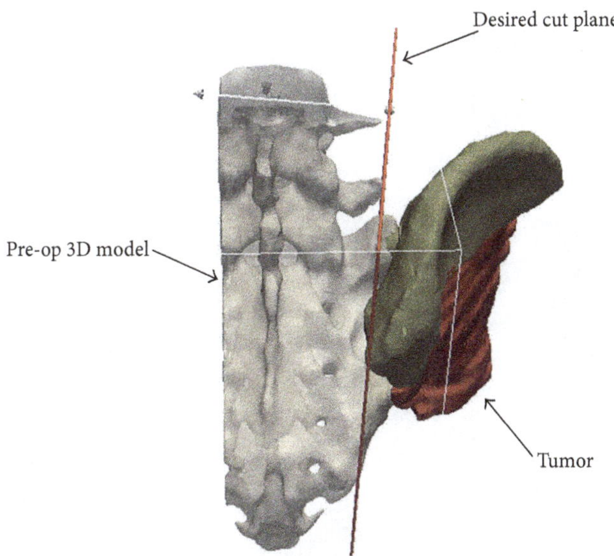

Figure 1: Preoperative planning for patient number 2. Preoperative CT images of the patient were segmented to construct the 3D virtual models of the patient and the tumor. The resection strategy consisted of one target plane defining the desired resection plane with a 6 mm safe margin.

in their clinical series). The value-added of the navigation technology has been recently investigated in an experimental study that demonstrated a significantly improved cutting accuracy during simulated bone tumor surgery of the pelvis [9].

Patient-specific instruments (PSI) have been developed as an alternative to navigation systems. PSI were developed originally for total knee arthroplasty [22, 23] with some residual controversy in terms of the achieved bone-cutting accuracy [24, 25]. Recently, other PSI-assisted applications such as pedicle screw insertion [26–28], hip arthroplasty [29, 30], and corrective osteotomy [31–33] have been described in the literature. PSI technology has been adapted also for bone tumor surgery [34–36]: the patient-specific cutting guides are equipped with bone-specific surfaces to fit into unique position on the patient and flat surfaces to materialize the desired resection planes. A recent experimental study has assessed quantitatively an equivalent value-added of both PSI and navigation technologies in terms of the achieved surgical margins during simulated bone tumor resections of the pelvis [37].

The present study aims to report a series of 11 clinical cases of PSI-assisted bone tumor surgery within the pelvis, with the specific goal of assessing how accurately a preoperative resection strategy can be replicated intraoperatively.

2. Materials and Methods

2.1. Patient Series. The prospective series was composed of 11 patients eligible for curative surgical resection of primary bone tumor of the pelvis (Table 1). Eight patients had a bone sarcoma of iliac bone involving the acetabulum, two patients had a sacral tumor, and one patient had a chondrosarcoma of proximal femur with intra-articular extension. During the same period, two more patients have been operated on by the same surgeon without PSI, the first because the short delay between the acquisition of CT and MRI images and the surgery did not allow to perform the preoperative planning and the PSI manufacturing and the second because the tumor was a chondrosarcoma arising around a total hip prosthesis that rendered the MRI images useless for the planning process.

2.2. Preoperative Planning of the Tumor Resections. The planning of the resection strategy, as described in [13], is based on the MRI and CT images. If these modalities have not been acquired during the diagnosis, a specific exam should be prescribed. Any scanning sequence of the acquired MRI can be used to perform the planning. The CT being crucial for PSI accuracy, its spatial resolution must be 1 mm or below in the Z direction. Tumor delineation is made by the surgeon with the aid of a radiologist on the 2D MRI slices using a segmentation software (ITK-Snap, version 2.0.0, Philadelphia) [38]. The set of MRI images was reconstructed in 3D and brought into the coordinate system of the CT images using a homemade multimodality registration algorithm. Then, the 3D model of the tumor volume was registered with the 3D bony structure extracted from the CT images.

The 3D model of the bony structure with the registered tumor volume was loaded into a visualization and computing software (Paraview, version 3.14.1, New York). This software enabled the surgeon to position target planes close to the boundary of the tumor (from 1 up to 6 planes; Figure 1). For each patient, the resection strategy consisted in several target planes defining the desired bone-cutting with a safe margin defined by the surgeon (namely, 10 to 15 mm). The safe margins have been decreased to 3 mm according to the possibility of preserving anatomic structures and the effectiveness of adjuvant therapy. For instance, for patient number 9, an unusual 3 mm safe margin was defined in order to preserve the sacroiliac joint.

Moreover, sometimes, no safe margin can be easily defined. For example, for patient number 6, the tumor was located in the proximal femur with intra-articular extension, and the resection planning consisted in a 3-plane bone-cutting around the acetabulum, free of tumor, to achieve an extra-articular resection of the hip. Consequently, no desired safe margin has been specifically defined for this case. There was no incidence on the postoperative analysis since the patient was not included because of artifacts created by the metallic implant.

2.3. Patient-Specific Instruments. Patient-specific instruments (PSI) were designed using computer-aided design (CAD) software (Blender version 2.65) according to the desired resection strategy. PSI were designed to have bone-specific contact surfaces to fit into unique position on the bony structure of the patient. These contact surfaces were defined by both surgeon and engineer accounting for surgical approach and bone exposure (described below). PSI were equipped with flat surfaces to indicate the target planes and cylindrical guides for 2 mm diameter Kirschner

Table 1: Patient series, tumor data, histopathological resection results and clinical outcomes.

Patient (gender (M/F), age (years))	Histology[1]	Enneking zones	Tumor size (mm)	Number of resection planes[2]	Closest desired safe margins[3] (mm)	Histological analysis	Neo and adjuvant treatment	Reconstruction	Complication	Follow-up (months)	Current status[4]
1 (F, 76)	CHS grade 2	I + II	200	1 (HER)	10	R0	—	Hip transposition	Deep infection	28	DF
2 (M, 54)	CHS grade 2	I + II + III	120	1 (HER)	6	R0	—	Prosthesis	—	19	DF
3 (M, 57)	CHS grade 2	II	140	3	10	R0	—	Prosthesis	—	17	DF
4 (M, 65)	CHS grade 2	II + III	160	2 (HER)	10	R0	—	Prosthesis	Deep infection	16	DF
5 (F, 69)	LMS	I + II	150	2	10	R0*	Chemotherapy	Prosthesis	ST LR***	22	DF
6 (M, 66)	CHS grade 2	II	140	3 (HER)	—	R0	—	Prosthesis	Deep infection	10	DF
7 (M, 60)	CHS grade 2	I + II + III	170	2	5	R0	—	Prosthesis	Deep infection; hip dislocation	12	DF
8 (F, 27)	CHS grade 2	IV	60	4	7	R2**	—	—	Scare desunion	8	DF
9 (M, 46)	CHS grade 2 LR of myxoid	I + II	270	1	3	R0	—	Prosthesis	Deep infection; hip dislocation	7	DF
10 (M, 17)	ES	II + III	100	3	10	R0	Chemotherapy; radiotherapy	Prosthesis	—	4	DF
11 (M, 54)	Bone sarcoma	IV	100	4	5	R0	Chemotherapy	—	—	0	DF

[1]CHS = chondrosarcoma; LMS = leiomyosarcoma; ES = Ewing's sarcoma; LR = local recurrence.
[2]HER = hip extra-articular resection.
[3]See Table 2 for detailed data on bone-cutting accuracy.
[4]DF = alive disease-free.
*R0 bone resection margin but R1 soft-tissue resection margin.
**R2 bone resection margin because tumor has been morselized for extraction.
***Soft-tissue local recurrence at 18 months; patient was reoperated on; now patient is free of disease.

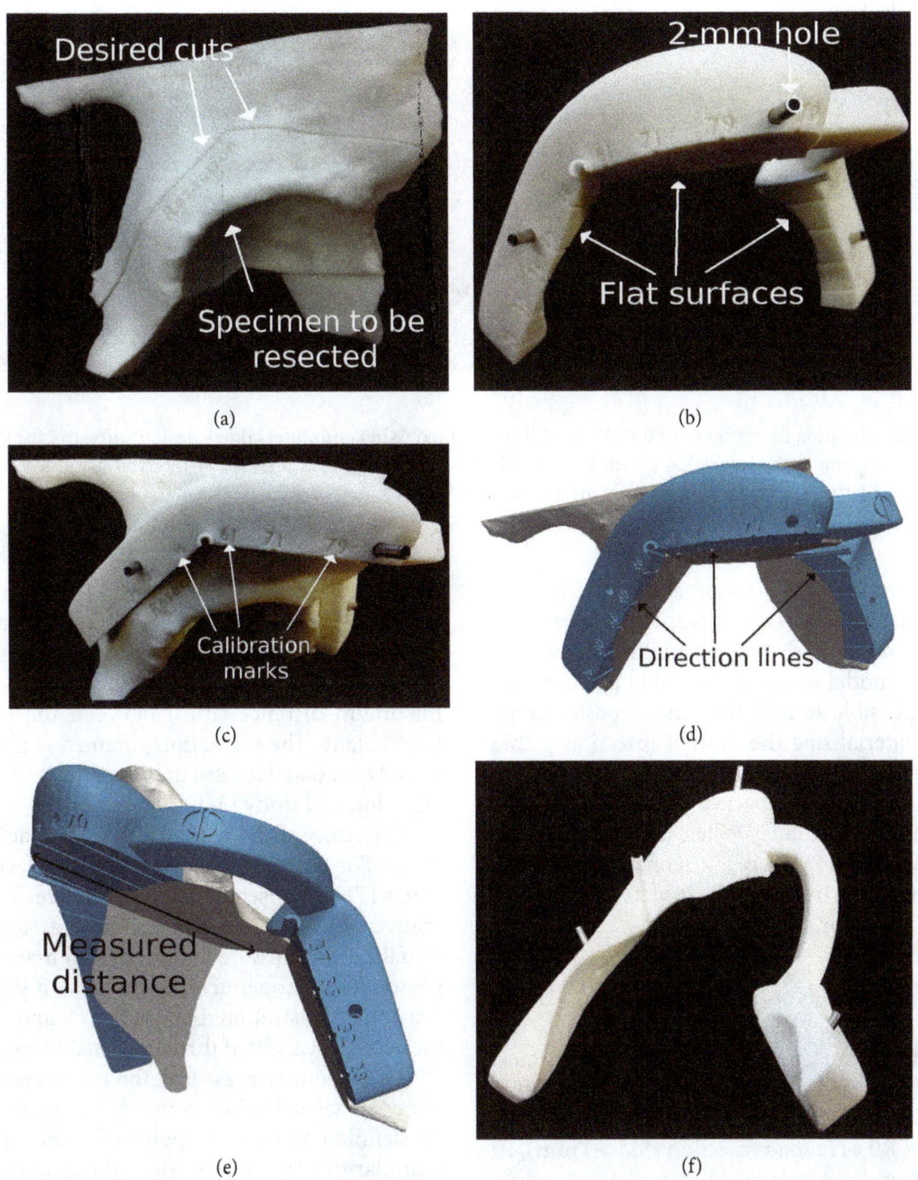

FIGURE 2: Bone models and PSI produced by additive manufacturing for patient number 6. (a) Bone model of the patient enables the visualization of the desired resection strategy and the tumor specimen to be resected. (b) PSI is equipped with flat surfaces to indicate the desired resection planes, holes to be pinned temporarily on the bone using Kirschner wires. (c) PSI has a position of best fit on the bone model. Calibration marks are engraved on the edge to provide visual control of the cutting depth. (d) Associated with a calibration mark direction lines indicate the depth of cutting. (e) The depth is measured from the outer edge of PSI to the deepest bone structure. (f) The direction lines engraved onto the flat surfaces of PSI.

wires to be pinned on the bony structure (Figure 2(b)). In addition, PSI provided calibration marks that provided a control over the cutting depth to prevent a soft tissue tear by the saw. The marks represented the distance along the associated direction line measured between the outer edge of the PSI and the deepest bone structure to be cut. The intended meaning is illustrated in Figure 2(e). PSI and bone models were manufactured by additive manufacturing with a dimensional tolerance of 0.2 mm using an ISO-certified biocompatible polyamide material [39]. PSI and bone models were sterilized using standard autoclave as recommended by polyamide provider.

2.4. PSI-Assisted Tumor Resections. The standard surgical approach has been used for each patient. Soft tissues were dissected following the surgeon's routine technique. Bone was exposed in the area of cuttings before actually performing the resection. The exact dissection areas were identified by using the bone models. PSI required a limited extra bone exposure (less than 10 mm) as their thickness did not exceed 20 mm specifically when positioned in critical area such as under the gluteus medius muscle for an iliac wing section.

PSI was positioned freehand by the surgeon and fixed on the bone surface using the K-wires (Figure 3). Positioning of PSI has been rated intraoperatively by the surgeon using a

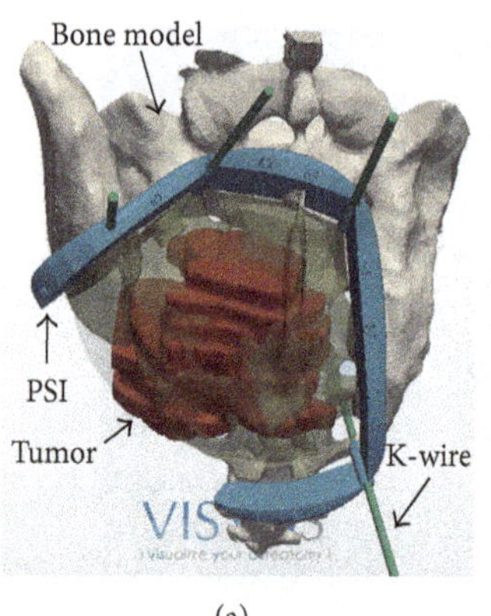

(a)

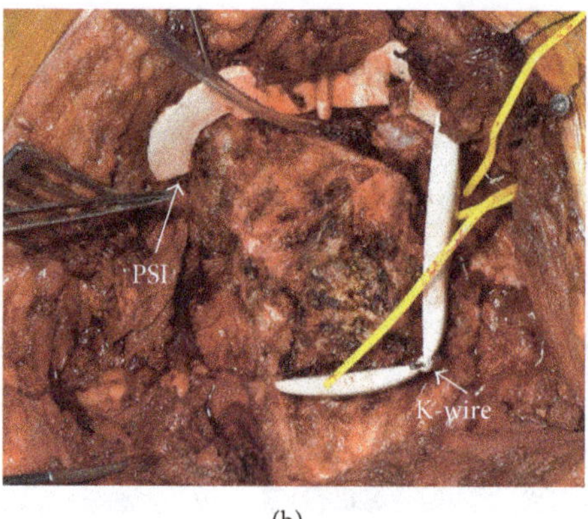

(b)

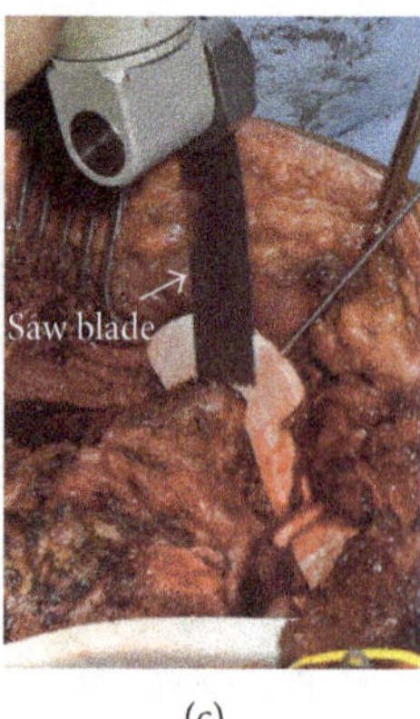

(c)

FIGURE 3: Intraoperative situation for patient number 11. (a) PSI is designed using computer-aided-design software. (b) PSI are sterilizable to be manipulated by the surgeon in the operating room. PSI is positioned on the bone and temporarily fixed using Kirschner wires. (c) Cuts are initiated with the oscillating saw guided by the flat surfaces of the PSI.

4-level scale: excellent (correct position at the first trial, in few seconds, without any doubt), good (easily positioned but not at the first trial), difficult (several trials with peroperative checks on the bone model to achieve a stable positioning), or ambiguous (impossible to find the unique positioning). The flat surfaces materializing the desired resection planes served as mechanical support for the cutting tools, such as an oscillating saw to initiate the bone cuts and then a bone chisel to complete the bone cuts. When the resection was achieved, both K-wires and PSI were taken off, the tumor was mobilized, and intrapelvic tissues were dissected for final *en bloc* extraction of the tumor.

2.5. Histopathological Analysis of Resected Specimens. Histopathological analysis of the resected tumor specimens was performed to evaluate the safety of the achieved surgical margins using the standardized classification by the Union for International Cancer Control (UICC). The UICC classification distinguishes R0 as *in sano* resection (SM > 1 mm), R1 as possible microscopic residuals (SM between 0 and 1 mm), and R2 as macroscopic residual disease [40].

2.6. Postoperative Follow-Up and Clinical Outcomes. Patients were clinically reviewed every 4 to 6 months. Patients underwent postoperative MRI and CT to assess local control and lung X-ray to control a potential distant spreading of the disease.

2.7. Quantitative Evaluation of Bone-Cutting Accuracy. Two parameters were used to evaluate the bone-cutting accuracy. First, the achieved surgical margin (SM) was used to evaluate the accuracy of the bone cut relative to the bone tumor. SM was defined as the minimum distance (mm) between the achieved cut plane and the boundary of the tumor. Consequently, the error in the desired safe margin (ESM) was defined as the difference (mm) between SM and the desired safe margin. Thus, negative values of ESM were found for cutting under the desired safe margin and positive values were found for cutting over the desired safe margin.

Second, the location accuracy (L) was used in accordance with the ISO1101 standard [41, 42] to evaluate the geometrical accuracy of the achieved cut plane with respect to the desired resection plane (the target plane). L was defined as the maximum distance (mm) between the cut plane and the target plane. The evaluation parameters SM and L have been already validated for use in bone tumor surgery in a previous experimental study [37].

CT-scans of the patients have been acquired postoperatively. For each CT-scan, the bone surfaces were extracted using ITK-Snap segmentation software. Then, each postoperative 3D model of the patient was loaded in Paraview visualization software and registered manually with the corresponding preoperative 3D model and planning (Figure 4). Accurate registration between pre- and postoperative 3D models was validated through visual inspection of the data.

One operator measured the parameters SM and L using Paraview visualization software. The operator measured SM by defining the closest point of each cut plane from the boundary of the tumor. Then the operator measured L by defining the most distant point of each cut plane from the corresponding target plane and measuring numerically the distance along the normal of the target plane. For patient number 2, the parameter L had to be corrected by the thickness of the saw blade to account for the loss of bone material (the kerf) during bone-cutting [43], because the PSI was positioned on the tumor side.

Results are presented as the mean and 95% confidence interval (CI).

3. Results

3.1. Histopathological Results and Clinical Outcomes. Positioning of the PSI on the bone surface was unambiguous for all cases. The positioning has been rated as excellent in seven patients, good in three patients, and difficult in one patient. Finally, the PSI was positioned within 5 minutes for each case.

All achieved surgical margins were classified R0, except in two patients. Patient number 5 suffered from a tumor in close contact with external iliac vessels. Although bone margins

TABLE 2: Achieved surgical margins SM and location accuracy L.

Resection plane (patient)	Desired safe margin (mm)	Achieved surgical margin SM (mm)	Error in safe margin ESM (mm)	Location accuracy L (mm)
1 (2)	6	5.2	−0.8	2.1
2 (4)	15	14.2	−0.8	2.5
3 (5)	10	6.6	−3.4	4.4
4 (7)	10	10.3	0.3	1.1
5 (9)	3	2.8	−0.2	2.8
6 (10)	12	12.1	0.1	2.7
7 (10)	10	8	−2	1.5
8 (11)	5	3.5	−1.5	2.7
9 (11)	5	5.7	0.7	2.6

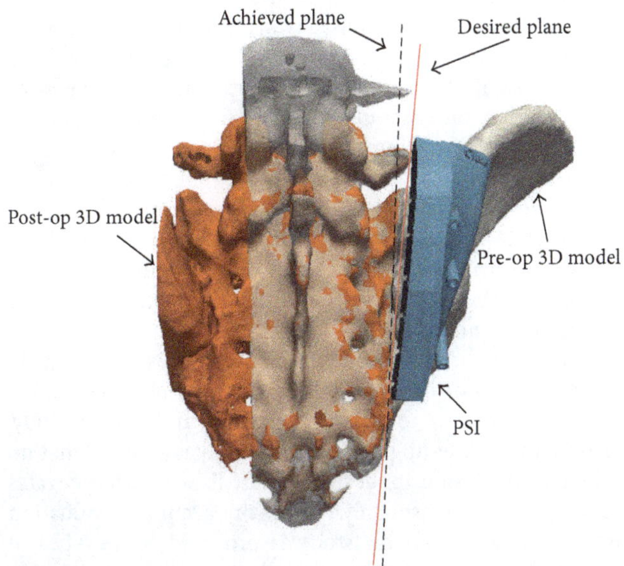

FIGURE 4: Quantitative evaluation of bone cuts for patient number 2. Postoperative 3D virtual model of the patient was constructed from the postoperative CT images and registered to the preoperative 3D model. The achieved cut plane was manually identified and compared to the desired cut plane. See text for details on the computation of location accuracy parameter L and surgical margin SM.

were classified R0, the resection was classified R1 because soft tissues margin was considered between 0 and 1 mm. Patient number 8 suffered intraoperatively from bad cardiovascular condition associated with severe bleeding requiring urgent extraction of the tumor which has been consequently morselized. The surgical margin was then classified R2.

The postoperative follow-up averaged 14 months with a range from 0 to 28 months. At the time of follow-up, patient number 5 had a recurrence at 18 months around iliac vessels. Reoperation was performed with soft tissue resection including vessels with allograft arterial reconstruction.

3.2. Bone-Cutting Accuracy. Of the 26 cut planes performed by the surgeon in this study, nine cut planes were eligible for the evaluation of the bone-cutting accuracy (Table 2). Twelve cut planes (all the cut planes of patients numbers 3, 6, and 8 and two cut planes of patient number 11) were excluded from the evaluation process because of no available postoperative CT-scan or inadequate resolution. One cut plane (patient number 1) was excluded because the presence of the bone autograft (reconstruction with hip transposition) in the postoperative CT images rendered the evaluation too inaccurate. Finally, four cut planes (one cut plane of patients numbers 4, 5, 7, and 10) were excluded because the presence of the metallic prosthesis rendered the postoperative CT images unsuitable for the evaluation of these bone cuts.

The errors in safe margin (difference between achieved and desired resection margins) averaged −0.8 mm (95% CI: −1.8 to 0.1 mm). The maximum positive error (cutting over the desired resection margin) was 0.3 mm (patient number 7), while the maximum negative error (cutting under the desired resection margin) was −3.4 mm (patient number 5).

The location accuracy of the achieved cut planes with respect to the desired target planes averaged 2.5 mm (95% CI: 1.8 to 3.2 mm). The maximum inaccuracy was found for patient number 5 with a difference of 4.4 mm between desired and achieved cut planes.

4. Discussion

This study reported a clinical series of 11 PSI-assisted bone tumor resections within the pelvis. The observed results showed that PSI-assisted bone-cutting can be performed safely with an accuracy clinically relevant for bone tumor surgery within the pelvis.

Histopathological results of the resected tumor specimens did not reveal any marginal or intralesional resection. However, for patient number 8, the resected tumor specimen had to be suddenly extracted because of severe intraoperative bleeding but could not have been removed *en bloc* because of its complex 3D shape, and the surgeon had to urgently morselize the specimen to be able to extract the tumor as soon as possible, inevitably inducing R2 bone resection margin. Adequate orientation of the desired resection planes should be optimized preoperatively during the planning process to guarantee intraoperative rapid *en bloc* extraction of the tumor. Moreover, for patient number 5, the iliac bone resection margin was classified R0 but the patient had a soft tissue local recurrence in the external iliac vessels that has been classified R1. In such case, achieving adequate soft tissue margin is highly challenging, especially as PSI is a technology that assists bone-cutting with no intended action on soft tissues.

By systematically achieving clear bone margins, it appears that PSI technology could have the potential to significantly reduce the risk of local recurrence. However, the short-term follow-up of the present study is not sufficient to state any improvement in terms of the oncological outcomes. A minimum 3-year follow-up should enable the drawing of more stringent conclusions about the presence or absence of local recurrence after bone tumor resections [44]. Moreover, local recurrence can appear even if safe margins are achieved, as it was recently demonstrated in several case series of navigation-assisted bone tumor surgeries [18, 44, 45].

Results in terms of the errors in safe margin ESM or the location accuracy L demonstrated how PSI enabled the surgeon to intraoperatively replicate the resection strategies with a very good cutting accuracy. These findings are consistent with the levels of bone-cutting accuracy already published in the literature on the clinical use of PSI and navigation technologies for bone tumor surgery. Wong et al. [35] reported a millimetric accuracy during a PSI-assisted bone tumor resection of the femur. Ritacco et al. [20] reported a series of 28 navigation-assisted bone tumor resections with an average cutting error of 2.5 mm between planned and achieved resection planes. Finally, Khan et al. [36] also investigated bone-cutting accuracy in accordance with the ISO1101 standard and reported a 2 mm location accuracy during a PSI-assisted multiplanar resection on a cadaveric femur.

Improvements in accuracy observed here are consistent with findings of a previous study on synthetic pelvic bone models [37]. The observed level of accuracy suggests that a 5 mm safe margin should be sufficient to obtain clear surgical margins when using PSI since the observed maximum error in safe margins is 3.4 mm. This decrease in the level of desired safe margins allows performing resections closer to the tumor boundary, offering the possibility of preserving either the sacroiliac or hip joint, a portion of bone, muscle insertions, or nerve roots. For example, in patient number 11, the 5 mm margin enabled preserving three sacral nerves, keeping organ functionalities of the patient.

PSI have several potential advantages that are more difficult to assess objectively. First, PSI are cost-effective since the technique is pay-per-use and does not require any intraoperative assistance. Second, in addition to the improvements in bone-cutting accuracy, the direct visual control of the cutting depth provided by the PSI through calibrated rulers allows for an easy mobilization of the resected tumor specimen, potentially increasing the safety of critical bone cuts such as posterior transsacral bone cuts.

PSI technology has some limitations. It requires a multidisciplinary team and, particularly, a technical person to perform the preoperative planning and design the instruments. PSI requires bone exposure to find a stable bone surface and to be accurately positioned. This can be a limit to the technique but somehow moderate since the bone exposure is also required before cutting bones with the conventional technique. Bone exposure was limited thanks to the visual support of the 3D bone model that was provided with the PSI. Finally, mispositioning of PSI can occur leading to an inaccuracy during the bone-cuttings.

PSI have to respect some technical requirements to meet relevant surgical performances. First, PSI must optimally fit into the bone surface without interfering with soft tissues (ligaments, muscles insertions, etc.). Then, the stability of PSI should be sufficient to ensure a safe and quick positioning on the bone surface. An interesting method to determine the stability of the PSI has been recently proposed in [46]. These authors have developed a quantitative stability score that provides an objective evaluation of the stability according to the contact surfaces between PSI and bone. This score can be computed before manufacturing to ensure an adequate stability. Finally, preoperative workflow requires sending images, defining surgical strategy, planning resection, and finally designing and manufacturing PSI. The timeframe for planning and manufacturing PSI is about 4 weeks, which fits with the clinical situation when patients undergo neochemotherapy and/or radiotherapy. When chondrosarcomas do not require neither chemotherapy nor radiotherapy, the complete process can be significantly shortened, requiring a high responsiveness of both surgeon and engineer. Anyway, a strong collaboration between surgeon and engineer as well as efficient communication tools are required.

This study has some limitations. First, this study has no randomization or control group. The rarity of bone tumors does not allow us to perform such a randomized study. Second, the follow-up period of this study is short so that no stringent conclusion about survival and local recurrence rates could be drawn reasonably. Third, the accuracy evaluation process proposed in this study is prone to some types of methodological errors that are hardly controllable. For example, the postoperative CT images can be unsuitable for evaluation purposes because the presence of a metallic implant (used for reconstruction) renders the identification of the cutting planes too inaccurate. Also, the 3D model reconstructed from the postoperative CT images has to be registered with the preoperative CT images and may lead to registration errors. Finally, bone formation may occur between the time of the surgery and the time of the postoperative CT acquisition, thus altering the identification of the achieved cut planes and potentially overestimating the cutting errors.

5. Conclusion

The present clinical study demonstrated that using PSI during bone tumor resection within the pelvis provides good cutting accuracy. Intraoperative use of PSI appeared to be quick and easy-to-handle and allowed obtaining bone clear margins. Follow-up should continue to observe local recurrence rate and draw stronger conclusion about the use of PSI technology during bone tumor resection within the pelvis and its effect on clinical outcomes.

References

[1] C. Delloye, X. Banse, B. Brichard, P. Docquier, and O. Cornu, "Pelvic reconstruction with a structural pelvic allograft after resection of a malignant bone tumor," *Journal of Bone and Joint Surgery A*, vol. 89, no. 3, pp. 579–587, 2007.

[2] I. Han, Y. M. Lee, H. S. Cho, J. H. Oh, S. H. Lee, and H. Kim, "Outcome after surgical treatment of pelvic sarcomas," *Clinics in Orthopedic Surgery*, vol. 2, no. 3, pp. 160–166, 2010.

[3] B. Fuchs, N. Hoekzema, D. R. Larson, C. Y. Inwards, and F. H. Sim, "Osteosarcoma of the pelvis: outcome analysis of surgical treatment," *Clinical Orthopaedics and Related Research*, vol. 467, no. 2, pp. 510–518, 2009.

[4] T. Ozaki, S. Flege, M. Kevric et al., "Osteosarcoma of the pelvis: experience of the Cooperative Osteosarcoma Study Group," *Journal of Clinical Oncology*, vol. 21, no. 2, pp. 334–341, 2003.

[5] C. Hoffmann, S. Ahrens, J. Dunst et al., "Pelvic Ewing sarcoma: a retrospective analysis of 241 cases," *Cancer*, vol. 85, no. 4, pp. 869–877, 1999.

[6] R. Gradinger, H. Rechl, and E. Hipp, "Pelvic osteosarcoma. Resection, reconstruction, local control, and survival statistics," *Clinical Orthopaedics and Related Research*, no. 270, pp. 149–158, 1991.

[7] M. Sluga, R. Windhager, S. Lang et al., "The role of surgery and resection margins in the treatment of Ewing's sarcoma," *Clinical Orthopaedics and Related Research*, no. 392, pp. 394–399, 2001.

[8] O. Cartiaux, P.-L. Docquier, L. Paul et al., "Surgical inaccuracy of tumor resection and reconstruction within the pelvis: an experimental study," *Acta orthopaedica*, vol. 79, no. 5, pp. 695–702, 2008.

[9] O. Cartiaux, X. Banse, L. Paul, B. G. Francq, C. Aubin, and P. Docquier, "Computer-assisted planning and navigation improves cutting accuracy during simulated bone tumor surgery of the pelvis," *Computer Aided Surgery*, vol. 18, no. 1-2, pp. 19–26, 2013.

[10] J. A. Abraham, "Recent advances in navigation-assisted musculoskeletal tumor resection," *Current Orthopaedic Practice*, vol. 22, no. 4, pp. 297–302, 2011.

[11] O. Cartiaux, L. Paul, P. Docquier, and X. Banse, "Computer- and robot-assisted resection and reconstruction of pelvic bone tumours—a review," *European Musculoskeletal Review*, vol. 6, no. 2, pp. 125–130, 2011.

[12] S. Fehlberg, S. Eulenstein, T. Lange, D. Andreou, and P. Tunn, "Computer-assisted pelvic tumor resection: fields of application, limits, and perspectives," *Recent Results in Cancer Research*, vol. 179, pp. 169–182, 2009.

[13] P. L. Docquier, L. Paul, O. Cartiaux, C. Delloye, and X. Banse, "Computer-assisted resection and reconstruction of pelvic tumor sarcoma," *Sarcoma*, vol. 2010, Article ID 125162, 8 pages, 2010.

[14] T. Y. C. So, Y. L. Lam, and K. L. Mak, "Computer-assisted navigation in bone tumor surgery: seamless workflow model and evolution of technique," *Clinical Orthopaedics and Related Research*, vol. 468, no. 11, pp. 2985–2991, 2010.

[15] H. S. Cho, H. G. Kang, H. S. Kim, and I. Han, "Computer-assisted sacral tumor resection. A case report," *Journal of Bone and Joint Surgery A*, vol. 90, pp. 1561–1566, 2008.

[16] C. Krettek, J. Geerling, L. Bastian et al., "Computer aided tumor resection in the pelvis," *Injury*, vol. 35, no. 1, pp. SA79–SA83, 2004.

[17] K. Wong, S. M. Kumta, K. Chiu et al., "Computer assisted pelvic tumor resection and reconstruction with a custom-made prosthesis using an innovative adaptation and its validation," *Computer Aided Surgery*, vol. 12, no. 4, pp. 225–232, 2007.

[18] L. Jeys, G. S. Matharu, R. S. Nandra, and R. J. Grimer, "Can computer navigation-assisted surgery reduce the risk of an intralesional margin and reduce the rate of local recurrence in patients with a tumour of the pelvis or sacrum?" *Bone and Joint Journal*, vol. 95, no. 10, pp. 1417–1424, 2013.

[19] K. C. Wong, S. M. Kumta, K. H. Chiu, G. E. Antonio, P. Unwin, and K. S. Leung, "Precision tumour resection and reconstruction using image-guided computer navigation," *Journal of Bone and Joint Surgery B*, vol. 89, no. 7, pp. 943–947, 2007.

[20] L. E. Ritacco, F. E. Milano, G. L. Farfalli, M. A. Ayerza, D. L. Muscolo, and L. A. Aponte-Tinao, "Accuracy of 3-D planning and navigation in bone tumor resection," *Orthopedics*, vol. 36, no. 7, pp. e942–e950, 2013.

[21] K. C. Wong and S. M. Kumta, "Joint-preserving tumor resection and reconstruction using image-guided computer navigation tumor," *Clinical Orthopaedics and Related Research*, vol. 471, no. 3, pp. 762–773, 2013.

[22] M. A. Hafez, K. L. Chelule, B. B. Seedhom, and K. P. Sherman, "Computer-assisted total knee arthroplasty using patient-specific templating," *Clinical Orthopaedics and Related Research*, no. 444, pp. 184–192, 2006.

[23] V. Y. Ng, J. H. DeClaire, K. R. Berend, B. C. Gulick, and A. V. Lombardi Jr., "Improved accuracy of alignment with patient-specific positioning guides compared with manual instrumentation in TKA," *Clinical Orthopaedics and Related Research*, vol. 470, no. 1, pp. 99–107, 2012.

[24] D. White, K. L. Chelule, and B. B. Seedhom, "Accuracy of MRI vs CT imaging with particular reference to patient specific templates for total knee replacement surgery," *The International Journal of Medical Robotics and Computer Assisted Surgery*, vol. 4, no. 3, pp. 224–231, 2008.

[25] R. M. Nunley, B. S. Ellison, J. Zhu, E. L. Ruh, S. M. Howell, and R. L. Barrack, "Do patient-specific guides improve coronal alignment in total knee arthroplasty?" *Clinical Orthopaedics and Related Research*, vol. 470, no. 3, pp. 895–902, 2012.

[26] E. Schkommodau, N. Decker, U. Klapper, K. Birnbaum, H. W. Staudte, and K. Radermacher, "Pedicle screw implantation using the DISOS template system," in *Navigation and Robotics in Total Joint and Spine Surgery*, J. B. Stiehl, W. H. Konermann, and R. G. Haaker, Eds., pp. 501–505, Springer, Berlin, Germany, 2003.

[27] S. Lu, Y. Q. Xu, Y. Z. Zhang et al., "A novel computer-assisted drill guide template for lumbar pedicle screw placement: a cadaveric and clinical study," *International Journal of Medical Robotics and Computer Assisted Surgery*, vol. 5, no. 2, pp. 184–191, 2009.

[28] V. Ferrari, P. Parchi, S. Condino et al., "An optimal design for patient-specific templates for pedicle spine screws placement," *International Journal of Medical Robotics and Computer Assisted Surgery*, vol. 9, no. 3, pp. 298–304, 2013.

[29] Y. Z. Zhang, B. Chen, S. Lu et al., "Preliminary application of computer-assisted patient-specific acetabular navigational template for total hip arthroplasty in adult single development dysplasia of the hip," *The International Journal of Medical Robotics and Computer Assisted Surgery*, vol. 7, no. 4, pp. 469–474, 2011.

[30] S. Takashi, H. Toshihisa, M. Tsuyoshi et al., "Validation of patient specific surgical guides in total hip arthroplasty," *The International Journal of Medical Robotics and Computer Assisted Surgery*, vol. 10, no. 1, pp. 113–120, 2013.

[31] J. G. G. Dobbe, J. C. Vroemen, S. D. Strackee, and G. J. Streekstra, "Patient-tailored plate for bone fixation and accurate 3D positioning in corrective osteotomy," *Medical and Biological Engineering and Computing*, vol. 51, no. 1-2, pp. 19–27, 2013.

[32] J. Victor and A. Premanathan, "Virtual 3D planning and patient specific surgical guides for osteotomies around the knee: a feasibility and proof-of-concept study," *Bone and Joint Journal*, vol. 95-B, no. 11, supplement A, pp. 153–158, 2013.

[33] K. Oka, T. Murase, H. Moritomo, and H. Yoshikawa, "Corrective osteotomy for malunited both bones fractures of the forearm with radial head dislocations using a custom-made surgical guide: two case reports," *Journal of Shoulder and Elbow Surgery*, vol. 21, no. 10, pp. e1–e8, 2012.

[34] L. Bellanova, L. Paul, and P. Docquier, "Surgical guides (patient-specific instruments) for pediatric tibial bone sarcoma resection and allograft reconstruction," *Sarcoma*, vol. 2013, Article ID 787653, 7 pages, 2013.

[35] K. C. Wong, S. M. Kumta, K. Y. Sze, and C. M. Wong, "Use of a patient-specific CAD/CAM surgical jig in extremity bone tumor resection and custom prosthetic reconstruction," *Computer Aided Surgery*, vol. 17, no. 6, pp. 284–293, 2012.

[36] F. A. Khan, J. D. Lipman, A. D. Pearle, P. J. Boland, and J. H. Healey, "Surgical technique: computer-generated custom jigs improve accuracy of wide resection of bone tumors," *Clinical Orthopaedics and Related Research*, vol. 471, no. 6, pp. 2007–2016, 2013.

[37] O. Cartiaux, L. Paul, B. G. Francq, X. Banse, and P. L. Docquier, "Improved accuracy with 3D planning and patient-specific instruments during simulated pelvic bone tumor surgery," *Annals of Biomedical Engineering*, vol. 42, no. 1, pp. 205–213, 2014.

[38] P. A. Yushkevich, J. Piven, H. C. Hazlett et al., "User-guided 3D active contour segmentation of anatomical structures: significantly improved efficiency and reliability," *NeuroImage*, vol. 31, no. 3, pp. 1116–1128, 2006.

[39] International Organization for Standardization, *Standard 10993:2009: Biological Evaluation of Medical Devices*, International Organization for Standardization, Geneva, Switzerland, 4th edition, 2009.

[40] C. Wittekind, C. C. Compton, F. L. Greene, and L. H. Sobin, "TNM residual tumor classification revisited," *Cancer*, vol. 94, no. 9, pp. 2511–2516, 2002.

[41] International Organization for Standardization, *Standard 1101: 2004: Geometrical Product Specifications (GPS)—Geometrical Tolerancing—Tolerances of Form, Orientation, Location and Run-out*, International Organization for Standardization, Geneva, Switzerland, 2nd edition, 2004.

[42] O. Cartiaux, L. Paul, P.-L. Docquier et al., "Accuracy in planar cutting of bones: an ISO-based evaluation," *The International Journal of Medical Robotics and Computer Assisted Surgery*, vol. 5, no. 1, pp. 77–84, 2009.

[43] J. A. Bailey, Y. Wang, F. R. W. van de Goot, and R. R. R. Gerretsen, "Statistical analysis of kerf mark measurements in bone," *Forensic Science, Medicine, and Pathology*, vol. 7, no. 1, pp. 53–62, 2011.

[44] H. S. Cho, J. H. Oh, I. Han, and H. Kim, "The outcomes of navigation-assisted bone tumour surgery: minimum three-year follow-up," *Journal of Bone and Joint Surgery B*, vol. 94, no. 10, pp. 1414–1420, 2012.

[45] K. C. Wong and S. M. Kumta, "Computer-assisted tumor surgery in malignant bone tumors," *Clinical Orthopaedics and Related Research*, vol. 471, no. 3, pp. 750–761, 2013.

[46] J. Van den Broeck, R. Wirix-Speetjens, and J. Vander Sloten, "Preoperative analysis of the stability of fit of a patient-specific surgical guide," *Computer Methods in Biomechanics and Biomedical Engineering*, 2013.

6

Homogenous Good Outcome in a Heterogeneous Group of Tumors: An Institutional Series of Outcomes of Superficial Soft Tissue Sarcomas

Valerie Francescutti,[1] Sartaj S. Sanghera,[1] Richard T. Cheney,[2] Austin Miller,[3] Kilian Salerno,[4] Rachel Burke,[5] Joseph J. Skitzki,[1] and John M. Kane III[1]

[1]*Department of Surgical Oncology, Roswell Park Cancer Institute, Buffalo, NY 14263, USA*
[2]*Department of Pathology and Laboratory Medicine, Roswell Park Cancer Institute, Buffalo, NY 14263, USA*
[3]*Department of Biostatistics and Bioinformatics, Roswell Park Cancer Institute, Buffalo, NY 14263, USA*
[4]*Department of Radiation Medicine, Roswell Park Cancer Institute, Buffalo, NY 14263, USA*
[5]*Naval Medical Center Portsmouth, Portsmouth, VA 23708, USA*

Correspondence should be addressed to Valerie Francescutti; valerie.francescutti@roswellpark.org

Academic Editor: Silvia Stacchiotti

Introduction. Superficial soft tissue sarcomas (S-STS) are generally amenable to wide excision. We hypothesized that local recurrence (LR) should be low, even without radiation therapy (RT), and sought to examine the contribution of depth to LR and OS. *Methods.* Patients with S-STS were retrospectively reviewed. Demographics, tumor features, treatment received, and outcomes were analyzed. *Results.* 103 patients were identified. Median age was 55 years; 53% of patients were female. Tumor site was 39% in trunk, 38% in the lower extremity, 14% in the upper extremity, and 9% in other locations. The most common histology was 36% leiomyosarcoma. Median tumor size was 2.8 cm (range 0.2–14 cm). Sixty-six percent of tumors were of intermediate/high grade. RT was administered preoperatively in 6% of patients and postoperatively in 15% of patients. An R0 resection was accomplished in 92%. At a median follow-up of 34.2 months (range 2.3–176), 9 patients had a LR (8.7%). Tumor size and grade were not associated with LR. OS was not associated with any tumor or patient variables on univariate analysis. *Conclusions.* LR was low for S-STS, even with large or high grade tumors and selective use of RT. Surgical resection alone may be adequate therapy for most patients. Superficial location seems to supersede other factors imparting a good prognosis for this group of tumors.

1. Introduction

Sarcomas are a heterogeneous group of solid tumors accounting for 1% of adult malignancies, with an annual incidence of soft tissue sarcoma (STS) of approximately 11,000 cases in the United States [1]. The heterogeneity of these tumors is significant with at least 50 different histologic subtypes of sarcoma identified, all of which have distinct biologic behavior and response to various treatments [2]. Further heterogeneity exists in that primary STS can occur in a myriad of anatomic locations including extremities, trunk, retroperitoneum, and head and neck [3].

Surgery, radiation, and systemic therapies are important treatment modalities in the treatment of patients with sarcoma. The aim of the local therapies includes negative margin resection with surgery and selective use of pre- or postoperative use of radiation therapy (RT) to decrease the rate of local recurrence (LR). There have been several factors that have been shown to predict risk for LR, including tumor size, tumor depth, histologic grade, surgical margin status, and the use of RT [4–9].

Superficial STS (S-STS) are a distinct group characterized by location above the superficial fascia, a factor that influences the T-stage in the AJCC Sarcoma Staging System

[10]. Superficial depth has been demonstrated in a number of studies to portend a good prognosis with respect to metastasis-free survival (MFS) [2, 3, 11–13]. Tumor depth in this group of sarcomas has been shown to be as predictive of behavior as size [11]. Retrospective series of S-STS have shown favorable prognosis, with overall low local recurrence (LR) rates and excellent overall survival (OS) rates [14–16]. In addition, many LRs are salvageable with further surgery and RT [17].

Although multimodality treatment including RT or chemotherapy may be appropriate in the management of select S-STS, the majority can be managed by surgical resection alone as resection with widely negative margins is technically feasible in a greater proportion of these cases than in deep STS [18]. Moreover, the timing of RT or chemotherapy with respect to surgery in S-STS is not as well defined as deep sarcomas and is generally the result of multidisciplinary discussion related to tumor histology and grade and the ability to achieve a resection with wide margins and pathologic features following resection.

The current study was undertaken to determine the outcomes of our series of patients with S-STS, including LR and OS rates. In addition, we sought to describe the use of therapies other than surgical resection such as RT and chemotherapy in the treatment of S-STS patients. For a more comprehensive evaluation of the management and outcomes of S-STS given the smaller numbers of patients in individual series, we also performed a comprehensive literature review of outcomes specific to S-STS to provide an overview of the management of this unique disease entity.

2. Methods

2.1. S-STS Patient Series

2.1.1. Patients. Institute ethics approval was obtained prior to study initiation. Charts of consecutive patients with S-STS undergoing definitive treatment from 1 January 1993 to 1 March 2011 at Roswell Park Cancer Institute (RPCI) were retrospectively reviewed. Patients were included in the study if they had a biopsy-proven sarcoma, superficial to fascia, and underwent treatment with curative intent (stages I–III). All initial biopsies (core needle or incisional) completed at outside institutions were reviewed by RPCI pathologist. Preoperative imaging generally included CT or MRI of the primary site at the discretion of the surgeon. Patients were excluded if tumor histology was dermatofibrosarcoma protuberans or if stage IV disease was identified at the time of planned initial surgical treatment. At the time of patient evaluation and treatment planning, malignant fibrous histiocytoma (MFH) was a histologic entity. Although presently this term is no longer used, patient cases were not reclassified at the time of the retrospective review and analysis to reflect this, as this diagnosis was used to make clinical decisions at the time of patient treatment. Surgical margins were defined as negative (free of microscopic or macroscopic tumor), close (margin was less than 2 cm, due to anatomic constraints), or positive (R1).

2.1.2. Data Collection. For each patient the following data were collected: age, sex, tumor location (upper or lower extremity, superficial trunk, and head and neck), tumor size, histology, grade, and stage. Data regarding surgical management, including details of resection, tissue defect closure, and margin status, were reviewed and collected. Use of multimodality therapy including RT and/or chemotherapy was assessed, and timing of each with respect to surgery was noted. Time to any event (LR and/or death) was determined from the date of diagnosis in months. All LRs were biopsy proven. For survival data, patients were censored at the date of last clinic visit. For date of death, this was obtained from patient charts or was determined from the RPCI death registry.

2.1.3. Outcomes. The primary outcome was local recurrence (LR) rate. Secondary outcomes included local recurrence free survival (LRFS) and overall survival (OS) rates.

2.1.4. Statistical Methods. To evaluate the effect of administration of RT, patients were classified as receiving or not receiving RT. In addition, the contribution of tumor size ($\leq$5 cm and >5 cm) and tumor grade on OS, LR, and LRFS was evaluated. Between-group comparisons of the distributions of continuous and categorical variables were assessed using the Wilcoxon Rank-Sum Test and Fischer's exact test, respectively. Patients were censored at the date of death or last follow-up. Differences in the time to LR were displayed in Kaplan-Meier plots. p values less than 0.05 were considered statistically significant.

3. Results

3.1. S-STS Patient Series. A total of 103 consecutive patients were identified for review. Table 1 includes demographic data for all patients, indicating a median age of 55 years, with an approximately equal sex distribution. The majority of S-STS was located in the lower extremity (37.9%) or trunk (38.8%) and was generally smaller in size ($\leq$5 cm). Median tumor size was 3.0 cm (range 0.15–14.0 cm). Approximately one-half of tumors were identified as either leiomyosarcomas or MFH, with other histologies represented in varying numbers.

Considering surgical management of S-STS, 92.2% of patients ($n = 95$) underwent an R0 resection (Table 1). Approximately one-third of patients required either a skin graft or flap for closure of the surgical site. Widely negative margins ($\geq$2 cm) were achieved in 75% of patients undergoing surgery. Close margins, considered as margins <2 cm but not positive, occurred in 20% of patients, with the majority of these having a close deep fascial margin.

Regarding multimodality therapy, a total of 8 patients received chemotherapy in the management of their disease; 5 of these patients had angiosarcoma. Of the patients that received chemotherapy preoperatively ($n = 5$), 3 had angiosarcoma, and 2 had "other" histologies. Of those receiving postoperative chemotherapy ($n = 3$), 2 had angiosarcoma, and 1 was noted to have lymph node metastases postoperatively. Concerning use of RT, 75% of patients received no RT. Of those patients receiving RT, the majority of RT was

TABLE 1: S-STS patient demographics, disease characteristics, and management.

	$n = 103$
Age, years	
Median (range)	55 (15–89)
Sex	
Male	48 (46.6%)
Tumor location	
Trunk	40 (38.8%)
Lower extremity	39 (37.9%)
Upper extremity	14 (13.6%)
Head and neck	8 (7.8%)
Vulva	2 (1.9%)
Tumor size	
≤5 cm	79 (76.6%)
>5 cm	21 (20.4%)
Unknown	3 (3.0%)
Histology	
Leiomyosarcoma	37 (35.9%)
MFH[1]	16 (15.5%)
Liposarcoma	8 (7.8%)
Pleomorphic sarcoma	8 (7.8%)
Myxofibrosarcoma	7 (6.8%)
Angiosarcoma	6 (5.8%)
Other[2]	21 (20.4%)
Grade	
Low	32 (31.0%)
Intermediate	7 (6.8%)
High	56 (54.4%)
Unknown	8 (7.8%)
Stage	
I	31 (30.0%)
II	49 (47.6%)
III	22 (21.4%)
Unknown	1 (1.0%)
Surgery, resection	
R0	95 (92.2%)
Wide (≥2 cm)	76 (80%)
Close (<2 cm)	19 (20%)
R1	6 (5.8%)
Unknown	2 (1.9%)
Surgery, closure of defect	
Skin graft	22 (21.4%)
Flap	14 (13.6%)
Radiation therapy	
Preoperative	6 (5.8%)
Postoperative	16 (15.5%)
None	77 (74.8%)
Other[3]	4 (3.9%)
Chemotherapy	
Preoperative	5 (4.9%)
Postoperative	3 (2.9%)
None	95 (92.2%)

[1]Malignant fibrous histiocytoma.
[2]Including epithelioid sarcoma, fibrosarcoma, synovial sarcoma, clear cell sarcoma, primitive neuroectodermal tumor (PNET), malignant peripheral nerve sheath tumor (MPNST), and not otherwise specified (NOS).
[3]Received after LR prior to excision.

TABLE 2: Outcome measures following treatment for S-STS.

Follow-up (months)	
Median (range)	34.2 (2.3–176.0)
Locoregional or distant metastasis site	
Lung	4 (3.9%)
Lymph node	2 (1.9%)
Liver	1 (1.0%)
Bone	1 (1.0%)
Local recurrence	9 (8.7%)
Overall survival	93.2%

administered in the postoperative period (n = 16). Of these 16 patients, most had a close surgical margin, especially deep (fascial).

Median follow-up for this cohort of patients was 34.2 months (range 2.3–176.0 months; Table 2). A total of 6 patients developed distant metastases in the follow-up period, with 4 developing lung metastases. Two patients developed lymph node metastases following resection of the primary S-STS. The overall LR rate was 8.7%. The OS for this cohort was 93.2%. LRFS and OS for the entire cohort can be found in Figures 1(a) and 1(b), respectively. Considering patients undergoing RT, LRFS was significantly lower in those patients undergoing RT (p = 0.03, Figure 2(a)), but there was no effect on OS compared with those not undergoing RT (Figure 2(b)).

Figure 2(c) indicates no effect of tumor size on LRFS (p = 0.46) and similarly no effect of tumor grade on LRFS (p = 0.79, Figure 2(d)).

4. Discussion

Tumor location exclusively above the fascia has been shown in prior reports to confer a favorable prognosis in studied cohorts of S-STS. S-STS account for 20–30% of all soft tissue sarcomas and as such it is important to have a more thorough understanding of their biological behavior to make informed treatment decisions.

This is a single institution series of S-STS managed surgically, with decisions on a case-by-case basis for the use of RT and chemotherapy. This series includes a variety of tumor locations and histologies very similar to other published series of S-STS, with the majority being T1a sarcoma (5 cm or smaller). It has been suggested that most series of S-STS include smaller, low grade tumors, which are detected earlier, and that these factors could account for the better outcomes [15, 19, 20]. However, in our series, the majority of tumors were of intermediate to high grade. This is in keeping with the findings of Salas and colleagues, who found no correlation between grade and LRFS on multivariate analysis [16]. Regarding the issue of superficial versus deep location and earlier detection, Pisters and colleagues prospectively evaluated surgery alone with selective use of RT in T1 sarcomas of the extremity and superficial trunk and noted an overall LR rate of 29% (8/28) for deep and 6.7% (4/60) for superficial sarcomas. These two groups, which were very

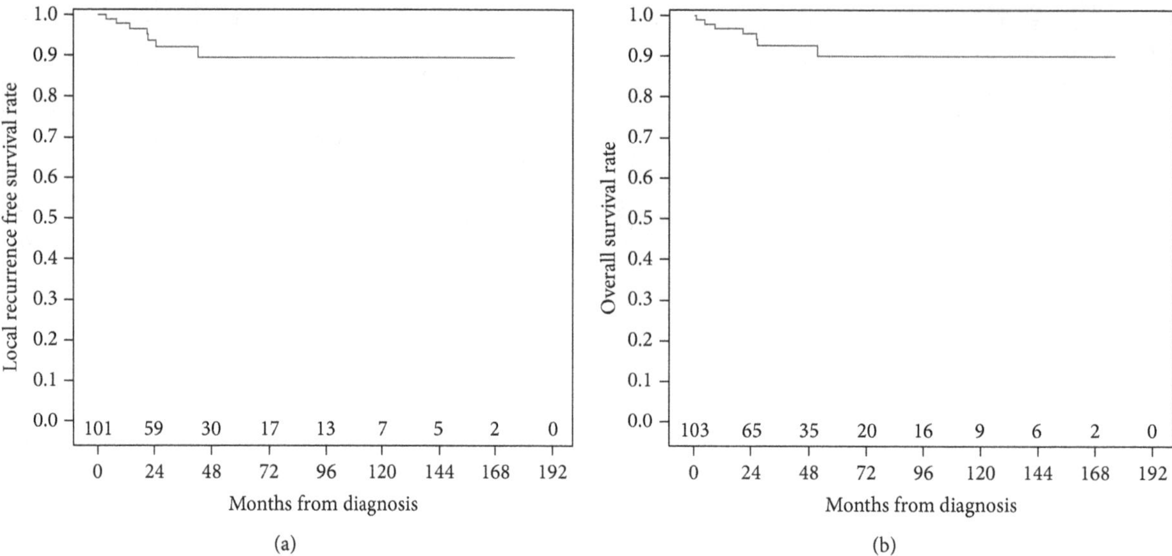

FIGURE 1: For all patients with S-STS, the local recurrence free survival (LRFS) rate was 93.2% (a), with median overall survival (OS) rate of 93.2% (b).

similar in terms of size and histology, still had discrepant LR rates [21]. This may be due to difficulty in achieving wide surgical margins in deep sarcomas as compared with those in superficial locations rather than a bias towards less aggressive smaller tumors that are detected earlier in the superficial group.

The approach to S-STS at our institution includes definitive surgical resection with wide margins. Wide margins were achieved in over 75% of patients. The LR rate in this series was low, at 8.7%, which compares favorably to other published series of S-STS [14–16, 19, 20]. Prior studies have indicated that the quality of surgical therapy is an independent prognostic factor for LRFS on multivariate analysis and this probably accounts for the favorable outcomes observed in our series [16, 20].

The local recurrence rate in our series was 8.7%. A total of 9 patients had a local recurrence. Of these 9 patients, 3 patients had wide margins (>/=2 cm), 2 had close margins (<2 cm), 2 had positive margins, and 2 had unknown margins. Four of the 9 patients with LR did not receive any RT. Both patients with positive margins received postoperative RT; one patient with close margins received postoperative RT. The second patient with close margins received RT postoperatively after resection of the local recurrence. Of those patients developing a LR, 6 patients had a single LR, while 3 had more than one LR (range 2-3). All LRs were managed with repeat surgical resection, some with the addition of RT. The overall low LR rate, in addition to the ability to successfully manage LR with surgical resection, is likely a reflection of more locally aggressive histology or tumor behavior in this small subset. In addition to surgery, consideration regarding the benefit of RT occurred on a case-by-case basis either by the treating physician or at the multidisciplinary team conference meeting. RT was used infrequently, in only 21.3% of patients in the pre- or postoperative period related to their initial resection. Chemotherapy was used most frequently in angiosarcoma patients, with a small number of other sarcoma patients receiving chemotherapy for treatment after the development of distant metastases.

Considering the effect of RT on OS and LRFS, it appears that those patients receiving RT had a poorer LRFS (p = 0.03), whereas OS was not affected. A total of 5 patients experiencing LR (55.6%) underwent RT treatment, 2 postoperatively after the initial resection and 3 after the LR. The poorer LRFS in the group receiving RT may be indicative of selective administration of RT in patients with known high-risk tumor biology or those in whom wide resection may be technically more difficult, with those more likely to develop a LR receiving RT. This is consistent with the findings of Coindre and colleagues, who noted a similar trend toward increased LR in the subset of patients to whom RT was administered because of a perceived high risk of recurrence based on the judgment of experienced clinicians [2].

Upon comprehensive review of the literature, only a small number of studies reported the outcomes of LR and OS in patients with S-STS separate from deep STS (Table 3). Overall, a total of 1024 cases in 6 series of S-STS have been documented, and results indicate a variable LR rate (8.0–24.8%). Of note, there is some variability in terms of S-STS included in each series, as two series included patients with DFSP, known to have a higher LR rate than other S-STS [15, 16]. The variable use of RT in these series, ranging from 8.5% to 52.8% of cases, indicates that no consensus exists on which patients may benefit most from this therapy. OS rates all fell within the same range for the various published series, although many had differing rates of histologic subtypes, tumor sizes, and proportion of patients receiving wide excision. Biau and colleagues evaluated the risk of LR in sarcoma based on several predictors in 1668 patients with localized STS of the extremity or trunk with a competition model.

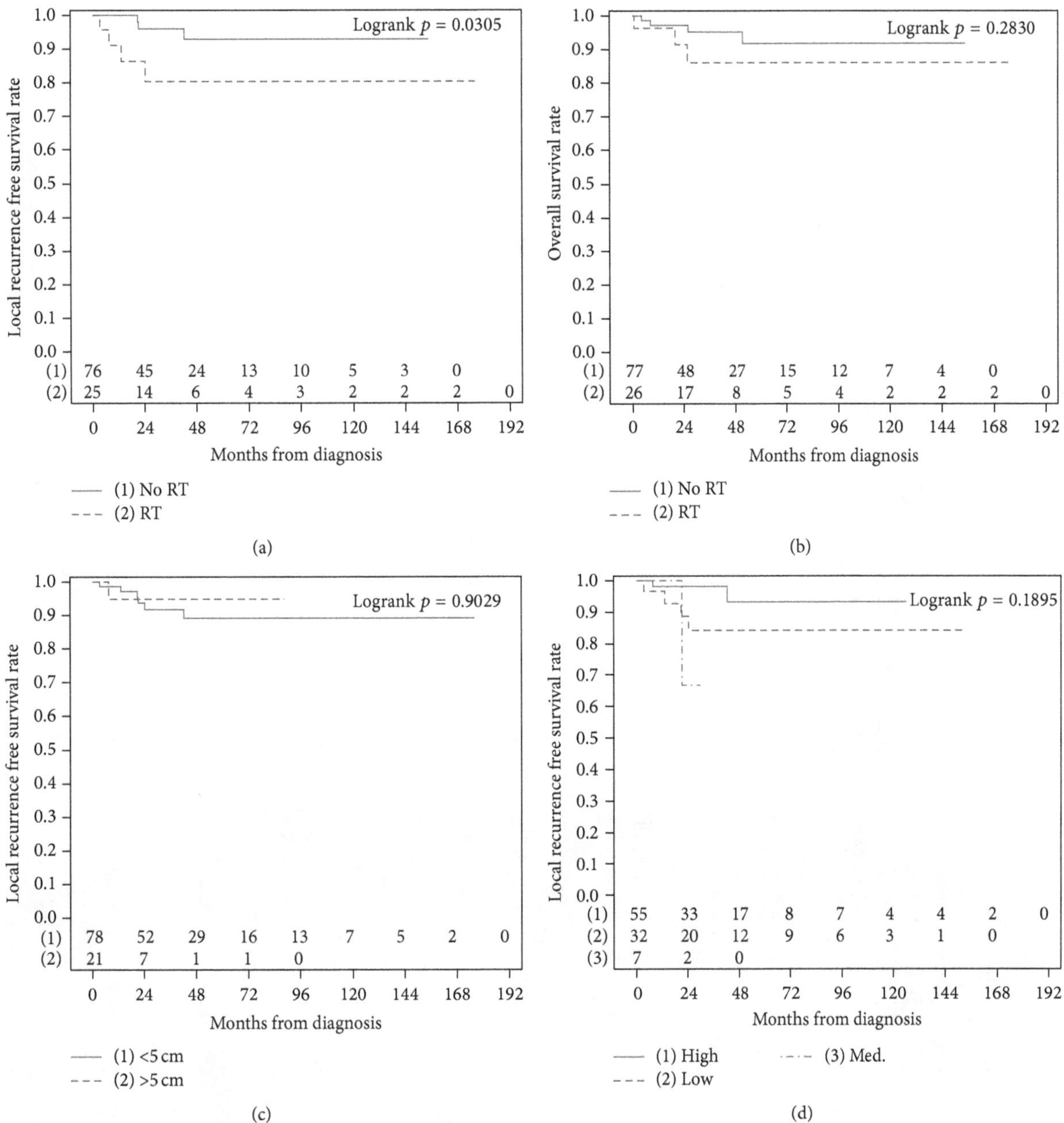

FIGURE 2: Dividing the cohort into those receiving radiation therapy (RT) either pre- or postoperatively, LRFS (a) was reduced in those patients undergoing RT as part of treatment ($p = 0.03$), whereas median OS (b) was not different between the two groups ($p = 0.28$). Both tumor size (c) and tumor grade (d) did not have an effect on recurrence free survival.

Their conclusions, similar to the practice at our institution, were the use of RT related to presentation status and surgical margins, with little influence of grade and tumor size [22].

These results taken together with our current series indicate that superficial anatomic location may supersede histology and size with respect to outcomes such as OS. One exception to this generalization is superficial angiosarcoma, where two larger series indicate a very different 5-year OS, between 34 and 45%, with very high LR rates (25–50%) [23, 24]. Although small numbers of angiosarcoma patients were included in most series, the rarity of this type of sarcoma did not affect OS rates, although contributing to the number of patients receiving chemotherapy.

The limitations of this study are related to its retrospective nature, including missing data, in particular related to overall tumor size when an excisional biopsy was completed at an outside facility. In addition, although this series involved low rates of RT use, information regarding surgical morbidities previously shown to be more frequent in STS such as surgical site infection and skin graft/flap failure was not collected.

Lastly, survival analysis may be limited by the fact that there were very few adverse outcomes. Only a univariate analysis of risk factors was performed, as a multivariate

Table 3: Literature review of treatment and outcomes for S-STS.

Series	n	Histologies	Location	Median size (range)	T-stage	Margin status	% receiving RT	Median follow-up (range)	LR rate	5-year OS
Rydholm et al., 1991 (Sweden) [19]	129	LMS, 18% MFH, 46% LPS, 10% AS, 0% Other, 26%	EX, 85% T, 15% H/N, 0% Other, 0%	4.3 cm (1–16 cm)	≤5 cm, 58% >5 cm, 38% Unknown, 4%	Wide, 58.1% Close, 41.9%	8.5%	NR	24.8%	80%
Brooks et al., 1998 (USA) [14]	215	LMS, 16% MFH, 43% LPS, 18% AS, 3% Other, 20%	EX, 100% T, 0% H/N, 0% Other, 0%	NR	<5 cm, 75% ≥5 cm, 25%	R0, 91.6% R1, 8.4%	25%	45 months (2 d–151 months)	14%	79%
Cany et al., 1999 (France) [15]	105	LMS, 20% MFH, 39% LPS, 3% AS, 5% Other[2], 33%	EX, 56.1% T, 27.7% H/N, 16.2% Other, 0%	3 cm (1–15 cm)	≤5 cm, 65.7% >5 cm, 34.3%	Wide, 85.4% Close, 14.6%	52.8%	111.9 months (19.2–321.9 months)	10.5%	75%
Salas et al., 2009 (France) [16]	367	LMS, 22.3% MFH[1], 9.0% AS, 14.4% Other[2], 54.3%	EX, 55.0% T, 35.4% H/N, 8.0% Other, 1.6%	NR	≤5 cm, 76.3% >5 cm, 21% Unknown, 2.7%	Wide, 76.3% Close, 21.2% Unknown, 2.5%	35.4%	74.2 months	23.4%	80.9%
Tsukushi et al., 2012 (Japan) [20]	105	LMS, 7.6% MFH, 24.8% LPS, 19.0% Other, 48.6%	EX, 73.3% T, 26.7%	NR	≤5 cm, 45.7% >5 cm, 54.3%	R0, 95.2% R1, 4.8%	4.8%	NR	8.0%	95.3%
Francescutti et al., 2015 (USA) [present study]	103	LMS, 35.9% MFH, 15.5% LPS, 7.8% AS, 5.8% Other, 35.0%	EX, 51.5% T, 38.8% H/N, 7.8% Other, 1.9%	3 cm (0.15–14 cm)	≤5 cm, 79.0% >5 cm, 21.0%	Wide, 75.2% Close, 18.8%	21.3%	34.2 months (2.3–176.0 months)	8.7%	93.2%
Total	**1024**									

[1]Myxofibrosarcoma in this series.
[2]Dermatofibrosarcoma protuberans (DFSP) in this series.
LMS, leiomyosarcoma; MFH, malignant fibrous histiocytoma; LPS, liposarcoma; AS, angiosarcoma; EX, upper or lower extremity; T, superficial trunk; H/N, head and neck; NR, not reported.

analysis was not possible due to the small number of events. Therefore the study was not adequately powered to accurately assess the impact of individual prognostic factors on survival.

Overall, the excellent outcomes for S-STS patients at our center highlight the importance of multidisciplinary management of such patients at specialized centers that can offer expertise through sarcoma pathology, surgical oncology, plastic surgery, radiation oncology, and medical oncology, for appropriate selection and timing of therapies for this group of patients.

5. Conclusion

Overall S-STS are well managed with surgical resection with wide margins as primary therapy. Selective use of RT in combination with appropriate surgical therapy has led to low LR rates, and these LRs are oftentimes managed adequately with repeat surgical resection. The treatment of sarcomas at centers experienced in multidisciplinary management through surgical resections and selective use of RT is integral to good outcome in this heterogeneous group of patients.

References

[1] R. Siegel, J. Ma, Z. Zou, and A. Jemal, "Cancer statistics, 2014," *CA Cancer Journal for Clinicians*, vol. 64, no. 1, pp. 9–29, 2014.

[2] J.-M. Coindre, P. Terrier, L. Guillou et al., "Predictive value of grade for metastasis development in the main histologic types of adult soft tissue sarcomas: a study of 1240 patients from the french federation of cancer centers sarcoma group," *Cancer*, vol. 91, no. 10, pp. 1914–1926, 2001.

[3] M. Tsujimoto, K. Aozasa, T. Ueda, Y. Morimura, Y. Komatsubara, and T. Doi, "Multivariate analysis for histologic prognostic factors in soft tissue sarcomas," *Cancer*, vol. 62, no. 5, pp. 994–998, 1988.

[4] J. M. Coindre, P. Terrier, N. B. Bui et al., "Prognostic factors in adult patients with locally controlled soft tissue sarcoma: a study of 546 patients from the French Federation of Cancer Centers Sarcoma Group," *Journal of Clinical Oncology*, vol. 14, no. 3, pp. 869–877, 1996.

[5] F. C. Eilber, G. Rosen, S. D. Nelson et al., "High-grade extremity soft tissue sarcomas: factors predictive of local recurrence and its effect on morbidity and mortality," *Annals of Surgery*, vol. 237, no. 2, pp. 218–226, 2003.

[6] A. Gronchi, P. G. Casali, L. Mariani et al., "Status of surgical margins and prognosis in adult soft tissue sarcomas of the extremities: a series of patients treated at a single institution," *Journal of Clinical Oncology*, vol. 23, no. 1, pp. 96–104, 2005.

[7] J. Weitz, C. R. Antonescu, and M. F. Brennan, "Localized extremity soft tissue sarcoma: improved knowledge with unchanged survival over time," *Journal of Clinical Oncology*, vol. 21, no. 14, pp. 2719–2725, 2003.

[8] G. K. Zagars, M. T. Ballo, P. W. T. Pisters et al., "Prognostic factors for patients with localized soft-tissue sarcoma treated with conservation surgery and radiation therapy: an analysis of 1225 patients," *Cancer*, vol. 97, no. 10, pp. 2530–2543, 2003.

[9] C. S. Trovik, H. C. F. Bauer, T. A. Alvegård et al., "Surgical margins, local recurrence and metastasis in soft tissue sarcomas: 559 surgically-treated patients from the Scandinavian Sarcoma Group Register," *European Journal of Cancer*, vol. 36, no. 6, pp. 710–716, 2000.

[10] S. B. Edge, D. R. Byrd, C. C. Compton, A. G. Fritz, F. Greene, and A. Trotti, *AJCC Cancer Staging Manual*, Springer, New York, NY, USA, 2010.

[11] A. Ravaud, N. B. Bui, J. M. Coindre et al., "Prognostic variables for the selection of patients with operable soft tissue sarcomas to be considered in adjuvant chemotherapy trials," *British Journal of Cancer*, vol. 66, no. 5, pp. 961–969, 1992.

[12] J. J. Gaynor, C. C. Tan, E. S. Casper et al., "Refinement of clinicopathologic staging for localized soft tissue sarcoma of the extremity: a study of 423 adults," *Journal of Clinical Oncology*, vol. 10, no. 8, pp. 1317–1329, 1992.

[13] P. W. Pisters, D. H. Leung, J. Woodruff, W. Shi, and M. F. Brennan, "Analysis of prognostic factors in 1,041 patients with localized soft tissue sarcomas of the extremities," *Journal of Clinical Oncology*, vol. 14, no. 5, pp. 1679–1689, 1996.

[14] A. D. Brooks, M. J. Heslin, D. H. Y. Leung, J. J. Lewis, and M. F. Brennan, "Superficial extremity soft tissue sarcoma: an analysis of prognostic factors," *Annals of Surgical Oncology*, vol. 5, no. 1, pp. 41–47, 1998.

[15] L. Cany, E. Stoeckle, J.-M. Coindre, G. Kantor, F. Bonichon, and B. N. Bui, "Prognostic factors in superficial adult soft tissue sarcomas: analysis of a series of 105 patients," *Journal of Surgical Oncology*, vol. 71, no. 1, pp. 4–9, 1999.

[16] S. Salas, E. Stoeckle, F. Collin et al., "Superficial soft tissue sarcomas (S-STS): a study of 367 patients from the French Sarcoma Group (FSG) database," *European Journal of Cancer*, vol. 45, no. 12, pp. 2091–2102, 2009.

[17] M. von Mehren, R. S. Benjamin, M. M. Bui et al., "Soft tissue sarcoma, version 2. 2012: featured updates to the NCCN guidelines," *Journal of the National Comprehensive Cancer Network*, vol. 10, no. 8, pp. 951–960, 2012.

[18] M. J. Heslin, J. Woodruff, and M. F. Brennan, "Prognostic significance of a positive microscopic margin in high-risk extremity soft tissue sarcoma: implications for management," *Journal of Clinical Oncology*, vol. 14, no. 2, pp. 473–478, 1996.

[19] A. Rydholm, P. Gustafson, B. Rooser, H. Willen, and N. O. Berg, "Subcutaneous sarcoma. A population-based study of 129 patients," *Journal of Bone and Joint Surgery B*, vol. 73, no. 4, pp. 662–667, 1991.

[20] S. Tsukushi, Y. Nishida, Y. Shido, J. Wasa, and N. Ishiguro, "Clinicopathological prognostic factors of superficial non-small round cell soft tissue sarcomas," *Journal of Surgical Oncology*, vol. 105, no. 7, pp. 668–672, 2012.

[21] P. W. T. Pisters, R. E. Pollock, V. O. Lewis et al., "Long-term results of prospective trial of surgery alone with selective use of radiation for patients with T1 extremity and trunk soft tissue sarcomas," *Annals of Surgery*, vol. 246, no. 4, pp. 675–682, 2007.

[22] D. J. Biau, P. C. Ferguson, P. Chung et al., "Local recurrence of localized soft tissue sarcoma: a new look at old predictors," *Cancer*, vol. 118, no. 23, pp. 5867–5877, 2012.

[23] M. B. Morgan, M. Swann, S. Somach, W. Eng, and B. Smoller, "Cutaneous angiosarcoma: a case series with prognostic correlation," *Journal of the American Academy of Dermatology*, vol. 50, no. 6, pp. 867–874, 2004.

[24] A. F. Nascimento, C. P. Raut, and C. D. Fletcher, "Primary angiosarcoma of the breast: clinicopathologic analysis of 49 cases, suggesting that grade is not prognostic," *The American Journal of Surgical Pathology*, vol. 32, no. 12, pp. 1896–1904, 2008.

7

Clinical Epidemiology of Low-Grade and Dedifferentiated Osteosarcoma in Norway during 1975 and 2009

Kjetil Berner,[1,2] Tom Børge Johannesen,[2] and Øyvind S. Bruland[1,3]

[1]*Department of Oncology, Oslo University Hospital, Norwegian Radium Hospital, 0424 Oslo, Norway*
[2]*The Norwegian Cancer Registry, 0304 Oslo, Norway*
[3]*Institute of Clinical Medicine, University of Oslo, 0318 Oslo, Norway*

Correspondence should be addressed to Øyvind S. Bruland; oyvind.bruland@medisin.uio.no

Academic Editor: Dae-Geun Jeon

Purpose. To describe epidemiological, clinical characteristics and treatment outcomes of low-grade osteosarcoma (LGOS), including dedifferentiated osteosarcoma (DLGOS). *Method.* We analysed a nationwide cohort comprised of patients with histologically verified LGOS and DLGOS between 1975 and 2009, based on registry sources supplemented with clinical records from hospitals involved in sarcoma management. *Results.* Fifty-four patients were identified, 12 of whom had DLGOS. The annual incidence for all patients was 0.3 per million, with the peak incidence in the third decade of the life. Fifteen patients experienced local relapses during follow-up and ten developed metastatic diseases, including three at primary diagnosis. Patients with DLGOS dominated the metastatic relapse group. The five-year sarcoma-specific survival rate was 91%, with no documented improvement over time. Free margin following surgical resection of the primary tumour had a positive impact on survival. As expected, both local relapse and metastasis during follow-up were associated with an unfavourable outcome. Radiotherapy predicted poor survival due to the selection of high-risk patients in need of such treatment. Neither higher age nor axial tumour localisation was adverse prognostic factors. *Conclusion.* LGOS has an excellent prognosis when surgically resected with a free margin; however, LGOS has the potential to dedifferentiate and metastasize with a poor outcome.

1. Introduction

Most osteosarcomas (OS) are high-grade lesions, while low-grade OSs (LGOS) are rare and include parosteal osteosarcoma (POS) and central LGOS (LGCOS) [1]. POS was first described in 1951 [2] and is characterised as a slow growing, low-grade malignancy arising from periosteal tissue directly adjacent to the cortex [1, 2]. LGCOS was first reported in 1977 [3] as a distinct entity of well-differentiated, intramedullary LGOS [1, 3, 4]. POS accounts for approximately 4% of all OS [5, 6] and LGCOS accounts for less than 2% [4, 7].

Most patients in the cohort were young adults with a peak incidence in the third decade of life in both subgroups of LGOSs [5–8]. There is no significant gender difference in the incidence of LGOS [6–9]. The majority of such primary tumours are located in the long bones, most often in the distal femur and proximal tibia, while flat bones are less likely to be affected [1, 4, 8].

In general, both subgroups of LGOSs have excellent prognoses when surgically resected with a wide margin [4, 7, 9]. However, LGOS has the potential to dedifferentiate to high-grade malignant lesions (DLGOS) upon recurrence [5–9]. Some LGOS will also show areas of high-grade malignancy already at primary diagnosis [1, 10]. Adjuvant chemotherapy is recommended in such circumstances [1, 8], due to the increased risk of subsequent metastasis [1, 8, 11].

The purpose of this study is to describe the epidemiological and clinical characteristics related to treatment outcomes in all LGOS and DLGOS from an unselected Norwegian population of OS patients between 1975 and 2009 [12]. To our knowledge, none of the previous nationwide studies [12–16] have specifically addressed this topic.

2. Material and Methods

2.1. Patient Cohort. Fifty-four cases of LGOS and DLGOS were identified based on histological reports from a population of 702 patients with OS and spindle cell non-OS in Norway between 1975 and 2009 [12, 17]. One hundred and thirty cases were retrieved from files and reexamined due to somewhat questionable pathological reports [12]; of these, 26 are included in the present study. Variables relevant to this study were retrospectively validated based on multiple and partly overlapping data and registry sources supplemented with clinical records from hospitals involved in sarcoma management. The DLGOS subgroup included all patients with dedifferentiated lesions, verified either at primary diagnosis or during follow-up. Malignancy grade was dichotomised between low-grade (grades I-II) and high-grade (grades III-IV) tumours [18]. Two patients had previously been reported with LGOS [12] but received chemotherapy due to small areas with documented grade III malignancy. Consequently, these cases are classified as "DLGOS at diagnosis" in the present study.

2.2. Clinicopathological Variables. We defined metastasis that occurred within six weeks of primary diagnosis as *primary metastatic disease* [12]. Information regarding metastasis or local recurrence was based on radiographic images and/or biopsy or fine needle aspiration cytology. *Tumour size* was defined as the maximum length of the tumour in cm and *duration of symptoms* referred to the interval in months between first symptom and time of biopsy [19]. The normal ranges for *serum alkaline phosphatase* (ALP) and *serum lactate dehydrogenase* (LDH) were measured in international units at the time of diagnosis [19].

2.3. Treatment Variables

Surgery. We dichotomised between amputation and other surgeries. The best local surgical margins were classified as free or positive margins. The former implied surgical removal of the primary tumour with wide or marginal margins (adequate surgery) [20] as defined by the surgeon and pathologist, while an intralesional margin and residual macroscopic tumour were categorized as positive margins. Patients with metastatic disease at the time of diagnosis must have achieved complete surgical remission for both their primary tumour and metastasis in order to be classified as having received adequate surgery. All patients treated with curettage were assumed to have a positive margin.

Chemotherapy. Adequate chemotherapy was defined as at least six courses of chemotherapy containing a minimum of two of the following drugs: high-dose methotrexate (at least 8 g/m^2), doxorubicin, cisplatin, or ifosfamide [19]. These four drugs are the most commonly used chemotherapy drugs worldwide [21, 22].

Radiotherapy. A curative treatment intent was defined as fractionated radiotherapy following surgery, for either the treatment of a primary tumour or a local recurrence, otherwise considered as palliative treatment.

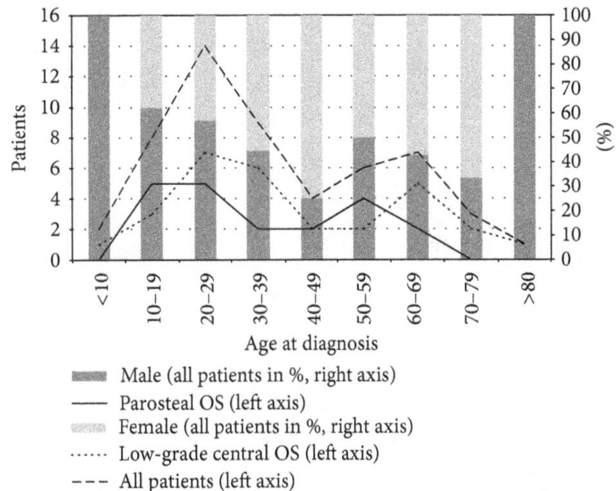

FIGURE 1: Gender (bar chart, right axis) and age at diagnosis (line diagram, left axis) of 54 patients with low-grade or dedifferentiated osteosarcoma (OS), including separate line diagrams for parosteal and low-grade central OS.

2.4. Statistical Analyses. A survival analysis using Kaplan-Meier estimates and a log-rank test were used to analyse sarcoma-specific survival (SSS) and event-free survival (EFS). For comparison, we also present SSS for all Norwegian high-grade OS patients between 1975 and 2009 [12, 17]. Overall survival was not used in these analyses since only about half of all deaths in the cohort were due to OS. Sarcoma-specific death or treatment-related deaths were the endpoints of SSS. The endpoints of EFS were date of first metastasis, local recurrence, or SSS, whichever occurred first. Patients with primary metastatic disease were not included in the EFS analysis. Follow-up was completed in July, 2013. Updated registries were used to prevent bias due to nonidentical follow-up of patients with few or frequent appointments [12]. The statistical analyses were conducted using SPSS version 22 (SPSS, Inc., Chicago, IL) and Stata version 13.1 (Stata Corporation, College Station, TX).

3. Results

3.1. Incidence. Fifty-four patients were diagnosed with LGOS or DLGOS between 1975 and 2009. These patients represent 11% of all OS during this period [12, 17]. The average annual incidence of 0.3 per million was bimodally distributed by age, with the dominant peak occurring in the patients' twenties (Figure 1). We report no significant gender differentiation of all patients in the cohort (Table 1 and Figure 1).

3.2. Clinicopathological Data. The LGCOS group was comprised of 29 patients, making it the largest subgroup in the present cohort (Tables 1 and 2). Interestingly, only 12 of these cases (41%) had tumours located in long bones, while 10 cases (34%) had tumours in the mandible or maxilla (Table 2). Jaw OS accounted for 7% of all skeletal OS, with a LGCOS to high-grade ratio of 32% [12]. With one exception, all 20 cases of POS were located in long bones (Table 2). Four

TABLE 1: Clinicopathological variables in 54 low-grade and dedifferentiated osteosarcoma (OS) patients.

	Low-grade OS[a] (%)	Dedifferentiated OS (%)	All patients[b] (%)
All patients	42	12	54
Gender			
Male	23 (55)	5 (42)	28 (52)
Female	19 (45)	7 (58)	26 (48)
Histological subgroups			
Parosteal OS	12 (29)	8 (67)	20 (37)
Low-grade central OS	25 (60)	4 (33)	29 (54)
Secondary low-grade OS	4 (10)		4 (7)
Extraskeletal low-grade OS	1 (2)		1 (2)
Tumour size			
≤6 cm	20 (67)	2 (25)	22 (58)
>6 cm	10 (33)	6 (75)	16 (42)
Median/mean size in cm	6/6	11/12	6/7
Range in cm	1–15	5–30	1–30
Symptom length			
≤6 months	16 (48)	5 (56)	21 (50)
>6 months	17 (52)	4 (44)	21 (50)
Median/mean length in months	7/18	6/27	7/20
Range in months	1–108	4–120	1–120

[a]No dedifferentiation at diagnosis or during follow-up. [b]Missing values equal the difference between the summarized number from each subgroup in the fourth column and the total number of patients in the study.

TABLE 2: Anatomical distribution of 54 patients with low-grade or dedifferentiated osteosarcoma (OS) combined. Separated between parosteal OS (POS), low-grade central OS (LGCOS), and other subgroups.

	POS (%)	LGCOS (%)	Other (%)[a]	All patients (%)
Humerus	4 (20)	1 (3)		5 (9)
Femur	11 (55)	5 (17)		16 (30)
Tibia	4 (20)	5 (17)	1 (20)	10 (19)
Fibula		1 (3)		1 (2)
Mandible, maxilla		10 (34)	3 (60)	13 (24)
Costa, scapula, clavicle		3 (10)		3 (6)
Columna vertebralis		1 (3)		1 (2)
Pelvis, sacrum	1 (5)	2 (7)		3 (6)
Other		1 (3)	1 (20)	2 (4)
Total	20 (100)	29 (100)	5 (100)	54 (100)

[a]Four cases of secondary low-grade OS and one case of extraskeletal low-grade OS (in the breast).

of the remaining five patients were classified as secondary LGOS (Table 1), with two cases arising from previous fibrous dysplasia, one case from a previous giant-cell tumour, and one due to previous radiotherapy. The fifth case of LGOS was located in the left breast of a young female [17, 23].

Twelve patients had DLGOS (Table 1), including six patients with high-grade POS at primary diagnosis. In addition, two cases of POS and four cases of LGCOS showed transformation to high-grade malignancy at the time of local recurrence, that is, five patients at time of first local relapse and the sixth one at time of a third local recurrence. These six DLGOS patients developed transformation to high-grade malignancy between 1 and 21 years after primary diagnosis (Table 3). Four of these six cases had previously undergone surgery with an intralesional surgical margin.

Median tumour size among DLGOSs was 11 cm and nearly twice as large as those of the rest of the cohort (Table 1). By contrast, approximately an equal duration of symptoms before biopsy was seen in both LGOS and DLGOS, that is, half a year in median length (Table 1). Six patients had symptoms for more than five years before an OS diagnosis was documented, due to very slow tumour growth. This explains the 13-month discrepancy between median and mean value for these patients (Table 1). About one-third of all patients had elevated ALP at diagnosis, in contrast to 20% with increased levels of LDH. Two patients had a pathologic fracture at time of diagnosis but only one had this in the weight-bearing lower extremity skeleton.

3.3. Local Recurrence and Metastases. Out of the 15 patients who experienced local recurrence, six revealed a high-grade morphology during follow-up (Table 3). Two patients with dedifferentiated POS and one with LGCOS had metastatic disease at time of primary diagnosis. In addition, seven patients developed metastases during follow-up. The patients

Table 3: Patients with local recurrence and/or metastasis at diagnosis or during follow-up among 54 low-grade or dedifferentiated osteosarcoma (OS) patients.

	Low-grade OS (%)	Dedifferentiated OS (%)	All patients (%)
Local recurrence			
No	33 (79)	6 (50)	39 (72)
Yes[a]	9 (21)	6 (50)	15 (28)
Median/mean in months	27/31	26/94	27/57
Range in months	7–62	15–255	7–255
Metastasis[b]			
No	40 (95)	4 (33)	44 (81)
Yes[c]	2 (5)	8 (67)[d]	10 (19)
Median/mean in months	59/59	33/78	33/74
Range in months	0–117	0–263	0–263

[a]Five with parosteal OS (POS), nine with low-grade central OS (LGCOS), and one with secondary low-grade OS. None of the six patients with high-grade malignancy at time of diagnosis experienced local recurrence during follow-up. [b]Metastasis at diagnosis or during follow-up. Three patients had primary metastatic disease: one with low-grade OS and two with dedifferentiated OS. [c]Five with POS and five with LGCOS. [d]Five patients with metastatic relapse during follow-up had previously experienced a local recurrence.

Table 4: Summary of treatment in 54 patients with low-grade or dedifferentiated osteosarcoma (OS).

	Low-grade OS (%)	Dedifferentiated OS (%)	All patients (%)
Surgery	42	12	54
Amputation	3 (7)	2 (17)	5 (9)
Other	39 (93)	10 (83)	49 (91)
Surgical margins[a]	40	12	52
Free margin	35 (87)	8 (67)	43 (83)
Positive margin	5 (13)	4 (33)	9 (17)
Chemotherapy	3	8	11
Adequate chemotherapy	2 (67)	7 (88)	9 (82)
At primary diagnosis	1 (33)[c]	5 (63)	6 (55)
Treatment of local relapse	1 (33)	2 (25)	3 (27)
Not adequate chemotherapy	1 (33)	1 (13)	2 (18)
Radiotherapy[b]	5	5	10
Curative treatment intention	4 (80)	2 (40)	6 (60)
Palliative treatment intention	1 (20)	3 (60)	4 (40)

[a]Surgical margins after last resection of primary tumour during primary treatment or later relapses. Two uncertain cases were not included. [b]Radiotherapy during primary treatment or later relapses. One patient that underwent radiotherapy with curative intent received later radiotherapy in a palliative setting. [c]The chemotherapy was terminated after an internal hemipelvectomy, since the operation specimen verified a LGOS. The patient was subsequently followed for ten years after primary surgery with no signs of recurrent disease.

with DLGOS dominated the group with metastatic relapse (Table 3); five of these eight DLGOS patients had previously experienced a local recurrence.

3.4. Treatment Modalities. Table 4 outlines the extent of treatment administered to LGOS and DLGOS patients and is discussed further in the following section.

Surgery. All 54 patients underwent at least one operation (Table 4). Only five patients were treated with amputation, including three whose amputations were part of their primary treatment. Information regarding surgical margins after resection of the primary tumour was available in 52 cases, including all cases of DLGOS (Table 4). The remaining two patients in the cohort both experienced local relapses during follow-up but did not develop metastasis.

Seven of the 43 patients that obtained *free surgical margins* after resection of the primary tumour (Table 4) experienced local recurrence during follow-up: four with LGOS and three with DLGOS. Furthermore, five patients with a similar margin status were diagnosed with metastases, including one in a primary metastatic setting. Only one of these five patients developed metastasis with a low-grade malignancy. The remaining nine patients in the cohort did not achieve adequate surgery due to *positive margins*, including four DLGOS patients (Table 4). Three of the four DLGOS patients developed local recurrence and subsequent metastases during follow-up, while the last patient had primary metastatic disease. In addition, three of the five LGOS patients with positive surgical margins experienced local relapse, while another underwent palliative surgery for a pathological humerus fracture due to primary metastatic disease.

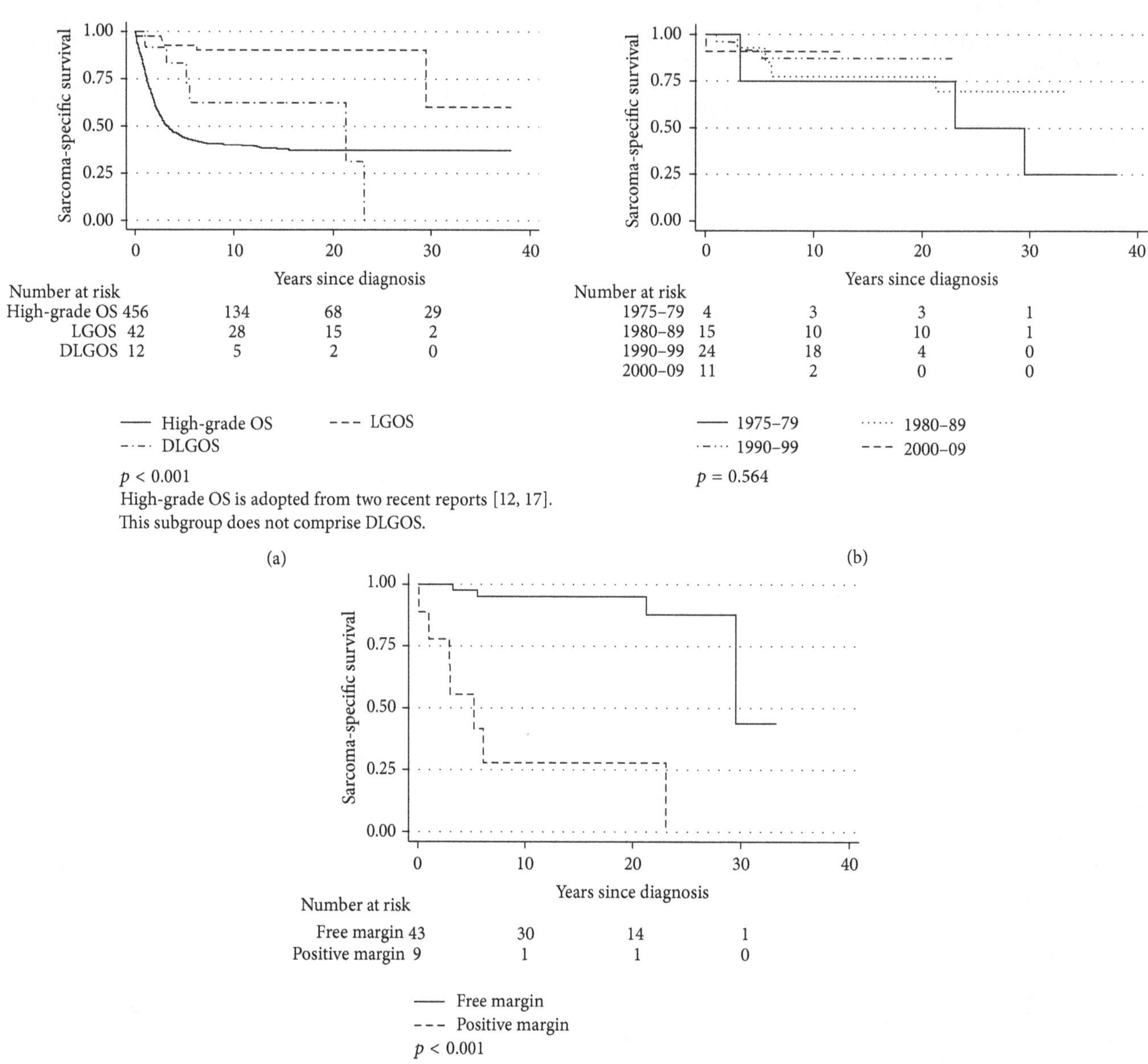

FIGURE 2: Sarcoma-specific survival of low-grade (LGOS) and dedifferentiated osteosarcoma (DLGOS) versus (a) high-grade OS, (b) dependent on time of diagnosis, 1975–2009, and (c) by best local surgical margin.

Chemotherapy. Adjuvant chemotherapy was, as expected, mainly reserved for patients with high-grade malignant lesions (Table 4). Only a 35-year-old man with LGOS received adequate chemotherapy, that is, after a second operation with decompression of the medulla due to a local relapse in the first lumbar vertebra [24].

Radiotherapy. Six patients received postoperative radiotherapy with curative intent (Table 4), including one case in which radiotherapy was used to treat the tumour in the appendicular skeleton. Fractionated radiotherapy was given due to marginal surgical margins in two cases and intralesional surgical margins in the remaining four cases. No signs of recurrent disease were later seen in the first two cases, whereas the other patients succumbed to their disease.

3.5. Cause of Death. Eight patients died of OS due to metastatic disease: two with LGOS and six with DLGOS. Another three LGOS patients died of OS due to local recurrence; in one case, there was a primary tumour in the mandible, and the other two cases developed tumours in the columna vertebralis. An additional 10 patients in the cohort died of other causes, which included other cancers (four cases), epilepsy (one case), infection (one case), gastric perforation (one case), heart disease (one case), "sudden death" (one case), and suicide (one case).

3.6. Survival Analyses. Patients with LGOS experienced an improved survival rate compared to both DLGOS and the high-grade OS cohorts (Figure 2(a)) [12, 17]. Five-year SSS was 91% for all patients in the present study and ten-year SSS

TABLE 5: Univariate Kaplan-Meier analyses of five-year sarcoma-specific survival and event-free survival according to different characteristics of 54 patients with low-grade or dedifferentiated osteosarcoma (OS).

	Sarcoma-specific survival			Event-free survival		
	Patients (%)	5 years in % (95% CI[a] in %)	p^b	Patients (%)	5 years in % (95% CI[a] in %)	p^b
Primary site of tumour			0.287			0.844
Extremity	33 (61)	91 (74–97)		30 (59)	80 (61–91)	
Axial	21 (39)	90 (74–96)		21 (41)	65 (41–82)	
Age			0.158			0.063
≤40 years	33 (61)	94 (77–98)		32 (63)	81 (62–91)	
>40 years	21 (39)	86 (62–95)		19 (37)	63 (37–80)	
Malignancy grade			<0.001			0.004
Low-grade	42 (78)	93 (79–98)		41 (80)	80 (64–90)	
Dedifferentiated	12 (22)	83 (48–96)		10 (20)	50 (18–75)	
Subgroup of OS			0.738			0.868
Parosteal OS	20 (37)	90 (66–97)		18 (35)	72 (46–87)	
Low-grade central OS	29 (54)	93 (75–98)		28 (55)	75 (55–87)	
Other	5 (9)	75 (13–96)		5 (10)	75 (13–96)	
Local recurrence			0.010			<0.001
No	40 (74)	92 (78–97)		37 (73)	97 (82–97)	
Yes	14 (26)	86 (54–96)		14 (27)	20 (5–42)	
Metastases at diagnosis or during follow-up			<0.001			0.001
No	44 (81)	95 (83–99)		44 (86)	79 (64–88)	
Yes	10 (19)	70 (33–89)		7 (14)	57 (17–84)	
Surgery[c]			<0.001			<0.001
Free margin	43 (83)	98 (83–100)		42 (86)	83 (52–95)	
Positive margin	9 (17)	56 (20–81)		7 (14)	29 (4–62)	
Adequate chemotherapy			0.091			0.447
No	45 (83)	93 (80–98)		44 (86)	74 (58–85)	
Yes	9 (17)	78 (36–94)		7 (14)	71 (26–92)	
Radiotherapy[d]			0.003			0.106
No	48 (89)	94 (82–98)		45 (88)	77 (62–87)	
Yes	6 (11)	67 (20–90)		6 (12)	50 (11–80)	

[a]Confidence interval. [b]Log-rank test. [c]Surgical margins after resection of primary tumour, last surgery performed. [d]Curative treatment intent.

was 85%. We found no improvement over time for all patients in the study, based on 10-year intervals (Figure 2(b)) and a cut-off in 1990 ($p = 0.31$, data not shown).

Table 5 presents the results of univariate analyses for five-year SSS and EFS according to a variety of characteristics. Gender ($p = 0.34/0.52$), tumour size ($p = 0.94/0.61$), symptom length ($p = 0.40/0.08$), ALP ($p = 0.49/0.47$), and LDH ($p = 0.84/0.62$) were not included in Table 5. Free margin following surgical resection of the primary tumour had a significant positive impact on survival for all patients (Figure 2(c) and Table 5), while local relapse or metastasis during follow-up was associated with a poor outcome (Table 5). Nevertheless, four patients died of metastases from OS despite a free surgical margin of the primary tumour, including three from the DLGOS subgroup. Radiotherapy predicted inferior SSS while chemotherapy had no significant impact on outcome (Table 5). Neither higher age nor axial tumour localisation was adverse prognostic factors.

4. Discussion

The patient material studied here is based on a nationwide cohort comprised of all Norwegian LGOS and DLGOS patients within a timeframe of 3-4 decades [12, 17]. To our knowledge, no previous nationwide study has specifically addressed topics related to clinical epidemiology and treatment results for these OS entities, except for separate incidence calculations [12, 15]. LGOS accounts for more than 10% of all OS in both Norway and Finland [12, 15], which is higher than usually reported [4–7]. Our result may be due to a broader patient base than normally reported, both as a consequence of the population-based nationwide approach, but also since we have included, for example, jaw OS, secondary OS, and extraskeletal OS in the present cohort. Since the diagnosis of LGOS in general is challenging, the lack of a systematic histological and radiological reevaluation of all cases in the gross study material analysed (see below) might also contribute to our findings.

The anatomical sites of POS in the present cohort (Table 2) were consistent with those in previous publications [1, 6, 8]. In contrast, the anatomical distribution of LGCOS, with the jaw as the single most frequent site, differs substantially from that of previously published studies in which long bones were the most commonly affected [3, 4]. This discrepancy may be due to chance, partly as a result of the relatively small sample size. For example, in the present cohort, about one-third of all jaw OSs [12] were LGOS, as compared to between 6% and 42% in previous studies [25–27]. Jaw OS accounted for less than 7% of all OSs in Norway [12], which is consistent with the findings from the Mayo Clinic [28].

The wide range in average duration of symptoms prior to diagnosis seemed reasonable due to the indolent tumour biology in most of these cases. We confirmed that patients may experience a slow growing tumour for years [6]. Such tumour growth may also explain why patients with low-grade histology had smaller tumour size at diagnosis (Table 1) than patients with high-grade OS [19].

It has been previously reported that up to 43% of all POS may contain areas of high-grade morphology [6, 29, 30] and develop de novo from low-grade lesions, either at diagnosis or during subsequent relapse. We confirmed these results. In addition, LGCOS has the potential to dedifferentiate [7–9]; four of our cases contained components with high-grade histology at the time of recurrence. As expected, DLGOS had a worse prognosis than LGOS due to the increased risk of metastasis, which is also confirmed in the literature [1, 6, 10, 31].

Overall, the prognosis for all patients in the present study was excellent following surgical removal with a free margin, which is consistent with the literature [6, 7, 10]. Five-year SSS for all patients in the cohort was 91%, with no improvement over time. Chemotherapy and radiotherapy are not routinely required for patients with LGOS [1, 7, 31], as confirmed in this report. Radiotherapy as a treatment modality predicted inferior SSS in the present analysis, probably due to the selection of high-risk patients in need of such treatment. OS is also known to be relatively resistant to radiotherapy [22, 32]. Neither higher age nor axial tumour localisation was adverse prognostic factors in the present study (Table 5), in contrast to the corresponding subgroups of high-grade OSs, which had a poor prognosis [19, 22, 33].

The strength of the present study, in our opinion, is the reliability of the database, which is validated by multiple and partially overlapping data and registry sources. As expected, we have not obtained complete clinical information for all patients in the present study. Nor has it been possible to obtain the same degree of detail regarding certain clinical variables with our approach as compared to a single institutional series and/or clinical trials. Furthermore, we cannot rule out that the quality could have been even better with a uniform histological reexamination of all 702 cases in the gross study material analysed, including immunohistochemical analyses as well as a retrospective review of the radiographic images in relevant cases. Nevertheless, a significant disadvantage of such an approach is the potential lack of histological specimens or radiographic images available for reexamination. This might be an even larger problem in nationwide studies than in studies based on, for example, an institutional series. For example, a previous Finnish study experienced a dropout rate of 34% due to missing original histological specimens [14], which is an unavoidable part of studies conducted in such a setting. Hence, we believe the potential disadvantage will exceed the potential gain of such an approach and that our key variables ensure the inclusion of an adequate amount of details in order to expand our knowledge regarding these rare OS entities.

5. Conclusion

To our knowledge, this is the first nationwide study addressing the clinicopathological features of LGOS and DLGOS. We confirmed that LGOS has an excellent prognosis when surgically resected with a free margin. LGOS also has the potential to dedifferentiate and metastasize with a poor outcome.

Disclaimer

The authors alone are responsible for the content and writing of the paper.

Acknowledgments

This project was supported by the South-Eastern Norway Regional Health Authority Research Program, with a pilot project supported by the National Resource Centre for Sarcomas in Norway. The authors thank all colleagues within the multidisciplinary sarcoma teams during 1975 and 2009 who reported the results of oncology, radiology, pathology, and orthopaedic surgery.

References

[1] C. D. M. Fletcher, J. A. Bridge, P. C. W. Hogendoorn, and F. Mertens, *WHO Classification of Tumours of Soft Tissue and Bone*, International Agency for Research on Cancer, Lyon, France, 4th edition, 2013.

[2] C. F. Geschickter and M. M. Copeland, "Parosteal osteoma of bone: a new entity," *Annals of surgery*, vol. 133, no. 6, pp. 790–807, 1951.

[3] K. K. Unni, D. C. Dahlin, R. A. McLeod, and D. J. Pritchard, "Intraosseous well-differentiated osteosarcoma," *Cancer*, vol. 40, no. 3, pp. 1337–1347, 1977.

[4] K. J. Andresen, M. Sundaram, K. K. Unni, and F. H. Sim, "Imaging features of low-grade central osteosarcoma of the long bones and pelvis," *Skeletal Radiology*, vol. 33, no. 7, pp. 373–379, 2004.

[5] K. Okada, F. J. Frassica, F. H. Sim et al., "Parosteal osteosarcoma. A clinicopathological study," *The Journal of Bone and Joint Surgery—American Volume*, vol. 76, no. 3, pp. 366–378, 1994.

[6] J.-F. Hang and P. C.-H. Chen, "Parosteal osteosarcoma," *Archives of Pathology and Laboratory Medicine*, vol. 138, no. 5, pp. 694–699, 2014.

[7] A. M. Malhas, V. P. Sumathi, S. L. James et al., "Low-grade central osteosarcoma: a difficult condition to diagnose," *Sarcoma*, vol. 2012, Article ID 764796, 7 pages, 2012.

[8] J. H. Schwab, C. R. Antonescu, E. A. Athanasian, P. J. Boland, J. H. Healey, and C. D. Morris, "A comparison of intramedullary and juxtacortical low-grade osteogenic sarcoma," *Clinical Orthopaedics and Related Research*, vol. 466, no. 6, pp. 1318–1322, 2008.

[9] A.-M. Kurt, K. K. Unni, R. A. McLeod, and D. J. Pritchard, "Low-grade intraosseous osteosarcoma," *Cancer*, vol. 65, no. 6, pp. 1418–1428, 1990.

[10] S. F. Bonar, "Central low-grade osteosarcoma: a diagnostic challenge," *Skeletal Radiology*, vol. 41, no. 4, pp. 365–367, 2012.

[11] K. Takeuchi, T. Morii, H. Yabe, H. Morioka, M. Mukai, and Y. Toyama, "Dedifferentiated parosteal osteosarcoma with well-differentiated metastases," *Skeletal Radiology*, vol. 35, no. 10, pp. 778–782, 2006.

[12] K. Berner, T. B. Johannesen, A. Berner et al., "Time-trends on incidence and survival in a nationwide and unselected cohort of patients with skeletal osteosarcoma," *Acta Oncologica*, vol. 54, no. 1, pp. 25–33, 2015.

[13] S. Harvei and O. Solheim, "The prognosis in osteosarcoma: norwegian national data," *Cancer*, vol. 48, no. 8, pp. 1719–1723, 1981.

[14] M. M. Sampo, M. Tarkkanen, A. H. Kivioja, M. H. Taskinen, R. Sankila, and T. O. Böhling, "Osteosarcoma in Finland from 1971 through 1990: a nationwide study of epidemiology and outcome," *Acta Orthopaedica*, vol. 79, no. 6, pp. 861–866, 2008.

[15] M. Sampo, M. Koivikko, M. Taskinen et al., "Incidence, epidemiology and treatment results of osteosarcoma in Finland—a nationwide population-based study," *Acta Oncologica*, vol. 50, no. 8, pp. 1206–1214, 2011.

[16] J. Whelan, A. McTiernan, N. Cooper et al., "Incidence and survival of malignant bone sarcomas in England 1979–2007," *International Journal of Cancer*, vol. 131, no. 4, pp. E508–E517, 2012.

[17] K. Berner, B. Bjerkehagen, O. S. Bruland, and A. Berner, "Extraskeletal osteosarcoma in Norway, between 1975 and 2009, and a brief review of the literature," *Anticancer Research*, vol. 35, no. 4, pp. 2129–2140, 2015.

[18] B. Bjerkehagen, J. Wejde, M. Hansson, H. Domanski, and T. Böhling, "SSG pathology review experiences and histological grading of malignancy in sarcomas," *Acta Orthopaedica*, vol. 80, no. 334, pp. 31–36, 2009.

[19] K. Berner, K. S. Hall, O. R. Monge, H. Weedon-Fekjær, O. Zaikova, and Ø. S. Bruland, "Prognostic factors and treatment results of high-grade osteosarcoma in Norway: a scope beyond the 'classical' patient," *Sarcoma*, vol. 2015, Article ID 516843, 14 pages, 2015.

[20] W. F. Enneking, S. S. Spanier, and M. Goodman, "A system for the surgical staging of musculoskeletal sarcoma," *Clinical Orthopaedics and Related Research*, vol. 153, pp. 106–120, 1980.

[21] J. K. Anninga, H. Gelderblom, M. Fiocco et al., "Chemotherapeutic adjuvant treatment for osteosarcoma: where do we stand?" *European Journal of Cancer*, vol. 47, no. 16, pp. 2431–2445, 2011.

[22] A. Luetke, P. A. Meyers, I. Lewis, and H. Juergens, "Osteosarcoma treatment—where do we stand? A state of the art review," *Cancer Treatment Reviews*, vol. 40, no. 4, pp. 523–532, 2014.

[23] O. T. Brustugun, W. Reed, J. P. Poulsen, and Ø. S. Bruland, "Primary osteosarcoma of the breast," *Acta Oncologica*, vol. 44, no. 7, pp. 767–770, 2005.

[24] Ø. S. Bruland, A. Skretting, Ø. P. Solheim, and M. Aas, "Targeted radiotherapy of osteosarcoma using ^{153}Sm-EDTMP: a new promising approach," *Acta Oncologica*, vol. 35, no. 3, pp. 381–384, 1996.

[25] E. H. Nissanka, E. A. P. D. Amaratunge, and W. M. Tilakaratne, "Clinicopathological analysis of osteosarcoma of jaw bones," *Oral Diseases*, vol. 13, no. 1, pp. 82–87, 2007.

[26] B. A. Guadagnolo, G. K. Zagars, A. K. Raymond, R. S. Benjamin, and E. M. Sturgis, "Osteosarcoma of the jaw/craniofacial region: outcomes after multimodality treatment," *Cancer*, vol. 115, no. 14, pp. 3262–3270, 2009.

[27] E. G. Demicco, V. Deshpande, G. P. Nielsen, S. V. Kattapuram, and A. E. Rosenberg, "Well-differentiated osteosarcoma of the jaw bones: a clinicopathologic study of 15 cases," *American Journal of Surgical Pathology*, vol. 34, no. 11, pp. 1647–1655, 2010.

[28] K. K. Unni and C. Y. Inwards, *Dahlin's Bone Tumors*, Lippincott Williams & Wilkins, Philadelphia, Pa, USA, 6th edition, 2010.

[29] F. Bertoni, K. K. Unni, J. W. Beabout, and F. H. Sim, "Parosteal osteoma of bones other than of the skull and face," *Cancer*, vol. 75, no. 10, pp. 2466–2473, 1995.

[30] D. S. Sheth, A. W. Yasko, A. K. Raymond et al., "Conventional and dedifferentiated parosteal osteosarcoma. Diagnosis, treatment, and outcome," *Cancer*, vol. 78, no. 10, pp. 2136–2145, 1996.

[31] S. O. Pintado, J. Lane, and A. G. Huvos, "Parosteal osteogenic sarcoma of bone with coexistent low- and high-grade sarcomatous components," *Human Pathology*, vol. 20, no. 5, pp. 488–491, 1989.

[32] R. Schwarz, O. Bruland, A. Cassoni, P. Schomberg, and S. Bielack, "The role of radiotherapy in oseosarcoma," *Cancer Treatment and Research*, vol. 152, pp. 147–164, 2009.

[33] P. C. W. Hogendoorn, N. Athanasou, S. Bielack et al., "Bone sarcomas: ESMO Clinical Practice Guidelines for diagnosis, treatment and follow-up," *Annals of Oncology*, vol. 21, supplement 5, pp. v204–v213, 2010.

8

A Patient-Derived Xenograft Model of Parameningeal Embryonal Rhabdomyosarcoma for Preclinical Studies

Jody E. Hooper,[1] Emma L. Cantor,[2,3] Macgregor S. Ehlen,[2,3] Avirup Banerjee,[2,3] Suman Malempati,[3] Peter Stenzel,[4] Randy L. Woltjer,[4] Regina Gandour-Edwards,[5] Neal C. Goodwin,[6,7] Yan Yang,[6,8] Pali Kaur,[6] Carol J. Bult,[6] Susan D. Airhart,[6] and Charles Keller[2,3,9]

[1]*Department of Pathology, Johns Hopkins Medicine, 600 N. Wolfe Street, Pathology B-106, Baltimore, MD 21287, USA*
[2]*Pediatric Cancer Biology Program, Papé Family Pediatric Research Institute, Oregon Health & Science University, 3181 S.W. Sam Jackson Park Road, Portland, OR 97239, USA*
[3]*Department of Pediatrics, Oregon Health & Science University, 3181 S.W. Sam Jackson Park Road, Portland, OR 97239, USA*
[4]*Department of Pathology, Oregon Health & Science University, 3181 S.W. Sam Jackson Park Road, Portland, OR 97239, USA*
[5]*University of California Davis School of Medicine and Cancer Center, Sacramento, CA 95817, USA*
[6]*The Jackson Laboratory, 1650 Santa Ana Avenue, Sacramento, CA 95838, USA*
[7]*Champions Oncology, Hackensack, NJ 07601, USA*
[8]*Leo Universal, Inc., Torrance, CA 90505, USA*
[9]*Children's Cancer Therapy Development Institute, Beaverton, OR 97005, USA*

Correspondence should be addressed to Jody E. Hooper; jhooper9@jhmi.edu and Charles Keller; charles@cc-tdi.org

Academic Editor: Manish Agarwal

Embryonal rhabdomyosarcoma (eRMS) is one of the most common soft tissue sarcomas in children and adolescents. Parameningeal eRMS is a variant that is often more difficult to treat than eRMS occurring at other sites. A 14-year-old female with persistent headaches and rapid weight loss was diagnosed with parameningeal eRMS. She progressed and died despite chemotherapy with vincristine, actinomycin-D, and cyclophosphamide plus 50.4 Gy radiation therapy to the primary tumor site. Tumor specimens were acquired by rapid autopsy and tumor tissue was transplanted into immunodeficient mice to create a patient-derived xenograft (PDX) animal model. As autopsy specimens had an ALK R1181C mutation, PDX tumor bearing animals were treated with the pan-kinase inhibitor lestaurtinib but demonstrated no decrease in tumor growth, suggesting that single agent kinase inhibitor therapy may be insufficient in similar cases. This unique parameningeal eRMS PDX model is publicly available for preclinical study.

1. Introduction

Rhabdomyosarcomas (RMS) are mesenchymal tumors showing skeletal muscle differentiation and represent the most common pediatric soft tissue sarcomas [1]. RMS are subdivided into alveolar (aRMS) and embryonal (eRMS) types, with each category showing distinct histologic appearance, behavior, and response to treatment. Approximately, 60% of RMS are the embryonal type [2]. eRMS presents commonly in the genitourinary and head and neck regions. Compared to aRMS, the average age of onset of embryonal rhabdomyosarcoma is younger, with a majority of cases diagnosed before age 10, and the prognosis is overall more favorable [3]. While the majority of aRMS show balanced translocation with fusion of *PAX3:FOX01* or *PAX7:FOX01*, recent publications suggest that driver mutations (e.g., *NRAS, KRAS, HRAS, FGFR4, PIK3CA, CTNNB1, FBXW7,* and *BCOR*) may underpin progression in the embryonal subtype of RMS (eRMS) [4, 5]. These studies have suggested that translocation negative aRMS may be more similar to eRMS than the histologic appearance might suggest [6, 7]. eRMS as currently defined overall shows a better prognosis than aRMS with 5-year survival of 80% versus 52% [8].

Besides histologic type, age of onset, and size of tumor, the site of the tumor is highly important for staging and prognosis of RMS [9]. Parameningeal rhabdomyosarcomas (PM-RMS) comprise half of head and neck RMS cases, which also include tumors located in the paranasal sinuses, nasal cavity, middle ear, and the infratemporal and pterygopalatine fossae [8]. Most PM-RMS are of the embryonal type, whereas those with alveolar features show a worse prognosis [10]. Patients with parameningeal eRMS had a 4-year failure-free survival rate of 68% on the most recent Children's Oncology Group study compared to 74% for similar eRMS with primary tumors at other sites [11]. The poorer prognosis of PM-RMS is mainly due to inaccessibility of the site and difficulty in achieving negative surgical margins [12]. Local recurrence is the most common form of relapse, and poor prognostic features include intracranial spread and meningeal involvement [10].

In genetically engineered mice, extra-axial eRMS and aRMS of the head and neck have been generated expressing the *Pax3:Foxo1* fusion gene and cooperating mutations [13–15]. Adult pleomorphic rhabdomyosarcomas have also been shown to develop spontaneously in aging A/J mice [16] or with expression of oncogenic KRAS [6, 7]. Constitutive activation of the Hedgehog pathway in the adipocyte lineage of mice has been associated with the formation of head and neck tumors resembling eRMS [17]. However, preclinical models of parameningeal eRMS tumors are still lacking. Xenograft models of cancer can reflect the heterogeneity of human tumors and create a stromal and vascular milieu not present in cell lines. Preservation of these relationships can more accurately mimic the behavior of human tumors, particularly in their responses to treatment. While immunocompromised test animals and subcutaneous implantation do not precisely mimic the environment within the human body, it is the nearest approximation available for research.

The rarity of PM-RMS and the clinically inaccessible site have made collection of biopsy tissue for xenografting difficult. Here we present an invaluable PDX model, the first such parameningeal eRMS preclinical model, for exploring the biology and preclinical therapeutic avenues in parameningeal RMS, created from tissue obtained at autopsy.

2. Case Presentation

A 14-year-old girl presented with a history of several weeks of persistent headache, hoarse voice, and 20 lb weight loss with tongue deviation on exam. A brain MRI scan showed a 1 × 2 cm enhancing right-sided skull based mass that was invading the hypoglossal nerve canal (Figure 1(a)). Biopsy of the mass showed poorly differentiated tumor with round to spindled cells in a myxoid background (Figure 1(b)). An extensive immunohistochemical panel including positive desmin and myogenin stains was consistent with rhabdomyosarcoma and cytogenetic testing was negative for (2; 13) and (1; 13) translocations, which would be more consistent with alveolar rhabdomyosarcoma. No anaplastic features were noted and the tumor was diagnosed as embryonal rhabdomyosarcoma. The tumor was not amenable to complete surgical resection, and thus the patient was diagnosed with IRS Stage 2, Group III eRMS. The patient received standard chemotherapy with vincristine, actinomycin-D, and cyclophosphamide. Local radiation therapy (RT) was initiated immediately for symptomatic treatment and 50.4 Gy RT to the local tumor produced slow improvement in the vocal cord paralysis and resolution of the tongue deviation.

Approximately 6 months after beginning chemotherapy and 4 months after the completion of RT, the patient developed lower extremity weakness, gait disturbance, incontinence, and headaches. Imaging revealed new diffuse leptomeningeal metastases involving the entire brain and spine. A ventriculoperitoneal shunt was placed, and, to address symptoms of lower extremity weakness and incontinence, the patient emergently received 30 Gy palliative RT to her lower thoracic spine. Shortly after completing RT, she developed difficulty in breathing, seizures, and altered mental status. With ongoing respiratory failure and neurologic deterioration, the family and medical team decided to transition the patient to comfort care only. The patient died shortly after extubation and permission to perform a complete autopsy was given by the family. The study was conducted with appropriate approval by the Institutional Review Board.

The autopsy was performed approximately 28 hours after death. Examination revealed numerous fleshy masses ranging from 1 to 6 cm involving the cerebrum (left frontal and occipital cortex and underlying white matter, cingulate gyrus bilaterally, genu of corpus callosum, left basal ganglia, hypothalamus and left thalamus, right hippocampus, and optic chiasm), cerebellum, and brainstem as well as the leptomeninges. Metastatic tumor was harvested sterilely from several brain sites and placed immediately in RPMI solution with sections fixed in 10% formalin for histology from the same anatomic sites. Histology showed poorly differentiated neoplasm with round to elongated spindled cells in a myxoid background, highly similar to those seen in the previous biopsy (Figure 1(c)).

3. Materials and Methods

3.1. PDX Model Creation. NSG (NOD.Cg-*Prkdcscid IL2rgtm1Wjl*/SzJ) mice were obtained from The Jackson Laboratory. These highly immune deficient mice have no mature T or B lymphocytes or functional natural killer cells and also have decreased cytokine signaling, rendering them excellent subjects for human tissue engraftment. All studies were done with the approval of The Jackson Laboratory Institutional Animal Care and Use Committee. Tumor pieces taken directly from the patient (50–125 mm^3) were implanted subcutaneously into the rear flanks of recipient female NSG mice using a trocar. Tumors were allowed to grow to approximately 1000 mm^3 when the tumors were collected and dissected into approximately 50 mm^3 fragments. The fragments were serially passaged in NSG mice to create cohorts of mice for drug-testing purposes. To maintain models and minimize genetic drift, fragments from the P0

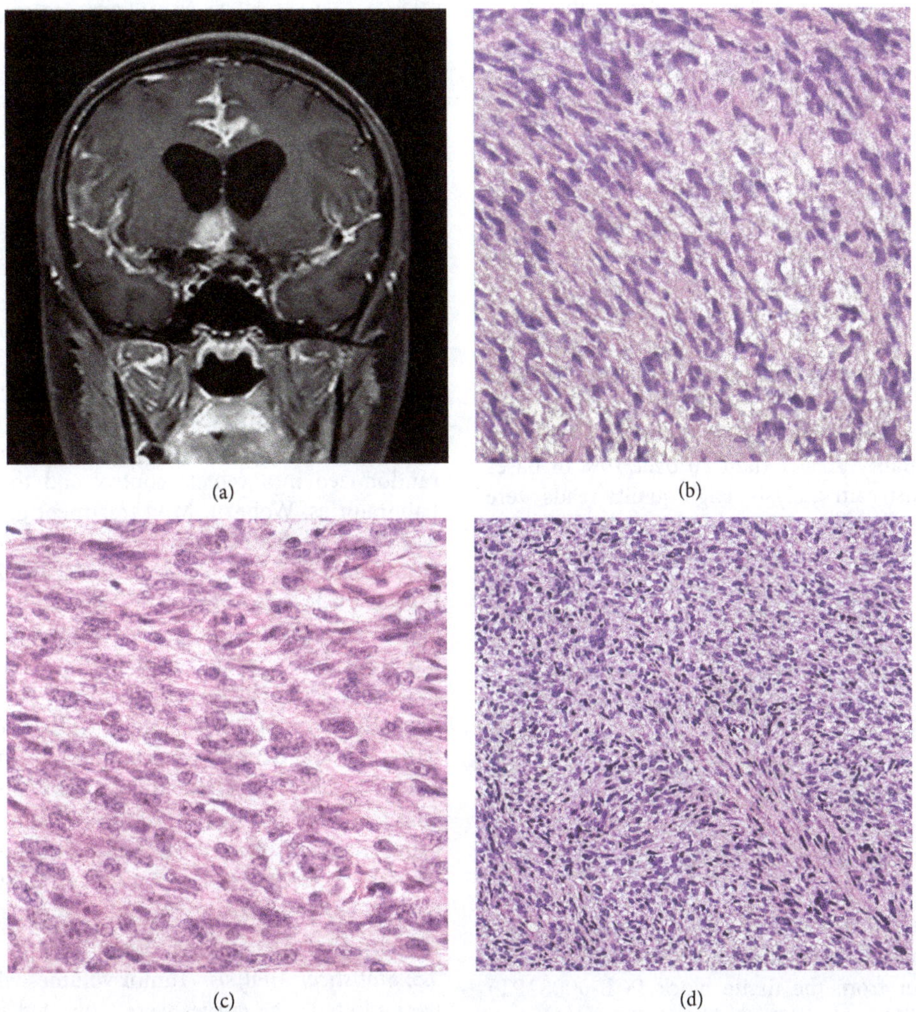

FIGURE 1: Radiographic imaging and comparative histology of human and PDX tumors: (a) 1 cm × 2 cm enhancing right-sided skull based mass that was invading the hypoglossal nerve canal. (b) H&E slide, 400x of brain biopsy showing sheets of elongated spindled cells with eosinophilic cytoplasm and a myxoid background, consistent with embryonal rhabdomyosarcoma. An H&E slide, 400x from the frontal lobe at autopsy (c), and a section of mouse xenograft, 200x (d), show highly similar morphologic features.

and P1 passages were frozen in 10% DMSO. These fragments are used to generate low passage number cohorts of tumor bearing mice as needed for study. PDX efficacy studies do not go beyond passage 6.

3.2. Genomics. Gene expression analysis was performed with the human exon 1.0 ST array (Affymetrix, Santa Clara, CA). Only the initial passaged tumor (P0) was characterized for gene expression because the patient sample could not be collected quickly enough to ensure data quality. PDX gene expression microarrays were processed in the R statistical programming environment [18]. First, arrays were loaded and grouped into probe sets with the BrainArray version 17 CDF [19] and Ensembl human gene annotations (annotation version 70 using the human assembly GRCh37). Individual probe intensities were quantile normalized, and log-transformed, but no background correction was performed. Summarized expression intensities were generated with the probe-level model as implemented by the AffyPLM R package [20], fitting a simple model of the logarithmic intensity for each probe as the sum of a sample effect, a probe effect, and a residual term, with the sample effect representing the summarized intensity of the entire transcript/gene. Mouse contamination effects on the arrays were assessed by hybridization of NSG mouse skin samples on triplicate arrays for the HuGene-1.0-st arrays.

Copy number variation for the patient tumor and the P0 PDX tumor were analyzed with the genome-wide human 6.0 SNP array (Affymetrix). The whole-genome allele-specific copy number profiles, fraction of aberrant cells, and tumor ploidy were estimated using ASCAT 2.2 [21, 22]. The input data for ASCAT was generated from the CEL files using the PennCNV-Affy package [23] which extracts the Log R Ratios (LRR) and B-Allele Frequency (BAF) and performs the GC correction. Ensemble genes (human genome annotation version 70) were then annotated with the segmented copy number of the major (CNVa) and minor (CNVb) alleles. Total copy number was computed by adding the values for the major and minor alleles. A segment was defined as loss of heterozygosity (LOH) if the major allele frequency was greater than 0.5 and the minor allele was less than 0.1.

TruSeq Amplicon Cancer Panel. Using the Illumina protocol, mutation hotspots from forty-eight (48) cancer-related genes were amplified and sequenced on the Illumina MiSeq sequencer. The TruSeq data were analyzed using a bioinformatics analysis pipeline developed at Jackson Laboratory. Briefly, sequencing reads generated by the platform were initially assessed for mouse contamination using Xenome v1.0.0 [24]. The human specific reads were further subjected to quality control using *NGSQCtoolkit v2.3* [25] and reads with base quality greater than 30 over 70% of bases were used in downstream analysis. High quality reads were mapped to human genome (Hg19) using *BWA* [26]. The resulting alignment was sorted by coordinates and further converted to binary alignment format by Picard tools (http://picard.sourceforge.net/). Subsequently, the *IndelRealigner* and *BaseRecalibrator* modules in the Genome Analysis tool kit (GATK) were used to preprocess the alignments [27, 28]. The realigned and recalibrated BAM file was used as an input to *GATK-UnifiedGenotyper* and the variant calls were restricted to the target region (Agilent sureSelect v4), soft filtered with read depth less than 140. Finally, *Pindel* [29] was used to identify microdeletions and all variants with allele frequency greater than 5% were reported.

3.3. Fluorescence In Situ Hybridization (FISH). FISH was performed with formalin-fixed paraffin embedded (FFPE) tissue sections (4 μM, cut from the tissue block PCB-00082PT) using the Standard Operational Procedures (SOP) established at the CLIA-certified Clinical Cytogenetics Laboratory at the Jackson Laboratory for Genomic Medicine. The FFPE slides were baked at 60°C overnight and then deparaffinized with xylene at room temperature for three times, 15 minutes each time. The slides were dehydrated with 100% ethanol at room temperature for 2 minutes and air-dried for approximately 15 minutes. The slides were treated with tissue pretreatment and digestion kits according to the instructions provided by the manufacturer (CytoCell). After digestion, the slides were dehydrated with 70%, 90%, and 100% ethanol, respectively, at room temperature for 2 minutes each, followed by air drying. For denaturation and hybridization, the slides were placed face-down onto a clean H&E slide and the unstained tissue section on paraffin slide was aligned with the corresponding tumor tissue area on the H&E slide. Using a diamond pen, the target tumor area was marked on the slide to be processed for FISH. 10 μL of PAX3 Breakapart probes was applied (Cytocell, LPS 012) and of PAX7 Breakapart probes (Cytocell, LPS 013) onto two separate marked areas, respectively, and the area was covered with a $22 \times 22\,mm^2$ glass cover slip. The area was sealed with rubber cement and the probes and slide were codenatured on the Hybrite at 94°C for 3 minutes. The slide was placed in a humidified chamber and incubated at the 37°C incubator for 48 hours. For posthybridization wash, the slides were immersed in 0.5X SSC at 72°C for 5 minutes. They were washed 3 times in 1XPBS with 0.025% Tween 20 at room temperature, 2 minutes each time. 10 μL of DAPI was applied to the marked area and it was covered with a $22 \times 22\,mm^2$ glass cover slip. The edges of the glass cover slip were sealed with nail polish to prevent slides from drying. In this study, we also performed interphase FISH with a normal human control cell line (GM12878) as a control test. The FISH slides were analyzed using the Leica GSL120 image scanner system.

3.4. Efficacy Evaluation in Tumor Bearing Mice. Because the patient's tumor sample harbored an ALK mutation, the potent, FDA-approved kinase inhibitor lestaurtinib was chosen for preclinical studies. NSG mice with PDX tumors at passage #2 and an average size of $250{\sim}300\,mm^3$ were randomized into vehicle control and the lestaurtinib (LC Laboratories, Woburn, MA) treatment groups. Lestaurtinib was prepared in 40% polyethylene glycol 100 (Spectrum New Brunswick, NJ), 10% povidone (ISP), and 2% benzyl alcohol (Spectrum,) as previously described [30]. A total of nine doses were given subcutaneously every 2 to 3 days over a 3-week dosing period at 10 mg/kg. Tumor volumes were measured with a digital caliper 3 times weekly and calculated using the formula: $0.5 \times \text{length} \times \text{width}^2$ (mm^3). Bodyweight, hair coat, and activity were monitored 3 times a week and animal welfare was checked daily. Animals were euthanized when tumors reached a $2{,}000\,mm^3$ tumor endpoint. The experiment was carried out twice. For the first experiment, the vehicle group enrolled 7 mice and the lestaurtinib group 6 mice. The second experiment had 6 mice in both groups.

3.5. Statistical Analysis. Tumor volumes with standard error were plotted. The curves were truncated when the number of animals currently on study in particular cohorts decreased to below 50% of the starting animal number for that cohort. The tumor growth delay (TGD) method was used to analyze drug treatment effects on time to tumor endpoint (TTE) for the therapeutic dosing regimen [11]. Statistical significance for median TTE values for treatment comparisons was determined by the Log-rank test with a 95% confidence value for two-tailed statistical analyses.

4. Results and Discussion

Five tumor fragments directly from the patient ($50–125\,mm^3$) were implanted into 5 recipient NSG mice to develop patient derived xenograft models. Within 4 months of tumor implantation, all five mice developed tumors with approximately $1000\,mm^3$ volume. Histology was analyzed on all xenografts and showed highly similar features to both the patient's prior premortem biopsy and autopsy specimens (Figure 1(d)). Ki-67 immunohistochemical staining was performed to confirm that human cells were proliferating within xenograft samples. This model and associated data are publicly available and represented in the JAX tumor model repository as PDX model TM00360 [31].

Copy number variation was only assessed for the patient tumor as the P0 PDX tumor failed quality control. Several

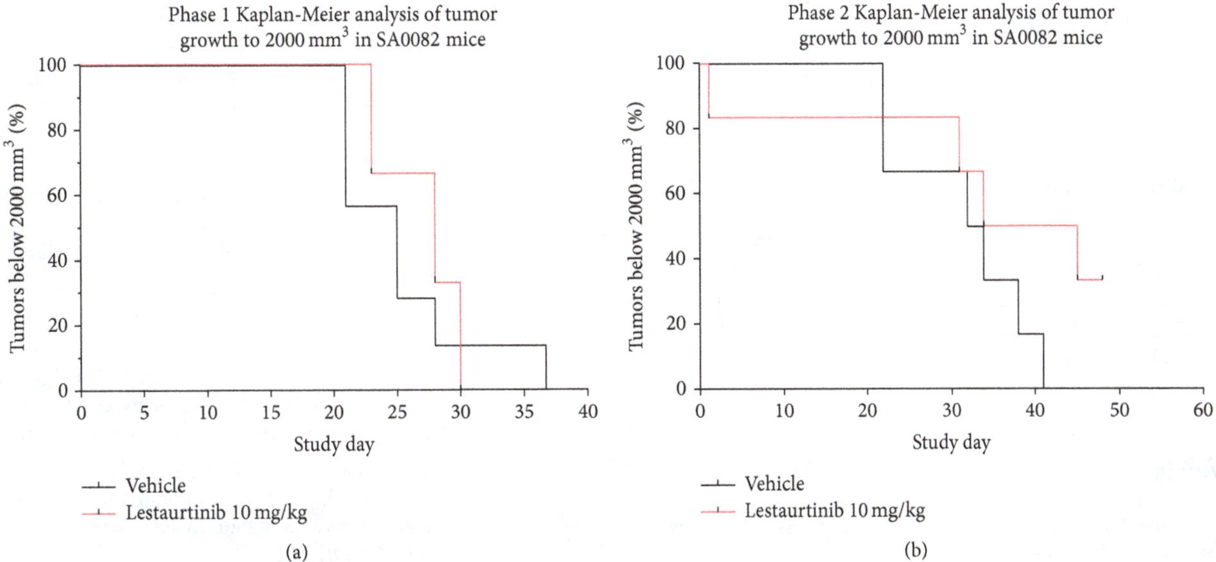

FIGURE 2: Preclinical testing of lestaurtinib in a parameningeal PDX. (a, b) Kaplan-Meier analysis of PDX mice from two different treatment cohorts.

regions of chromosomal amplification and deletion were observed consistent with previous analyses of rhabdomyosarcomas including gains in chromosomes 2, 8, 11, 12, and 20 [32]. Additionally, gains in chromosomes 5 and 19 were observed. Losses were observed for chromosomes 2, 9, 10, and 11. Genes in the amplified regions included several frequently amplified in soft tissue tumors: CDK4, MDM2, GLI4, and MYC [33].

TruSeq cancer panel targeted amplicon sequencing in both patient and P0 PDX tumor samples revealed an ALK R1181C mutation and no other mutations in the 48 gene panel including the *NRAS*, *KRAS*, *HRAS*, *PIK3CA*, *CTNNB1*, and *FBXW7* genes. The *BCOR* and *FGFR4* genes were not analyzed as they are not included in the TruSeq cancer panel. FISH assay revealed no break-apart involving PAX3 or PAX7.

All mice equally tolerated the treatments with body weights and clinical observations remaining stable for both the vehicle and lestaurtinib treated mice. Tumors grew progressively for both treatments as indicated by mean tumor volumes over time. There was no statistical significance in tumor growth between vehicle and lestaurtinib treatment groups and the Kaplan-Meier survival curves did not differ significantly between vehicle and lestaurtinib treatment groups ($p > 0.05$; Figure 2).

Chemotherapy is a mainstay of treatment for rhabdomyosarcoma, particularly in cases such as our patient when surgical resection is not feasible [34]. Monsma et al. previously utilized a PDX model of alveolar rhabdomyosarcoma, first identifying potential therapies by gene expression profiling and then testing the efficacy of agents *in vivo* [35]. This approach is similar to the one taken in our study. Prior mouse models of eRMS have shown varied pathways to tumorigenesis with individual pathways correlated to specific sites, suggesting that generation of site specific xenografts could lend insight into treatment of rare variants such as PM-RMS [36].

5. Conclusions

To our knowledge, this is the first patient-derived xenograft for parameningeal rhabdomyosarcoma. We and others have previously described the importance of research autopsy [37, 38]. This patient succumbed to fulminant eRMS with mass effect after completing radiation and while still receiving multiagent chemotherapy. The ability to obtain treatment resistant eRMS tumor tissue at autopsy and generate PDX is critical to our ability to understand the mechanisms of resistance and to evaluate the impact of novel therapies directed at identified targets. It is of particular interest that while this tumor did demonstrate an *ALK* R1181C mutation, lestaurtinib (which has a 71 nM Kd for ALK) still had no effect [39]. It is possible that this mutation may not drive response to therapy or that most recurrent cancers will not respond to single agent treatment. While our study did not demonstrate response of the xenograft tumors to a pan-kinase inhibitor, generation of the PDX from autopsy tissue provides a tool for identification of potential novel targeted therapies, as well as treatments which might target lestaurtinib resistant tumors in humans.

Disclosure

All authors have approved the paper for submission.

Authors' Contribution

All authors have contributed significantly to the work.

Acknowledgments

This work was funded by a Nylund Family bequeath, the Rally Foundation Legacy Gift Pilot Program, and a gift from Braver, Stronger, Smarter Fighting Childhood Cancer Foundation. The authors are also deeply indebted to the family who made this selfless tissue gift possible.

References

[1] S. Malempati and D. S. Hawkins, "Rhabdomyosarcoma: review of the Children's Oncology Group (COG) soft-tissue Sarcoma committee experience and rationale for current COG studies," *Pediatric Blood & Cancer*, vol. 59, no. 1, pp. 5–10, 2012.

[2] B. Belyea, J. G. Kephart, J. Blum, D. G. Kirsch, and C. M. Linardic, "Embryonic signaling pathways and rhabdomyosarcoma: contributions to cancer development and opportunities for therapeutic targeting," *Sarcoma*, vol. 2012, Article ID 406239, 13 pages, 2012.

[3] S. Ognjanovic, A. M. Linabery, B. Charbonneau, and J. A. Ross, "Trends in childhood rhabdomyosarcoma incidence and survival in the United States, 1975–2005," *Cancer*, vol. 115, no. 18, pp. 4218–4226, 2009.

[4] J. F. Shern, L. Chen, J. Chmielecki et al., "Comprehensive genomic analysis of rhabdomyosarcoma reveals a landscape of alterations affecting a common genetic axis in fusion-positive and fusion-negative tumors," *Cancer Discovery*, vol. 4, no. 2, pp. 216–231, 2014.

[5] X. Chen, E. Stewart, A. Shelat et al., "Targeting oxidative stress in embryonal rhabdomyosarcoma," *Cancer Cell*, vol. 24, no. 6, pp. 710–724, 2013.

[6] S. Hettmer, J. Liu, C. M. Miller et al., "Sarcomas induced in discrete subsets of prospectively isolated skeletal muscle cells," *Proceedings of the National Academy of Sciences of the United States of America*, vol. 108, no. 50, pp. 20002–20007, 2011.

[7] J. M. Blum, L. Añó, Z. Li et al., "Distinct and overlapping sarcoma subtypes initiated from muscle stem and progenitor cells," *Cell Reports*, vol. 5, no. 4, pp. 933–940, 2013.

[8] K. T. Montone, F. G. Barr, P. J. Zhang, M. D. Feldman, and V. A. LiVolsi, "Embryonal and alveolar rhabdomyosarcoma of parameningeal sites in adults: a report of 13 cases," *International Journal of Surgical Pathology*, vol. 17, no. 1, pp. 22–30, 2009.

[9] E. Davicioni, M. J. Anderson, F. G. Finckenstein et al., "Molecular classification of rhabdomyosarcoma—genotypic and phenotypic determinants of diagnosis: a report from the Children's Oncology Group," *The American Journal of Pathology*, vol. 174, no. 2, pp. 550–564, 2009.

[10] S. K. Childs, K. R. Kozak, A. M. Friedmann et al., "Proton radiotherapy for parameningeal rhabdomyosarcoma: clinical outcomes and late effects," *International Journal of Radiation Oncology, Biology, Physics*, vol. 82, no. 2, pp. 635–642, 2012.

[11] C. A. S. Arndt, J. A. Stoner, D. S. Hawkins et al., "Vincristine, actinomycin, and cyclophosphamide compared with vincristine, actinomycin, and cyclophosphamide alternating with vincristine, topotecan, and cyclophosphamide for intermediate-risk rhabdomyosarcoma: children's oncology group study D9803," *Journal of Clinical Oncology*, vol. 27, no. 31, pp. 5182–5188, 2009.

[12] J. H. M. Merks, G. L. De Salvo, C. Bergeron et al., "Parameningeal rhabdomyosarcoma in pediatric age: results of a pooled analysis from North American and European cooperative groups," *Annals of Oncology*, vol. 25, no. 1, pp. 231–236, 2014.

[13] M. Geltzeiler, G. Li, J. Abraham, and C. Keller, "The case for primary salivary rhabdomyosarcoma," *Frontiers in Oncology*, vol. 5, article 74, 2015.

[14] J. Abraham, Y. Nuñez-Álvarez, S. Hettmer et al., "Lineage of origin in rhabdomyosarcoma informs pharmacological response," *Genes and Development*, vol. 28, no. 14, pp. 1578–1591, 2014.

[15] B. P. Rubin, K. Nishijo, H.-I. H. Chen et al., "Evidence for an unanticipated relationship between undifferentiated pleomorphic sarcoma and embryonal rhabdomyosarcoma," *Cancer Cell*, vol. 19, no. 2, pp. 177–191, 2011.

[16] R. B. Sher, G. A. Cox, K. D. Mills, and J. P. Sundberg, "Rhabdomyosarcomas in aging A/J mice," *PLoS ONE*, vol. 6, no. 8, Article ID e23498, 2011.

[17] M. E. Hatley, W. Tang, M. R. Garcia et al., "A mouse model of rhabdomyosarcoma originating from the adipocyte lineage," *Cancer Cell*, vol. 22, no. 4, pp. 536–546, 2012.

[18] Gentleman RIaR, "R: a language for data analysis and graphics," *Journal of Computational and Graphical Statistics*, vol. 5, no. 3, pp. 299–314, 1996.

[19] R. Sandberg and O. Larsson, "Improved precision and accuracy for microarrays using updated probe set definitions," *BMC Bioinformatics*, vol. 8, article 48, 2007.

[20] L. Gautier, L. Cope, B. M. Bolstad, and R. A. Irizarry, "Affy—analysis of *Affymetrix GeneChip* data at the probe level," *Bioinformatics*, vol. 20, no. 3, pp. 307–315, 2004.

[21] P. Van Loo, G. Nilsen, S. H. Nordgard et al., "Analyzing cancer samples with SNP arrays," *Methods in Molecular Biology*, vol. 802, pp. 57–72, 2012.

[22] P. Van Loo, S. H. Nordgard, O. C. Lingjærde et al., "Allele-specific copy number analysis of tumors," *Proceedings of the National Academy of Sciences of the United States of America*, vol. 107, no. 39, pp. 16910–16915, 2010.

[23] K. Wang, M. Li, D. Hadley et al., "PennCNV: an integrated hidden Markov model designed for high-resolution copy number variation detection in whole-genome SNP genotyping data," *Genome Research*, vol. 17, no. 11, pp. 1665–1674, 2007.

[24] T. Conway, J. Wazny, A. Bromage et al., "Xenome—a tool for classifying reads from xenograft samples," *Bioinformatics*, vol. 28, no. 12, pp. i172–i178, 2012.

[25] R. K. Patel and M. Jain, "NGS QC toolkit: a toolkit for quality control of next generation sequencing data," *PLoS ONE*, vol. 7, no. 2, Article ID e30619, 2012.

[26] H. Li and R. Durbin, "Fast and accurate short read alignment with Burrows-Wheeler transform," *Bioinformatics*, vol. 25, no. 14, pp. 1754–1760, 2009.

[27] A. McKenna, M. Hanna, E. Banks et al., "The Genome Analysis Toolkit: a MapReduce framework for analyzing next-generation DNA sequencing data," *Genome Research*, vol. 20, no. 9, pp. 1297–1303, 2010.

[28] M. A. Depristo, E. Banks, R. Poplin et al., "A framework for variation discovery and genotyping using next-generation DNA

sequencing data," *Nature Genetics*, vol. 43, no. 5, pp. 491–498, 2011.

[29] K. Ye, M. H. Schulz, Q. Long, R. Apweiler, and Z. Ning, "Pindel: a pattern growth approach to detect break points of large deletions and medium sized insertions from paired-end short reads," *Bioinformatics*, vol. 25, no. 21, pp. 2865–2871, 2009.

[30] R. Iyer, A. E. Evans, X. Qi et al., "Lestaurtinib enhances the antitumor efficacy of chemotherapy in murine xenograft models of neuroblastoma," *Clinical Cancer Research*, vol. 16, no. 5, pp. 1478–1485, 2010.

[31] C. J. Bult, D. M. Krupke, D. A. Begley et al., "Mouse Tumor Biology (MTB): a database of mouse models for human cancer," *Nucleic Acids Research*, vol. 43, no. 1, pp. D818–D824, 2015.

[32] J. A. Bridge, J. Liu, S. J. Qualman et al., "Genomic gains and losses are similar in genetic and histologic subsets of rhabdomyosarcoma, whereas amplification predominates in embryonal with anaplasia and alveolar subtypes," *Genes Chromosomes & Cancer*, vol. 33, no. 3, pp. 310–321, 2002.

[33] P. Ragazzini, G. Gamberi, L. Pazzaglia et al., "Amplification of CDK4, MDM2, SAS and GLI genes in leiomyosarcoma, alveolar and embryonal rhabdomyosarcoma," *Histology and Histopathology*, vol. 19, no. 2, pp. 401–411, 2004.

[34] J. Radzikowska, W. Kukwa, A. Kukwa, A. Czarnecka, and A. Krzeski, "Rhabdomyosarcoma of the head and neck in children," *Contemporary Oncology*, vol. 19, no. 2, pp. 98–107, 2015.

[35] D. J. Monsma, D. M. Cherba, P. J. Richardson et al., "Using a rhabdomyosarcoma patient-derived xenograft to examine precision medicine approaches and model acquired resistance," *Pediatric Blood and Cancer*, vol. 61, no. 9, pp. 1570–1577, 2014.

[36] V. P. Kashi, M. E. Hatley, and R. L. Galindo, "Probing for a deeper understanding of rhabdomyosarcoma: insights from complementary model systems," *Nature Reviews Cancer*, vol. 15, no. 7, pp. 426–439, 2015.

[37] J. A. Jarzembowski and M. J. Hicks, "Pediatric autopsy consent: helping families create hope out of despair," *Pediatric Blood and Cancer*, vol. 60, no. 2, pp. 173–174, 2013.

[38] J. L. Alabran, J. E. Hooper, M. Hill et al., "Overcoming autopsy barriers in pediatric cancer research," *Pediatric Blood and Cancer*, vol. 60, no. 2, pp. 204–209, 2013.

[39] M. I. Davis, J. P. Hunt, S. Herrgard et al., "Comprehensive analysis of kinase inhibitor selectivity," *Nature Biotechnology*, vol. 29, no. 11, pp. 1046–1051, 2011.

Costs Associated with Intravenous Cancer Therapy Administration in Patients with Metastatic Soft Tissue Sarcoma in a US Population

Mei Sheng Duh,[1] Michelle D. Hackshaw,[2] Jasmina I. Ivanova,[1] Gregory Kruse,[3] Lesley-Ann N. Miller,[2] Patrick Lefebvre,[1] Paul Karner,[1] and Bruce Wong[4]

[1] *Analysis Group, Inc., 111 Huntington Avenue, Tenth Floor, Boston, MA 02199, USA*
[2] *GlaxoSmithKline, Philadelphia, PA 19102, USA*
[3] *University of Pennsylvania, Philadelphia, PA 19104, USA*
[4] *Bruce Wong and Associates, Inc., Wayne, PA 19087, USA*

Correspondence should be addressed to Mei Sheng Duh; mduh@analysisgroup.com

Academic Editor: Luca Sangiorgi

Background. The most common chemotherapies in metastatic soft tissue sarcoma (mSTS) require intravenous (IV) administration. This often requires patients to make multiple outpatient visits per chemotherapy cycle, possibly impeding patients' daily activities and increasing caregiver burden and medical costs. This study investigated costs associated with IV cancer therapy administration in mSTS from the payer perspective of the health care system. *Patients and Methods.* From the Experian Healthcare database, 1,228 mSTS patients were selected. Data were analyzed on outpatient visits during 2005–2012 involving IV cancer therapy administration. Costs were estimated on a per patient per visit (PPPV) and per patient per month (PPPM) basis. *Results.* The mean (median) cost of IV therapy was $2,427 ($1,532) PPPV and $5,468 ($4,310) PPPM, of which approximately 60% was IV drug costs. IV administration costs averaged $399 PPPV and $900 PPPM, representing 16.5% of total visit costs. Anthracycline and alkylating-agents-based therapies had the highest PPPV and PPPM IV administration costs, respectively (mean $479 and $1,336, resp.). Patients with managed care insurance had the highest IV administration costs (mean $504 PPPV; $1,120 PPPM). *Conclusions.* IV administration costs constitute a considerable proportion of the total costs of receiving an IV cancer therapy to treat mSTS.

1. Introduction

Soft tissue sarcomas (STS) are a rare, complex group of childhood and adult neoplasms with differentiation towards mesenchymal tissue, which may arise almost anywhere in the body [1]. STS account for approximately 1% of malignant tumours in adults and 2% of total cancer mortality [2]. It is estimated that in 2012 approximately 10,280 people were diagnosed with STS in the United States (USA) [3]. STS exhibit remarkable histologic diversity and consist of a heterogeneous group of tumours with over 50 subtypes [2]. In a recent study of 17,364 cases of STS, malignant fibrous histiocytoma (24.1%), leiomyosarcoma (14.8%), sarcoma (12.8%), and myxoid liposarcoma (5.9%) were the most prevalent histological subtypes [4]. Although local control can be obtained through the use of surgery and radiotherapy, in patients who experience recurrence at distant sites (~50% of all patients), >90% will ultimately die of this malignancy [5]. The five-year survival rate for patients with advanced/metastatic disease is also low (e.g., 8% in patients with lung metastasis [6]).

The most commonly used chemotherapies in metastatic soft tissue sarcoma (mSTS) are intravenously (IV) administered agents [7]. Although the cost burden of IV cancer therapy (e.g., cost of IV administration and the cost of IV drugs) has been studied for specific cancer types (e.g., breast and small cell lung cancer) [8, 9] and other conditions, such as rheumatoid arthritis [10], no study to date has assessed the costs associated with IV cancer therapy administration in a mSTS population.

This study reports estimates of the total and component costs associated with IV cancer therapy administration in patients with mSTS from the payer perspective of the US health care system, based on an analysis of claims data from a large contract and claims management system.

2. Methods

2.1. Data Sources. Data for this study were obtained from the Experian Healthcare (Experian) database, which maintains a contract and claims management system that supports 350 general/oncology clinics in the US. The database contains a complete history of diagnoses (ICD-9-CM codes), procedures, and drug therapies received by both publicly and privately insured patients within the clinics, as well as patient demographics (e.g., age, gender, and geographic region) and insurance type (e.g., managed care, indemnity, Medicare, and Medicaid). For every patient clinic visit, Experian records the service dates, total charged, total contracted payments, and total allowed, with individual services, procedures, and drugs broken out by line item (Current Procedural Terminology, Fourth Edition [CPT-4] and Healthcare Common Procedure Coding System [HCPCS] codes). The Experian dataset used in this study covers the period from January 1, 2005, to April 30, 2012.

2.2. Study Design. This study employed a retrospective, longitudinal cohort design. The index date was defined as the date of the first IV cancer therapy infusion for mSTS treatment. Therapy windows were calculated as a patient-drug combination for the purposes of reporting study outcomes on a per month basis. The observation period for each patient-drug window begins at the index date and ends with either the last IV cancer therapy administration (if the patient only remains on one therapy) or the last visit of that IV cancer therapy before a patient switches to a different IV cancer therapy, plus a therapeutic effect. The therapeutic effect for patients that do not switch therapies is the average interval between administrations across the entire dataset for that particular IV cancer therapy. For patients who received a single IV therapy, the observation period length was calculated as the length of the therapy plus the average interval across the entire dataset for that particular IV cancer therapy. For patients that switch IV cancer therapies, the therapeutic effect is defined as the minimum of either the time between the last visit of that therapy and the start of the new therapy or average therapy interval across the entire dataset.

2.3. Study Population. The selection of patients in the study sample is depicted in Figure 1. The population of patients with mSTS receiving IV therapy was determined by a claims algorithm [11] that required patients to have (1) at least one diagnosis of a distant secondary malignant neoplasm (ICD-9-CM 196.XX-199.0); (2) a diagnosis of mSTS between January 1, 2005, and April 30, 2012; and (3) at least one claim of an IV cancer therapy used to treat mSTS (defined according to NCCN treatment guidelines [7]) following mSTS diagnosis. (For the purposes of this study, IV cancer therapies used to treat mSTS included actinomycinD, bevacizumab, carboplatin, cisplatin, cyclophosphamide, dacarbazine, docetaxel, doxorubicin, epirubicin, etoposide, gemcitabine, ifosfamide, interferon, irinotecan, mesna, oxaliplatin, paclitaxel, temozolomide, topotecan, vincristine, and vinorelbine.) Diagnosis of mSTS was defined as at least two medical claims with an ICD-9-CM diagnosis code of 171, or the following combination of IV cancer therapies and other selected ICD-9-CM diagnoses:

(i) a combination therapy of ifosfamide (HCPCS: J9208, J9209, C9427) and doxorubicin or liposomal doxorubicin (HCPCS: J9000, J9001, C9415) (both agents to be administered within 30 days), except if also diagnosed with osteosarcoma (ICD-9-CM: 170), nasopharyngeal carcinoma (ICD-9-CM: 147), lung cancer (ICD-9-CM:162.3-162.9), uterine cancer (ICD-9-CM: 179, 180, 182), breast cancer (ICD-9-CM:174), prostate cancer (ICD-9-CM: 185), renal cancer (ICD-9-CM: 189), or malignant neoplasm of lymphatic and hematopoietic tissue (ICD-9-CM: 200-208) at any time, or

(ii) at least 1 medical claim for retroperitoneal or peritoneal cancer (ICD-9-CM: 158), except if also diagnosed with renal cell carcinoma (ICD-9-CM: 189.0, 198.0), transitional cell carcinoma (ICD-9-CM: 189.1, 189.2), mesothelioma (ICD-9-CM: 163), gastrointestinal stromal tumors (ICD-9-CM: 159.0, 159.8, 159.9), uterine cancer (ICD-9-CM: 179, 180, 182), ovarian cancer (ICD-9-CM: 183), or other and unspecified female genital-organ cancer (ICD-9-CM: 184) at any time.

2.4. Treatment Costs and IV Administration Related Costs. Treatment costs were estimated using the contracted allowed payment for a claim rather than the practice charges, based on adjudication of the claim by the patient's third-party insurance plan. A contracted payment is defined as the amount that the provider is eligible to receive from all parties, including primary and secondary payers and the patient, based on the contractual agreement with the payer. Because the contracted payment represents the actual payment to providers from payers, it depicts a more accurate and detailed view of the true economic burden to payers of IV cancer therapy administration in mSTS patients.

Treatment costs included all costs incurred on eligible IV cancer therapy dates of service. Costs were categorized as (i) IV cancer therapy administration procedure costs, (ii) IV cancer therapy drug costs for mSTS, and (iii) costs associated with other visit-related drugs and services provided on the day of the IV cancer therapy visit. Claim codes used to identify IV infusion administration costs are consistent with those used in previous research [8–10].

Treatment costs were calculated per patient per IV visit (PPPV) and per patient per month (PPPM). PPPM costs were calculated by first computing average per month treatment costs for each patient, defined as the sum of all costs on days with IV cancer therapy administrations during the observation period divided by the length of the observation period

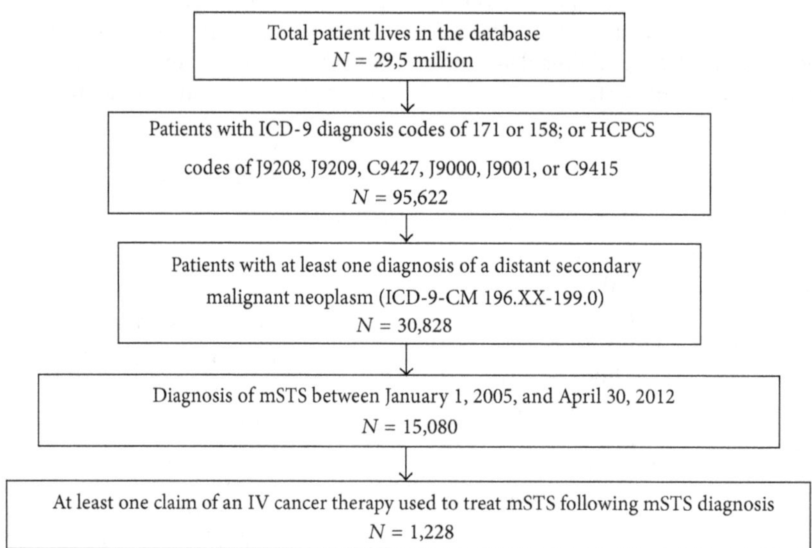

FIGURE 1: Sample selection.

for each patient in person-months. Average PPPM treatment costs for the overall sample were then calculated as a weighted average of the average per month cost, using the length of the observation period as the weight. Reporting PPPM costs is an approach commonly used in nonexperimental study settings to account for different lengths of observation periods among study patients.

2.5. Statistical Analyses. Patient characteristics as of the index date were obtained from the Experian dataset. Age was standardized as patient age in 2009 and divided into five categories: less than 25, from 25 to 39, from 40 to 54, from 55 to 64, and greater than 64 years. Insurance type was defined at the time of the index mSTS diagnosis and was held constant during the study period. Patient characteristics were reported as frequencies and percentages for categorical variables and sample size, means, standard deviations, medians, and ranges for continuous variables.

Medians, means, standard deviations, and quartile ranges of PPPV and PPPM treatment costs were reported for the overall mSTS patient sample. The total and component IV administration costs were further stratified by patient cohorts based on age, gender, region, insurance status, IV drugs, and number of administered drugs during the visit. Cost data was adjusted based on the medical consumer price index (CPI) [12] and reported in 2011 in US dollars. Two sensitivity analyses were performed to assess potential biases arising from patient selection and outliers: (i) analyses were repeated based on an alternative definition of mSTS diagnosis in which patients were only required to have at least two medical claims with an ICD-9-CM diagnosis code of 171; (ii) analyses were repeated after excluding IV administration visits with administration costs in the top 1%. Analyses were performed using SAS 9.3 (SAS Institute, Inc., Cary, NC, USA).

3. Results

A total of 1,228 patients with mSTS were identified. Baseline patient characteristics are presented in Table 1. The sample included a broad range of the patient age groups with almost a quarter of patients with ages greater than 64 years. Gender was not consistently recorded on all claims; only about half (48%) of patients had gender recorded. The numbers of reported male and female patients in the sample were similar. About half (50.7%) of the patients were insured by managed care, and another quarter (25.0%) were covered by Medicare (either traditional FFS or Medicare HMOs). The South was the most represented region which contained about half (49.7%) of the patient sample, with fewer patients residing in the Northeast (3.3%) and Southwest (8.7%).

3.1. PPPV Costs. Per patient per IV visit costs (PPPV) in which an IV cancer therapy was administered, subdivided into IV drug costs, IV administration costs, and other visit-related service costs, are presented in Table 2. The mean (median) cost per IV visit across the entire mSTS patient sample was $2,427 ($1,532). IV administration costs represented 16.5% of these costs with a mean of $399 per visit. About three-quarters (74.5%) of the IV administration costs were associated with direct administration of the cancer therapy (infusion time), with the remaining quarter of costs associated with therapeutic, diagnostic, and prophylactic administration (24.1%) and hydration administration (1.4%).

Mean IV drug costs were $1,450 and represented 59.7% of the total cost of the visit. The remaining 23.8% of the visit costs ($578) were attributed to other visit-related services. Evaluation and management office visits, supplies and equipment, and other miscellaneous administration comprised a small part of these costs with a mean of $22

TABLE 1: Patient characteristics for mSTS sample.

Patient characteristic	Count (N = 1,228)	Percent
Age[1]		
Less than 25	117	9.5%
25 to 39	152	12.4%
40 to 54	316	25.7%
55 to 64	345	28.1%
Greater than 64	298	24.3%
Gender[2]		
Female	289	23.5%
Male	295	24.0%
Insurance type[3]		
Managed care	622	50.7%
Medicare	283	23.0%
Medicare HMO	24	2.0%
Medicaid	67	5.5%
Medicaid HMO	10	0.8%
Indemnity	68	5.5%
Other[4]	154	12.5%
Region		
Midwest	240	19.5%
Northeast	41	3.3%
South	610	49.7%
Southwest	107	8.7%
West	230	18.7%

1: Age of the patient in 2009.
2: 644 patients were missing gender information.
3: Insurance type is defined at the time of the index mSTS diagnosis.
4: Other includes workers' compensation, Tricare, and self-pay.

(3.7% of other visit-related services). The remaining 96.2% of other visit-related costs were other IV drugs and specially administered oral drugs. Drugs to treat the symptoms of the disease and side effects comprised the largest part of these other drugs: colony-stimulating factors mean cost of $160 per visit, antiemetic agents mean cost of $171 per visit, and antihypercalcemic agents mean cost of $30 per visit. The other large cost categories were off-label chemotherapy agents (mean cost of $50 PPPV) and monoclonal antibody agents (mean cost of $84 PPPV).

IV visit costs on a PPPV basis, broken down by age, gender, region, type of insurance, IV drug used to treat mSTS, and number of IV drugs administered per visit, are presented in Table 3(a). IV administration costs ranged from $311 to $457 (13.9% to 28.1% of total IV visit costs) across age groups. Patients with ages less than 25 years and greater than 64 years had the lowest administration costs. IV administration costs and costs of other visit-related services were very similar between females and males. Patients in the Southwest region reported the lowest IV administration costs ($308) and other visit-related services ($341), and patients in the West reported the highest IV administration costs ($489) and other visit-related services ($646).

The largest differences in IV administration costs were found by insurance status. Managed care patients had the highest IV administration costs (mean $504 per visit) while Medicaid patients had the lowest (mean $92 per visit). The most expensive IV drugs in terms of IV administration costs were anthracycline-based therapies at $479 per visit and the cheapest were angiogenesis-based therapies at $301 per visit. Finally, costs of IV administration tended to increase with the number of IV drugs administered in a visit. Administering a single therapy cost an average of $304, increasing to $693 for three therapies and $936 for four therapies.

3.2. PPPM Costs. Total mean PPPM costs, subdivided into IV drug costs, IV administration costs, and other visit-related service costs, are presented in Table 2. Total mean (median) PPPM cost for the entire sample was $5,468 ($4,310) with quartile ranges from $2,066 to $7,431. Mean IV administration costs were $900 PPPM, of which $671 was due to chemotherapy administration, $217 was due to therapeutic, diagnostic, and prophylactic administration, and $12 was due to hydration administration. Mean PPPM cost per IV drug was $3,268 with quartile ranges between $427 and $4,704. Other visit-related costs were $1,300 PPPM. Supplies/equipment, evaluation and management office visits, and miscellaneous administration costs accounted for about $50 PPPM. Among other (i.e., non-mSTS) IV drugs administered during the visits, the costliest were those used to control side effects, including antiemetic agents ($384 PPPM) and colony-stimulating factors ($359 PPPM). Other high-cost categories include monoclonal antibody agents ($190 PPPM), off-label chemotherapy ($111 PPPM), and other miscellaneous agents ($113 PPPM).

IV visit costs on a PPPM basis, broken down by age, gender, region, type of insurance, IV drug used to treat mSTS, and number of IV drugs administered per visit, are presented in Table 3(b). Administration costs were similar across most age groups except for patients greater than 64 years, who had average administration costs about two-thirds ($623 PPPM) the size of the other age categories. Similar to the trend in total costs, patients in the Midwest and the West reported much higher IV administration costs PPPM at $1,080 and $1,030, respectively. Patients in the Northeast and Southwest reported much lower other visit-related costs than other regions.

Large variations in PPPM IV administration and other visit-related service costs were observed by insurance status. The highest IV administration PPPM costs were found in managed care patients and indemnity patients at $1,121 and $1,052, respectively. These patients also experienced higher other visit-related service costs compared to other insurance types. As with the PPPV results, other visit-related service costs were highest among patients with workers' compensation, Tricare, or self-pay insurance. In contrast to the PPPV where anthracycline-based agents were reported to have higher IV administration costs, the alkylating-based agents had much higher PPPM IV administration costs compared to the other therapies. Finally, the step-like trend of increasing IV administration costs based on the number of administered IV drugs during the visit was also observed in the PPPM analysis.

TABLE 2: IV visit costs per patient per visit (PPPV) and per patient per month (PPPM) by cost categories.

Cost category	Sum ($)[2]	%	Costs PPPV ($)[1] Median	Mean	Std. dev.	1st quartile	3rd quartile	Costs PPPM ($)[1] Median	Mean	Std. dev.	1st quartile	3rd quartile
No. of visits												
PPPV	13,583											
PPPM	6,025											
Total	**32,970,401**	**100.0%**	**1,532.11**	**2,427.33**	**2,674.95**	**720.50**	**3,187.80**	**4,310.20**	**5,467.61**	**133.01**	**2,065.64**	**7,430.99**
IV administration	**5,425,305**	**16.5%**	**342.01**	**399.42**	**291.78**	**226.62**	**513.84**	**678.54**	**899.57**	**24.91**	**395.94**	**1,130.75**
Chemotherapy administration	4,044,094	74.5%	253.53	297.73	227.91	163.67	379.00	489.72	670.50	19.34	282.65	832.90
Hydration administration	75,244	1.4%	0.00	5.54	23.55	0.00	0.00	0.00	12.45	1.26	0.00	2.55
Therapeutic, diagnostic, prophylactic admin.	1,305,967	24.1%	77.40	96.15	100.63	31.94	130.82	156.15	216.61	7.12	72.72	276.57
IV drug (for mSTS)	**19,693,317**	**59.7%**	**537.77**	**1,449.85**	**2,175.31**	**98.59**	**1,828.55**	**2,236.07**	**3,268.45**	**102.50**	**427.21**	**4,703.56**
Other visit-related services	**7,851,778**	**23.8%**	**190.55**	**578.06**	**1,178.00**	**42.31**	**483.00**	**725.44**	**1,299.60**	**51.60**	**294.02**	**1,573.49**
Miscellaneous administration	112,606	1.4%	0.00	8.29	72.83	0.00	0.00	0.00	18.68	1.52	0.00	15.69
Supplies/equipment	14,537	0.2%	0.00	1.07	13.76	0.00	0.00	0.00	2.39	0.57	0.00	0.00
Office visit/evaluation and mgmt. services	168,391	2.1%	0.00	12.40	41.77	0.00	0.00	0.00	27.90	2.00	0.00	4.18
Other IV drugs/specially admin. oral drugs	7,556,244	96.2%	185.76	556.30	1,167.77	17.25	468.02	688.65	1,250.63	51.33	241.48	1,498.94
Antihypercalcemic agents	407,395	5.4%	0.00	29.99	260.40	0.00	0.00	0.00	67.62	7.25	0.00	0.00
Colony-stimulating factor	2,175,927	28.8%	0.00	160.19	699.58	0.00	0.00	0.00	358.66	27.14	0.00	58.14
Antiemetic	2,317,729	30.7%	95.85	170.63	220.46	0.71	254.66	291.67	384.22	11.32	54.81	556.62
Use for IV infusion	90,036	1.2%	0.00	6.63	15.56	0.00	2.72	0.21	14.94	1.25	0.00	5.39
Corticosteroid for hypersensitivity	53,693	0.7%	1.09	3.95	16.74	0.00	2.33	2.67	8.91	0.91	0.98	6.32
Used to clear (flush) IV lines or catheters	6,515	0.1%	0.00	0.48	5.49	0.00	0.00	0.00	1.08	0.39	0.00	0.00
H2 antagonists for hypersensitivity	3,533	0.0%	0.00	0.26	2.54	0.00	0.00	0.00	0.59	0.08	0.00	0.00
For anemia	4,987	0.1%	0.00	0.37	7.79	0.00	0.00	0.00	0.83	0.23	0.00	0.00
Anticancer agent monoclonal antibody	1,143,295	15.1%	0.00	84.17	713.08	0.00	0.00	0.00	189.76	32.30	0.00	0.00
Anticancer agent chemotherapy	674,420	8.9%	0.00	49.65	319.96	0.00	0.00	0.00	111.43	21.30	0.00	0.00
Misc. other drugs	678,714	9.0%	0.00	49.97	358.51	0.00	1.34	1.93	112.59	10.55	0.00	26.98

1: Treatment costs derived from the contracted allowed payment for a claim.
2: Sum over all visits/months and patients.

Table 3: (a) Cost categories breakdown per patient per visit (PPPV) by demographic characteristics, IV drug, and number of drugs administered per visit[1]. (b) Cost categories breakdown per patient per month (PPPM) by demographic characteristics, IV drug, and number of drugs administered per visit[1].

(a)

Category	No. of patients	No. of visits	Total Average costs ($)	%	IV drug Average costs ($)	%	IV administration Average costs ($)	%	Other visit-related services Average costs ($)	%
Total	**1,228**	**13,583**	**2,427.33**	**100.0%**	**1,449.85**	**59.7%**	**399.42**	**16.5%**	**578.06**	**23.8%**
Age										
Less than 25	117	1,944	1,117.32	100.0%	462.60	41.4%	314.53	28.1%	340.19	30.4%
25 to 39	152	2,001	2,228.42	100.0%	1,276.28	57.3%	447.07	20.1%	505.07	22.7%
40 to 54	316	3,471	2,632.44	100.0%	1,531.81	58.2%	435.10	16.5%	665.52	25.3%
55 to 64	345	3,351	3,292.29	100.0%	2,057.09	62.5%	457.14	13.9%	778.06	23.6%
Greater than 64	298	2,816	2,190.91	100.0%	1,431.09	65.3%	311.49	14.2%	448.33	20.5%
Gender[2]										
Female	289	3,367	2,149.91	100.0%	1,282.05	59.6%	341.70	15.9%	526.16	24.5%
Male	295	3,617	2,082.48	100.0%	1,162.35	55.8%	360.57	17.3%	559.56	26.9%
Region										
Midwest	240	2,653	2,471.90	100.0%	1,485.45	60.1%	424.76	17.2%	561.69	22.7%
Northeast	41	342	2,240.14	100.0%	1,348.44	60.2%	391.31	17.5%	500.39	22.3%
South	610	7,112	2,140.51	100.0%	1,166.50	54.5%	373.68	17.5%	600.33	28.0%
Southwest	107	1,064	1,675.80	100.0%	1,026.85	61.3%	308.40	18.4%	340.56	20.3%
West	230	2,412	3,582.08	100.0%	2,447.14	68.3%	488.75	13.6%	646.19	18.0%
Insurance type[3]										
Managed care	622	6,874	2,936.17	100.0%	1,783.86	60.8%	504.22	17.2%	648.10	22.1%
Medicare	283	2,763	1,879.52	100.0%	1,182.80	62.9%	271.84	14.5%	424.88	22.6%
Medicare HMO	24	251	1,543.22	100.0%	880.70	57.1%	241.51	15.6%	421.01	27.3%
Medicaid	67	787	859.31	100.0%	344.74	40.1%	91.61	10.7%	422.96	49.2%
Medicaid HMO	10	145	709.35	100.0%	334.71	47.2%	185.94	26.2%	188.70	26.6%
Indemnity	68	1,036	2,199.25	100.0%	1,359.22	61.8%	371.24	16.9%	468.80	21.3%
Other[4]	154	1,727	2,402.50	100.0%	1,281.98	53.4%	384.41	16.0%	736.11	30.6%
IV drug (for mSTS)[5]										
Gemcitabine-based	429	3,315	3,302.95	100.0%	2,447.16	74.1%	358.70	10.9%	497.09	15.0%
Anthracycline-based	434	2,005	2,344.63	100.0%	1,024.02	43.7%	479.23	20.4%	841.38	35.9%
Alkylating-agents-based	424	3,772	1,469.59	100.0%	474.53	32.3%	433.81	29.5%	561.25	38.2%
Angiogenesis inhibitors	58	374	5,249.94	100.0%	4,291.45	81.7%	301.03	5.7%	657.47	12.5%
Taxane-based	172	1,123	2,184.18	100.0%	1,323.34	60.6%	409.22	18.7%	451.62	20.7%
Other	352	2,994	2,458.42	100.0%	1,552.03	63.1%	356.33	14.5%	550.06	22.4%
Number of administered IV drugs[6]										
One	998	8,016	1,855.27	100.0%	1,007.91	54.3%	304.23	16.4%	543.13	29.3%
Two	680	4,336	3,423.98	100.0%	2,348.01	68.6%	481.76	14.1%	594.21	17.4%
Three	161	1,049	2,515.14	100.0%	1,058.61	42.1%	693.36	27.6%	763.17	30.3%
Four	47	182	3,372.39	100.0%	1,771.78	52.5%	935.96	27.8%	664.65	19.7%

(b) Continued.

Category	No. of patients	No. of months	Total Average costs ($)	%	IV drug Average costs ($)	%	IV administration Average costs ($)	%	Other visit-related services Average costs ($)	%
Total	**1,228**	**6,025.0**	**5,467.61**	**100.0%**	**3,268.45**	**59.8%**	**899.57**	**16.5%**	**1,299.60**	**23.8%**
Age										
Less than 25	117	623.3	3,476.65	100.0%	1,442.50	41.5%	978.12	28.1%	1,056.03	30.4%
25 to 39	152	836.2	5,338.35	100.0%	3,054.94	57.2%	1,070.62	20.1%	1,212.80	22.7%
40 to 54	316	1,513.3	6,030.91	100.0%	3,511.16	58.2%	997.38	16.5%	1,522.37	25.2%
55 to 64	345	1,650.8	6,686.45	100.0%	4,181.94	62.5%	928.28	13.9%	1,576.23	23.6%
Greater than 64	298	1,401.4	4,386.23	100.0%	2,869.85	65.4%	623.09	14.2%	893.29	20.4%
Gender[2]										
Female	289	1,588.8	4,544.31	100.0%	2,712.88	59.7%	721.32	15.9%	1,110.11	24.4%
Male	295	1,563.7	4,819.57	100.0%	2,689.15	55.8%	835.49	17.3%	1,294.93	26.9%
Region										
Midwest	240	1,040.6	6,289.83	100.0%	3,784.40	60.2%	1,079.88	17.2%	1,425.55	22.7%
Northeast	41	207.8	3,687.44	100.0%	2,219.64	60.2%	644.12	17.5%	823.67	22.3%
South	610	3,200.9	4,753.24	100.0%	2,590.95	54.5%	830.59	17.5%	1,331.70	28.0%
Southwest	107	434.6	4,106.94	100.0%	2,531.00	61.6%	754.76	18.4%	821.18	20.0%
West	230	1,141.2	7,563.95	100.0%	5,170.11	68.4%	1,030.27	13.6%	1,363.58	18.0%
Insurance type[3]										
Managed care	622	3,088.9	6,532.36	100.0%	3,971.37	60.8%	1,120.58	17.2%	1,440.41	22.1%
Medicare	283	1,374.0	3,764.41	100.0%	2,374.73	63.1%	544.94	14.5%	844.73	22.4%
Medicare HMO	24	113.4	3,415.78	100.0%	1,949.36	57.1%	534.56	15.6%	931.86	27.3%
Medicaid	67	375.7	1,804.71	100.0%	722.61	40.0%	196.05	10.9%	886.05	49.1%
Medicaid HMO	10	37.9	2,716.27	100.0%	1,281.66	47.2%	712.02	26.2%	722.59	26.6%
Indemnity	68	365.1	6,232.59	100.0%	3,853.04	61.8%	1,051.79	16.9%	1,327.76	21.3%
Other[4]	154	670.0	6,191.80	100.0%	3,305.31	53.4%	991.86	16.0%	1,894.63	30.6%
IV drug (for mSTS)										
Gemcitabine-based	429	1,577.9	7,021.77	100.0%	5,208.74	74.2%	761.17	10.8%	1,051.86	15.0%
Anthracycline-based	434	1,243.0	3,752.46	100.0%	1,629.15	43.4%	768.24	20.5%	1,355.07	36.1%
Alkylating-agents-based	424	1,221.5	4,753.73	100.0%	1,559.65	32.8%	1,365.87	28.7%	1,828.21	38.5%
Angiogenesis inhibitors	58	321.6	7,532.36	100.0%	6,191.35	82.2%	460.33	6.1%	880.67	11.7%
Taxane-based	172	575.0	4,253.79	100.0%	2,563.94	60.3%	802.76	18.9%	887.08	20.9%
Other[5]	352	1,086.0	6,006.84	100.0%	3,755.13	62.5%	907.76	15.1%	1,343.95	22.4%

(b) Continued.

Category	No. of patients	No. of months	Total		IV drug		IV administration		Other visit-related services	
			Average costs ($)	%	Average costs ($)	%	Average costs ($)	%	Average costs ($)	%
Number of administered IV drugs[6]										
One	998	2,492.2	3,950.35	100.0%	2,105.69	53.3%	610.28	15.4%	1,234.38	31.2%
Two	680	2,781.1	6,616.14	100.0%	4,463.78	67.5%	954.84	14.4%	1,197.52	18.1%
Three	161	514.1	6,725.12	100.0%	2,888.23	42.9%	1,631.79	24.3%	2,205.10	32.8%
Four	47	237.6	5,218.13	100.0%	2,296.07	44.0%	1,702.72	32.6%	1,219.34	23.4%

1: Treatment costs derived from the contracted allowed payment for a claim.
2: 644 patients were missing gender information.
3: Insurance type is defined at the time of the index mSTS diagnosis.
4: Other includes workers' compensation, Tricare, and self-pay.
5: Gemcitabine-based includes gemcitabine monotherapy and combination therapies. Anthracycline-based includes doxorubicin and epirubicin monotherapies and combination therapies. Alkylating-agents-based includes monotherapies and combination therapies with cisplatin, cyclophosphamide, dacarbazine, etoposide, ifosfamide, temozolomide, and topotecan. Angiogenesis inhibitors include bevacizumab monotherapy. Taxane-based includes docetaxel and paclitaxel monotherapies and combination therapies. Other includes actinomycin D, carboplatin, irinotecan, interferon, oxaliplatin, vincristine, and vinorelbine.
6: Number of mSTS treatments that were administered during the visit.

TABLE 4: (a) Cost categories breakdown per patient per visit (PPPV) by demographic characteristics, IV drug, and number of drugs administered per visit: sensitivity analyses using alternative definition of mSTS diagnosis[1]. (b) Cost categories breakdown per patient per visit (PPPV) by demographic characteristics, IV drug, and number of drugs administered per visit: sensitivity analyses excluding visits with administration costs in the top 1%[1].

(a)

Category	No. of patients	No. of visits	Total		IV drug		IV administration		Other visit-related services	
			Average costs ($)	%	Average costs ($)	%	Average costs ($)	%	Average costs ($)	%
Total	**1,023**	**11,777**	**2,293.60**	**100.0%**	**1,334.09**	**58.2%**	**392.81**	**17.1%**	**566.71**	**24.7%**
Age										
Less than 25	112	1,872	1,067.78	100.0%	435.96	40.8%	304.44	28.5%	327.38	30.7%
25 to 39	138	1,897	2,077.10	100.0%	1,153.72	55.5%	439.82	21.2%	483.56	23.3%
40 to 54	266	2,999	2,569.69	100.0%	1,486.01	57.8%	442.27	17.2%	641.41	25.0%
55 to 64	282	2,833	3,159.29	100.0%	1,941.58	61.5%	438.70	13.9%	779.01	24.7%
Greater than 64	225	2,176	2,029.35	100.0%	1,263.70	62.3%	299.93	14.8%	465.72	22.9%
Gender[2]										
Female	234	2,882	1,971.97	100.0%	1,135.12	57.6%	332.27	16.8%	504.58	25.6%
Male	234	3,156	1,856.48	100.0%	970.27	52.3%	347.30	18.7%	538.91	29.0%
Region										
Midwest	189	2,235	2,206.58	100.0%	1,292.76	58.6%	423.45	19.2%	490.38	22.2%
Northeast	19	199	2,733.61	100.0%	1,665.07	60.9%	367.43	13.4%	701.11	25.6%
South	513	6,204	2,001.71	100.0%	1,021.93	51.1%	367.81	18.4%	611.97	30.6%
Southwest	95	985	1,620.03	100.0%	1,021.50	63.1%	308.51	19.0%	290.02	17.9%
West	207	2,154	3,491.98	100.0%	2,388.44	68.4%	473.90	13.6%	629.64	18.0%
Insurance type[3]										
Managed care	530	6,076	2,773.41	100.0%	1,646.46	59.4%	492.05	17.7%	634.91	22.9%
Medicare	217	2,200	1,756.68	100.0%	1,073.70	61.1%	271.13	15.4%	411.86	23.4%
Medicare HMO	19	181	1,808.04	100.0%	959.11	53.0%	274.88	15.2%	574.05	31.7%
Medicaid	61	756	814.99	100.0%	282.49	34.7%	93.08	11.4%	439.42	53.9%
Medicaid HMO	9	141	614.82	100.0%	233.36	38.0%	187.46	30.5%	193.99	31.6%
Indemnity	55	881	2,003.24	100.0%	1,200.97	60.0%	373.60	18.6%	428.67	21.4%
Other[4]	132	1,542	2,270.35	100.0%	1,211.04	53.3%	365.92	16.1%	693.39	30.5%
IV drug (for mSTS)[5]										
Gemcitabine-based	374	2,926	3,438.08	100.0%	2,551.62	74.2%	366.02	10.6%	520.44	15.1%
Anthracycline-based	406	1,904	2,304.97	100.0%	1,006.55	43.7%	483.34	21.0%	815.08	35.4%
Alkylating-agents-based	383	3,416	1,494.70	100.0%	498.44	33.3%	430.76	28.8%	565.51	37.8%
Angiogenesis inhibitors	33	250	5,499.09	100.0%	4,413.94	80.3%	276.56	5.0%	808.59	14.7%
Taxane-based	141	945	2,280.97	100.0%	1,371.47	60.1%	416.92	18.3%	492.59	21.6%
Other	260	2,336	1,681.11	100.0%	953.29	56.7%	299.76	17.8%	428.06	25.5%

(a) Continued.

Category	No. of patients	No. of visits	Total Average costs ($)	Total %	IV drug Average costs ($)	IV drug %	IV administration Average costs ($)	IV administration %	Other visit-related services Average costs ($)	Other visit-related services %
Number of administered IV drugs[6]										
One	831	6,874	1,717.75	100.0%	890.29	51.8%	295.14	17.2%	532.32	31.0%
Two	581	3,779	3,245.44	100.0%	2,178.48	67.1%	467.91	14.4%	599.05	18.5%
Three	148	963	2,449.85	100.0%	1,097.77	44.8%	696.15	28.4%	655.92	26.8%
Four	44	161	3,603.77	100.0%	1,876.43	52.1%	985.49	27.3%	741.85	20.6%

1: mSTS diagnosis defined as at least two medical claims with an ICD-9-CM diagnosis code of 171 and at least one medical claims with a diagnosis of a distant secondary malignant neoplasm (ICD-9-CM 196.XX-199.0). Treatment costs derived from the contracted allowed payment for a claim.

2: 644 patients were missing gender information.

3: Insurance type is defined at the time of the index mSTS diagnosis.

4: Other includes workers' compensation, Tricare, and self-pay.

5: Gemcitabine-based includes gemcitabine monotherapy and combination therapies. Anthracycline-based includes doxorubicin and epirubicin monotherapies and combination therapies. Alkylating-agents-based includes monotherapies and combination therapies with cisplatin, cyclophosphamide, dacarbazine, etoposide, ifosfamide, temozolomide, and topotecan. Angiogenesis inhibitors include bevacizumab monotherapy. Taxane-based includes docetaxel and paclitaxel monotherapies and combination therapies. Other includes actinomycin D, carboplatin, irinotecan, interferon, oxaliplatin, vincristine, and vinorelbine.

6: Number of mSTS treatments that were administered during the visit.

(b)

Category	No. of patients	No. of visits	Total Average costs ($)	Total %	IV drug Average costs ($)	IV drug %	IV administration Average costs ($)	IV administration %	Other visit-related services Average costs ($)	Other visit-related services %
Total	**1,221**	**13,325**	**2,363.53**	**100.0%**	**1,417.87**	**60.0%**	**376.94**	**15.9%**	**568.72**	**24.1%**
Age										
Less than 25	116	1,934	1,104.42	100.0%	459.15	41.6%	307.88	27.9%	337.38	30.5%
25 to 39	151	1,953	2,170.22	100.0%	1,251.49	57.7%	423.35	19.5%	495.38	22.8%
40 to 54	313	3,377	2,565.44	100.0%	1,521.19	59.3%	402.53	15.7%	641.72	25.0%
55 to 64	344	3,274	3,227.77	100.0%	2,021.82	62.6%	429.45	13.3%	776.50	24.1%
Greater than 64	297	2,787	2,112.86	100.0%	1,365.08	64.6%	299.66	14.2%	448.12	21.2%
Gender[2]										
Female	289	3,352	2,143.16	100.0%	1,278.43	59.7%	337.16	15.7%	527.57	24.6%
Male	295	3,604	2,073.06	100.0%	1,158.90	55.9%	357.01	17.2%	557.15	26.9%
Region										
Midwest	240	2,636	2,454.05	100.0%	1,478.01	60.2%	417.56	17.0%	558.48	22.8%
Northeast	41	339	2,242.53	100.0%	1,357.27	60.5%	383.64	17.1%	501.61	22.4%
South	604	6,969	2,084.97	100.0%	1,150.36	55.2%	347.76	16.7%	586.85	28.1%
Southwest	107	1,062	1,669.85	100.0%	1,023.82	61.3%	306.28	18.3%	339.75	20.3%
West	229	2,319	3,433.15	100.0%	2,342.75	68.2%	449.85	13.1%	640.56	18.7%
Insurance type[3]										
Managed care	615	6,647	2,838.48	100.0%	1,737.24	61.2%	468.51	16.5%	632.73	22.3%
Medicare	283	2,759	1,875.14	100.0%	1,180.06	62.9%	270.15	14.4%	424.93	22.7%
Medicare HMO	24	251	1,543.22	100.0%	880.70	57.1%	241.51	15.6%	421.01	27.3%
Medicaid	67	787	859.31	100.0%	344.74	40.1%	91.61	10.7%	422.96	49.2%
Medicaid HMO	10	145	709.35	100.0%	334.71	47.2%	185.94	26.2%	188.70	26.6%
Indemnity	68	1,036	2,199.25	100.0%	1,359.22	61.8%	371.24	16.9%	468.80	21.3%
Other[4]	154	1,700	2,357.83	100.0%	1,259.37	53.4%	364.05	15.4%	734.42	31.1%

(b) Continued.

Category	No. of patients	No. of visits	Total Average costs ($)	Total %	IV drug Average costs ($)	IV drug %	IV administration Average costs ($)	IV administration %	Other visit-related services Average costs ($)	Other visit-related services %
IV drug (for mSTS)[5]										
Gemcitabine-based	429	3,305	3,290.15	100.0%	2,439.82	74.2%	354.74	10.8%	495.59	15.1%
Anthracycline-based	423	1,925	2,275.39	100.0%	1,022.92	45.0%	432.97	19.0%	819.50	36.0%
Alkylating-agents-based	419	3,686	1,396.09	100.0%	441.77	31.6%	405.93	29.1%	548.39	39.3%
Angiogenesis inhibitors	58	367	5,217.74	100.0%	4,275.64	81.9%	281.20	5.4%	660.90	12.7%
Taxane-based	172	1,106	2,141.45	100.0%	1,300.21	60.7%	392.87	18.3%	448.37	20.9%
Other	348	2,936	2,319.72	100.0%	1,439.00	62.0%	334.77	14.4%	545.96	23.5%
Number of administered IV drugs[6]										
One	997	7,994	1,842.21	100.0%	998.14	54.2%	300.77	16.3%	543.30	29.5%
Two	670	4,229	3,333.67	100.0%	2,291.94	68.8%	456.61	13.7%	585.11	17.6%
Three	156	966	2,353.14	100.0%	1,023.01	43.5%	613.09	26.1%	717.04	30.5%
Four	39	136	2,913.93	100.0%	1,714.22	58.8%	699.57	24.0%	500.14	17.2%

1: Treatment costs derived from the contracted allowed payment for a claim.
2: 644 patients were missing gender information.
3: Insurance type is defined at the time of the index mSTS diagnosis.
4: Other includes workers' compensation, Tricare, and self-pay.
5: Gemcitabine-based includes gemcitabine monotherapy and combination therapies. Anthracycline-based includes doxorubicin and epirubicin monotherapies and combination therapies. Alkylating-agents-based includes monotherapies and combination therapies with cisplatin, cyclophosphamide, dacarbazine, etoposide, ifosfamide, temozolomide, and topotecan. Angiogenesis inhibitors include bevacizumab monotherapy. Taxane-based includes docetaxel and paclitaxel monotherapies and combination therapies. Other includes actinomycin D, carboplatin, irinotecan, interferon, oxaliplatin, vincristine, and vinorelbine.
6: Number of mSTS treatments that were administered during the visit.

3.3. Sensitivity Analyses. Tables 4(a) and 4(b) report the results of two sensitivity analyses undertaken to assess the extent of any potential biases in the results arising from patient selection and outliers. In Table 4(a), total and subdivided PPPV costs were based on an alternative definition of mSTS diagnosis in which patients were only required to have at least two medical claims with an ICD-9-CM diagnosis code of 171. IV administration costs were generally similar and in fact represented a slightly larger percentage of total IV visit costs (17.1%), compared to those based on the primary definition of mSTS diagnosis presented in Table 3(a).

In Table 4(b), total and subdivided PPPV costs are reported after excluding visits with administration costs in the top 1%. Again, results were generally similar to those based on all IV administration visits, presented in Table 3(a). In particular, IV administration costs represented 15.9% of total IV visit costs.

4. Discussion

This retrospective analysis assessed costs associated with the administration of IV cancer therapies in mSTS patients from 2005 to 2012 using Experian data. IV administration costs accounted for about 16.5% of costs per IV visit among patients with mSTS. Other visit-related service costs accounted for about 23.8% of the cost PPPV. These results indicate that non-IV drug costs represent a considerable proportion of the total costs when receiving an IV cancer therapy to treat mSTS.

Cost estimates stratified by patient characteristics indicate that some of the largest differences in IV administration costs across patients exist between patients with different types of insurance. Patients with managed care had the highest IV administration costs ($504 PPPV), while Medicaid patients had the lowest ($92 PPPV). IV administration costs also varied widely across regions, as well as by the type of IV cancer drug and number of IV cancer drugs administered.

The share of total treatment costs related to IV administration reported in this study of mSTS patients is similar to estimates reported in both malignant and nonmalignant diseases where drugs are administered by IV infusion. A 2008 study of treatment costs in patients with metastatic breast cancer reported average total treatment costs of $2,477 PPPV, 10.2% of which were IV administration costs [9]. In a separate 2008 study of patients with small cell lung cancer, IV administration costs were estimated to be 11.8% of average total costs [8]. Finally, in a 2011 study of costs in rheumatoid arthritis patients, IV administration costs were 7.9% of average total costs [10].

This study did not account for indirect costs, such as those associated with patient and caregiver time (e.g., travel time) and lost productivity, which by their nature are more difficult to collect and suffer from greater variability. By only examining direct healthcare-system-related costs of IV cancer therapy administration in an mSTS sample, this study likely understates the true total cost of IV therapy to society.

As with all retrospective studies using claims data, identification of mSTS patients relies on the accuracy of diagnosis coding. No clinical information was available to ascertain stage. Advanced STS was identified based on a claims algorithm that has not been validated. To address this concern, a sensitivity analysis was performed where costs were calculated using an alternative claims algorithm. Results of this sensitivity analysis were similar to those reported here. In addition, costs related to IV cancer therapy administration were determined only from clinic claims and were limited to services identified on the claim as an infusion administration cost. This method may underestimate true medical infusion costs since it does not capture costs related to late infusion reactions and complications that require medical care on days following the infusion. Clinic claims also exclude any additional costs of oral drugs or drugs administered in an inpatient setting.

Other study limitations included limited information about patient enrollment and disease progression. Patients appear in the dataset through clinic visits, but the date of initial diagnosis of mSTS may have occurred earlier. In addition, it was not possible to determine why patients may have stopped visiting the clinic. It was also not possible to assess disease progression. To address these limitations, costs were estimated on the basis of actual clinic visits and reported both PPPV and PPPM.

5. Conclusion

Using data from the Experian database, this study found that the mean cost of receiving IV cancer therapy in an mSTS patient population was $2,427 PPPV and $5,468 PPPM. IV administration costs accounted for 16.5% of these costs and other visit-related services accounted for 23.8% of these costs. Thus, nonstudy drug related costs are about 40% of the costs associated with administration of IV cancer therapy for mSTS patients. There was substantial variation in the cost of IV administration by insurance type, region, type of anticancer drug, and the number of anticancer drugs administered in a single visit.

This study contributes to the understanding of IV therapy administration costs in mSTS patients. Further research is needed to investigate the association between IV administration costs and mSTS cancer stage and to estimate indirect costs of IV administration associated with mSTS patient and caregiver time.

Acknowledgments

Research support was provided to Analysis Group, Inc., and Bruce Wong and Associates, Inc., by GlaxoSmithKline (GSK). Mei Sheng Duh, Jasmina I. Ivanova, Patrick Lefebvre, and Paul Karner are employees of Analysis Group, Inc. Bruce Wong is an employee of Bruce Wong and Associates, Inc. Gregory Kruse is a doctoral student at The Wharton School, University of Pennsylvania. Michelle D. Hackshaw and Lesley-Ann N. Miller are employees of and own stock in GSK. None of the authors have a direct financial interest in SAS Institute, Inc.

References

[1] Mayo Clinic, "Soft tissue sarcoma: definition," January 2012, http://www.mayoclinic.com/health/soft-tissue-sarcoma/DS00601.

[2] C. Fletcher, K. Unni, and F. Mertens, *Pathology and Genetics of Tumors of Soft Tissue and Bone*, International Agency for Research on Cancer Press, Lyon, France, 2002.

[3] R. Siegel, D. Naishadham, and A. Jemal, "Cancer statistics, 2012," *CA: Cancer Journal for Clinicians*, vol. 62, no. 1, pp. 10–29, 2012.

[4] R. J. Canter, S. Beal, D. Borys, S. R. Martinez, R. J. Bold, and A. S. Robbins, "Interaction of histologic subtype and histologic grade in predicting survival for soft-tissue sarcomas," *Journal of the American College of Surgeons*, vol. 210, no. 2, pp. 191.e2–198.e2, 2010.

[5] N. Penel, M. van Glabbeke, S. Marreaud, M. Ouali, J. Y. Blay, and P. Hohenberger, "Testing new regimens in patients with advanced soft tissue sarcoma: analysis of publications from the last 10 years," *Annals of Oncology*, vol. 22, no. 6, pp. 1266–1272, 2011.

[6] J.-Y. Blay, M. van Glabbeke, J. Verweij et al., "Advanced soft-tissue sarcoma: a disease that is potentially curable for a subset of patients treated with chemotherapy," *European Journal of Cancer*, vol. 39, no. 1, pp. 64–69, 2003.

[7] National Comprehensive Care Network, "NCCN clinical practice guidelines in onclogy: soft tissue sarcoma," June 2012, http://www.nccn.org/professionals/physician_gls/pdf/sarcoma.pdf.

[8] M. S. Duh, J. R. Weiner, P. Lefebvre, M. Neary, and A. T. Skarin, "Costs associated with intravenous chemotherapy administration in patients with small cell lung cancer: a retrospective claims database analysis," *Current Medical Research and Opinion*, vol. 24, no. 4, pp. 967–974, 2008.

[9] G. B. Kruse, M. M. Amonkar, G. Smith, D. C. Skonieczny, and S. Stavrakas, "Analysis of costs associated with administration of intravenous single-drug therapies in metastatic breast cancer in a U.S. population," *Journal of Managed Care Pharmacy*, vol. 14, no. 9, pp. 844–857, 2008.

[10] B. J. Wong, M. A. Cifaldi, S. Roy, D. C. Skonieczny, and S. Stavrakas, "Analysis of drug and administrative costs allowed by U.S. Private and public third-party payers for 3 intravenous biologic agents for rheumatoid arthritis," *Journal of Managed Care Pharmacy*, vol. 17, no. 4, pp. 313–320, 2011.

[11] J. E. Butrynski, M. S. Duh, A. A. Fournier et al., "Soft tissue sarcoma (STS): challenges identification, treatment patterns, and cost of disease management in the U.S.," *Journal of Clinical Oncology*, vol. 26, no. 15, ASCO Annual Meeting Proceedings, Chicago, Ill, USA, Abstract 10573, 2008.

[12] Bureau of Labor Statistics, "U.S. medical care services," http://data.bls.gov.

10

Long-Term Clinical Responses of Neoadjuvant Dendritic Cell Infusions and Radiation in Soft Tissue Sarcoma

Shailaja Raj,[1] Marilyn M. Bui,[1] Gregory Springett,[1] Anthony Conley,[2] Sergio Lavilla-Alonso,[3] Xiuhua Zhao,[1] Dungsa Chen,[1] Randy Haysek,[1] Ricardo Gonzalez,[1] G. Douglas Letson,[1] Steven Eric Finkelstein,[4] Alberto A. Chiappori,[1] Dmitry I. Gabrilovitch,[3] and Scott J. Antonia[1]

[1]*H. Lee. Moffitt Cancer Center, Tampa, FL 33612, USA*
[2]*MD Anderson Cancer Institute, Houston, TX 77030, USA*
[3]*The Wistar Institute, Philadelphia, PA 19104, USA*
[4]*21st Century Oncology, Scottsdale, AZ 85251, USA*

Correspondence should be addressed to Shailaja Raj; skrimuno@gmail.com

Academic Editor: Ajay Puri

Purpose. Patients with large >5 cm, high-grade resectable soft tissue sarcomas (STS) have the highest risk of distant metastases. Previously we have shown that dendritic cell (DC) based vaccines show consistent immune responses. *Methods.* This was a Phase I single institution study of neoadjuvant radiation with DC injections on 18 newly diagnosed high-risk STS patients. Neoadjuvant treatment consisted of 50 Gy of external beam radiation (EBRT), given in 25 fractions delivered five days/week, combined with four intratumoral injections of DCs followed by complete resection. The primary endpoint was to establish the immunological response to neoadjuvant therapy and obtain data on its clinical safety and outcomes. *Results.* There were no unexpected toxicities or serious adverse events. Twelve out of 18 (67%) patients were alive, of which an encouraging 11/18 (61%) were alive with no systemic recurrence over a period of 2–8 years. Favorable immunological responses correlated with clinical responses in some cases. *Conclusions.* This study provides clinical support to using dendritic cell injections along with radiation in sarcomas, which when used optimally in combination can help clinical outcomes in soft tissue sarcoma. Study registration number is NCT00365872.

1. Introduction

Although sarcomas are relatively rare neoplasms, more than 8,000 new cases of soft tissue sarcomas (STS) occur in the United States every year, making this disease a significant health problem affecting all age groups [1]. Despite appropriate curative therapies, patients with localized high-grade STS larger than 5 cm remain at significant risk of treatment failure and death from metastatic disease, with prognosis becoming ever more dismal with increased tumor size and higher grade [2–5].

Multimodality therapy, including radiation and at times systemic chemotherapy, in properly selected patients, can improve local control rate, decrease the morbidity associated with surgery and increase the duration of relapse-free survival [3–5]. Coindre et al. found that high-grade tumors had a metastasis-free survival rate of 44% [6] Earlier on, a meta-analysis of 14 trials comprising 1,568 patients, with localized resectable extremity and nonextremity primary STS [7], showed that the overall survival was not improved significantly by the use of chemotherapy. There was a trend towards improved survival with an absolute potential benefit of 4%, which translated to an overall survival improvement from 50% to 54%. An Italian Study showed that adjuvant chemotherapy in high-grade, over 5 cm, soft tissue sarcomas had a disease-free survival of 48 months with use of epidoxorubicin and ifosfamide [8]. This demonstrated a 41% relative reduction in the risk of disease relapse, translating to an absolute benefit of 27% from chemotherapy at two years and 13% at four years.

One potential approach to decrease the risk of recurrence in large, high-grade, soft tissue sarcomas is immunotherapy using vaccines. Vaccines can deliver tumor-associated immunogenic factors (antigens) that provide a Trojan horse effect [9]. The use of dendritic cells holds promise for sarcoma patients who are often resistant to chemotherapy. Intratumoral injection of dendritic cells is one of the methods that can utilize a large number of antigens from tumors without the need for their selection based on HLA typing or expression. Manipulation of the tumor microenvironment by ionizing radiation is also an important contributing factor in addition to the antitumor effects caused by the dendritic cells. Radiation therapy on its own can induce an immune response; for example, external beam radiotherapy can trigger signals that stimulate Toll-like receptor four on DCs [10, 11]. Radiation also has a direct effect on tumors by rendering them more susceptible to vaccine-mediated T-cell killing or releasing cytokines and inflammatory proteins. Finally, it can alter the tumor microenvironment to promote greater infiltration of immune effector cells [12–14].

We tested the hypothesis that the combination of dendritic cell vaccine and radiation would augment immune and antitumor responses in a preclinical murine model. This was done using dendritic cell administration in two well-characterized mouse tumor models, MethA sarcoma and C3 tumor, which carry defined MHC class I-restricted tumor-specific antigens. The study first found that the number of labeled dendritic cells trafficking to the tumors dramatically increased if the tumor was irradiated before subcutaneous administration of the dendritic cells. Next, it showed that when dendritic cell vaccination and radiation were combined in the MethA sarcoma mouse group, by day 14, 10 of 12 mice rejected their tumors completely. In the C3 tumor model, the combination resulted in significantly reduced tumor growth, with 4 of 10 mice rejecting their tumors and the remainder showing slowed tumor growth [15]. Other preclinical studies have also shown that combining local tumor irradiation with intratumoral DC administration resulted in potent antitumor immune responses that translated into an antitumor effect [16]. Immune escape has been demonstrated both in GIST [17] and Ewing's sarcoma [18, 19].

We then sought to translate these preclinical findings into a Phase I trial, to focus on the feasibility, safety, and immunological responses of dendritic cell vaccine with radiation followed by surgery. The primary endpoint was immunological responses that have been previously reported. Here, our primary aim is to provide an update of the long-term clinical results of this neoadjuvant trial that treated newly diagnosed, high-risk soft tissue sarcoma patients with a combination of DC injections and radiation. Our second aim is to compare immune responses to the clinical responses to DC injections with radiation combined in the treatment of high-grade sof t tissue sarcomas over 5 cm in size.

2. Methods

2.1. Patient Selection. Patients over age 18 with histologically confirmed > 5 cm intermediate or high-grade STS of the extremity/trunk/chest wall were eligible for enrollment. Patients were required to have a World Health Organization (WHO) performance status of 0 or 1, no exposure to steroids in the first four weeks, adequate organ function, no coagulation disorders, and no contraindication to resection. A radiation oncologist had to confirm that each patient had a 2-3 cm strip of skin that could be spared from radiation before the start of treatment. Patients with severe allergic reactions, GIST, retroperitoneal sarcomas, metastatic disease and chronic intercurrent illness, prior radiation therapy, severe immunosuppressive disease or HIV, or previous autoimmune disease were all excluded. All patients were clinically confirmed Stage III, with a significant risk of progressing to distant metastases.

2.2. Preparation and Administration of DCs. Expanded autologous DC can be routinely obtained from mononuclear cell fraction progenitors obtained from individuals using leukapheresis, followed by *ex vivo* expansion with standardized protocols [20]. DCs collected in this manner are HLA-matched (autologous) and are competent to take up tumor-derived apoptotic bodies and present tumor antigens to lymphocytes. DCs (10^7 cells) with a phenotype lineage (CD3, CD14, CD19, CD20, and CD56) negative and HLA-DR positive were injected in a total volume of 1 mL.

2.3. Evaluation of DC Migration. DCs labeled with ^{111}In and 5×10^6 cells were injected intratumorally before surgery. DC labeling and imaging were published previously [12].

2.4. Study Design and Treatment. We had enrolled eighteen patients at Moffitt Cancer Center, who were analyzed for clinical and immunological outcomes. They were required to provide written informed consent to a University of South Florida Institutional Review Board that previously approved the protocol.

Patients were treated with external beam radiation (EBRT) 50 Gy in 25 equal fractions, delivered five days per week (Monday–Friday), combined with 10^7 dendritic cells in a total volume of 1 mL, and injected intratumorally, three times on the second, third, and fourth Fridays during the radiation. One additional DC injection was given several days before surgery. Surgical resection of tumors occurred 3–6 weeks after completion of radiation.

2.5. Coordinating Radiation Therapy and Dendritic Cell Injections. To maximize the immunological response, the radiation therapy was coordinated to ensure that adequate apoptosis (forming apoptotic bodies for uptake into DCs with subsequent tumor antigen presentation) was ongoing within the soft tissue sarcoma at the time of intratumoral dendritic cell injection. No studies of serial sarcoma tumor biopsies after external-beam radiation to establish the time course of apoptosis have been published to our knowledge. In our protocol, dendritic cell injections were given after 18, 27, 36, and 50.40 Gy of radiation. Dendritic cells were injected on Friday morning after completing the radiation fraction for that day as this ensured that there was a period of 48 hours before the next radiation treatment, thus minimizing the risk of inactivation of DCs.

2.6. Evaluation of Immune Responses. Survivin is an anti-apoptotic protein that preferentially blocks mitochondrial-dependent apoptosis by targeting caspase 9 [20, 21]. Overexpression of this protein has been documented in many tumors including soft tissue sarcomas. Survivin-specific immune responses in healthy individuals and prostate-cancer patients have been measured by our group previously [20]. We planned to evaluate the survivin-specific responses in this trial. For this, peripheral blood mononuclear cells (PBMC), tumor cells harvested through core biopsies, and tumor cell lysates (TCL) prepared by repeated snap freeze-thawing cycles were stored in liquid nitrogen, as described [22]. Two sources of tumor-associated antigens (TAAs) were used to evaluate comparatively the immune response in patients: whole tumor cell lysate (TCL) and survivin. T-cell responses to TCL were assessed using IFN-γ ELISPOT [23] and proliferation assays. To evaluate T-cell response to survivin, DCs were infected with adenovirus-survivin (Ad-surv), as described previously, to serve as stimulator cells [23].

The immune response of an individual patient was considered to be positive if 2 criteria were met: first, if at any time point the response in the IFN-γ ELISPOT assay was higher than 30 spots per 2×10^5 cells or if the 3[H]-thymidine counts in the proliferation assay were greater than 3000 CPM; second, when the response in the IFN-γ ELISPOT assay or proliferation assay was greater than two standard deviations than the control lysate at the same time point and two standard deviations greater than the response at baseline before the start of treatment.

2.7. Statistical Analysis. We used GraphPad Prism Software 6 for statistical analysis. Univariate Chi-square tests were used to test differences in demographics or clinical characteristics; Kaplan-Meier and log-rank tests were employed for determining survival outcomes.

3. Results

3.1. Study Characteristics. From May 2007 to January 2009, we enrolled a total of 18 patients (ClinicalTrials.gov identifier NCT00365872). The demographics and patient characteristics are described in Table 1. The median age group was 20–80 years with 77% male and 23% female.

3.2. Safety. The overall toxicities are summarized in Table 2. With the four doses of dendritic cell injections, we recorded injection site reactions, fatigue, nausea, pain, and constipation. There were no grades 4 or 5 toxicities and hepatic or renal events and no treatment-related deaths observed. Additionally no unexpected serious adverse reactions including autoimmune events were reported. Overall the intratumoral method of dendritic cell injections was well tolerated and together with radiation was a feasible mode of treatment.

TABLE 1: Demographics and clinical characteristics of patients enrolled on combined treatment of neoadjuvant radiation and dendritic cell injections.

Demographics	Phase I
Age	
<61	10
>61	8
Gender	
Female	4
Male	14
Primary site	
Upper extremity	7
Lower extremity	11
Histology	
Epithelioid sarcomas	2
Sarcomas with myxoid features	2
Pleomorphic sarcomas	10
Others	4
Stage	
T2N0M0 Stage IIB	1
T2NxM0 G3 Stage III	17

3.3. Clinical Outcomes. Clinical follow-up was available for all individuals for a minimum period of twenty-four months after primary DC immunization and those who were alive, to over eight years. Amongst the eighteen vaccinated patients twelve (67%) remain alive with no disease recurrence. Eight patients (45%) are alive between 6 and nine years and three over four years, while one patient was lost to follow-up after three years. Interestingly one patient, who progressed with lung metastases in 2 years, remains alive for eight years, being treated on other protocols. The remaining six (33%) died of progressive metastatic disease to the lung between seven months and three years after treatment.

The disease-free survival at two years is 83% and at four years is 67%. The log-rank tests for trend showed a significant trend at $p = 0.04$, whereas, by Gehan-Wilcoxon test, the results were not statistically significant. The median survival was 57 months.

Of the 18 eligible patients, 6 had progressed, and 5 have died. Of the deaths, 5/30 (17%) were confirmed deaths from progressive metastatic disease to the lung. Of the 12 patients, last known to be alive as of April 28, 2015, the median follow-up is 4.4 years (range 0.7–8.7 years).

Figure 1(a) displays DFS of study patients. A total of 7 patients have had disease progression and the DFS estimate at two years is 83% and at four years is 67%. Figure 1(b) displays OS of study patients. A total of 6 patients have died, and the median time to progression was 142 days. We observed clinical responses in high-grade soft tissue sarcomas over 5 cm in size to be 67% from this study that is superior to the previously published outcomes of 45–55% [1, 3, 7, 8].

Table 2: Common adverse events of Phase I trial combining neoadjuvant radiation and dendritic cell injections subdivided by grades 1–5 and total number of events during the course of the treatment.

	Grade 1	Grade 2	Grade 3	Grade 4	Grade 5	Total
Pain	33	22	5	0	0	61
Rash	16	0	0	0	0	16
Erythema	19	0	0	0	0	19
Hyperglycemia	16	5	0	0	0	22
Limb edema	16	5	0	0	0	22
Hyper pigmentation	5	0	0	0	0	5
Injection site reactions	11	5	0	0	0	16
Pruritus	5	0	0	0	0	5
Fatigue	66	33	0	0	0	99
Back pain	5	11	0	0	0	16
Nausea	38	11	5	0	0	54
Bruising	5	0	0	0	0	5
Constipation	44	11	0	0	0	55
Allergic reaction/hypersensitivity	5	0	0	0	0	5

Of the eight patients that show disease-free survival between six and eight years, five had positive immune responses either to tumor cell lysate and/or survivin. Comparing survival in immune responders versus none responders using a two-tailed unpaired t-test showed that there was no difference between the two groups (p = 0.16, CI = −27.68 to 55.18).

3.4. Accumulation of Myeloid-Derived Suppressor Cells and Regulatory T Lymphocytes. The primary endpoint of the study was to examine the immunologic T-cell response to stimulation with specific tumor associated antigens (tumor cell lysate and survivin) as published before [12].

3.5. Correlation of Immunological with Clinical Response. Ten out of 18 individuals (56%) demonstrated evidence of an immune response to either tumor cell lysates (TCL) or survivin, at least at one point after the start of the treatment. Seven patients showed a response to only TCL, two patients to only survivin, and four to both TCL and survivin (Table 3). Tumor necrosis did not correlate with survival using log-rank test (Mantel-Cox) p = 0.08 (Table 3, Figures 2(a) and 2(b)). We found that there were some patients whose immune responses correlated with prolonged survival (Table 3). Due to their small numbers, this was not statistically significant and warrants further evaluation through prospective randomized controlled clinical trials.

3.6. Case Report. A 46-year-old lady, who received neoadjuvant radiation and DC vaccine, had minimal side effects from the vaccine and a positive immune response to tumor antigens and survivin. Subsequent CAT scans a year later showed lung nodules suspicious for metastatic disease. These were surgically resected showing fibrosis, hyalinization, and infiltration of reactive lymphocytes on histopathological analysis (Figures 3(a), 3(b), and 3(c)).

4. Discussion

From this neoadjuvant clinical trial, we find that the dendritic cell injections were well tolerated with minimal side effects. Durable clinical responses were seen in these preliminary trials when compared to standard treatments with previously published results [1, 3, 4, 7].

First of all, these exploratory trials were designed with the intention of piloting DC injections for safety and immune response assessment in STS. In this study 12 out of 18 patients (67%) were alive with no systemic recurrence at eight years, while 6 out of 18 (33%) progressed to metastatic disease to the lung in 3 years. The fact that significant clinical responses are seen in these patients led to this report, indicating that the DC vaccines warrant further clinical evaluation by prospective randomized clinical trials. The immune change in the tumor microenvironment correlating with such prolonged remissions is what we need to focus on with appropriate correlative research while designing clinical trials in the future.

In these studies, leukapheresis followed by *ex vivo* expansion with standardized protocols was utilized to obtain expanded autologous DCs from mononuclear cell fraction progenitors that are HLA-matched (autologous) and competent to take up tumor-derived apoptotic bodies and present tumor antigens to lymphocytes. Bridging the gap in the DC maturational pathway caused by tumors defeats the tumor-induced immune tolerance seen in cancer patients. In our murine model, there was a direct relationship between acquisition of detectable tumor-specific cytotoxic T lymphocyte activity and clinical cure.

Dendritic cell (DC) therapy has not yet been validated, as there is no standardized method for its preparation [20, 21], timing of administration, and lineages of dendritic cells used (mononuclear or plasmacytoid) [24]. Several vaccine-based trials have been reported but have limited efficacy.

Traditionally radiation therapy has been viewed as immunosuppressive, but its immune functions can be

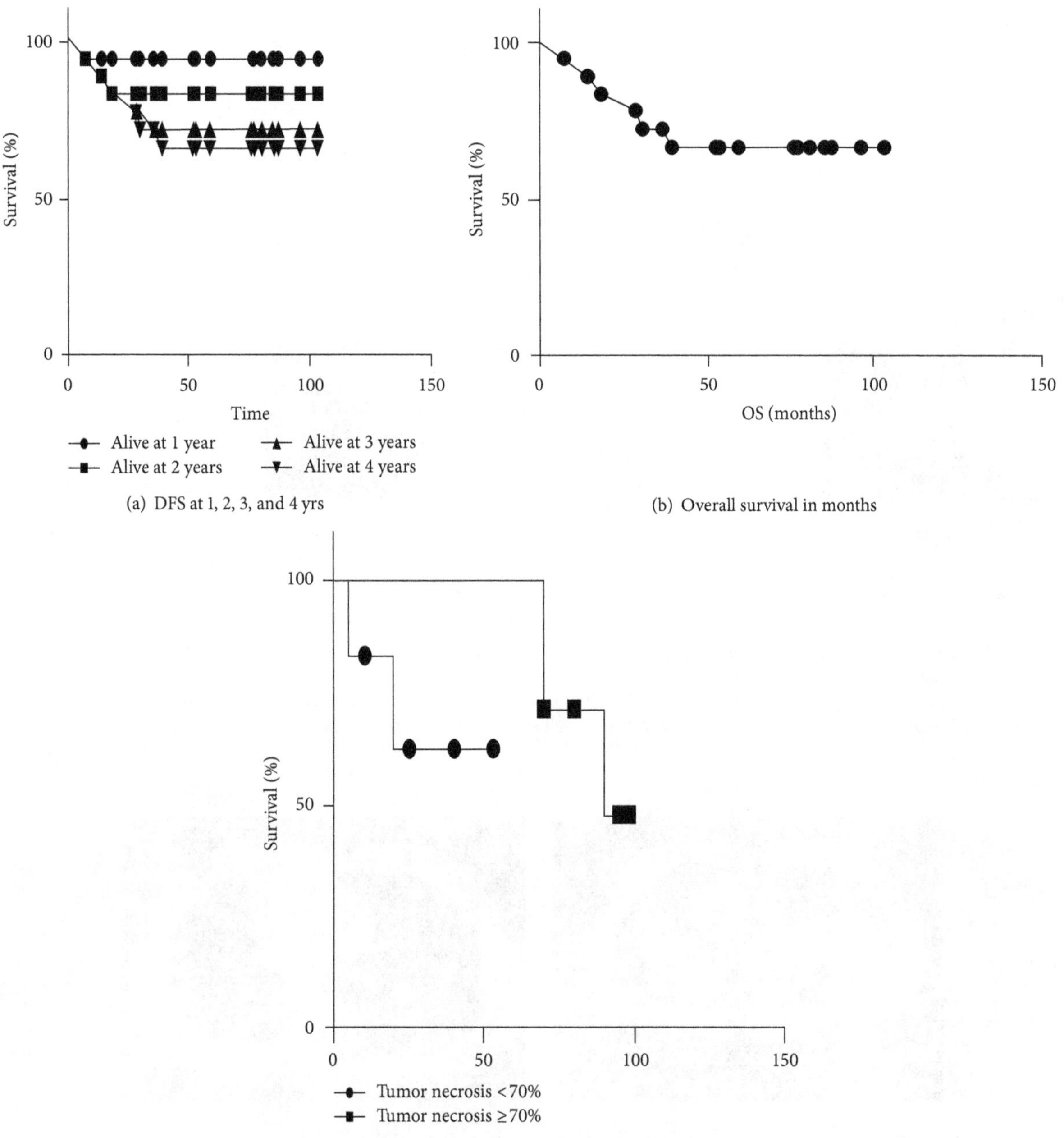

(a) DFS at 1, 2, 3, and 4 yrs

(b) Overall survival in months

(c) Tumor necrosis correlated with survival

FIGURE 1: (a) Kaplan Meir curves showing the disease-free survival at 1, 2, 3, and 4 years (94%, 83%, 72%, and 66%, resp.) of patients who received neoadjuvant intratumoral injection of dendritic cells and radiation in high-grade soft tissue sarcomas over 5 cm. (b) Kaplan Meir curve showing overall survival of patients in months on patients who received neoadjuvant intratumoral injection of dendritic cells and radiation in high-grade soft tissue sarcomas over 5 cm. (c) Kaplan Meir curves showing tumor necrosis less than 70% or ≥70% in patients who received intratumoral dendritic cell injections followed by radiation and then surgery with resection of tumors to determine the percentage of necrosis after surgery $p = 0.76$.

complex. There is published data that radiation doses below 20 Gy do not affect the antigen-presenting function of DCs *in vitro* [15]. Thus, it is unlikely that the radiation at 2 Gy per fraction would have any significant effect on DC functions, even if the cells were very slow to migrate. The exact dose and delivery method of radiation with DC vaccine are still unknown and currently under evaluation.

This exploratory analysis is one of the first attempts at initiating DC vaccine therapy for soft tissue sarcoma. The primary objective of establishing immunological responses following DC therapy combined with radiation in soft tissue sarcoma was confirmed along with significant clinical responses in these patients, which warrants comparative trials with controlled treatment groups that will help define therapeutic efficacy.

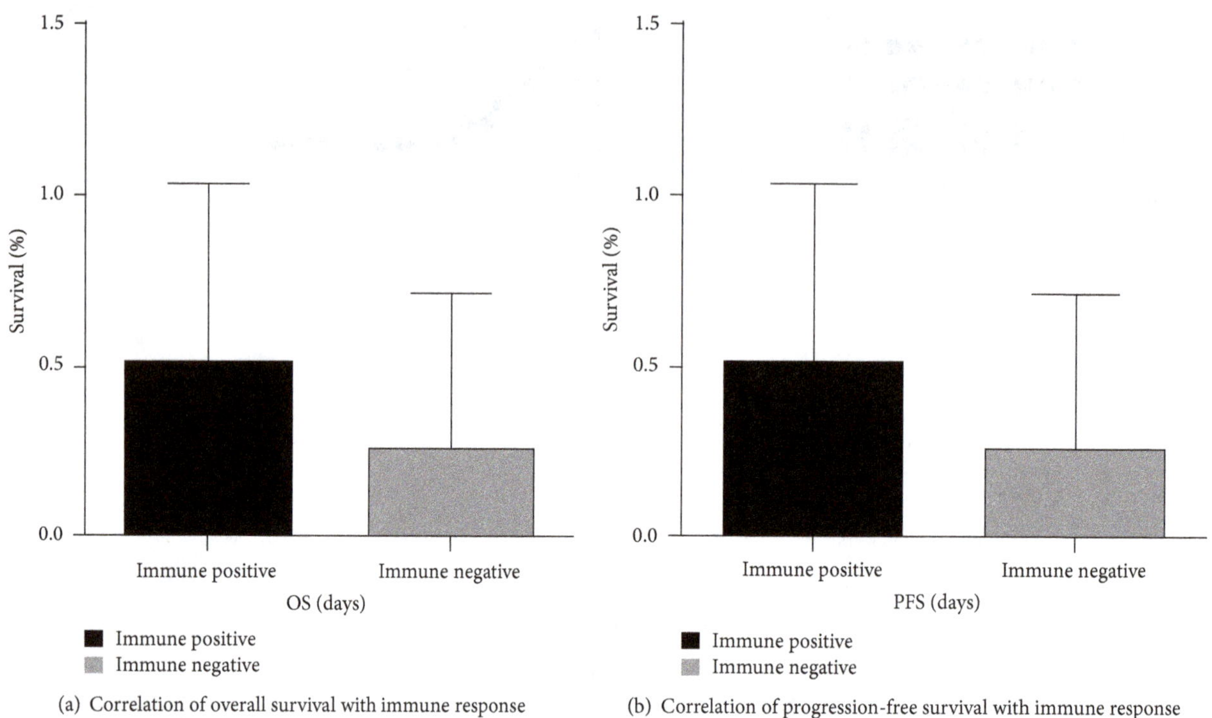

(a) Correlation of overall survival with immune response

(b) Correlation of progression-free survival with immune response

FIGURE 2: The eighteen patients who received neoadjuvant radiation and DC vaccine were divided into two groups based on their immune response (positive and negative) and then correlated with the overall survival in days and progression free survival.

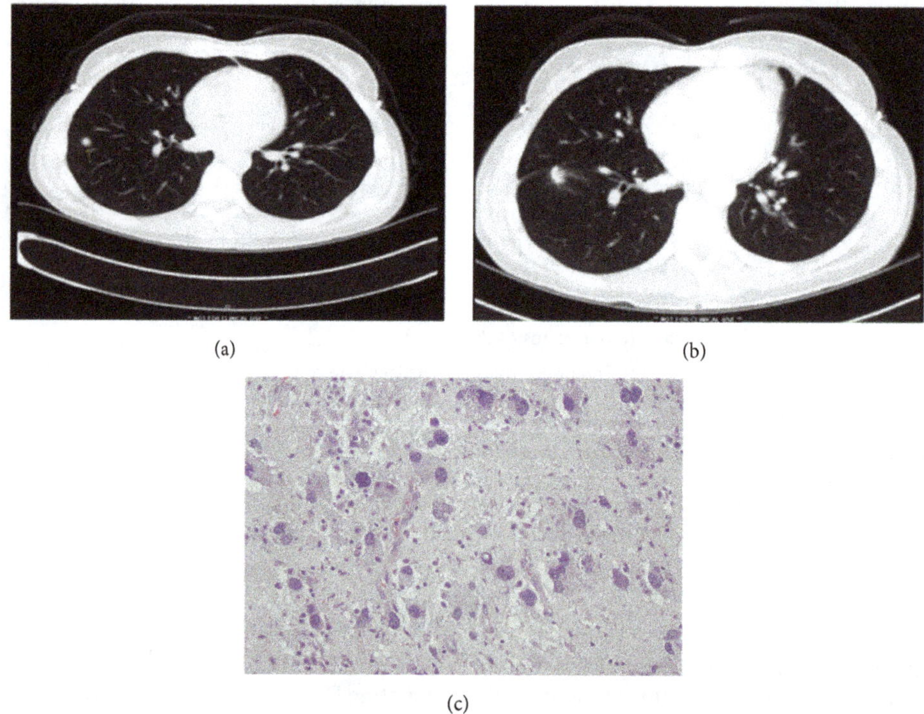

(a) (b) (c)

FIGURE 3: Pre- and postsurgery CAT scan of a 46-year-old lady with history of dedifferentiated liposarcoma patient who completed the DC vaccine + RT treatment, underwent surgical resection, and approximately 10 months later presented with (a and b) pre- and post-CT scans showing the presence of the lung nodules (two) and then postsurgical imaging study after its resection. (c) Pathological analysis showed tissue necrosis, hyalinization, and infiltration of lymphocytes and is currently free of systemic or local recurrence over 8 years.

TABLE 3: Histological type, immune responses to tumor cell lysates, and proliferation and immune response to survivin, percentage of tumor necrosis, and survival in months data of 18 patients recieving neoadjuvant radiation and dendritic cell vaccine treatment.

ID	Histology	Age	Gender	Location	Survival in months	Tumor necrosis in %	Progression to lung metastases in days	Immune response to TCL proliferation	Immune response to TCL (IFN/Elispot)	Immune response to survivin
1	Myxoid liposarcoma	41	M	Groin	103	NA		Positive	Positive	Negative
2	Synovial sarcoma	53	M	Right shoulder	96	NA	951	Negative	Positive	NA
3	Dedifferentiated liposarcoma	46	F	Right thigh	103	70%		Negative	Negative	Positive
4	Spindle/ pleomorphic	69	F	Left knee	59	98%		NA	NA	NA
5	Undifferentiated pleomorphic sarcoma	64	F	Left pelvis	80	80%		Negative	Negative	Negative
6	Sarcoma with myxoid and chondroid features	73	F	Lumbar spine	53	53%		Negative	Negative	Negative
7	Pleomorphic sarcoma	79	M	Left arm	76	25%		Positive	Negative	Negative
8	Undifferentiated pleomorphic sarcoma	71	M	Left thigh	14	70%	142	Negative	Negative	Positive
9	Myxoid liposarcoma	55	M		52	NA		Positive	Positive	Negative
10	Fibrosarcoma	73	M	Back	85	NA		Positive	Positive	Negative
11	Spindle cell sarcoma	81	M	Right flank	77	10%		Negative	Negative	NA
12	Synovial sarcoma	25	M	Left thigh	28	NA	146	Positive	Negative	NA
13	Fibrosarcoma	52	M	Right thigh	30	20%	132	Positive	Negative	NA
14	Undifferentiated pleomorphic sarcoma	58	M	Left thigh	7	90%	48	NA	NA	NA
15	Synovial sarcoma	34	M	Left knee	39	70%	947	NA	NA	NA
16	Undifferentiated pleomorphic sarcoma	60	M	Right leg	87	40%		Negative	Negative	NA
17	Spindle cell sarcoma	81	M	Right flank	36	95%		NA	NA	NA
18	Undifferentiated pleomorphic sarcoma	50	M	Right paraspinal	18	5%	102	Positive	Negative	NA

Acknowledgments

The authors acknowledge Robert Maki, David Barker, Cristina Iclozan, David Noyes, and Noel Clarke.

References

[1] A. I. Spira and D. S. Ettinger, "The use of chemotherapy in soft-tissue sarcomas," *The Oncologist*, vol. 7, no. 4, pp. 348–359, 2002.

[2] M. F. Brennan, E. S. Casper, L. B. Harrison, M. H. Shiu, J. Gaynor, and S. I. Hajdu, "The role of multimodality therapy in soft-tissue sarcoma," *Annals of Surgery*, vol. 214, no. 3, pp. 328–336, 1991.

[3] S. A. Rosenberg, J. Tepper, E. Glatstein et al., "The treatment of soft-tissue sarcomas of the extremities: prospective randomized evaluations of (1) limb-sparing surgery plus radiation therapy compared with amputation and (2) the role of adjuvant chemotherapy," *Annals of Surgery*, vol. 196, no. 3, pp. 305–315, 1982.

[4] P. W. Pisters, L. B. Harrison, D. H. Leung, J. M. Woodruff, E. S. Casper, and M. F. Brennan, "Long-term results of a prospective randomized trial of adjuvant brachytherapy in soft tissue sarcoma," *Journal of Clinical Oncology*, vol. 14, no. 3, pp. 859–868, 1996.

[5] B. Rooser, P. Gustafson, and A. Rydholm, "Is there no influence of local control on the rate of metastases in high-grade soft tissue sarcoma?" *Cancer*, vol. 65, no. 8, pp. 1727–1729, 1990.

[6] J.-M. Coindre, P. Terrier, L. Guillou et al., "Predictive value of grade for metastasis development in the main histologic types of adult soft tissue sarcomas," *Cancer*, vol. 91, no. 10, pp. 1914–1926, 2001.

[7] J. F. Tierney, "Adjuvant chemotherapy for localised resectable soft-tissue sarcoma of adults: meta-analysis of individual data," *The Lancet*, vol. 350, no. 9092, pp. 1647–1654, 1997.

[8] S. Frustaci, F. Gherlinzoni, A. De Paoli et al., "Adjuvant chemotherapy for adult soft tissue sarcomas of the extremities and girdles: results of the Italian randomized cooperative trial," *Journal of Clinical Oncology*, vol. 19, no. 5, pp. 1238–1247, 2001.

[9] D. Nelson, S. Fisher, and B. Robinson, "The 'trojan Horse' approach to tumor immunotherapy: targeting the tumor microenvironment," *Journal of Immunology Research*, vol. 2014, Article ID 789069, 14 pages, 2014.

[10] J. Banchereau and R. M. Steinman, "Dendritic cells and the control of immunity," *Nature*, vol. 392, no. 6673, pp. 245–252, 1998.

[11] G. Schreibelt, J. Tel, K. H. E. W. J. Sliepen et al., "Toll-like receptor expression and function in human dendritic cell subsets: implications for dendritic cell-based anti-cancer immunotherapy," *Cancer Immunology, Immunotherapy*, vol. 59, no. 10, pp. 1573–1582, 2010.

[12] S. E. Finkelstein, C. Iclozan, M. M. Bui et al., "Combination of external beam radiotherapy (EBRT) with intratumoral injection of dendritic cells as neo-adjuvant treatment of high-risk soft tissue sarcoma patients," *International Journal of Radiation Oncology, Biology, Physics*, vol. 82, no. 2, pp. 924–932, 2012.

[13] M. Chakraborty, S. I. Abrams, C. N. Coleman, K. Camphausen, J. Schlom, and J. W. Hodge, "External beam radiation of tumors alters phenotype of tumor cells to render them susceptible to vaccine-mediated T-cell killing," *Cancer Research*, vol. 64, no. 12, pp. 4328–4337, 2004.

[14] B. Park, C. Yee, and K.-M. Lee, "The effect of radiation on the immune response to cancers," *International Journal of Molecular Sciences*, vol. 15, no. 1, pp. 927–943, 2014.

[15] E. Nikitina and D. I. Gabrilovich, "Combination of γ-irradiation and dendritic cell administration induces a potent antitumor response in tumor-bearing mice: approach to treatment of advanced stage cancer," *International Journal of Cancer*, vol. 94, no. 6, pp. 825–833, 2001.

[16] S. Teitz-Tennenbaum, Q. Li, S. Rynkiewicz et al., "Radiotherapy potentiates the therapeutic efficacy of intratumoral dendritic cell administration," *Cancer Research*, vol. 63, no. 23, pp. 8466–8475, 2003.

[17] S. Rusakiewicz, M. Semeraro, M. Sarabi et al., "Immune infiltrates are prognostic factors in localized gastrointestinal stromal tumors," *Cancer Research*, vol. 73, no. 12, pp. 3499–3510, 2013.

[18] P. Brinkrolf, S. Landmeier, B. Altvater et al., "A high proportion of bone marrow T cells with regulatory phenotype (CD4+CD25^{hi}FoxP3+) in Ewing sarcoma patients is associated with metastatic disease," *International Journal of Cancer*, vol. 125, no. 4, pp. 879–886, 2009.

[19] D. Berghuis, S. J. Santos, H. J. Baelde et al., "Pro-inflammatory chemokine-chemokine receptor interactions within the Ewing sarcoma microenvironment determine CD8^{+} T-lymphocyte infiltration and affect tumour progression," *The Journal of Pathology*, vol. 223, no. 3, pp. 347–357, 2011.

[20] V. Pisarev, B. Yu, R. Salup, S. Sherman, D. C. Altieri, and D. I. Gabrilovich, "Full-length dominant-negative survivin for cancer immunotherapy," *Clinical Cancer Research*, vol. 9, no. 17, pp. 6523–6533, 2003.

[21] D. C. Altieri, "Validating survivin as a cancer therapeutic target," *Nature Reviews Cancer*, vol. 3, no. 1, pp. 46–54, 2003.

[22] J. D. Geiger, R. J. Hutchinson, L. F. Hohenkirk et al., "Vaccination of pediatric solid tumor patients with tumor lysate-pulsed dendritic cells can expand specific T cells and mediate tumor regression," *Cancer Research*, vol. 61, no. 23, pp. 8513–8519, 2001.

[23] S. E. Finkelstein, T. Carey, I. Fricke et al., "Changes in dendritic cell phenotype after a new high-dose weekly schedule of interleukin-2 therapy for kidney cancer and melanoma," *Journal of Immunotherapy*, vol. 33, no. 8, pp. 817–827, 2010.

[24] W. J. Lesterhuis, I. J. M. De Vries, G. Schreibelt et al., "Route of administration modulates the induction of dendritic cell vaccine-induced antigen-specific T cells in advanced melanoma patients," *Clinical Cancer Research*, vol. 17, no. 17, pp. 5725–5735, 2011.

11

Cell Senescence in Myxoid/Round Cell Liposarcoma

Christina Kåbjörn Gustafsson,[1] Anders Ståhlberg,[1] Katarina Engtröm,[2] Anna Danielsson,[1] Ingela Turesson,[3] and Pierre Åman[1]

[1] *Sahlgrenska Cancer Center, Department of Pathology, Institute of Biomedicine, University of Gothenburg, Box 425, 40530 Gothenburg, Sweden*
[2] *Department of Oncology, Institute of Medical Sciences, University of Gothenburg, Blå stråket 2, 41345 Gothenburg, Sweden*
[3] *Department of Oncology, Institute of Medical Sciences, Uppsala University, 75185 Uppsala, Sweden*

Correspondence should be addressed to Pierre Åman; pierre.aman@gu.se

Academic Editor: Charles Catton

Myxoid/round cell liposarcoma (MLS/RCLS) is the second most common liposarcoma type and characterized by the fusion oncogenes *FUS-DDIT3* or *EWSR1-DDIT3*. Previous analysis of cell cycle regulatory proteins revealed a prominent expression of G1-cyclins, cyclin dependent kinases, and their inhibitors but very few cells progressing through the G1/S boundary. Here, we extend the investigation to proteins involved in cell senescence in an immunohistochemistry based study of 17 MLS/RCLS cases. Large subpopulations of tumor cells expressed the RBL2 pocket protein and senescence associated heterochromatin 1γ and IL8 receptor β. We conclude that MLS/RCLS tissues contain major populations of senescent tumor cells and this may explain the slow growth rate of this tumor type.

1. Introduction

Liposarcoma is the most common soft tissue tumor in humans and myxoid/round cell liposarcoma (MLS/RCLS) is the second most common liposarcoma type. In a majority of the cases MLS/RCLS develops in large muscles, most often in the thigh [1]. MLS/RCLS tissue is composed of round to oval shaped mesenchymal cells and a variable number of lipoblasts, set in a myxoid matrix with a fine piped capillary network. Most cases of MLS tumors are relatively slow growing but 10–15% show a hyper cellular round cell morphology (RCLS) with less myxoid component that is associated with an unfavourable prognosis [1].

The fusion oncogenes *FUS-DDIT3* or *EWSR1-DDIT3* are present in almost all cases of MLS/RCLS. They result from *t*(12; 16) or *t*(12; 22) chromosome translocation and have causative roles in development of MLS/RCLS [2–5]. *FUS-DDIT3* and *EWSR1-DDIT3* encode abnormal transcription factors that deregulate the expression of target genes [6–8]. For example, we previously showed that *FUS-DDIT3* directly induces production of IL6 and IL8 by binding to the *IL6* and *IL8* promoters [9, 10].

A recent study reports that most MLS/RCLS cases also carry TERT promoter mutations, suggesting an increased TERT activity and extended cellular life span [11]. The RCLS variant is also associated with additional mutations, most commonly in PIK3CA [12].

Previous studies of cell cycle regulating proteins in MLS/RCLS revealed a prominent expression of growth promoting G1 cyclins and cyclin dependent kinases (CDK), coexpressed with cyclin dependent kinase inhibitors P16, P19, and P27 (also known as CDKN2A, CDKN2D, and CDKN1B, resp.) [13]. This pattern suggested that the growth promoting cyclin/CDK activity was counteracted by CDK inhibitors and this could explain the low frequency of proliferating cells identified by Ki67 and cyclin A staining (typically less than 8 and 4 percent, resp.) [13].

Recent results from investigations of senescent cells suggest that they express G1 cyclins, CDKs, and their inhibitors

TABLE 1: Cases and immunohistochemistry data.

Case	Age		Site	RB1[1] (%)	HP1γ[1] (%)	RBL2[1] (%)	IL8R[1] (%)	KI67[1] (%)	FUS/DDIT3 rearrangement[2]	Histological classification
1	42	im	Hip	35	50	79	55	nd	+	MLS
2	45	im	Thigh	23	66	77	86	<1	+	MLS
3	37	im	Thigh	73	50	69	69	4	+	MLS
4	36	im	Thigh	60	56	55	86	<1	+	MLS
5	80	im	Thigh	62	60	93	91	2	+	MLS
6	34	im	Thigh	58	44	91	79	3	+	MLS
7	56	im	Thigh	72	47	76	64	<1	+	MLS
8	46	sc	Thigh	65	51	85	86	1	+	MLS
9	73	im	Lower leg	75	49	83	83	<1	nd	MLS
10	45	other	Peritoneal	73	54	80	80	3	nd	MLS
11	49	sc	Thorax met	94	56	93	90	nd	+	MLS
12	33	other	Peritoneal	25	76	87	50	<1	+	MLS/RCLS
13	37	im	Leg	9	14	69	62	nd	nd	MLS/RCLS
14	38	im	Thigh	81	47	68	85	6	+	MLS/RCLS
15	76	sc	Back	73	50	82	54	<1	+	MLS/RCLS
16	46	im	Hip	85	45	0	74	8	+	RCLS
17	19	im	Shoulder	77	51	78	79	7	nd	RCLS

[1]Percent cells expressing respective protein.
[2]*FUS-DDIT3* rearrangement status as determined by FISH. [+]Indicates presence of *FUS-DDIT3* rearrangements. nd: not determined due to technical problems or lack of material.
im: intramuscular; sc: subcutaneous; nd: not determined; met: metastasis.

as well as a typical expression signature of cytokines and their receptors [14–17]. These new data and concepts provide a possible explanation for the expression patterns observed in MLS/RCLS and prompted a renewed investigation with focus on senescence markers. In the present study, we have employed immunohistochemistry (IHC) and analysed a cohort of 17 MLS/RCLS cases for expression of proteins associated with growth control and senescence. The results suggest that substantial proportions of MLS/RCLS tumor cells are senescent.

2. Materials and Methods

2.1. Tissue Samples. The clinicopathological characteristics of all tumors are presented in Table 1. Formalin-fixed tissues taken at surgery from previously untreated cases with MLS/RCLS were embedded in paraffin using routine procedures and stored at room temperature. Use of tissue samples for this study was examined and approved by the Ethical Board associated with the University of Gothenburg. All selected MLS cases were examined by two clinical pathologists specialized in soft tissue tumors and by the first author, also a clinical pathologist.

2.2. Cell Cultures. Human foreskin derived fibroblasts (passage 8) were cultured in RPMI1640 with 5% fetal calf serum. Immunofluorescence studies were made 5 days after a 10 Gy dose of X-ray radiation. MLS cell lines 402-91, 1765-92, and 2645-94 and HT1080 clones [4, 18, 19] were cultured in RPMI1640 with GlutaMAX and 8% fetal bovine serum, 100 U/mL penicillin, and 100 μg/mL streptomycin. All media and supplements were obtained from Life Technologies. All cells were maintained at 37°C with air containing 5% CO_2.

2.3. IL-6 Dependence Assay. MLS cell lines 402-91, 1765-92, and 2645-94 were seeded to 96 well microtiter plates at 2000 cells/well and allowed to settle for 8 hours. The culture medium was replaced with medium supplemented with 3% fetal bovine serum, with and without 1 unit/mL of recombinant IL6 and with or without 0.5 μg/mL of monoclonal IL6 antibody mAB 206 (R&D systems). Trypan blue excluding cells were counted in an inverted microscope after 48 hours of incubation. An Epstein-Barr virus immortalized lymphoblastoid cell line was included as positively responding control [20].

2.4. Immunohistochemistry and Immunofluorescence Microscopy. Series of 5 μm tissue sections were cut from each biopsy, deparaffinised, rehydrated, boiled in microwave oven for 10 minutes for epitope retrievement, and stained with the antibodies listed in Table 2. Bound antibodies were visualized using the LSAB secondary antibody streptavidin biotin peroxidase system (DAKO). Stained sections were examined on a light microscope.

For immunofluorescence analysis, cultures of human fibroblasts were washed twice with PBS and fixed in 4%

TABLE 2: Antibodies used for immunohistochemistry and immunofluorescence.

Antigen	Antibody	Dilution	Retrievement
IL8Rβ	SC-23811	1:50	PH6
RBL2	SC-53641	1:50	PH9
RB1	BD #5544136	1:20	PH9
TP53	Calbio.OP43A	1:100	
CCNA	NM MS1061-S1	1:15	
P21	Millipore OP64	1:25	
P15	SC-56327	1:20	
HP1γ	Millipore 05-690	1:100	PH6
KI67	Dako IR-626	1:1	PH6

SC: SantaCruz Biotechnology; BD: Becton Dickinson and Company; Calbio: calbiochem; NM: neomarker; epitope retrievement was performed at indicated PH by boiling for 5 minutes.

TABLE 3: Senescence markers in irradiated fibroblasts.

Marker	Control	Irradiated
IL8R	Negative	100^{++}
RBL2	8, 12 (mitotic)$^{++}$	94, 96^{+}
RB1	100^{++}	30, 33^{+}
P53	Negative	100^{++}
CCNA	17, 20^{++}	Negative
P21	Negative	100^{+++}
P15	Negative	100^{+}
HP1γ	$<1^{++}$	100^{+++}

Percentage positive cells for respective marker are shown. $^{+,++,+++}$ indicate weak, medium, and strong expression, respectively. Mitotic: expression seen only in mitotic cells. Results from two experiments are shown. Two values are shown when there was variation between the experiments.

paraformaldehyde in PBS. After two more washes in PBS, the slides were mounted in an antifade mount containing the DNA binding dye DAPI (4,6-diamidino-2-phenylindole dihydrochloride) (Olink Bioscience) and examined on a fluorescence microscope. Several antibodies were tested for each antigen and evaluated by IHC staining of tissue sections containing published positive and negative cell populations. The selected primary antibodies were also tested by western blot analysis of MLS cell lines and other reference cell lines as described elsewhere [13]. Irradiated fibroblasts were used as a control for the senescence markers used (Table 3). Detection of RB1 expression worked satisfactorily only with the antibody and protocol detailed in Table 2. Evaluation of IHC stains was made by Christina Kåbjörn, specialist pathologist, and Pierre Åman.

2.5. Flow Cytometric Analysis of Cell Cycle Phase Distribution. Paraffin-embedded, formalin-fixed tissues were dewaxed, and single-cell suspensions were prepared and labeled with propidium iodide (Life Technology, catalogue number P3566) according to the providers protocol and as previously described [21]. Flow cytometric analysis of DNA content was evaluated using the FACS calibur system (BD Biosciences). The ModFit LT software (Verity Software House) was used for analysis and peak detection to identify distributions of G1, S, and G2 cells.

2.6. FISH Analysis. Interphase FISH analysis of FUS-DDIT3 and EWSR1-DDIT3 rearrangements [22] was performed on formalin-fixed 1–4 μm paraffin tissue sections. Three break-apart probes, DDIT3, FUS,and EWSR1 (Vysis Inc.), were used according to protocols supplied by the manufacturer. Nuclei were counterstained with 10 μL 4′,6′,-diamidino-2′-phenylindole dihydrochloride (DAPI). The sections were analyzed and reanalyzed by two independent reviewers. At least 100 nuclei per section were scored. The interpretation of intact, fusion, and split signals was based on guidelines recommended by the manufacturer and from other clinical laboratories using this method.

3. Results

Irradiated fibroblasts were used as a control for the senescence markers and antibodies used. Our data showed a very strong expression of all investigated senescence associated markers in irradiated cells compared to control cultured cells (Table 3).

Our Ki67 IHC staining results (Table 1) and previous data [13] showed that most MLS cases contain very few Ki 67 positive cells, typically less than 4%, but some RCLS tissues contained smaller tissue regions with up to 8% positive cells. A previous investigation also showed only few cells expressing the S-G2 phase specific cyclin A, suggesting that a majority of the cells are arrested in the G1 phase [13]. Here, our flow cytometry analysis of cell nuclei from two human MLS/RCLS tissues showed 94% and 96% G1-phase cells, respectively (Figure 1), supporting our conclusion that most MLS/RCLS tumor cells were arrested in the G1 phase of the cell cycle.

IHC analysis of pocket proteins showed that 9–94% of the cells expressed the proliferation associated RB1 and 0–93% expressed the rest of phase protein RBL2. It is thus obvious that there are overlaps in expression of the RB1 and RBL2 proteins.

Our IHC analysis showed only weak signals for the RB1 protein in MLS tissues compared to control tissue samples from other tumor types. This prompted a further analysis of RB1 protein expression in MLS cells. Western blot analysis showed a strong expression of a normal sized RB1 protein in all three investigated MLS derived cell lines (Figure 2). Forced expression of FUS-DDIT3 gave no effects on RB1 expression in the human HT1080 fibrosarcoma cell line (Figure 2).

Between 14 and 76% of the tumor cells stained positive for heterochromatin protein (HP1γ) (Table 1 and Figure 1). Together with the pocket protein results, these data suggest that a large proportion of the MLS/RCLS cells are arrested in the G1 phase and that the tumors contain a substantial fraction of senescent cells.

Cell senescence is associated with a distinct cytokine and cytokine receptor expression signature and FUS-DDIT3 is known to induce IL6 and IL8 expression in the tumor cells. IHC analysis of MLS/RCLS tissues showed that the

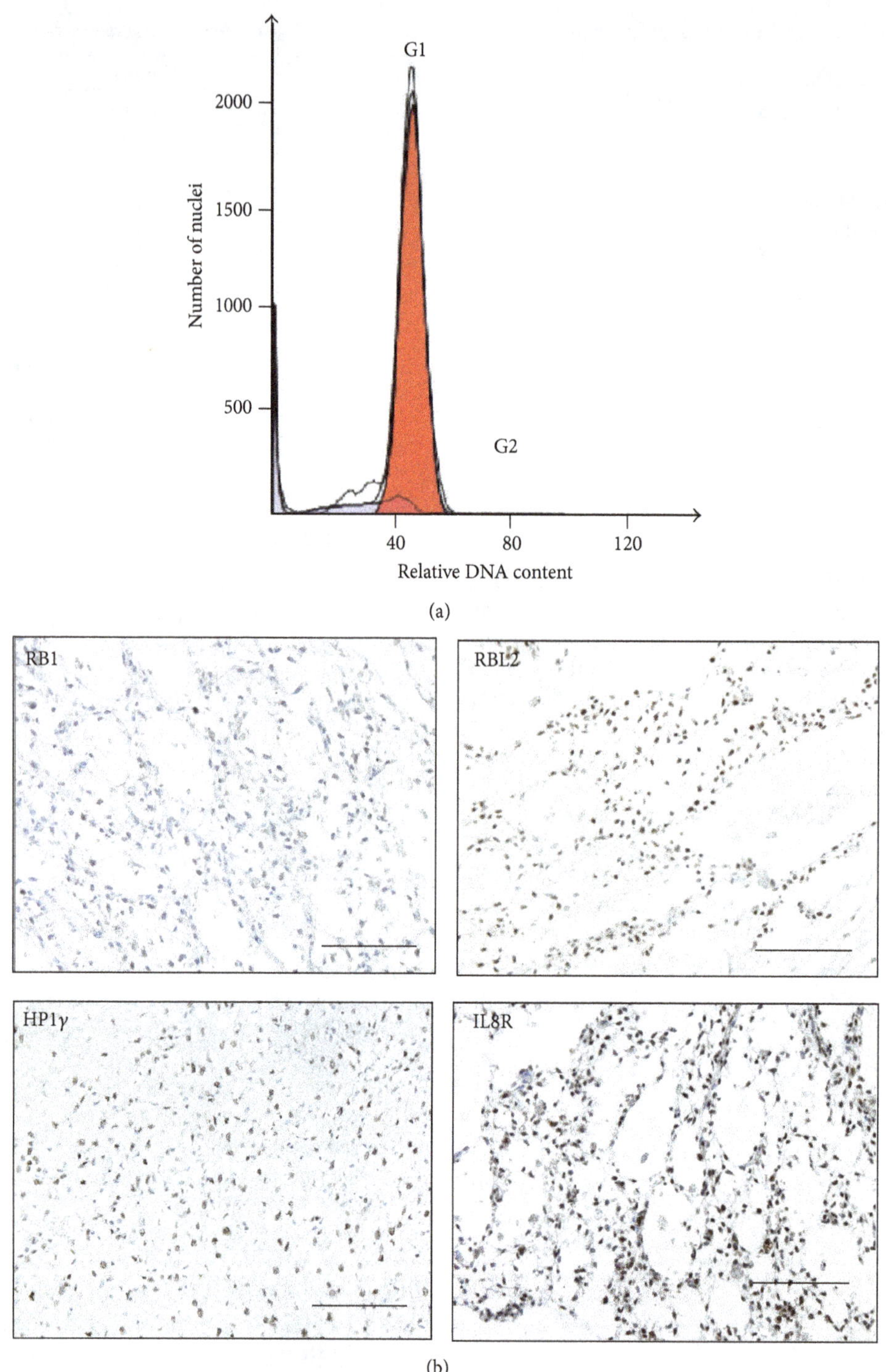

FIGURE 1: (a) Flow cytometry histogram of cell nuclei extracted from paraffin embedded MLS/RCLS tumor tissue (Cases 8) showing more than 95% of the cells in the G1 phase of the cell cycle (red). (b) Immunohistochemistry analysis of RB1, RBL2, HP1γ, and IL8R in MLS/RCLS tumor tissues. Brown staining shows reactivity with the specific antibodies. Bars are 100 μm.

senescence associated IL8 receptor beta (also known as CXCR2) was expressed in 50–91% of the tumor cells (Table 1 and Figure 1). We tested MLS/RCLS tumor cell lines for in vitro growth and survival dependence on IL6, but no effects of treatment with IL6 or IL6 blocking antibodies were detected (data not shown).

4. Discussion

Our previous analysis of cell cycle regulator expression in MLS/RCLS suggested that a majority of the tumor cells were arrested in the G1 phase of the cell cycle [13]. Only a few percent of the cells escape this arrest as detected by low numbers of Ki67 and cyclin A positive cells. This conclusion is supported here by the present Ki67 IHC analysis of 17 MLS/RCLS cases and by flow cytometry analysis of two cases.

The Ki67 and cytometry analysis was complemented by an IHC based investigation of the pocket proteins RB1 and RBL2 (also known as P105 and P130). RB1 and RBL2 are important control hubs for cell cycle regulation and proliferation driving transcription factors. RB1 is expressed in proliferating cells and is also necessary for induction of senescence, while RBL2 is expressed in resting and senescent cells. Consequently, the levels of RB1 decrease and the levels of RBL2 increase, as cells enter a nonproliferative or senescent cell state [23–27]. Our IHC results for RB1 and RBL2 support the previous conclusion that large subpopulations of tumor cells are in a resting state.

IHC staining of RB1 in MLS/RCLS tissues gave generally weak signals calling for further analysis. Six different RB1 specific antibodies and various staining/antigen retrieving conditions were tested (data not shown). Compared to the staining intensities for RBL2 and HP1γ, the signal was always found weaker in MLS tumor tissues and RB1 staining was also weaker in MLS tissues compared to reference tumor tissues of other entities. Analysis of MLS/RCLS derived cell lines showed RB1 protein expression in level with other tumor cell lines and much stronger than the expression in cultured normal fibroblasts (Figure 2). Comparison of HT1080 fibrosarcoma cells with and without the *FUS-DDIT3* showed that the fusion protein has no direct effect on RB1 expression (Figure 2). Taken together, our data suggest that MLS/RCLS cells are capable of normal expression of RB1. The fading RB1 expression in MLS/RCLS may thus result from a normal downregulation in connection with growth cessation of many tumor cells.

Some senescent cell types are characterized by nuclear heterochromatin foci that can be visualized by DNA-stains and the increased expression of heterochromatin protein 1 gamma (HP1γ) [28, 29]. The IHC analysis of HP1γ in MLS/RCLS tissues showed a heterogeneous pattern with large numbers of strongly stained cells. This suggests that large subpopulations of the tumor cells are senescent with expanded heterochromatin formation and thus they may be permanently excluded from further proliferation.

FUS-DDIT3 binds the promoter regions of the *IL8* and *IL6* encoding genes leading to expression of these genes [9, 10]. IL6 is reported as an autocrine growth or survival factor in several tumor types [30–33]. Our results suggested, however, that IL6 is not a growth/survival factor for MLS/RCLS cells. More recently IL6 and IL8 were reported to be parts of a cytokine expression profile (IL6 and IL8) that is typical for senescent cells [34–36]. Instead of acting as growth factors, IL6 together with IL8 may thus be part of a senescence mechanism in MLS/RCLS. Our data showing IL8 receptor expression in many of the tumor cells is in line with this interpretation. The IL8 receptor beta expression also indicates a possible senescence associated IL8 autocrine activity as the tumor cells also are producing IL8 [7]. A schematic presentation of the investigated senescence associated factors in MLS/RCLS is shown in Figure 3.

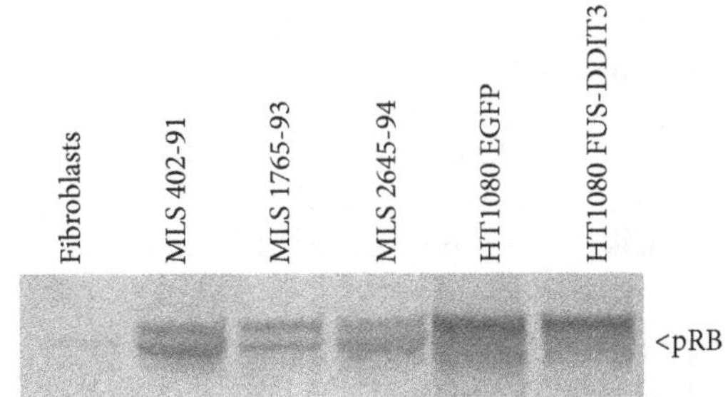

FIGURE 2: Western blot analysis of RB1 expression in cultured normal human fibroblasts, MLS cell lines, and FUS-DDIT3 or EGFP transfected HT1080 cells.

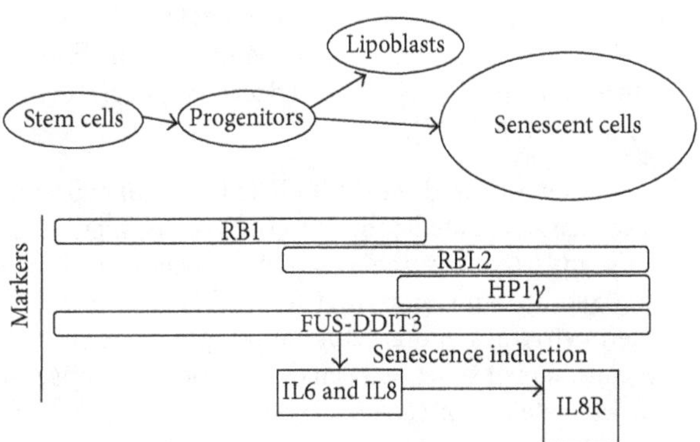

FIGURE 3: Schematic presentation of tumor populations and factors involved in senescence. A small population of proliferating cells arises from a hypothetical tumor stem cell population. Most of these cells enter senescence and a few percent differentiates into lipoblasts. RB1 and RBL2 proteins are central factors involved in growth regulation and entry/maintenance of cell senescence. RB1 is expressed in proliferating cells and is also necessary for differentiation and senescence. RBL2 is expressed in resting and senescent cells. Increased HP1γ expression is typical for senescent cells. IL6 and IL8 are produced by the tumor cells and IL8 may bind to the IL8β receptor expressed by senescent tumor cells.

Our hypothesis that major subpopulations of MLS/RCLS cells are senescent may seem contradictory to the recent report that MLS/RCLS tumors carry TERT promoter mutations. Such mutations may indicate an increased TERT activity and immortalization of the tumor cells [11]. The large numbers of senescent cells in MLS/RCLS tumors may, however, be caused by oncogene induced stress responses resulting in senescence. This hypothesis is supported by our previous in vitro experiments with FUS-DDIT3 transfection into various cell types. Forced FUS-DDIT3 expression caused cell death and senescence in most cell types and only very few cells in permissive cell lines maintained proliferative capacity [18]. Surviving FUS-DDIT3 transfected cells also had a slower in vivo and in vitro growth rate compared to wild-type cells [18]. Oncogenic stress induced senescence has been reported for many oncogenes and is thought to serve as a major barrier against tumor development in vivo [14–17]. This mechanism may also explain the observed low growth rate and abundance of senescent cells in MLS/RCLS tumors.

Ten to fifteen percent of MLS/RCLS cases show round cell morphology and this is associated with increased growth rate and unfavorable prognosis. Inspection of our limited cohort of cases failed to detect any correlation between the RCLS morphology and expression data of the analyzed markers. A possible association between RCLS morphology and number of senescent cells has to be tested in a larger tumor material.

Irradiated fibroblasts showed a very strong expression of all investigated senescence associated markers. In a clinical study, we have previously reported that irradiation of MLS/RCLS tumors results in transformation to a lipoma like morphology with highly differentiated adipocyte like cells [37]. Further investigations of irradiated MLS/RCLS tumors will show if this treatment causes maturation of senescent cells into adipocyte like cells. Such effects have been reported in other tumor types [38].

We have investigated 17 MLS/RCLS tumors for expression of senescence associated proteins. The results suggest that large subpopulations of tumor cells are in a senescent cell state characterized by expression of HP1γ, RBL2, and senescence associated cytokines and a cytokine receptor. The presence of large numbers of senescent cells may explain the observed slow growth rate of this sarcoma type.

Acknowledgments

This work was supported by grants from the Swedish Cancer Society, Swedish Research Council, LUA/ALF grants, Västra Götaland, Assar Gabrielssons Research Foundation, Johan Jansson Foundation for Cancer Research, Swedish Society for Medical Research, BioCARE National Strategic Research Program at University of Gothenburg, and Wilhelm and Martina Lundgren Foundation for Scientific Research.

References

[1] C. D. Fletcher, K. K. Unni, and F. Mertens, *Tumors of Soft Tissue and Bone. WHO Classification Pathology and Genetics*, IARCPress, Lyon, France, 2000.

[2] A. Crozat, P. Aman, N. Mandahl, and D. Ron, "Fusion of CHOP to a novel RNA-binding protein in human myxoid liposarcoma," *Nature*, vol. 363, no. 6430, pp. 640–644, 1993.

[3] T. H. Rabbitts, A. Forster, R. Larson, and P. Nathan, "Fusion of the dominant negative transcription regulator CHOP with a novel gene FUS by translocation t(12;16) in malignant liposarcoma," *Nature Genetics*, vol. 4, no. 2, pp. 175–180, 1993.

[4] P. Åman, D. Ron, N. Mandahl et al., "Rearrangement of the transcription factor gene CHOP in myxoid liposarcomas with t(12;16)(q13;p11)," *Genes Chromosomes and Cancer*, vol. 5, no. 4, pp. 278–285, 1992.

[5] I. Panagopoulos, M. Höglund, F. Mertens, N. Mandahl, F. Mitelman, and P. Åman, "Fusion of the EWS and CHOP genes in myxoid liposarcoma," *Oncogene*, vol. 12, no. 3, pp. 489–494, 1996.

[6] N. Riggi, L. Cironi, P. Provero et al., "Expression of the FUS-CHOP fusion protein in primary mesenchymal progenitor cells gives rise to a model of myxoid liposarcoma," *Cancer Research*, vol. 66, no. 14, pp. 7016–7023, 2006.

[7] H. Zinszner, R. Albalat, and D. Ron, "A novel effector domain from the RNA-binding protein TLS or EWS is required for oncogenic transformation by CHOP," *Genes and Development*, vol. 8, no. 21, pp. 2513–2526, 1994.

[8] H. Zinszner, D. Immanuel, Y. Yin, F.-X. Liang, and D. Ron, "A topogenic role for the oncogenic N-terminus of TLS: nucleolar localization when transcription is inhibited," *Oncogene*, vol. 14, no. 4, pp. 451–461, 1997.

[9] M. Göransson, M. K. Andersson, C. Forni et al., "The myxoid liposarcoma FUS-DDIT3 fusion oncoprotein deregulates NF-κB target genes by interaction with NFKBIZ," *Oncogene*, vol. 28, no. 2, pp. 270–278, 2009.

[10] M. Göransson, E. Elias, A. Ståhlberg, A. Olofsson, C. Andersson, and P. Åman, "Myxoid liposarcoma FUS-DDIT3 fusion oncogene induces C/EBP β-mediated interleukin 6 expression," *International Journal of Cancer*, vol. 115, no. 4, pp. 556–560, 2005.

[11] P. J. Killela, Z. J. Reitmana, Y. Jiao et al., "TERT promoter mutations occur frequently in gliomas and a subset of tumors derived from cells with low rates of self-renewal," *Proceedings of the National Academy of Sciences of the United States of America*, vol. 110, no. 15, pp. 6021–6026, 2013.

[12] J. Barretina, B. S. Taylor, S. Banerji et al., "Subtype-specific genomic alterations define new targets for soft-tissue sarcoma therapy," *Nature Genetics*, vol. 42, no. 8, pp. 715–721, 2010.

[13] A. Olofsson, H. Willén, M. Göransson et al., "Abnormal expression of cell cycle regulators in FUS-CHOP carrying liposarcomas," *International Journal of Oncology*, vol. 25, no. 5, pp. 1349–1355, 2004.

[14] M. Braig, S. Lee, C. Loddenkemper et al., "Oncogene-induced senescence as an initial barrier in lymphoma development," *Nature*, vol. 436, no. 7051, pp. 660–665, 2005.

[15] J. Bartkova, N. Rezaei, M. Liontos et al., "Oncogene-induced senescence is part of the tumorigenesis barrier imposed by DNA damage checkpoints," *Nature*, vol. 444, no. 7119, pp. 633–637, 2006.

[16] M. Braig and C. A. Schmitt, "Oncogene-induced senescence: putting the brakes on tumor development," *Cancer Research*, vol. 66, no. 6, pp. 2881–2884, 2006.

[17] P. Yaswen and J. Campisi, "Oncogene-induced senescence pathways weave an intricate tapestry," *Cell*, vol. 128, no. 2, pp. 233–234, 2007.

[18] K. Engström, H. Willén, C. Kåbjörn-Gustafsson et al., "The myxoid/round cell liposarcoma fusion oncogene FUS-DDIT3 and the normal DDIT3 induce a liposarcoma phenotype in transfected human fibrosarcoma cells," *American Journal of Pathology*, vol. 168, no. 5, pp. 1642–1653, 2006.

[19] S. Thelin-Jarnum, C. Lassen, I. Panagopoulos, N. Mandahl, and P. Aman, "Identification of genes differentially expressed in TLS-CHOP carrying myxoid liposarcomas," *International Journal of Cancer*, vol. 83, no. 1, pp. 30–33, 1999.

[20] T. Yokoi, T. Miyawaki, A. Yachie, K. Kato, Y. Kasahara, and N. Taniguchi, "Epstein-Barr virus-immortalized B cells produce IL-6 as an autocrine growth factor," *Immunology*, vol. 70, no. 1, pp. 100–105, 1990.

[21] I. Köpf, C. Hanson, U. Delle, I. Verbiené, and A. Weimarck, "A rapid and simplified technique for analysis of archival formalin-fixed, paraffin-embedded tissue by fluorescence in situ hybridization (FISH)," *Anticancer Research*, vol. 16, no. 5, pp. 2533–2536, 1996.

[22] H. Yoshida, K. Nagao, H. Ito, K. Yamamoto, and S. Ushigome, "Chromosomal translocations in human soft tissue sarcomas by interphase fluorescence in situ hybridization," *Pathology International*, vol. 47, no. 4, pp. 222–229, 1997.

[23] H. Helmbold, W. Deppert, and W. Bohn, "Regulation of cellular senescence by Rb2/p130," *Oncogene*, vol. 25, no. 38, pp. 5257–5262, 2006.

[24] F. P. Fiorentino, C. E. Symonds, M. MacAluso, and A. Giordano, "Senescence and p130/Rbl2: a new beginning to the end," *Cell Research*, vol. 19, no. 9, pp. 1044–1051, 2009.

[25] S. Haferkamp, S. L. Tran, T. M. Becker, L. L. Scurr, R. F. Kefford, and H. Rizos, "The relative contributions of the p53 and pRb pathways in oncogene-induced melanocyte senescence," *Aging*, vol. 1, no. 6, pp. 542–556, 2009.

[26] H. Helmbold, N. Kömm, W. Deppert, and W. Bohn, "Rb2/p130 is the dominating pocket protein in the p53-p21 DNA damage response pathway leading to senescence," *Oncogene*, vol. 28, no. 39, pp. 3456–3467, 2009.

[27] H. Helmbold, U. Galderisi, and W. Bohn, "The switch from pRb/p105 to Rb2/p130 in DNA damage and cellular senescence," *Journal of Cellular Physiology*, vol. 227, no. 2, pp. 508–513, 2012.

[28] P. D. Adams, "Remodeling chromatin for senescence," *Aging Cell*, vol. 6, no. 4, pp. 425–427, 2007.

[29] R. Zhang, W. Chen, and P. D. Adams, "Molecular dissection of formation of senescence-associated heterochromatin foci," *Molecular and Cellular Biology*, vol. 27, no. 6, pp. 2343–2358, 2007.

[30] D. Giri and M. Ittmann, "Interleukin-8 is a paracrine inducer of fibroblast growth factor 2, a stromal and epithelial growth factor in benign prostatic hyperplasia," *American Journal of Pathology*, vol. 159, no. 1, pp. 139–147, 2001.

[31] D. Giri, M. Ozen, and M. Ittmann, "Interleukin-6 is an autocrine growth factor in human prostate cancer," *American Journal of Pathology*, vol. 159, no. 6, pp. 2159–2165, 2001.

[32] M. M. Kawano, H. Ishikawa, N. Tsuyama et al., "Growth mechanism of human myeloma cells by interleukin-6," *International Journal of Hematology*, vol. 76, supplement 1, pp. 329–333, 2002.

[33] H. Nakanishi, K. Yoshioka, S. Joyama et al., "Interleukin-6/soluble interleukin-6 receptor signaling attenuates proliferation and invasion, and induces morphological changes of a newly established pleomorphic malignant fibrous histiocytoma cell line," *American Journal of Pathology*, vol. 165, no. 2, pp. 471–480, 2004.

[34] J. C. Acosta, A. O'Loghlen, A. Banito et al., "Chemokine signaling via the CXCR2 receptor reinforces senescence," *Cell*, vol. 133, no. 6, pp. 1006–1018, 2008.

[35] J. C. Acosta, A. O'Loghlen, A. Banito, S. Raguz, and J. Gil, "Control of senescence by CXCR2 and its ligands," *Cell Cycle*, vol. 7, no. 19, pp. 2956–2959, 2008.

[36] T. Kuilman and D. S. Peeper, "Senescence-messaging secretome: SMS-ing cellular stress," *Nature Reviews Cancer*, vol. 9, no. 2, pp. 81–94, 2009.

[37] K. Engström, P. Bergh, C.-G. Cederlund et al., "Irradiation of myxoid/round cell liposarcoma induces volume reduction and lipoma-like morphology," *Acta Oncologica*, vol. 46, no. 6, pp. 838–845, 2007.

[38] K.-H. von Wangenheim, H.-P. Peterson, and K. Schwenke, "A major component of radiation action: interference with intracellular control of differentiation," *International Journal of Radiation Biology*, vol. 68, no. 4, pp. 369–388, 1995.

12

Desmoplastic Small Round Blue Cell Tumor: A Review of Treatment and Potential Therapeutic Genomic Alterations

Ajaz Bulbul,[1,2] Bridget Noel Fahy,[3] Joanne Xiu,[4] Sadaf Rashad,[5] Asrar Mustafa,[6] Hatim Husain,[7] and Andrea Hayes-Jordan[8]

[1]*Department of Hematology/Oncology, Kymera Independent Physicians, Carlsbad, NM, USA*
[2]*Division of Internal Medicine, Department of Hematology/Oncology, Texas Tech University Health Sciences Center School of Medicine, Lubbock, TX, USA*
[3]*Department of Surgery, University of New Mexico, Albuquerque, NM, USA*
[4]*Caris Life Sciences, Phoenix, AZ, USA*
[5]*All Saints University School of Medicine, Roseau, Dominica*
[6]*Acharya Shri Chander College of Medical Sciences and Hospital, Jammu, India*
[7]*Moores Cancer Center, University of California, San Diego, La Jolla, CA, USA*
[8]*Department of Pediatric Surgical Oncology, University of Texas MD Anderson Cancer Center, Houston, TX, USA*

Correspondence should be addressed to Ajaz Bulbul; ajazbulbul@gmail.com

Academic Editor: Chandrajit Premanand Raut

Desmoplastic small round blue cell tumors (DSRCTs) originate from a cell with multilineage potential. A molecular hallmark of DSRCT is the EWS-WT1 reciprocal translocation. Ewing sarcoma and DSRCT are treated similarly due to similar oncogene activation pathways, and DSRCT has been represented in very limited numbers in sarcoma studies. Despite aggressive therapy, median survival ranges from 17 to 25 months, and 5-year survival rates remain around 15%, with higher survival reported among those undergoing removal of at least 90% of tumor in the absence of extraperitoneal metastasis. Almost 100% of these tumors contain t(11;22) (p13;q12) translocation, and it is likely that EWS-WT1 functions as a transcription factor possibly through WT1 targets. While there is no standard protocol for this aggressive disease, treatment usually includes the neoadjuvant HD P6 regimen (high-dose cyclophosphamide, doxorubicin, and vincristine (HD-CAV) alternating with ifosfamide and etoposide (IE) chemotherapy combined with aggressively attempted R0 resection). We aimed to review the molecular characteristics of DSRCTs to explore therapeutic opportunities for this extremely rare and aggressive cancer type.

1. Background

Desmoplastic small round blue cell tumors (DSRCTs) are a highly aggressive and rare mesenchymal tumor, of which approximately 200–450 cases have been described so far [1, 2]. DSRCT was first reported as a separate identity in 1989 by Gerald and Rosai [3] who proposed that DSRCT arose during development from a progenitor cell with potential for multiphenotypic differentiation [4].

2. Clinical Presentation

Young men comprise the vast majority of cases with a mean age at diagnosis of 22 years [2, 5, 6]. Clinically, DSRCT has been shown to have a predilection for developing in the abdominal and pelvic cavity with extra-abdominal involvement being much less common [5].

In the majority of cases, patients with DSRCT present with advanced disease. Most patients remain asymptomatic for extended periods of time, and diagnosis is made when tumor burden is significant [2]. The most common symptoms are abdominal pain and weight loss [5]. Constipation due to mass effect caused by the tumor and bowel obstruction have also been reported [2]. Due to a significant burden of peritoneal disease, some patients will present with an abdominal mass alone, but the most common presentation is abdominal distension from ascites. Liver metastases are seen both at the time of diagnosis and with relapse. Other distant sites include lymph nodes, lungs, and bones [2, 7, 8]. Omental and hepatic metastases can also be seen.

3. Histopathology

Histologically, the tumors consist of solid sheets, large nests, small clumps, or cords of cohesive, small, round, ovoid, or spindled cells lying in a hypocellular, desmoplastic, collagenous stroma [5]. Immunohistochemical staining demonstrates the divergent differentiation of the neoplastic cells. Neoplastic cells typically express epithelial (keratin and epithelial membrane antigen (EMA)), mesenchymal (vimentin), neural (CD56 and neuron-specific enolase (NSE)), and muscle (desmin) markers [4, 9]. The molecular hallmark of DSRCT is the EWS-WT1 fusion protein. The t(11;22) (p13;q12) translocation is present in virtually all cases [10–12]. The WT1 protein is a transcriptional activator of genes involved in renal and gonadal differentiation; it regulates the mesenchymal to epithelial transition that occurs in renal development. Most of these tumors contain t(11;22) (p13;q12) translocation, and it is possible that EWS-WT1 functions as a transcription factor, possibly through WT1 targets [13, 14].

4. Diagnostic Studies

CT scan with oral and intravenous contrast is the imaging modality of choice when evaluating patients with known or suspected DSRCT. Characteristic findings in DSRCT include soft tissue masses which are often bulky (mean, 6 cm; range, 1–28 cm), lobulated, and heterogeneous with hypodense areas; these findings are present in up to three-quarters of patients [15], and a significant desmoplastic reaction differentiates DSRCTs from other small round cell tumors [16]. Adenopathies are present in approximately half of patients at the time of diagnosis (intraperitoneal, retroperitoneal, and pelvic) [15, 17]. In a radiological review of 13 cases of abdominal DSRCT, the most common finding was the presence of several lobulated peritoneal soft tissue masses (mean number of masses/patient = 4). The main sites of peritoneal involvement were the pelvis, omentum, retroperitoneum, and small bowel mesentery. In six cases, moderate ascites was seen. Five of 13 patients had liver metastases, with an average of four lesions per case. Associated thoracic metastases were found in three patients [18].

MRI findings include heterogeneous T1 low signal and heterogeneous T2 high signal. After gadolinium administration, there is heterogeneous contrast enhancement. Subtle hypointense foci are sometimes seen on T2-weighted images representing desmoplastic reaction. Hyperintense T1 signal and fluid/fluid levels may suggest recent hemorrhage in a tumor [19].

FDG-PET scanning has been shown to impart important additional information and has a relevant impact on treatment planning when used in concert with CT scan [20, 21]. FDG-PET is sometimes obtained at diagnosis and during surveillance. FDG-PET/CT has been found to be superior to CT in detection of lymph node involvement (sensitivity, 95% versus 25%, resp.), bone lesions (sensitivity, 90% versus 57%, resp.), and renal lesions [20]. In a study of 65 patients, FDG uptake was seen in all primary intra-abdominal and pelvic tumors [22] and accurately detected 97% of all DSRCT lesions with sensitivity, specificity, positive, and negative predictive values of 96%, 99%, 98%, and 97%, respectively. However, CT is more reliable than FDG-PET in depicting lung metastases [20].

Core biopsy specimens are preferred to acquire sufficient sample. Fine-needle aspiration specimens, although commonly employed, are not adequate during the workup of DSRCT due to issues with low cellularity of the sample, necrosis, and predominantly a desmoplastic reaction. Fine-needle aspiration is challenging and requires pathological expertise in the utilization of ancillary techniques such as immunocytochemistry and flow cytometric immunophenotyping. The absence of the characteristic desmoplastic stroma in DSRCT and its cytologic features make cytologic interpretation difficult [23]. Characteristic cytologic features are seen in the right clinical context of small round blue cells with cytoplasmic densities and purple-stained connective stroma [24] and should raise suspicion of DSRCT that should be confirmed by its unique cytogenetic abnormality. The cells include granular chromatin and smooth to irregular nuclear membranes and show nuclear molding, cytoplasmic vacuoles, pseudorosettes, and metachromatic stroma [25] compared to other potential diagnoses like Ewing sarcoma. RT-PCR for EWS-WT1 transcript detection is a way of increasing diagnostic accuracy [26]. However, using a combination of both techniques, 86.4% of DSRCT can be typed accurately [26, 27].

5. Staging

The UICC staging of sarcoma is inadequate for DSRCT as it classifies nearly all patients as metastatic [2]. Several staging methods have been proposed for DSRCT, and there is currently no validated staging system. Due to the extensive nature of the peritoneal disease frequently present, the Peritoneal Cancer Index is often used. In this system, the abdominal cavity is divided into 13 regions, and each region is assigned a lesion size score ranging from 0 (no tumor seen) to 3 (tumor >5 cm or confluence) [28]. The MD Anderson group has suggested the inclusion of liver and extra-abdominal metastases into this staging system to adjust for the use of hyperthermic intraperitoneal chemotherapy (HIPEC) and the finding that extra-abdominal metastasis correlated with poor survival [29]. It is unclear if this strategy applies to the adult population since the median age in that study was 12 years in few who underwent HIPEC. The estimated median overall 3-year survival for patients not undergoing surgery or HIPEC was 26% compared with 71% in patients who underwent HIPEC and surgery compared with 62% who only received debulking surgery [7].

6. Imaging

CT scan with contrast is the imaging of choice for staging and surveillance. CT is more reliable than FDG-PET in depicting lung metastases [20]. Soft tissue masses seen are often bulky (mean, 6 cm; range, 1–28 cm), lobulated, and heterogeneous with hypodense areas up to three-quarters of patients. Adenopathy is present in about half the time of the diagnosis (intraperitoneal, retroperitoneal, and pelvic). Occasionally, moderate ascites is seen [18]. FDG-PET scanning has been shown to impart important additional information and has a relevant impact on changing treatment planning when used in concert with CT scan [20, 30]. FDG-PET can be used at diagnosis and during surveillance and has been found to be superior to CT in detection of lymph node involvement (sensitivity, 95% versus 25%, resp.) and bone metastases (sensitivity, 90% versus 57%, resp.) [20].

7. Molecular Findings

As in certain other tumors, the function of the Wilms tumor protein (WT1) in repressing gene transcription is lost in DSRCT [31]. There is reported loss of the zinc finger region of WT1 in EWS-WT1 which serves to convert WT1 from a repressor of transcription to a dominant transcriptional activator oncogene including some 35 target genes [14, 32]. Some of these are growth factor genes such as *PDGFα*; growth factor receptor genes such as IGF-1 receptor, EGFR, and *IL-2/15Rβ* [13, 33]; transcriptional regulators including *c-MYC, n-MYC, PAX2-2, ENT4*, and *WT-1*; and extracellular protein-encoding genes such as e-Syndecan, E-cadherin, and TALLA-1 which is a tetraspanin-family genes that encodes transmembrane proteins responsible for regulating cell adhesion, migration, and metastasis [34]. CCN2 (connective tissue growth factor) is highly expressed in DSRCT and may have autocrine or paracrine roles in disease progression [31]; however, the precise contribution of these molecular events and their potential as a therapeutic target remain poorly understood and applied.

Embryologically, WT1 is involved in urogenital development [35]. Normal WT1 protein is expressed in tissues which undergo mesenchymal-epithelial conversion from mesoderm [36] and may have a role in mesothelial formation in embryonic development [37]. This may explain the mesenchymal propensity of the tumor and some usage of the name "mesothelioblastoma." Variant fusion isoforms generated due to alternative mRNA splicing have led to discovery of two protein isoforms. Some of these cases express full-length WT1 or have variant transcripts (KTS+), resulting in atypical staining patterns. The KTS+ variant has different transcriptional targets than the KTS– isoform [38].

Neither isoform of EWS-WT1 is sufficient to transform wild-type murine embryonic fibroblasts (MEFs). The oncogenic potential of both can be unmasked by p53 loss as seen by nuclear localization of p53, and copy-number amplification and gene-set enrichment analysis demonstrated augmentation of the WNT pathway [39]. In the absence of intact p53 protein, WT1 acts as a transcriptional activator [40].

Genomic analysis on LMS, UPS, and MPNST has shown novel genetic alterations; however, DSRCT has been represented in very limited numbers [41]. Limited sequencing studies have been performed on DSRCT because of the small number of cases shown. Protein biomarkers show c-kit in 19% of cases, and HER2/neu overexpression (3+) is also seen but uncommon in desmoplastic small round cell tumors [42]. EGFR gene amplification occurs at a rate of 16.9% by FISH. This was also true for LMS, MPNST, osteosarcoma, and UPS [41].

Molecular profiling on 35 DSRCTs sampled from patients having surgery for DSRCT (Caris Life Sciences, Phoenix, AZ) that were compared with Ewing sarcoma revealed low immunogenicity (<10 mutations/Mb) and low frequency of actionable mutations including PD-L1 in both tumor types. High AR expression could present as a potential therapeutic target for DSRCT while taxanes may be more effective in Ewing sarcoma compared to DSRCT based on TUBB3 expression [43]. Given the male predominance of this subset of disease, it is not surprising that, when compared to Ewing sarcoma, no significant difference was seen in protein expressions with the exception of a significantly higher overexpression of AR in DSRCT (59% versus 3%, $p = 1.7E\text{-}10$) and TUBB3 (56% versus 29%, $p = 0.03$) [43].

There is known to be relatively low concordance across platforms and for individual genes or proteins. cKIT overexpression by IHC in one study did not associate with *cKIT* mutations [41]. This is in contrast to GIST, where more than 80% of cases carry an activating mutation in the KIT gene and more concordance is seen [44]. There is in fact quite a low frequency of actionable mutations detected in series that looked at genomic alterations which overall included only 9 patients of DSRCT [41].

Given the interest in immunotherapy, currently, most of the interest lies with PD-1 and PD-L1 inhibitors. Previous work has shown that both PD-1 positivity and PD-L1 positivity were independent prognostic indicators of OS and EFS in sarcoma [45]. Intratumoral infiltration of PD-1-positive lymphocytes and PD-L1 expression have been seen in 65% and 58% of STS, respectively [45]. PD-1 positivity and PD-L1 expression are associated with advanced clinicopathological parameters and presence of distant metastasis, and both PD-1 positivity and PD-L1 positivity are independent prognostic indicators of overall survival (OS) [45, 46]. Over 150 sarcoma subtypes have been analyzed for PD-L1 tumor expression and the presence of PD-1+ tumor-infiltrating lymphocytes (TILs): up to 65% of sarcomas expressed PD-L1 which, along with PD-1 TIL positivity, correlates with poorer overall survival and aggressive tumor features [47]. DSRCT, however, is not very well represented in these studies.

We now know that a higher mutational rate is observed in melanoma (median of 13.2 mutations per Mb) and in NSCLC, reflecting their high responses to immunotherapy. The median of somatic mutations per Mb is 10.5 for smokers and 0.6 for nonsmokers, in which mutations are known to be secondary caused by selective pressures such as UV light and tobacco smoke exposure, respectively.

Mutational loads are lower in MSS colorectal tumors (3.2 mutations per Mb), with higher mutational loads in MSI-high tumors [48] reflecting their response to PD-1 inhibitors [49]. Low mutational loads of 1.53 mutations per Mb in RCC may reflect why PD-1 staining was not suggestive of activity to nivolumab [50]. Cytokine-based immunotherapies have also shown limited benefit in the advanced setting of sarcomas. A large randomized trial of adjuvant interferon maintenance in resected osteosarcoma patients did not provide significant improvement [51]. DSRCT is not a very immunogenic tumor. Some soft tissue and bone sarcomas have been shown to express PD-1 ligand, and additional information is emerging about the role of somatic mutations in predicting response [46, 51, 52].

There is recent evidence showing SLFN11 mRNA transcript and protein levels in DSRCT-1 are comparable to EWS cell lines. Schlafen-11 (SLFN11), a putative biomarker for defective DNA damage repair, and SCRT-1 demonstrated sensitivity to PARPi as single agent or in combination with either the topoisomerase I inhibitor irinotecan or ionizing radiation [53].

8. Treatment

Aggressive attempts at R0 resection have been a cornerstone of any curative intent strategy for DSRCT. HIPEC has been shown to optimize outcomes in single-center retrospective studies for disease in the abdomen [54]. Complete cytoreduction is performed prior to HIPEC using cisplatin. Because of large tumor sizes on clinical presentation and unresectable metastatic disease, surgery is usually preceded by induction of neoadjuvant HD chemotherapy, which is followed by consolidation treatment with either radiation or myeloablative treatment (Table 1) [6, 29, 55, 56].

The surgical goal is to remove >90% of the tumor [56], and resection to less than 1.0 cm tumor size [7]. This mostly requires omentectomy, peritoneal stripping, splenectomy for hilar involvement, and local resection of the diaphragmatic peritoneum [55, 56]. Microscopic negative margins are difficult to achieve because of the desmoplastic nature of the tumor; therefore consolidative 30 Gy WAP-RT [57]/IMRT [58], HIPEC [29], [^{90}Y]yttrium microspheres radioembolotherapy [59], myeloablative chemotherapy (rarely used now) [55, 56, 60], or consolidative chemotherapy has been employed in most of these studies, and relapses occur early without consolidation. R0 resection and HIPEC to sterilize extensive peritoneal metastasis can lead to median survival of up to 63 months [54].

DSRCT is somewhat alkylator sensitive, and response seems to be dose responsive [55]. Doxorubicin is a common thread in the treatment of patients who either achieved long-term survival or had response to a standard consolidative radiotherapy dose of 30 Gy when delivered by external beam to the whole abdomen and pelvis [57, 58]. Myeloablative chemotherapy with thiotepa and carboplatin, etoposide followed by autologous bone marrow, or peripheral stem cell rescue has been employed with limited success [56, 61]. Case report of [^{90}Y]yttrium microspheres radioembolotherapy leading to a dramatic sustained reduction in the hepatic metastatic load has also been reported [59, 62].

Most of the early case reports in the last 2 decades have used standard dose alkylating agents, Adriamycin-based treatment with less than favorable responses [3, 9, 63]. Irinotecan and temozolomide combination has shown up to 68% objective response in recurrent Ewing sarcoma during early retrospective studies [64]. Phase II study (TEMIRI) of temozolamide 100–125 mg/m^2/day (days 1–5) and irinotecan 10 mg/m^2/day (days 1–5 and 8–12) every 3 weeks show responses between 33% in a familiar tumor histology of medulloblastoma with some of the patients having a desmoplastic variant [65].

Kushner et al. reported 10 patients prospectively that were the first to use high-dose alkylator-based therapy (Table 1) in an alternating 7 courses of chemotherapy regimen in 1996. The P6 regimen consisted of high-dose cyclophosphamide, doxorubicin, and vincristine (HD-CAV) on cycles 1, 2, 3, and 6 given with cyclophosphamide (4200 mg/m^2), doxorubicin (75 mg/m^2), and vincristine (HD-CAV) alternating with ifosfamide (9 to 12 mg/m^2) and etoposide (500 to 1000 mg/m^2) on cycles 4, 5, and 7. The regimen was chosen due to its prior effectiveness and experience of use in Ewing sarcomas and metastatic neuroblastoma in children and young adults where it was called the "N6" protocol; N likely represents neuroblastoma [66, 67].

A modified P6 regimen and a modified PAVEP regimen [63, 68] (cyclophosphamide, pirarubicin, etoposide, and cisplatin) have been employed to decrease severe adverse events and to improve the completion rate of chemotherapy. These modified regimens use Cytoxan of 4 g/m^2 and replace Adriamycin with pirarubicin. The modified P6 regimen use higher ifosfamide dose (12 g/m^2 divided for five days) instead of 9 g/m^2 in the original P6 regimen. The addition of irinotecan, topotecan, carboplatin, and cisplatin leads to few months of stable disease at best in selected patients [56, 57].

The insensitivity of the tumor to high-dose chemotherapy may implicate a stem cell hypothesis in DSRCT [69, 70]. This may reflect on the heterogeneity of the tumor and contribute to the general difficulty in eradicating the tumor. Unlike Ewing sarcoma, the putative CD133+ stem cell has not been identified to date [69, 70]. Quantitative real-time PCR analysis of putative stem cell maintenance revealed that CD133+ ESFT cells express significantly higher levels [70]. This could certainly explain tumor characteristics and lead to the identification of new targets for more effective therapies [70]. Radiation is more easily tolerated in pediatric patients and may improve local control [57, 58]. Most relapses are intraperitoneal and/or hepatic WAP-RT. Acute toxicities are approximately 80%, and almost a third of patients experience acute hematologic toxicity, with grade 4 thrombocytopenia seen in 76% of patients. Small bowel obstruction occurred in 7 patients (33%) after surgery and WAPI [57]. In one study, postoperative WAP-RT was predictive of 3-year overall survival, as were the absence of EPM and complete surgical resection. Heated intraperitoneal chemoinfusion with cisplatin had no impact on overall survival in that analysis [1].

9. Targeted Agents

It is unclear if, despite poor long-term outcomes, we should continue treating these patients with HD chemotherapy [2] and prolonged in-patient hospital protocols. A standard Ewing sarcoma alternating VAC/IE protocol with standard alkylator doses (Cytoxan 1200 mg/m^2 over 60 min) and 1800 mg of ifosfamide per square meter per day for five days [71], given with mesna, could be evaluated since oncogene

Table 1: Summary of patients' characteristics, treatments, and outcome in DSRCT.

Study	Number of patients	Type of study	Age range	Chemo	Cytoxan dose	Response	Survival	Additional Rx	Comment
Kushner et al. [55]	10 (untreated patients)	Prospective	7–22 (median, 14 yrs)	P6	4.2 g/m^2 over 2 days	PR 70%; CR 20% (no path CR)	Median OS 19 mo (22 for 7 pts in CR). 5 remained in CR at 38 mo	40% RT; 30% BMT; 30% ABMT[#]	1 tumor-related Budd-Chiari death. Carboplatin/ thiotepa for myeloablative transplant
Hayes-Jordan et al. [29]	24	Retrospective	8–43 (median, 12 yrs)	P6	4.2 g/m^2 over 2 days	RR not reported. Complete resection to less than 1.0 cm tumor size was achieved in all 8 patients who underwent HIPEC	3 yr OS: HIPEC + Sx = 71%; chemo/RT = 26%; Sx alone = 62%**	HIPEC cisplatin	HIPEC only used in 5–25 yr age group. Thoracic metastasis suggested poor prognosis
Lal et al. [56] (MSKCC)	66	Retrospective	7–58 (median, 19 yrs)	P6	4.2 g/m^2 over 2 days	Not reported	3 yr OS 44%; 5 yr OS 15%; 3 yr OS 58% with GTR*	CPT-11, topotecan, carboplatin, cisplatin were added in selected patients	In 71%, greater than 90% tumor resection was possible. 71% underwent Rx with P6 regimen
Farhat et al. [63]	5	Retrospective	16–26 (median 22 yrs)	PA(E)VP	900 mg/m^2 over 3 days	4 stable disease 1 CR	Mean survival 24 mo	ABMT (carboplatin, 800 mg/m^2; etoposide, 1200 mg/m^2; and ifosfamide, 6 g/m^2) in 1 patient	Chemotherapy was given adjuvantly. 1 CR was reported to have tunica vaginalis (primary)
Pinnix et al. [58]	8	Retrospective	5–20 (median, 11 yrs)	P6	4.2 g/m^2 over 2 days	5/8 had complete resection; 2/8 had near complete (>90%) resection	At 30 mo, three patients died of PD, four were alive with active disease, and one was in CR	7/8 patients had HIPEC	25% had extra-abdominal metastasis. Mean time to IMRT failure 6.6 mo. 70–80% Gr 2 GI toxicity. Limited Gr ½ hematological toxicity mostly anemia

Table 1: Continued.

Study	Number of patients	Type of study	Age range	Chemo	Cytoxan dose	Response	Survival	Additional Rx	Comment
Goodman et al. [57] (MSKCC)	21	Retrospective	8–34 (median, 16.5 yrs)	P6	4.2 g/m^2 over 2 days	Not reported. Maximal debulking in all but 1 patient	3 yr OS 48%; 3 yr RFS 14%; median OS 32 mo	Cisplatin, carboplatin, topotecan, irinotecan, and vinorelbine were also used. 30 Gy WA-XRT	Grade 4 thrombocytopenia, leukopenia, and anemia in 76%, 29%, and 33%, respectively. Bowel obstruction in 33%
Wong et al. [98]	41	Retrospective	16–45 (median, 27 yrs)	Vincristine + ifosfamide + doxorubicin + etoposide (VIDE) in a 1/3rd of 1st line Rx	Ifos 3 g/m^2 over 3 days	Not reported	3 yr OS 27%; 5 yr OS 16%	6/41 received XRT	VIDE chemotherapy appeared to confer the longest TTP (median, 14.6 months)
Aguilera et al. [73]	1 (5 yr old, only outpatient regimen)	Case report	5 yrs	VIDE (vincristine (1.5 mg/m^2), dexrazoxane/ doxorubicin (750/75 mg/m^2), and etoposide (150 mg/m^2))	Ifos 3 g/m^2 over 3 days (outpatient)	R0 resection with microscopic residual disease	Relapse at 18 months. Alive at 2 yrs after Dx	HIPEC cisplatin 100 mg/m^2 and aggressive tumor debulking. Followed by Temodar/ irinotecan maintenance x12 followed by IMRT (30 Gy)	Ifosfamide infusions were done at home with bag changes by home health nursing. Retroperitoneal relapse treated with IMRT with bevacizumab (5 mg/kg) and 2 perihepatic metastases with radiofrequency ablation/ cryoablation followed by chronic outpatient maintenance chemotherapy (valproic acid, cyclophosphamide, and rapamycin)

#ABMT = autologous myeloablative transplant. *GTR = gross tumor resection. **There was no statistical difference in estimated OS for those who received debulking surgery compared with HIPEC, in those who did not receive HIPEC. There were no survivors greater than 3 years.

activation pathways in DSRCT may be similar to those in Ewing sarcoma [72]. Some centers are using a modified P6 protocol [2, 68] which is similar to VDC/IE (vincristine, total dose of 2 mg; Adriamycin, 75 mg/m^2; and cyclophosphamide, 1200 mg/m^2 with mesna). Dactinomycin at 1.25 mg per square meter per dose is substituted for doxorubicin when a total doxorubicin dose of 375 mg per square meter is reached. Ifosfamide and etoposide are administered (1800 mg/m^2 of ifosfamide for five days, given with mesna, and 100 mg/m^2 of etoposide over five days) [71]. The Ewing sarcoma regimen whether used in a dose-dense or three weekly schedule also provides a maintenance phase of treatment of up to 49 weeks [71]. There is suggestion of longer outcomes with an outpatient maintenance therapy that consisted of irinotecan and temozolomide followed by XRT and HIPEC in a 5-year-old patient [73].

Small molecule TKIs have shown dismal results so far including sorafenib and sunitinib. In a DSRCT cell line, the mTOR inhibitor induces apoptosis [74]; in practice, however, rapamycin and temsirolimus have had limited PFS [75, 76]. Therefore, mTOR inhibition may only have a role in a combination setting rather than as single therapy. In a retrospective review of patients who received pazopanib within EORTC trials, a clinical benefit rate (PR + SD >12 weeks) of 78% was reported among patients who had progressed on prior treatments among 9 patients [77].

Recently, olaratumab, a novel PDGFRa inhibitor, was approved with doxorubicin in soft tissue sarcomas (STS) with a histology subtype for which an anthracycline-containing regimen may be appropriate; however, in the study, DSRCT was not represented [78]. DSRCT had more limited representation with pazopanib approval in the PALETTE trial [79], with eribulin [80], and with the approval of trabectedin [81].

Eribulin has shown activity in pretreated patients with L-sarcomas and recently showed a 2-month survival benefit in the phase III study compared to dacarbazine [80]; however, outcomes in pretreated patients with synovial sarcoma and other types of soft tissue sarcoma did not meet the prespecified primary efficacy endpoint for activity [82]. Ewing family tumors were excluded in the study; however, three-quarters of patients were still alive at 6 months [82], suggesting that microtubule inhibition may warrant further study since vinca alkaloids have historically shown activity with Ewing family tumors [83, 84]. We must perform tumor biomarker evaluations in these clinical trials comparing responding patients with nonresponders to understand who may truly benefit or not from these therapies [83].

Gemcitabine and docetaxel have been used as an outpatient regimen for STS other than leiomyosarcoma and could have benefit in patients unable to tolerate very aggressive chemotherapy [85–87]. A clinical trial undergoing (NCT01532687) is currently looking at gemcitabine with or without pazopanib and is currently recruiting.

IGF-1R inhibition has been seen to mitigate mTOR activation and is supported by preclinical data supporting its additive antitumor effects by combining them [88]. Cixutumumab at 6 mg/kg IV weekly was combined with temsirolimus in heavily pretreated patients with Ewing family tumors that included DSRCT with one-third of the patients achieving relatively durable CR/PR [89]. This was well tolerated, with preliminary evidence of durable antitumor activity, and attempts to evaluate response in a phase II study for STS after stratifying for the expression of IGF-1R on tumor tissue [90]. Other DSRCT targeted agents include GD2 [91] and ganitumab, a fully human monoclonal antibody against type-1 insulin-like growth factor receptor (IGF-1R), showing 6% ORR and 17 (49%) SD rate in an open label phase II trial [92]. These novel clinical trials with biomarker and molecular data-driven interventions reflect the direction this field is moving with the availability of newer diagnostic tools.

10. Role of Immunotherapy

Tumor mutational load (TML) may affect response rates to immunotherapy as seen in NSCLC and melanoma. Higher TML tumors are more responsive to immune checkpoint inhibition [52]. Single-agent anti-PD-1 antibodies have had limited efficacy across sarcomas to date. A phase II study (SARC028) is evaluating the role of pembrolizumab across various sarcoma histologies (NCT02301039) [47]. None of the patients in a recently reported DSRCT cohort had identifiable tumoral PD-L1 expression by SP142 antibody testing, and the significance of PD-1-positive TILs is unclear at this time [43]. The composite of tumoral PD-L1 positivity and PD-1 positivity among tumor-infiltrating lymphocytes has been suggested as an indicator of prognosis in soft tissue sarcoma patients [45]. Another small, but heterogeneous, patient cohort at MSKCC demonstrated no association between PD-L1 expression, TIL and clinicopathological features, and overall survival using the DAKO 5H-1 antibody [93]. DSRCT patients, however, were not represented in these small data sets. B7H3, an immunomodulatory cell surface molecule, is seen in >90% DSRCTs. In a phase I study, a radioimmunoconjugate showed promise in an ongoing clinical trial (NCT01099644).

11. Future Directions

An ongoing NCT01189643 trial is looking at addition of two cycles of irinotecan, temozolomide, and bevacizumab followed by a standard P6 protocol utilizing the data, suggesting that VEGFR-2 and VEGFA overexpress in DSRCT cell lines and xenograft models [94]. A pilot study evaluating the combination of irinotecan, temozolomide, and bevacizumab is active in patients with DSRCT, and it is feasible to combine these agents with standard chemotherapy without greater than expected toxicity with response rates around 27% [95].

A phase I/II clinical trial is studying the side effects and the most effective dose of the notch signaling pathway inhibitor RO4929097 when given together with vismodegib in DSRCT patients (NCT01154452). A study looking at intraperitoneal radioimmunotherapy with a novel antibody 8H9 for patients with DSRCT is also recruiting (NCT01099644).

A current study which is ongoing but not recruiting adds irinotecan, temozolomide, and bevacizumab to the chemotherapy regimen currently used in DSRCT. An ongoing phase II study (SARC028) is looking at the role of pembrolizumab in

TABLE 2: Clinical trials recently completed in DSRCT.

Clinical trial (ID); phase	Drugs	Status	Assigned intervention
NCT01154452; phase 1B/II	Vismodegib (hedgehog inhibitor) and NOTCH inhibitor RO4929097	Completed	Vismodegib and Gamma-Secretase/Notch Signalling Pathway Inhibitor RO4929097 in Treating Patients with Advanced or Metastatic Sarcoma
NCT00563680; phase II	Drug: AMG 479 (IGF-R1 Ab)	Completed	QUILT-3.025: A Phase 2 Study of AMG 479 in Relapsed or Refractory Ewing's Family Tumor and Desmoplastic Small Round Cell Tumors
NCT00062205; phase I, II	Drug: imatinib mesylate	Completed	Imatinib Mesylate in Treating Patients With Recurrent Ewing's Family of Tumors or Desmoplastic Small Round Cell Tumor
NCT00055952; phase II	Drug: exatecan mesylate (camptothecin)	Completed	Exatecan Mesylate in Treating Patients With Ewing's Sarcoma, Primitive Neuroectodermal Tumor, or Desmoplastic Small Round Cell Tumor
NCT00720174; phase I	Biological: cixutumumab (IGF-1R Ab); drug: doxorubicin hydrochloride; other: laboratory biomarker analysis	Completed	Cixutumumab and Doxorubicin Hydrochloride in Treating Patients With Unresectable, Locally Advanced, or Metastatic Soft Tissue Sarcoma
NCT00436657; phase I	Drug: CHPP of cisplatin; procedure: abdominal surgery	Completed	Continuous Hyperthermic Peritoneal Perfusion (CHPP) With Cisplatin for Children With Peritoneal Cancer
NCT00093821; phase I	Drug: tanespimycin (HSP90 inhibitor)	Completed	Tanespimycin in Treating Young Patients With Recurrent or Refractory Leukemia or Solid Tumors

TABLE 3: Ongoing clinical trials in DSRCT.

Clinical trial (ID); phase	Drugs	Current status	Assigned intervention
NCT01189643; pilot study	CPT-11, TMZ, bevacizumab	Ongoing but not recruiting	Two cycles of the investigational combination irinotecan, temozolomide, and bevacizumab will be given followed by conventional chemotherapy with a modified P6 approach and surgical local control. Completion of modified P6 chemotherapy will be followed by a second-look surgery
NCT01099644; phase I	Biological: ^{131}I-8H9	Recruiting	Intraperitoneal Radioimmunotherapy With ^{131}I-8H9 for Patients With Desmoplastic Small Round Cell Tumors and Other Solid Tumors Involving the Peritoneum
NCT02173093; phase I	Biological: IL-2 | biological: GD2Bi-aATC | biological: GM-CSF	Recruiting	Activated T Cells Armed With GD2 Bispecific Antibody in Children and Young Adults With Neuroblastoma and Osteosarcoma, DSRCT
NCT02982941; phase I	Drug: enoblituzumab	Recruiting	Enoblituzumab (MGA271) in Children With B7-H3-expressing Solid Tumors
NCT01532687; phase II	Gemcitabine ± pazopanib	Recruiting	Gemcitabine Hydrochloride With or Without Pazopanib Hydrochloride in Treating Patients With Refractory Soft Tissue Sarcoma
NCT00089245; phase I	Radiation: iodine I-131 monoclonal antibody 8H9	Recruiting	Radiolabeled Monoclonal Antibody Therapy in Treating Patients with Refractory, Recurrent, or Advanced CNS or Leptomeningeal Cancer/Sarcomas

sarcoma (NCT01189643). Similar to many general sarcoma studies, DSRCT is not represented in this study because of the limited number of patients with this disease.

12. Conclusion

Because of the rarity of DSRCT, limited data are available regarding the impact of various treatment modalities on survival. Aggressive surgery, radiotherapy, and chemotherapy have all been used to control DSRCT. Unfortunately, durable responses are limited, and the prognosis for patients with DSRCT remains poor [1]. The largest available single-institution study of 66 patients with DSRCT reported a 3-year and 5-year overall survival rate of 44% and 15%, respectively. Use of a combined surgery and a Ewing-based chemotherapy regimen of vincristine, doxorubicin, and cyclophosphamide (VAC) and ifosfamide + etoposide (IE) in various combinations achieves a maximal tumor debulking and is associated with improved overall survival relative to other chemotherapy regimens. Greater than 90% tumor resection was highly significant in prolonging overall survival compared to lesser resections [56]. The impact of optimal debulking was also confirmed in these studies [7, 29].

High-dose chemotherapy, radiotherapy to high-risk sites, and myeloablative chemotherapy with stem cell rescue have been described in selected cases [55]. Some investigators have described the use of cytoreduction and hyperthermic intraperitoneal chemotherapy using cisplatin for treatment of carcinomatosis and yttrium microspheres for treatment of liver metastasis from DSRCT [7]. Consolidative IMRT after debulking and/or HIPEC although used can lead to suboptimal outcomes secondary to GI and hematological toxicities and inferior DFS [96, 97]. Based upon the available data, the treatment strategy currently associated with the best overall survival includes optimal resection of ≥90% of the tumor and high-dose chemotherapy regimens. Given the significant tumor response seen in many patients following systemic chemotherapy, deferring resection until a maximal response to systemic therapy is achieved is currently advocated by some clinical investigators [62].

Little progress has been made in the field of small molecule TKIs for sarcomas since the approval of imatinib for GIST in 2002, and despite the recent FDA approval of the multi-tyrosine kinase inhibitor pazopanib, any direct efficacy for DSRCT is limited and from small retrospective studies. Rather than pursuing different chemotherapy combinations without a solid genomic basis, the field has moved to patient selection based on identifying the optimal combination of targeted therapy, chemotherapy based on chemotherapy sensitivity studies and possibly for high mutational load patient checkpoint inhibitors, or immunotherapy using a tumor signature to determine an approach so as to improve outcomes in clinically applicable ways.

A collaborative effort to include DSRCTs in clinical trials with targeted agents is crucial to determine if there truly is a clinical benefit from this novel treatment option. Recently concluded trials are eagerly awaiting to provide insight into these questions (Table 2) to show a hitherto unsurpassed survival benefit of 26.5 months in SRS with the drug olaratumab and have prompted an accelerated FDA approval in October 2016.

It is unlikely that combinational chemotherapy will significantly improve outcomes in DSRCT. Surgery should remain the cornerstone of treatment. Extended genome sequencing and immunotherapy are being assessed in future clinical trials (Table 3), and it remains to be determined what the role will be in the future for many of the emerging agents.

References

[1] C. Honore, K. Amroun, L. Vilcot et al., "Abdominal desmoplastic small round cell tumor: multimodal treatment combining chemotherapy, surgery, and radiotherapy is the best option," *Annals of Surgical Oncology*, vol. 22, no. 4, pp. 1073–1079, 2015.

[2] A. Dufresne, P. Cassier, L. Couraud et al., "Desmoplastic small round cell tumor: current management and recent findings," *Sarcoma*, vol. 2012, Article ID 714986, 5 pages, 2012.

[3] W. L. Gerald and J. Rosai, "Case 2 desmoplastic small cell tumor with divergent differentiation," *Pediatric Pathology*, vol. 9, no. 2, pp. 177–183, 1989.

[4] W. L. Gerald and J. Rosai, "Desmoplastic small cell tumor with multi-phenotypic differentiation," *Zentralblatt für Pathologie*, vol. 139, no. 2, pp. 141–151, 1993.

[5] M. E. Lae, P. C. Roche, L. Jin, R. V. Lloyd, and A. G. Nascimento, "Desmoplastic small round cell tumor: a clinicopathologic, immunohistochemical, and molecular study of 32 tumors," *American Journal of Surgical Pathology*, vol. 26, no. 7, pp. 823–835, 2002.

[6] R. E. Schwarz, W. L. Gerald, B. H. Kushner, D. G. Coit, M. F. Brennan, and M. P. La Quaglia, "Desmoplastic small round cell tumors: prognostic indicators and results of surgical management," *Annals of Surgical Oncology*, vol. 5, no. 5, pp. 416–422, 1998.

[7] A. Hayes-Jordan and P. M. Anderson, "The diagnosis and management of desmoplastic small round cell tumor: a review," *Current Opinion in Oncology*, vol. 23, no. 4, pp. 385–389, 2011.

[8] E. A. Albano and J. Kanter, "Images in clinical medicine. Sister Mary Joseph's nodule," *New England Journal of Medicine*, vol. 352, no. 18, p. 1913, 2005.

[9] W. L. Gerald, H. K. Miller, H. Battifora, M. Miettinen, E. G. Silva, and J. Rosai, "Intra-abdominal desmoplastic small round-cell tumor. Report of 19 cases of a distinctive type of high-grade polyphenotypic malignancy affecting young individuals," *American Journal of Surgical Pathology*, vol. 15, no. 6, pp. 499–513, 1991.

[10] C. R. Antonescu, W. L. Gerald, M. S. Magid, and M. Ladanyi, "Molecular variants of the EWS-WT1 gene fusion in desmoplastic small round cell tumor," *Diagnostic Molecular Pathology*, vol. 7, no. 1, pp. 24–28, 1998.

[11] W. L. Gerald, J. Rosai, and M. Ladanyi, "Characterization of the genomic breakpoint and chimeric transcripts in the EWS-WT1 gene fusion of desmoplastic small round cell tumor," *Proceedings of the National Academy of Sciences of the United States of America*, vol. 92, no. 4, pp. 1028–1032, 1995.

[12] J. Liu, M. M. Nau, J. C. Yeh, C. J. Allegra, E. Chu, and J. J. Wright, "Molecular heterogeneity and function of EWS-WT1 fusion transcripts in desmoplastic small round cell tumors," *Clinical Cancer Research*, vol. 6, no. 9, pp. 3522–3529, 2000.

[13] S. B. Lee, K. A. Kolquist, K. Nichols et al., "The EWS-WT1 translocation product induces PDGFA in desmoplastic small round-cell tumour," *Nature Genetics*, vol. 17, no. 3, pp. 309–313, 1997.

[14] B. S. Worley, L. T. van den Broeke, T. J. Goletz et al., "Antigenicity of fusion proteins from sarcoma-associated chromosomal translocations," *Cancer Research*, vol. 61, no. 18, pp. 6868–6875, 2001.

[15] J. Chen, Z. Wu, B. Sun et al., "Intra-abdominal desmoplastic small round cell tumors: CT and FDG-PET/CT findings with histopathological association," *Oncology Letters*, vol. 11, no. 5, pp. 3298–3302, 2016.

[16] R. Thomas, G. Rajeswaran, K. Thway, C. Benson, K. Shahabuddin, and E. Moskovic, "Desmoplastic small round cell tumour: the radiological, pathological and clinical features," *Insights into Imaging*, vol. 4, no. 1, pp. 111–118, 2013.

[17] B. Kis, K. N. O'Regan, A. Agoston, O. Javery, J. Jagannathan, and N. H. Ramaiya, "Imaging of desmoplastic small round cell tumour in adults," *British Journal of Radiology*, vol. 85, no. 1010, pp. 187–192, 2012.

[18] M. Chouli, J. Viala, C. Dromain, K. Fizazi, P. Duvillard, and D. Vanel, "Intra-abdominal desmoplastic small round cell tumors: CT findings and clinicopathological correlations in 13 cases," *European Journal of Radiology*, vol. 54, no. 3, pp. 438–442, 2005.

[19] R. A. Vicens, M. Patnana, O. Le et al., "Multimodality imaging of common and uncommon peritoneal diseases: a review for radiologists," *Abdominal Imaging*, vol. 40, no. 2, pp. 436–456, 2015.

[20] T. Volker, T. Denecke, I. Steffen et al., "Positron emission tomography for staging of pediatric sarcoma patients: results of a prospective multicenter trial," *Journal of Clinical Oncology*, vol. 25, no. 34, pp. 5435–5441, 2007.

[21] A. Ostermeier, M. B. McCarville, F. Navid, S. E. Snyder, and B. L. Shulkin, "FDG PET/CT imaging of desmoplastic small round cell tumor: findings at staging, during treatment and at follow up," *Pediatric Radiology*, vol. 45, no. 9, pp. 1308–1315, 2015.

[22] V. C. Arora, A. P. Price, S. Fleming et al., "Characteristic imaging features of desmoplastic small round cell tumour," *Pediatric Radiology*, vol. 43, no. 1, pp. 93–102, 2013.

[23] N. P. Caraway, C. V. Fanning, R. J. Amato, N. G. Ordóñez, and R. L. Katz, "Fine-needle aspiration of intra-abdominal desmoplastic small cell tumor," *Diagnostic Cytopathology*, vol. 9, no. 4, pp. 465–470, 1993.

[24] J. Klijanienko, P. Colin, J. Couturier et al., "Fine-needle aspiration in desmoplastic small round cell tumor: a report of 10 new tumors in 8 patients with clinicopathological and molecular correlations with review of the literature," *Cancer Cytopathology*, vol. 122, no. 5, pp. 386–393, 2014.

[25] J. P. Crapanzano, M. Cardillo, O. Lin, and M. F. Zakowski, "Cytology of desmoplastic small round cell tumor," *Cancer*, vol. 96, no. 1, pp. 21–31, 2002.

[26] Z. Pohar-Marinsek, "Difficulties in diagnosing small round cell tumours of childhood from fine needle aspiration cytology samples," *Cytopathology*, vol. 19, no. 2, pp. 67–79, 2008.

[27] U. Gautam, R. Srinivasan, A. Rajwanshi, D. Bansal, and R. K. Marwaha, "Comparative evaluation of flow-cytometric immunophenotyping and immunocytochemistry in the categorization of malignant small round cell tumors in fine-needle aspiration cytologic specimens," *Cancer*, vol. 114, no. 6, pp. 494–503, 2008.

[28] R. L. Harmon and P. H. Sugarbaker, "Prognostic indicators in peritoneal carcinomatosis from gastrointestinal cancer," *International Seminars in Surgical Oncology*, vol. 2, no. 1, p. 3, 2005.

[29] A. Hayes-Jordan, H. Green, N. Fitzgerald, L. Xiao, and P. Anderson, "Novel treatment for desmoplastic small round cell tumor: hyperthermic intraperitoneal perfusion," *Journal of Pediatric Surgery*, vol. 45, no. 5, pp. 1000–1006, 2010.

[30] S. M. Schuetze, "Utility of positron emission tomography in sarcomas," *Current Opinion in Oncology*, vol. 18, no. 4, pp. 369–373, 2006.

[31] A. W. Rachfal, M. H. Luquette, and D. R. Brigstock, "Expression of connective tissue growth factor (CCN2) in desmoplastic small round cell tumour," *Journal of Clinical Pathology*, vol. 57, no. 4, pp. 422–425, 2004.

[32] V. Scharnhorst, A. J. van der Eb, and A. G. Jochemsen, "WT1 proteins: functions in growth and differentiation," *Gene*, vol. 273, no. 2, pp. 141–161, 2001.

[33] J. C. Wong, S. B. Lee, M. D. Bell et al., "Induction of the interleukin-2/15 receptor beta-chain by the EWS-WT1 translocation product," *Oncogene*, vol. 21, no. 13, pp. 2009–2019, 2002.

[34] E. Ito, R. Honma, J. Imai et al., "A tetraspanin-family protein, T-cell acute lymphoblastic leukemia-associated antigen 1, is induced by the Ewing's sarcoma-Wilms' tumor 1 fusion protein of desmoplastic small round-cell tumor," *American Journal of Pathology*, vol. 163, no. 6, pp. 2165–2172, 2003.

[35] T. A. Natoli, J. A. Alberta, A. Bortvin et al., "Wt1 functions in the development of germ cells in addition to somatic cell lineages of the testis," *Developmental Biology*, vol. 268, no. 2, pp. 429–440, 2004.

[36] J. F. Armstrong, K. Pritchard-Jones, W. A. Bickmore, N. D. Hastie, and J. B. Bard, "The expression of the Wilms' tumour gene, WT1, in the developing mammalian embryo," *Mechanisms of Development*, vol. 40, no. 1-2, pp. 85–97, 1993.

[37] A. K. Charles, S. Mall, J. Watson, and P. J. Berry, "Expression of the Wilms' tumour gene WT1 in the developing human and in paediatric renal tumours: an immunohistochemical study," *Molecular Pathology*, vol. 50, no. 3, pp. 138–144, 1997.

[38] A. J. Murphy, K. Bishop, C. Pereira et al., "A new molecular variant of desmoplastic small round cell tumor: significance of WT1 immunostaining in this entity," *Human Pathology*, vol. 39, no. 12, pp. 1763–1770, 2008.

[39] P. Bandopadhayay, A. M. Jabbour, C. Riffkin et al., "The oncogenic properties of EWS/WT1 of desmoplastic small round cell tumors are unmasked by loss of p53 in murine embryonic fibroblasts," *BMC Cancer*, vol. 13, no. 1, p. 585, 2013.

[40] A. A. Sandberg and J. A. Bridge, "Updates on the cytogenetics and molecular genetics of bone and soft tissue tumors. desmoplastic small round-cell tumors," *Cancer Genetics and Cytogenetics*, vol. 138, no. 1, pp. 1–10, 2002.

[41] S. Movva, W. Wen, W. Chen et al., "Multi-platform profiling of over 2000 sarcomas: identification of biomarkers and novel therapeutic targets," *Oncotarget*, vol. 6, no. 14, pp. 12234–12247, 2015.

[42] P. J. Zhang, J. R. Goldblum, B. R. Pawel, C. Fisher, T. L. Pasha, and F. G. Barr, "Immunophenotype of desmoplastic small round cell tumors as detected in cases with EWS-WT1 gene fusion product," *Modern Pathology*, vol. 16, no. 3, pp. 229–235, 2003.

[43] J. Xiu, A. Bulbul, and S. Rashad, "Potential therapeutic genomic alterations in desmoplastic small round blue cell tumor," *Journal of Clinical Oncology*, vol. 35, no. 15, p. 11066, 2017.

[44] S. Hirota, K. Isozaki, Y. Moriyama et al., "Gain-of-function mutations of c-kit in human gastrointestinal stromal tumors," *Science*, vol. 279, no. 5350, pp. 577–580, 1998.

[45] J. R. Kim, Y. J. Moon, K. S. Kwon et al., "Tumor infiltrating PD1-positive lymphocytes and the expression of PD-L1 predict poor prognosis of soft tissue sarcomas," *PLoS One*, vol. 8, no. 12, p. e82870, 2013.

[46] L. Paoluzzi, M. V. Ghesani, A. Cacavio, A. Rapkiewicz, and G. Rosen, "Anti-PD1 therapy with nivolumab in sarcoma," *Journal of Clinical Oncology*, vol. 34, no. 15, p. 11047, 2016.

[47] M. A. Burgess, J. Crowley, D. K. Reinke et al., "SARC 028: a phase II study of the anti-PD1 antibody pembrolizumab (P) in patients (Pts) with advanced sarcomas," *Journal of Clinical Oncology*, vol. 33, no. 15, p. TPS10578, 2015.

[48] B. Timmermann, M. Kerick, C. Roehr et al., "Somatic mutation profiles of MSI and MSS colorectal cancer identified by whole exome next generation sequencing and bioinformatics analysis," *PLoS One*, vol. 5, no. 12, p. e15661, 2010.

[49] D. T. Le, J. N. Uram, H. Wang et al., "PD-1 blockade in tumors with mismatch-repair deficiency," *New England Journal of Medicine*, vol. 372, no. 26, pp. 2509–2520, 2015.

[50] R. J. Motzer, B. Escudier, D. F. McDermott et al., "Nivolumab versus everolimus in advanced renal-cell carcinoma," *New England Journal of Medicine*, vol. 373, no. 19, pp. 1803–1813, 2015.

[51] M. Burgess and H. Tawbi, "Immunotherapeutic approaches to sarcoma," *Current Treatment Options in Oncology*, vol. 16, no. 6, p. 26, 2015.

[52] S. Champiat, C. Ferté, S. Lebel-Binay, A. Eggermont, and J. C. Soria, "Exomics and immunogenics: bridging mutational load and immune checkpoints efficacy," *Oncoimmunology*, vol. 3, no. 1, p. e27817, 2014.

[53] M. Mellado-Lagarde, S. M. Federico, C. Tinkle, A. Shelat, and E. Stewart, "PARP inhibitor combination therapy in desmoplastic small round cell tumors," *Journal of Clinical Oncology*, vol. 35, no. 15, p. e23212, 2017.

[54] A. Hayes-Jordan, H. L. Green, H. Lin et al., "Complete cytoreduction and HIPEC improves survival in desmoplastic small round cell tumor," *Annals of Surgical Oncology*, vol. 21, no. 1, pp. 220–224, 2014.

[55] B. H. Kushner, M. P. LaQuaglia, N. Wollner et al., "Desmoplastic small round-cell tumor: prolonged progression-free survival with aggressive multimodality therapy," *Journal of Clinical Oncology*, vol. 14, no. 5, pp. 1526–1531, 1996.

[56] D. R. Lal, W. T. Su, S. L. Wolden, K. C. Loh, S. Modak, and M. P. La Quaglia, "Results of multimodal treatment for desmoplastic small round cell tumors," *Journal of Pediatric Surgery*, vol. 40, no. 1, pp. 251–255, 2005.

[57] K. A. Goodman, S. L. Wolden, M. P. La Quaglia, and B. H. Kushner, "Whole abdominopelvic radiotherapy for desmoplastic small round-cell tumor," *International Journal of Radiation Oncology, Biology, Physics*, vol. 54, no. 1, pp. 170–176, 2002.

[58] C. C. Pinnix, H. P. Fontanilla, A. Hayes-Jordan et al., "Whole abdominopelvic intensity-modulated radiation therapy for desmoplastic small round cell tumor after surgery," *International Journal of Radiation Oncology, Biology, Physics*, vol. 83, no. 1, pp. 317–326, 2012.

[59] V. Subbiah, R. Murthy, and P. M. Anderson, "[^{90}Y]Yttrium microspheres radioembolotherapy in desmoplastic small round cell tumor hepatic metastases," *Journal of Clinical Oncology*, vol. 29, no. 11, pp. e292–e294, 2011.

[60] M. Mazuryk, A. H. Paterson, W. Temple, K. Arthur, T. Crabtree, and D. A. Stewart, "Benefit of aggressive multimodality therapy with autologous stem cell support for intra-abdominal desmoplastic small round cell tumor," *Bone Marrow Transplantation*, vol. 21, no. 9, pp. 961–963, 1998.

[61] G. Bisogno, A. Ferrari, A. Rosolen et al., "Sequential intensified chemotherapy with stem cell rescue for children and adolescents with desmoplastic small round-cell tumor," *Bone Marrow Transplantation*, vol. 45, no. 5, pp. 907–911, 2010.

[62] A. Hayes-Jordan, M. P. LaQuaglia, and S. Modak, "Management of desmoplastic small round cell tumor," *Seminars in Pediatric Surgery*, vol. 25, no. 5, pp. 299–304, 2016.

[63] F. Farhat, S. Culine, C. Lhomme et al., "Desmoplastic small round cell tumors: results of a four-drug chemotherapy regimen in five adult patients," *Cancer*, vol. 77, no. 7, pp. 1363–1366, 1996.

[64] D. A. Casey, L. H. Wexler, M. S. Merchant et al., "Irinotecan and temozolomide for Ewing sarcoma: the Memorial Sloan-Kettering experience," *Pediatric Blood & Cancer*, vol. 53, no. 6, pp. 1029–1034, 2009.

[65] J. Grill, B. Geoerger, L. Gesner et al., "Phase II study of irinotecan in combination with temozolomide (TEMIRI) in children with recurrent or refractory medulloblastoma: a joint ITCC and SIOPE brain tumor study," *Neuro-Oncology*, vol. 15, no. 9, pp. 1236–1243, 2013.

[66] B. H. Kushner, P. A. Meyers, W. L. Gerald et al., "Very-high-dose short-term chemotherapy for poor-risk peripheral primitive neuroectodermal tumors, including Ewing's sarcoma, in children and young adults," *Journal of Clinical Oncology*, vol. 13, no. 11, pp. 2796–2804, 1995.

[67] B. H. Kushner, M. P. LaQuaglia, M. A. Bonilla et al., "Highly effective induction therapy for stage 4 neuroblastoma in children over 1 year of age," *Journal of Clinical Oncology*, vol. 12, no. 12, pp. 2607–2613, 1994.

[68] T. Watanabe, S. Miyamoto, K. Kitagori et al., "A case of long-term survival of metastatic desmoplastic small round cell tumor treated with multimodal therapy," *Oncology Letters*, vol. 3, no. 1, pp. 30–34, 2012.

[69] J. E. Visvader and G. J. Lindeman, "Cancer stem cells in solid tumours: accumulating evidence and unresolved questions," *Nature Reviews Cancer*, vol. 8, no. 10, pp. 755–768, 2008.

[70] M. L. Suva, N. Riggi, J. C. Stehle et al., "Identification of cancer stem cells in Ewing's sarcoma," *Cancer Research*, vol. 69, no. 5, pp. 1776–1781, 2009.

[71] H. E. Grier, M. D. Krailo, N. J. Tarbell et al., "Addition of ifosfamide and etoposide to standard chemotherapy for Ewing's sarcoma and primitive neuroectodermal tumor of bone," *New England Journal of Medicine*, vol. 348, no. 8, pp. 694–701, 2009.

[72] H. Werner, G. Idelman, M. Rubinstein, P. Pattee, S. R. Nagalla, and C. T. Roberts Jr., "A novel EWS-WT1 gene fusion product in desmoplastic small round cell tumor is a potent transactivator of the insulin-like growth factor-I receptor (IGF-IR) gene," *Cancer Letters*, vol. 247, no. 1, pp. 84–90, 2007.

[73] D. Aguilera, A. Hayes-Jordan, P. Anderson, S. Woo, M. Pearson, and H. Green, "Outpatient and home chemotherapy with novel local control strategies in desmoplastic small round cell tumor," *Sarcoma*, vol. 2008, Article ID 261589, 9 pages, 2008.

[74] O. M. Tirado, S. Mateo-Lozano, and V. Notario, "Rapamycin induces apoptosis of JN-DSRCT-1 cells by increasing the Bax : Bcl-xL ratio through concurrent mechanisms dependent and independent of its mTOR inhibitory activity," *Oncogene*, vol. 24, no. 20, pp. 3348–3357, 2005.

[75] A. M. Thijs, W. T. van der Graaf, and C. M. van Herpen, "Temsirolimus for metastatic desmoplastic small round cell tumor," *Pediatric Blood & Cancer*, vol. 55, no. 7, pp. 1431-1432, 2010.

[76] A. Dimitrakopoulou-Strauss, P. Hohenberger, P. Strobel, A. Marx, and L. G. Strauss, "A recent application of fluoro-18-deoxyglucose positron emission tomography, treatment monitoring with a mammalian target of rapamycin inhibitor: an example of a patient with a desmoplastic small round cell tumor," *Hellenic Journal of Nuclear Medicine*, vol. 10, no. 2, pp. 77–79, 2007.

[77] A. M. Frezza, C. Benson, I. R. Judson et al., "Pazopanib in advanced desmoplastic small round cell tumours: a multi-institutional experience," *Clinical Sarcoma Research*, vol. 4, p. 7, 2014.

[78] W. D. Tap, R. L. Jones, B. A. Van Tine et al., "Olaratumab and doxorubicin versus doxorubicin alone for treatment of soft-tissue sarcoma: an open-label phase 1b and randomised phase 2 trial," *Lancet*, vol. 388, no. 10043, pp. 488–497, 2016.

[79] W. T. van der Graaf, J. Y. Blay, S. P. Chawla et al., "Pazopanib for metastatic soft-tissue sarcoma (PALETTE): a randomised,

double-blind, placebo-controlled phase 3 trial," *Lancet*, vol. 379, no. 9829, pp. 1879–1886, 2012.

[80] P. Schoffski, S. Chawla, R. G. Maki et al., "Eribulin versus dacarbazine in previously treated patients with advanced liposarcoma or leiomyosarcoma: a randomised, open-label, multicentre, phase 3 trial," *Lancet*, vol. 387, no. 10028, pp. 1629–1637, 2016.

[81] G. D. Demetri, M. von Mehren, R. L. Jones et al., "Efficacy and safety of trabectedin or dacarbazine for metastatic liposarcoma or leiomyosarcoma after failure of conventional chemotherapy: results of a phase III randomized multicenter clinical trial," *Journal of Clinical Oncology*, vol. 34, no. 8, pp. 786–793, 2016.

[82] P. Schoffski, I. L. Ray-Coquard, A. Cioffi et al., "Activity of eribulin mesylate in patients with soft-tissue sarcoma: a phase 2 study in four independent histological subtypes," *Lancet Oncology*, vol. 12, no. 11, pp. 1045–1052, 2011.

[83] R. G. Maki, "Eribulin in soft-tissue sarcomas," *Lancet Oncology*, vol. 12, no. 11, pp. 988-989, 2011.

[84] E. K. Rowinsky and R. C. Donehower, "The clinical pharmacology and use of antimicrotubule agents in cancer chemotherapeutics," *Pharmacology & Therapeutics*, vol. 52, no. 1, pp. 35–84, 1991.

[85] M. L. Hensley, R. Maki, E. Venkatraman et al., "Gemcitabine and docetaxel in patients with unresectable leiomyosarcoma: results of a phase II trial," *Journal of Clinical Oncology*, vol. 20, no. 12, pp. 2824–2831, 2002.

[86] K. M. Leu, L. J. Ostruszka, D. Shewach et al., "Laboratory and clinical evidence of synergistic cytotoxicity of sequential treatment with gemcitabine followed by docetaxel in the treatment of sarcoma," *Journal of Clinical Oncology*, vol. 22, no. 9, pp. 1706–1712, 2004.

[87] J. O. Bay, I. Ray-Coquard, J. Fayette et al., "Docetaxel and gemcitabine combination in 133 advanced soft-tissue sarcomas: a retrospective analysis," *International Journal of Cancer*, vol. 119, no. 3, pp. 706–711, 2006.

[88] R. T. Kurmasheva, L. Dudkin, C. Billups, L. V. Debelenko, C. L. Morton, and P. J. Houghton, "The insulin-like growth factor-1 receptor-targeting antibody, CP-751,871, suppresses tumor-derived VEGF and synergizes with rapamycin in models of childhood sarcoma," *Cancer Research*, vol. 69, no. 19, pp. 7662–7671, 2009.

[89] A. Naing, P. LoRusso, S. Fu et al., "Insulin growth factor-receptor (IGF-1R) antibody cixutumumab combined with the mTOR inhibitor temsirolimus in patients with refractory Ewing's sarcoma family tumors," *Clinical Cancer Research*, vol. 18, no. 9, pp. 2625–2631, 2012.

[90] S. P. D'Angelo, A. N. Shoushtari, N. P. Agaram et al., "PD-L1 expression and immune infiltrates in sarcoma," *Journal of Clinical Oncology*, vol. 32, no. 15, p. 10522, 2014.

[91] S. Modak, W. Gerald, and N. K. Cheung, "Disialoganglioside GD2 and a novel tumor antigen: potential targets for immunotherapy of desmoplastic small round cell tumor," *Medical and Pediatric Oncology*, vol. 39, no. 6, pp. 547–551, 2002.

[92] W. D. Tap, G. Demetri, P. Barnette et al., "Phase II study of Ganitumab, a fully human anti-type-1 insulin-like growth factor receptor antibody, in patients with metastatic Ewing family tumors or desmoplastic small round cell tumors," *Journal of Clinical Oncology*, vol. 30, no. 15, pp. 1849–1856, 2016.

[93] S. P. D'Angelo, A. N. Shoushtari, N. P. Agaram et al., "Prevalence of tumor infiltrating lymphocytes and PD-L1 expression in the soft tissue sarcoma microenvironment," *Human Pathology*, vol. 46, no. 3, pp. 357–365, 2015.

[94] H. D. Magnan, T. Chou, M. P. LaQuaglia, W. Gerald, M. Ladanyi, and M. S. Merchant, "Elevated expression of VEGFR-2 and VEGFA in desmoplastic small round cell tumor (DSRCT) and activity of bevacizumab and irinotecan in a xenograft model of DSRCT," *Journal of Clinical Oncology*, vol. 27, no. 15, p. 20, 2016.

[95] H. D. Magnan, A. Price, A. J. Chou et al., "A pilot trial of irinotecan, temozolomide and bevacizumab (ITB) for treatment of newly diagnosed patients with desmoplastic small round cell tumor (DSRCT)," in *Proceedings of American Society of Clinical Oncology Annual Meeting Abstracts ASCO'17*, Chicago, IL, USA, July 2017.

[96] N. B. Desai, N. F. Stein, M. P. LaQuaglia et al., "Reduced toxicity with intensity modulated radiation therapy (IMRT) for desmoplastic small round cell tumor (DSRCT): an update on the whole abdominopelvic radiation therapy (WAP-RT) experience," *International Journal of Radiation Oncology, Biology, Physics*, vol. 85, no. 1, pp. e67–e72, 2013.

[97] E. M. Osborne, T. M. Briere, and A. Hayes-Jordan, "Survival and toxicity following sequential multimodality treatment including whole abdominopelvic radiotherapy for patients with desmoplastic small round cell tumor," *Radiotherapy and Oncology*, vol. 119, no. 1, pp. 40–44, 2017.

[98] H. H. Wong, H. M. Hatcher, C. Benson et al., "Desmoplastic small round cell tumour: characteristics and prognostic factors of 41 patients and review of the literature," *Clinical Sarcoma Research*, vol. 3, no. 1, p. 14, 2013.

Histopathological Diagnostic Discrepancies in Soft Tissue Tumours Referred to a Specialist Centre: Reassessment in the Era of Ancillary Molecular Diagnosis

Khin Thway, Jayson Wang, Taka Mubako, and Cyril Fisher

Sarcoma Unit, Department of Histopathology, The Royal Marsden NHS Foundation Trust, 203 Fulham Road, London SW3 6JJ, UK

Correspondence should be addressed to Khin Thway; khin.thway@rmh.nhs.uk

Academic Editor: Chandrajit Premanand Raut

Introduction. Soft tissue tumour pathology is a highly specialised area of surgical pathology, but soft tissue neoplasms can occur at virtually all sites and are therefore encountered by a wide population of surgical pathologists. Potential sarcomas require referral to specialist centres for review by pathologists who see a large number of soft tissue lesions and where appropriate ancillary investigations can be performed. We have previously assessed the types of diagnostic discrepancies between referring and final diagnosis for soft tissue lesions referred to our tertiary centre. We now reaudit this 6 years later, assessing changes in discrepancy patterns, particularly in relation to the now widespread use of ancillary molecular diagnostic techniques which were not prevalent in our original study. *Materials and Methods.* We compared the sarcoma unit's histopathology reports with referring reports on 348 specimens from 286 patients with suspected or proven soft tissue tumours in a one-year period. *Results.* Diagnostic agreement was seen in 250 cases (71.8%), with 57 (16.4%) major and 41 (11.8%) minor discrepancies. There were 23 cases of benign/malignant discrepancies (23.5% of all discrepancies). 50 ancillary molecular tests were performed, 33 for aiding diagnosis and 17 mutational analyses for gastrointestinal stromal tumour to guide therapy. Findings from ancillary techniques contributed to 3 major and 4 minor discrepancies. While the results were broadly similar to those of the previous study, there was an increase in frequency of major discrepancies. *Conclusion.* Six years following our previous study and notably now in an era of widespread ancillary molecular diagnosis, the overall discrepancy rate between referral and tertiary centre diagnosis remains similar, but there is an increase in frequency of major discrepancies likely to alter patient management. A possible reason for the increase in major discrepancies is the increasing lack of exposure to soft tissue cases in nonspecialist centres in a time of subspecialisation. The findings support the national guidelines in which all suspected soft tissue tumour pathology specimens should be referred to a specialist sarcoma unit.

1. Introduction

Soft tissue tumours are rare with an annual incidence of 2.5 per 100000 population [1] but represent a heterogeneous group of neoplasms that can occur at virtually any anatomic site and thereby occur in the surgical pathology workload of all histopathologists. In the United Kingdom, the National Institute of Clinical Excellence (NICE) and Royal College of Pathologists (RCPath) recommend that patients with a provisional histological and/or radiological diagnosis of bone or soft tissue sarcoma should be referred to specialist multidisciplinary units for evaluation and diagnostic review by a specialist sarcoma pathologist and/or radiologist who are part of a sarcoma multidisciplinary team (MDT) and that there should be a formal system for second opinions and review of difficult cases, with access to diagnostic molecular and cytogenetic facilities [2, 3]. The Royal Marsden Hospital is a tertiary cancer centre whose Sarcoma Unit takes approximately 1500 new histopathology accessions per year, of which about 350 are referral cases. This department has previously published a comparative study of referral and final histological diagnoses of soft tissue tumour specimens referred to the Unit in 2005 [4]. Since then, two developments have occurred: (a) comprehensive adoption of the NICE and RCPath recommendations to routinely refer patients with potential sarcomas to specialist centres and (b) the widespread routine use of ancillary molecular and molecular cytogenetic diagnostic techniques. In this study, we determined areas of diagnostic discrepancy in the reporting of cases of soft tissue tumours referred to a specialist sarcoma unit in 2011, to assess changes in discrepancy patterns in light of these new developments in the interval of 6 years.

2. Materials and Methods

2.1. Patient Cases. A retrospective reaudit was performed for patients referred with soft tissue lesions to a specialist soft tissue sarcoma unit over a one-year period. The record files within the Department of Histopathology at the Royal Marsden Hospital were examined for a period of 12 months from the 1st of January to the 31st of December 2011. Patients were either surgical or oncological referrals. Referrals to the surgical unit were usually patients with a new histological diagnosis after biopsy, or with recurrent lesions referred for further surgery. Patients were referred to the medical or clinical oncology units for planning of (neo) adjuvant treatment. All second opinion cases (including those sent for pathological opinion, where the patient was not referred to our centre) were excluded, as were cases without referring reports. All cases included in the study had been reviewed by one or both of the specialist soft tissue pathologists (K.T. and C.F.). The material sent comprised either paraffin blocks, unstained slides, and stained slides or a mixture of each. Where blocks or sufficient stained slides were available, additional tests were performed as necessary, including immunohistochemistry, fluorescence in situ hybridisation (FISH), and quantitative real time reverse transcription polymerase chain reaction (RQ-PCR).

2.2. Pathology Review. These methods are as previously outlined [4]. Each referring report was compared with the subsequent Sarcoma Unit report for differences in diagnosis and grading. Grading was assigned according to the system by the French Federation of Cancer Centres Sarcoma Group (FNCLCC) [5, 6]. Grading categories were defined as (1) not applicable, (2) not done, (3) no difference in grade, (4) difference by one grade, and (5) difference by two grades. For gastrointestinal stromal tumour (GIST), assessment of potential biological behaviour into low, intermediate, and high risk was also compared as for grading. Tumours, for which the referring pathologist had identified tumour type, performed a mitotic count, and reported on the absence or amount of necrosis but had not given a numerical grade, were retrospectively graded on review and recorded as "graded." Tumours for which the mitotic count had not been performed, or the presence or absence of necrosis not indicated or where neither had been done, were not retrospectively graded. Tumours which the referring pathologist had assigned as low, intermediate, and high grade were interpreted as grades 1, 2, and 3, respectively. Grading was deemed as "not applicable" (1) in certain sarcomas considered routinely to display aggressive or "high grade" behaviour, (2) in metastatic tumours, (3) in tumours not formally graded, such as dermatofibrosarcoma protuberans (DFSP), (4) in benign lesions, (5) if there was a difference in diagnosis between the referring and specialist unit report, making grading noncomparable, or (6) if there was insufficient material for grading.

2.3. Classification of Discrepancies. Major discrepancies were defined as those that could lead to significant change in clinical management, with ensuing under- or overtreatment, and were divided into six groups: (1) malignant > malignant (resulting in significant management change), (2) malignant > benign, (3) benign > malignant, (4) mesenchymal > non-mesenchymal, (5) other (e.g., benign > benign, but resulting in significant management change), and (6) major grading discrepancies, comprising tumours in which there was any interchange of grade between grades 2-3 and grade 1 (as this could lead to management change). Minor discrepancies were divided into those of diagnosis, classification, or grading, but they were those in which the discrepancy was not thought to provoke significant management change. Minor changes in which the discrepancy was purely semantic, or in Sarcoma Unit reports in which subcategorisation was chiefly for special or academic interest (e.g., the addition of a finding of myofibroblastic differentiation within pleomorphic sarcoma), were disregarded. The reasons for discrepancy were analysed, by further assessing reports and reviewing slides where appropriate or possible, to look for sources of error such as interpretation of morphology or immunohistochemistry.

3. Results

3.1. Patient and Tumour Characteristics. A total of 350 specimens were received from 288 patients in the 1-year period. No review could be made on 2 cases which were excluded from the study: 1 was where only blocks were available and the material was cut out on sectioning and the other was where the wrong slides were sent and no subsequent material was provided. 203 cases were resection specimens and 145 were biopsies (most commonly needle core biopsies). There were 230 cases from district general hospitals, 83 from teaching hospitals, 27 from overseas hospitals, and 8 from private laboratories. There were 167 oncological referrals and 181 surgical referrals. 175 patients were female and 111 were male (ratio 1.57 : 1), and median age at diagnosis was 57.5 years (range 2–96 years). Where available from the gross specimen or cross-sectional imaging, median tumor size was 7 cm (range 1–37 cm). Detailed patient and tumour characteristics are shown in Table 1.

3.2. Summary of Discrepancies. Of the 348 cases, 250 (71.8%) were diagnostically concordant or had minimal diagnostic discrepancies. 201 were completely concordant, while 47 were not graded by the referring pathologist, with a grade assigned at our institute. Two cases reported as spindle cell sarcomas were refined at our centre to spindle cell sarcomas with myoid differentiation. Of the 250 cases, 201 were malignant diagnoses, 30 were benign, and 19 were of uncertain or intermediate malignant potential (the majority of which were fibromatosis or inflammatory myofibroblastic tumours (IMT)).

Table 1: Patient and tumour characteristics.

Patient/tumour characteristics	Total
Male	111 (38.8%)
Female	175 (61.2%)
Median age	57.5 years (range 2–96 years)
Tumor size	7 cm (range 1–37 cm)
Tumor location	
Intra-abdominal	125
Uterus	39
Vagina/vulva	5
Pelvic/perineum	14
Retroperitoneum	13
Stomach	7
Small bowel	5
Colon/rectum	7
Mesenteries/peritoneum	13
Adrenal	1
Kidney	2
Bladder	5
Prostate	2
Liver	6
Abdomen NOS	6
Trunk	63
Breast	14
Chest wall	9
Abdominal wall/flank	9
Back	8
Buttock	6
Paraspinal region	6
Pubic	2
Sternum	1
Lower limb	45
Thigh	21
Groin/spermatic cord/scrotum	6
Knee	2
Calf/shin	5
Foot	6
Leg (not otherwise specified, NOS)	5
Upper limb	23
Axilla	4
Shoulder	8
Forearm	3
Wrist/finger	2
Arm NOS	6
Head and neck	23
Scalp	6
Orbit	2

Table 1: Continued.

Patient/tumour characteristics	Total
Parotid	2
Nose	1
Cheek	3
Maxilla	1
Mandible	2
Oral/tongue	2
Neck	4
Thoracic cavity	11
Mediastinum	1
Trachea	1
Heart	1
Lung	8
Others (lymph nodes/skin/bone marrow)	4

NOS: not otherwise specified.

There were 41 minor discrepancies (11.8%) (summarised in Table 2), of which 3 were minor grading differences (i.e., grades 2 to 3 and vice versa). Seven cases were diagnosed as benign lesions, while 31 were malignant diagnoses. There were 57 major discrepancies (16.4%) (summarised in Table 3), of which 10 were reclassified from benign to malignant (including intermediate malignant potential) and 13 were reclassified from malignant (including intermediate) to benign. Overall, these 23 benign-malignant discrepancies accounted for 23.5% of all discrepant cases. Of the remaining 34 cases, 11 were malignant-malignant reclassifications, 1 was a benign-benign reclassification, 8 were major discrepancies in grading, 13 were mesenchymal-nonmesenchymal discrepancies, and 1 was a major discrepancy involving reclassification of a carcinoma. Overall, of the 57 cases, 14 were finally diagnosed as benign, 3 as intermediate malignant potential, and 40 as malignant.

3.3. Analysis of Discrepant Cases by Histology. There were 7 total discrepancies involving GIST, with 5 major discrepancies (2 of initial GIST rediagnosed as other spindle cell sarcomas and 1 of initial GIST rediagnosed as fibrous tissue and 2 being major grading discrepancies) and 2 minor grading discrepancies. 19 cases of discrepancy involved leiomyosarcomas, with 5 benign-malignant discordances (3 cases of diagnosis changed from benign entities to leiomyosarcoma, and 2 of leiomyosarcomas changed to benign tumours), 4 major classification discrepancies (involving leiomyosarcomas and other spindle cell tumours), 3 major discrepancies involving grade, and 7 minor classification discrepancies (leiomyosarcomas versus pleomorphic sarcomas with myoid differentiation). Four major discrepancies involved fibromatosis (2 originally diagnosed as benign entities and reclassified as fibromatosis and 2 originally diagnosed as fibromatosis and reclassified as benign). One case was originally diagnosed as IMT but was rediagnosed as Wegener's granulomatosis. Finally, 5 discrepancies involved liposarcomas: 2 major (2 of initial atypical lipomatous tumour/well-differentiated

Table 2: Summary of cases showing minor discrepancy.

Referral diagnosis	Final diagnosis	n
Malignant	Malignant	
DFSP	DFSP with fibrosarcoma	5
DFSP with fibrosarcoma	Fibrosarcoma	1
DFSP with fibrosarcoma	Spindle cell sarcoma	1
Malignant SFT	Fibrosarcoma	1
Fibrosarcoma	MPNST	1
Myxoinflammatory fibrosarcoma	Myxofibrosarcoma	1
Myxoid liposarcoma	Myxofibrosarcoma	1
Spindle cell sarcoma	Myxofibrosarcoma	1
RMS NOS	Embryonal RMS	1
RMS NOS	Pleomorphic RMS	1
RMS NOS	Myoid sarcoma	1
Myoid sarcoma	Pleomorphic RMS	1
Leiomyosarcoma	Myoid sarcoma	4
Leiomyosarcoma	Spindle cell sarcoma	1
Leiomyosarcoma	Undifferentiated neoplasm	1
Leiomyosarcoma	Myofibrosarcoma	1
MPNST	Clear cell sarcoma	1
Undifferentiated neoplasm	Clear cell sarcoma	1
PEComa, ?atypical features	PEComa, malignant	2
DDL	Spindle cell sarcoma	1
Sarcoma	Malignant neoplasm	2
Extraskeletal myxoid chondrosarcoma	Malignant neoplasm	1
Benign	Benign	
Spindle cell lesion	Myxoma	1
Myxoid lesion	Myxoma	1
Benign neoplasm	Ossifying fibromyxoid tumour	1
Spindle cell lesion	Neurofibroma	1
Giant cell tumour of tendon sheath	Ossifying fibroma	1
SFT	Schwannoma	1
Fibrosis	Benign smooth muscle tumour	1
Grade	Grade	
GIST 2	GIST 3	1
GIST 3	GIST 2	1
Spindle cell sarcoma 3	Myxofibrosarcoma 2	1

DFSP: dermatofibrosarcoma protuberans; DDL: dedifferentiated liposarcoma; GIST: gastrointestinal stromal tumour; MPNST: malignant peripheral nerve sheath tumour; NOS: not otherwise specified; RMS: rhabdomyosarcoma; SFT: solitary fibrous tumour.

liposarcoma (ALT/WDL) rediagnosed as lipoma, 1 of dedifferentiated liposarcoma (DDL) diagnosed originally as low grade fibromyxoid sarcoma, and 1 of WDL regraded as DDL, grade 2) and 1 minor, originally diagnosed as DDL but reclassified as spindle cell sarcoma after results of FISH.

3.4. Contribution of Immunohistochemistry to Diagnoses. Additional immunohistochemistry contributed to change in final diagnosis in 23 cases: in 9/41 minor and 14/57 major discrepancies. Of these 23 cases, the contributory tests had not been performed by the referring centre (rather than these being instances of repeat testing which gave a different pattern or intensity of staining). These were 7 tests for h-caldesmon (for leiomyosarcoma), 3 CDK4 (for WDL/DDL), 2 DOG1 (for GIST), 2 beta-catenin (for fibromatosis), 1 each of CD34 (DFSP), desmin, myogenin (rhabdomyosarcoma (RMS)), p63 (sarcomatoid carcinoma), PSAP (prostatic carcinoma), and TLE1 (synovial sarcoma). In 3 cases, a wide panel of antibodies was used.

3.5. Contribution of Molecular and Molecular Cytogenetic Tests to Diagnoses. Of the 348 cases, 50 had FISH or molecular studies performed here. 17 were mutational analyses for *c-kit* and *PDGFRA* genes in GIST, which were performed to guide targeted therapy decisions and which were not contributory to the final histological diagnosis. In 6/50 cases, FISH or RQ-PCR was unsuccessful (technical fails), likely due to DNA and RNA degradation due to differences in tissue fixation in the referral laboratories; 4 of these had no discrepancies between referral and final diagnoses. Two had minor discrepancies: 1 was minor involving grading of GIST, and, in the other, the requested test was for alveolar rhabdomyosarcoma (ARMS). The diagnosis was changed from myoid sarcoma to pleomorphic RMS, and the histologic features were not wholly typical for ARMS, so the failure of the test did not have significant bearing on diagnosis. In the remaining 27 cases, FISH and/or RT-PCR were performed as follows: (1) 12 for *EWSR1* gene rearrangement, of which 9 did not result in discrepancies and 3 resulted in minor discrepancies (1: extraskeletal myxoid chondrosarcoma to poorly differentiated neoplasm, 1: malignant peripheral nerve sheath tumour (MPNST) to clear cell sarcoma, and 1: malignant neoplasm to clear cell sarcoma); (2) 3 for *MDM2* gene amplification, resulting in 2 major discrepancies (1 myxoid liposarcoma to DDL and 1 ALT to lipoma) and 1 minor (DDL to spindle cell sarcoma); (3) 3 for *ALK1* gene rearrangements with no discrepancies involved; (4) 3 for *SS18-SSX1/2* fusion genes with 2 resulting in no discrepancies and 1 resulting in minor discrepancy to which the test did not contribute (leiomyosarcoma to spindle cell sarcoma); (5) 2 for *FUS-CREB3L1/2* fusion genes with no discrepancies; (6) 2 for *PAX3/7-FOXO1* gene fusions, with 1 resulting in no discrepancies and 1 case of major discrepancy to which the test did not contribute (GIST to spindle cell RMS); and (7) 2 for *JAZF1-SUZ12* gene fusion, with 1 major discrepancy (pleomorphic sarcoma to endometrial stromal sarcoma (ESS)) and 1 minor discrepancy in which the test was not contributory (metastatic sarcoma to metastatic undifferentiated neoplasm). Overall, there were 7 cases in which FISH or PCR techniques contributed to the final diagnosis which resulted in either major or minor discrepancies.

TABLE 3: Summary of cases showing major discrepancy.

Referral diagnosis	Final Diagnosis	n
Benign	Malignant (Including locally aggressive, although non-metastasising neoplasms)	
Angiomyxoma	Fibromatosis	1
Nerve sheath tumour	Fibromatosis	1
Granular cell tumour (benign)	Granular cell tumour (malignant)	4 (1 patient)
Haemangiopericytoma	DDL	1
Leiomyoma	Leiomyosarcoma	2
Reactive tissue	Leiomyosarcoma	1
Malignant (Including locally aggressive although non-metastasising neoplasms)	Benign	
Fibromatosis	Scar	1
Fibromatosis	Nuchal-type fibroma	1
ALT	Lipoma	2
MPNST	Atypical neurofibroma	1
Leiomyosarcoma	BFH	1
DFSP	BFH	1
Metastatic renal carcinoma	Clear cell BFH	1
Angiosarcoma	Haemangioma	1
GIST	Fibrous tissue only	1
Leiomyosarcoma	Schwannoma	1
IMT	Wegener's granulomatosis	1
Malignant	Malignant	
STUMP	Leiomyosarcoma (grade 2)	2
ESS	Leiomyosarcoma	1
ESS	Osteosarcoma	1
GIST	Spindle cell sarcoma	1
GIST	Spindle RMS	1
Leiomyosarcoma	MPNST	1
LGFMS	Fibromatosis	1
LGFMS	DDL	1
Synovial sarcoma	Malignant neoplasm	1
Benign	Benign	
Schwannoma	Benign naevus	1
Mesenchymal	Non-mesenchymal	
UPS	Carcinosarcoma	4
Synovial sarcoma	Carcinosarcoma	1
Chondrosarcoma	Carcinosarcoma	1
Leiomyosarcoma	Carcinosarcoma	1
Sarcoma	Seminoma	1
MPNST	Melanoma	2

TABLE 3: Continued.

Referral diagnosis	Final Diagnosis	n
Non-mesenchymal	Mesenchymal	
Carcinoma	Pleomorphic RMS	1
Carcinoma	Spindle cell sarcoma	1
Lymphoma	SFT	1
Non-mesenchymal	Non-mesenchymal	
Undifferentiated carcinoma	Prostatic carcinoma	1
Grade	Grade	
GIST grade 2/3	GIST 1	2
Leiomyosarcoma 2/3	Leiomyosarcoma 1	2
Leiomyosarcoma 1	Leiomyosarcoma 2	1
Myxofibrosarcoma 2	Myxofibrosarcoma 1	1
WDL	DDL grade 2	1
High grade sarcoma	ESS	1

Abbreviations: ALT atypical lipomatous tumour; BFH benign fibrous histiocytoma; DFSP dermatofibrosarcoma protuberans; DDL dedifferentiated liposarcoma; ESS endometrial stromal sarcoma; GIST gastrointestinal stromal tumour; IMT inflammatory myofibroblastic tumour; LGFMS low grade fibromyxoid sarcoma; MPNST malignant peripheral nerve sheath tumour; RMS rhabdomyosarcoma; SFT solitary fibrous tumour; STUMP smooth muscle tumour of uncertain malignant potential; UPS undifferentiated pleomorphic sarcoma; WDL well differentiated liposarcoma.

4. Discussion

In our previous audit of referral cases to our institution in 2005, there were 349 specimens from 277 patients [4], of which diagnostic agreement was seen in 73.4% and diagnostic discrepancy in 27.5% (15.7% minor, 10.9% major, and 5% of the discrepant cases being benign-malignant discordances). In comparison, two decades, previously the Southeastern Cancer Study Group, reported a 28% disagreement rate between primary institutional diagnosis and reviewer diagnosis [7]. In 1989, the Scandinavian Sarcoma Group reported that 25% of reviewed sarcomas were reclassified, with grade changed in 40% [8]. The North West England peer review in 1991 showed a discrepancy rate of approximately 35% (disagreement in subtype in 17% and change in diagnosis to non-sarcomatous tumours in 18%), with an agreement rate of sarcoma subtype of 53%, and the remaining cases accounted for tumours where subtype could not be further specified, where classification was only possible as "malignant tumour NOS," or where diagnosis could not be given [9]. The 2001 audit of soft tissue second opinion cases by Arbiser et al. showed major discrepancy in 25% of cases and minor discrepancy in 7% [10]. Finally, a three-centre analysis of French and Italian referrals showed a concordance rate of 56%, partial concordance of 35%, and complete discordance of 8% [11]. In our current study, there were similar frequencies of discrepancy to those described in our previous audit and to the other studies above. The slight variations encountered might be due to different criteria for classification of discrepancies. For example, we placed tumours which were not graded within the concordant group, as no error was actually made by the referring pathologist, but other studies have categorised these as minor discrepancies. We wished in particular to compare our current results with our previous findings, using identical criteria to define discrepancies. While the overall frequency of discrepant cases here (28.2%) was similar to our previous audit (26.6%) [4], in this study, we found more major discrepancies (16.4% in 2011 compared with 10.9% in 2005) and fewer minor discrepancies (11.8% in 2011 compared with 15.7% in 2005) compared with 2005. Furthermore, this increase in proportion of major discrepancies appeared to be mainly due to the number of benign-malignant discordances (23.5% compared with 5%).

This might in part be due to the increasing use of ancillary molecular and molecular cytogenetic testing, which has become commonplace in the diagnosis of soft tissue neoplasms since the previous study of 2005. A recent study assessing impact of molecular analysis on final sarcoma diagnosis in 763 cases found that such ancillary tests contributed to diagnosis of up to 4% of GISTs and 31% of ALT/WDL/DDL [12]. At our centre, the routine molecular and cytogenetics service for soft tissue sarcomas was established in 2006. In 2011, the year of this study, the service performed 405 FISH and 270 PCR analyses for soft tissue neoplasms. Of these, only 50 tests were performed on our referral cohort and contributed to 7 discrepancies. The most useful tests in reevaluating diagnosis were FISH (for assessing *MDM2* amplification status to determine whether differentiated lipomatous tumours or pleomorphic tumours were ALT/WDL or DDL, resp.) and for assessment of *EWSR1* gene rearrangement (for diagnosis of a variety of tumours, such as clear cell sarcoma).

However, this is still insufficient to explain the increase in proportion of major discrepancies, especially benign-malignant discordances. In our original audit, the commonest cause of discrepancies was found to be due to differences between the referring pathologist's interpretation of morphology or immunophenotype and that of the tertiary centre pathologist's, rather than the lack of or inappropriate use of immunohistochemical tests at the referring centre. Similarly, in this study, we found that the majority of referral cases had appropriate immunohistochemistry tests performed but that, in 23 cases, additional immunohistochemical tests contributed to the cases of diagnostic discrepancy of which the commonest antibodies omitted at referral centres were h-caldesmon for leiomyosarcoma, CDK4 for WDL/DDL, DOG1 for GIST, and beta-catenin for fibromatosis. It can certainly be argued that CDK4 is not sufficiently in widespread use in general pathology laboratories, although the other three antibodies, as well as others contributing to discrepancy, are in common use in the majority of diagnostic laboratories. It therefore appears that most discrepancies uncovered by immunohistochemistry are interpretational, due to unfamiliarity by the referring pathologist of either specific disease entities or antibodies, rather than due to the use by the tertiary centre of crucial rare antibodies not in common use in most laboratories.

Looking more specifically at discordant cases, there were fewer discrepancies related to GIST compared with 2005. Previously, pitfalls in the diagnosis of GIST existed due to inconsistent staining with CD34 and CD117 [13, 14], but now there is increasing familiarity with this neoplasm and its pattern of immunohistochemical staining, including the use of DOG1 antibody [15] as recommended in national guidelines. In contrast, there was no significant decrease in discrepancies involving leiomyosarcomas, fibromatosis, and liposarcomas, which were among the commonest causes of discrepancy. While in some cases this was due to lack of use of antibodies such as h-caldesmon and beta-catenin, in many the appropriate antibodies were used, but interpretation of morphologic features and immunohistochemical staining patterns led to discordant referring and tertiary centre diagnoses. Common sources of error included (a) diagnosing leiomyosarcoma based on focal expression of smooth muscle actin (SMA) and desmin alone, without the use of more specific smooth muscle markers [16] (as SMA can be diffusely expressed in myofibroblasts in both reactive and neoplastic conditions, and desmin is a broad spectrum marker of muscle lineage and is also expressed in other lesions such as myofibroblastoma), (b) interpreting cytoplasmic and especially paranuclear beta-catenin staining as positive for fibromatosis [17], and (c) interpreting overstaining or background staining of some antibodies, such as cytokeratins or CD31.

Therefore, in the majority of cases, as with our previous study, the major cause of discrepancies appears attributable to differences in interpretation by the referral and tertiary centre pathologists. The particular increase in benign-malignant interpretational differences might, in turn, be a result of (a) the increasing impetus to refer potential soft tissue cases to specialist centres with a subsequent deskilling of general pathologists in working up these cases and (b) increasing pressure on pathologists to reduce laboratory costs and turnaround times. In summary, we found that while overall rates of histological diagnostic discrepancy between referring and tertiary centre have remained stable 6 years following the previous study, there has been an increase in the proportion of major discrepancies. While this study is of a time period in which molecular and molecular cytogenetic ancillary diagnosis are commonplace, access to these investigations at the tertiary centre only contributed to a small fraction of diagnostic discrepancies, while, as before, interpretational differences contributed to the largest proportion of discrepancies, and this might be in part due to increasing lack of expertise in this specialist area, in the age of subspecialisation.

Acknowledgment

The authors acknowledge support from the NIHR Royal Marsden/ICR Biomedical Research Centre.

References

[1] A. L. Hartley, V. Blair, M. Harris et al., "Sarcomas in North West England: II incidence," *The British Journal of Cancer*, vol. 64, no. 6, pp. 1145–1150, 1991.

[2] "Improving Outcomes for People with Sarcoma," http://www.nice.org.uk/nicemedia/pdf/SarcomaFullGuidance.pdf.

[3] C. Fisher, "Dataset for cancer histopathology reports on soft tissue sarcomas," Royal College of Pathologists, 2012, http://www.rcpath.org/Resources/RCPath/Migrated%20Resources/Documents/G/G094_DatasetSoftTissue_Mar14.pdf.

[4] K. Thway and C. Fisher, "Histopathological diagnostic discrepancies in soft tissue tumours referred to a specialist centre," *Sarcoma*, vol. 2009, Article ID 741975, 7 pages, 2009.

[5] J. M. Coindre, M. Trojani, G. Contesso et al., "Reproducibility of a histopathologic grading system for adult soft tissue sarcoma," *Cancer*, vol. 58, no. 2, pp. 306–309, 1986.

[6] L. Guillou, J. M. Coindre, F. Bonichon et al., "Comparative study of the National Cancer Institute and French Federation of Cancer Centers Sarcoma Group grading systems in a population of 410 adult patients with soft tissue sarcoma," *Journal of Clinical Oncology*, vol. 15, no. 1, pp. 350–362, 1997.

[7] C. A. Presant, W. O. Russell, R. W. Alexander, and Y. S. Fu, "Soft-tissue and bone sarcoma histopathology peer review: The frequency of disagreement in diagnosis and the need for second pathology opinions. The Southeastern Cancer Study Group experience," *Journal of Clinical Oncology*, vol. 4, no. 11, pp. 1658–1661, 1986.

[8] T. A. Alvegard and N. O. Berg, "Histopathology peer review of high-grade soft tissue sarcoma: the Scandinavian Sarcoma Group experience," *Journal of Clinical Oncology*, vol. 7, no. 12, pp. 1845–1851, 1989.

[9] M. Harris, A. L. Hartley, V. Blair et al., "Sarcomas in North West England: I. Histopathological peer review," *British Journal of Cancer*, vol. 64, no. 2, pp. 315–320, 1991.

[10] Z. K. Arbiser, A. L. Folpe, and S. W. Weiss, "Consultative (expert) second opinions in soft tissue pathology: analysis of problem-prone diagnostic situations," *The American Journal of Clinical Pathology*, vol. 116, no. 4, pp. 473–476, 2001.

[11] I. Ray-coquard, M. C. Montesco, J. M. Coindre et al., "Sarcoma: concordance between initial diagnosis and centralized expert review in a population-based study within three European regions," *Annals of Oncology*, vol. 23, no. 9, Article ID mdr610, pp. 2442–2449, 2012.

[12] A. Neuville, D. Ranchère-Vince, A. P. Dei Tos et al., "Impact of molecular analysis on the final sarcoma diagnosis: a study on 763 cases collected during a European epidemiological study," *The American Journal of Surgical Pathology*, vol. 37, no. 8, pp. 1259–1268, 2013.

[13] N. D. Riddle, R. J. Gonzalez, J. A. Bridge, S. Antonia, and M. M. Bui, "A CD117 and CD34 immunoreactive sarcoma masquerading as a gastrointestinal stromal tumor: diagnostic pitfalls of ancillary studies in sarcoma," *Cancer Control*, vol. 18, no. 3, pp. 152–159, 2011.

[14] M. Sabah, M. Leader, and E. Kay, "The problem with KIT: clinical implications and practical difficulties with CD117 immunostaining," *Applied Immunohistochemistry and Molecular Morphology*, vol. 11, no. 1, pp. 56–61, 2003.

[15] I. Espinosa, C. H. Lee, M. K. Kim et al., "A novel monoclonal antibody against DOG1 is a sensitive and specific marker for gastrointestinal stromal tumors," *American Journal of Surgical Pathology*, vol. 32, no. 2, pp. 210–218, 2008.

[16] K. Watanabe, T. Kusakabe, N. Hoshi, A. Saito, and T. Suzuki, "h-Caldesmon in leiomyosarcoma and tumors with smooth muscle cell-like differentiation: its specific expression in the smooth muscle cell tumor," *Human Pathology*, vol. 30, no. 4, pp. 392–396, 1999.

[17] J. W. Carlson and C. D. M. Fletcher, "Immunohistochemistry for β-catenin in the differential diagnosis of spindle cell lesions: Analysis of a series and review of the literature," *Histopathology*, vol. 51, no. 4, pp. 509–514, 2007.

Genomic, Epigenomic, and Transcriptomic Profiling towards Identifying Omics Features and Specific Biomarkers that Distinguish Uterine Leiomyosarcoma and Leiomyoma at Molecular Levels

Tomoko Miyata,[1,2] Kenzo Sonoda,[2] Junko Tomikawa,[1] Chiharu Tayama,[1] Kohji Okamura,[3] Kayoko Maehara,[1,4] Hiroaki Kobayashi,[2,5] Norio Wake,[2] Kiyoko Kato,[2] Kenichiro Hata,[1] and Kazuhiko Nakabayashi[1]

[1] *Department of Maternal-Fetal Biology, National Research Institute for Child Health and Development, 2-10-1 Okura, Setagaya, Tokyo 157-8535, Japan*
[2] *Department of Obstetrics and Gynecology, Graduate School of Medical Sciences, Kyushu University, 3-1-1 Maidashi, Higashi-ku, Fukuoka 812-8582, Japan*
[3] *Department of Systems BioMedicine, National Research Institute for Child Health and Development, 2-10-1 Okura, Setagaya, Tokyo 157-8535, Japan*
[4] *Department of Health Nutrition, Faculty of Health Science, Kio University, 4-2-4 Umami-naka, Koryo-cho, Kitakatsuragi-gun 635-0832, Japan*
[5] *Department of Obstetrics and Gynecology, Faculty of Medicine, Kagoshima University, 8-35-1 Sakuragaoka, Kagoshima 890-0075, Japan*

Correspondence should be addressed to Kenichiro Hata; hata-k@ncchd.go.jp and Kazuhiko Nakabayashi; nakabaya-k@ncchd.go.jp

Academic Editor: Eugenie S. Kleinerman

Uterine leiomyosarcoma (LMS) is the worst malignancy among the gynecologic cancers. Uterine leiomyoma (LM), a benign tumor of myometrial origin, is the most common among women of childbearing age. Because of their similar symptoms, it is difficult to preoperatively distinguish the two conditions only by ultrasound and pelvic MRI. While histopathological diagnosis is currently the main approach used to distinguish them postoperatively, unusual histologic variants of LM tend to be misdiagnosed as LMS. Therefore, development of molecular diagnosis as an alternative or confirmatory means will help to diagnose LMS more accurately. We adopted omics-based technologies to identify genome-wide features to distinguish LMS from LM and revealed that copy number, gene expression, and DNA methylation profiles successfully distinguished these tumors. LMS was found to possess features typically observed in malignant solid tumors, such as extensive chromosomal abnormalities, overexpression of cell cycle-related genes, hypomethylation spreading through large genomic regions, and frequent hypermethylation at the polycomb group target genes and protocadherin genes. We also identified candidate expression and DNA methylation markers, which will facilitate establishing postoperative molecular diagnostic tests based on conventional quantitative assays. Our results demonstrate the feasibility of establishing such tests and the possibility of developing preoperative and noninvasive methods.

1. Introduction

Uterine sarcoma is a malignant mesenchymal tumor composed of cells derived from uterine myometrium and represents the worst prognostic disease in gynecologic malignancies. The incidence of uterine sarcoma has been estimated to account for 8% of primary uterine malignancies [1]. Three major subtypes of uterine sarcomas are carcinosarcoma, endometrial stromal sarcoma, and leiomyosarcoma (LMS), all of which are resistant to surgery, chemotherapy, and radiotherapy. Although patients' prognosis is dependent on histopathological subtype and stage, 5-year relative survival

TABLE 1: Clinical features of nine samples analyzed in this study.

Sample	Clinical diagnosis	Tissue-type obtained	Age	Major axis of tumor (cm)	Preoperative therapy
NM1	Cervical cancer, stage Ib1	Normal myometrium	43	—	None
NM2	Cervical cancer, stage Ib2	Normal myometrium	38	—	None
NM3	Cervical cancer, stage Ib2	Normal myometrium	49	—	None
LM1	Interstitial myoma	Leiomyoma	52	18	None
LM2	Submucosal myoma	Leiomyoma	48	6	None
LM3	Submucosal myoma	Leiomyoma	53	6	GnRHa
LMS1	Leiomyosarcoma, stage IV	Leiomyosarcoma	49	25	None
LMS2	Leiomyosarcoma, stage I	Leiomyosarcoma	54	20	None
LMS3	Leiomyosarcoma, stage I	Leiomyosarcoma	83	10	None

GnRHa, gonadotrophin-releasing hormone analogues.

rates of uterine sarcoma are 63–73%, 24–43%, 32–38%, and 6% at stages I, II, III, and IV, respectively, of the staging system determined by the International Federation of Gynecology and Obstetrics (FIGO) [2, 3]. LMS represents the most common subtype and mostly occurs in menopausal women over 40 years of age, who usually present symptoms such as abnormal vaginal bleeding, palpable pelvic mass, and pelvic pain. As these symptoms resemble those of the far more common uterine leiomyoma (LM), particularly degenerated LM, it is difficult to preoperatively distinguish LMS and LM by ultrasound and pelvic MRI [1]. A meta-analysis of 133 studies showed that the prevalence of occult LMS at surgery for presumed LM was estimated to be approximately 1 in 2000 [4]. Occult LMS cases tend to be discovered at their late stages, since they are often observed (as presumed leiomyoma) in outpatient clinics. Histopathological diagnosis after surgery is the only currently available means to distinguish the two conditions. However, some LM variants, such as the mitotically active type and LM with massive lymphoid infiltration, may be misdiagnosed as LMS during histopathological examination. In fact, in a previous population-based study of uterine sarcoma, of the 356 cases initially classified in the study as LMS, 97 cases (27%) were reclassified as LM or LM variants after review [5]. Introduction of confirmatory molecular diagnosis in addition to histopathological diagnosis is an option to be considered to decrease the risk of making inaccurate diagnoses. Identification of novel molecular markers highly specific to LMS will help to further improve the diagnostic accuracy of LMS.

"Cancer genomics" refers to the profiling of tumor genomes using various strategies such as DNA copy number, DNA methylation, transcriptome, and whole-genome sequencing [6]. Such omics data have been successfully utilized to identify genes and pathways perturbed in cancer and to discover novel diagnostic, prognostic, and therapeutic markers in several cancer types [7–9]. Such precedent and successful cases of cancer omics approaches at various phases suggest the necessity and importance of collecting omics datasets for gynecologic cancers as a basis towards identifying their diagnostic and prognostic markers and therapeutic targets. However, due to the rare incidence of LMS (0.4 in 100,000 [10]), the available omics profiles for LMS have been very limited so far. In the present study, we aimed at comprehensively understanding the differences between LM and LMS at the molecular level by analyzing the genomic, epigenomic, and transcriptomic profiles of these benign and malignant uterine tumors and also at extracting candidate expression and DNA methylation markers, which are potentially useful to establish molecular diagnostic tests using conventional assays.

2. Materials and Methods

2.1. Samples. We obtained three samples each of normal uterus myometrium tissue (NM1, NM2, and NM3), leiomyoma tissue (LM1, LM2, and LM3), and leiomyosarcoma tissue (LMS1, LMS2, and LMS3) from nine patients, whose clinical features are summarized in Table 1. Although NM samples were collected from cervical cancer patients, cancerous tissues were not mixed. Both LM and LMS samples were obtained from the center of the nidus. In three LMS cases, the LMS area was observed not to be associated with any LM-like areas by eye examination at surgery. The present study was approved by the Ethics Committee of the National Center for Child Health and Development (#234) and the Ethics Committee of Kyushu University (#231). All participating patients signed informed consent forms. All specimens were isolated during primary surgery at the Department of Obstetrics and Gynecology in the Kyushu University Hospital, immediately frozen in liquid nitrogen, and stored at −80°C. The cell lines examined in this study were SKN (RBRC-RCB0513) obtained from the RIKEN BRC and SK-UT1 (HTB-114) and SK-UT1B (HTB-115) obtained from the American Type Culture Collection.

2.2. Cell Culture. All cells were cultured under standard culture conditions (at 37°C, 5% CO_2 in air) in a medium supplemented with 15% fetal bovine serum and Penicillin-Streptomycin-Glutamine Liquid (final 1x, GIBCO 10378-016). HamF12 medium was used for SKN cells and Eagle medium was used for SK-UT1 and SK-UT1B cells.

2.3. Genomic DNA and Total RNA Preparation. Genome DNA and total RNA were isolated from tissues and cells using the AllPrep Mini Kit (Qiagen) according to the manufacturer's protocol.

2.4. Single Nucleotide Polymorphism (SNP) Array Analysis for the Detection of Chromosomal Abnormalities. DNA amplification, labeling, and hybridization were performed according to the manufacturer's protocol of the HumanCytoSNP-12 BeadChip (Illumina). Two hundred ng of genomic DNA was subjected to DNA amplification for each of the samples. After hybridization and washing, the array slides were scanned on an iScan system (Illumina). Log R ratios (LRR) and B allele frequencies (BAF) were calculated using GenomeStudio version 2010.1 and visualized using KaryoStudio Data Analysis Software version 1.0 (Illumina). LRR and BAF represented the normalized signal intensity and the normalized ratio of the quantity of the B allele to the total quantity of both A and B alleles, respectively. Detection of copy neutral loss of heterozygosity (CNLOH) and copy number alterations (gain and loss) was performed using CNVpartition V3.0.7.0 (Illumina) and R-GADA (R-genome alteration detection analysis) [11], respectively, with default parameters.

2.5. Gene Expression Array Analysis. Total RNA samples were subjected to gene expression microarray analysis using the Whole Human Genome Microarray Kit, 4 × 44 K (Agilent), by following the manufacturer's instructions. This array contains a total of 41,093 probes covering 19,596 genes. Total RNAs (200 ng each) were amplified and labelled with Cy3 using the Low Input QuickAmp Labeling Kit (Agilent). The resultant cRNAs were fragmented at 60°C for 30 min in the dark, 600 ng of which was hybridized on the microarray at 65°C for 17 h. After washing, slides were then scanned using the Agilent microarray scanner G2505B. Signal intensities from the scanned images were determined using feature extraction software (version 10.7.3.1). Raw intensity data were then transferred to the GeneSpring software version 12.6 (Agilent), normalized (quantile normalization), and analyzed further using principal component analysis (PCA) and a selection of differentially expressed genes. The hierarchical clustering analysis for 1,036 differentially expressed genes was performed using Heatmap2 in the R package, gplots (https://cran.r-project.org/web/packages/gplots/gplots.pdf), with default parameters (complete linkage with Euclidean distance). The aforementioned 1,036 differentially expressed genes were selected as follows: Of 40,093 probes, 1,680 probes that were differentially expressed in at least one of the four groups of NM, LM, LMS, and LMS cell lines were selected by one-way ANOVA analysis (multiple testing correction, Benjamini-Hochberg; threshold, corrected $P < 0.05$) for log 2-transformed normalized signal intensity values; of these, 1,324 probes with a fold-change value of >2 or <0.5 in the group comparison between LMS and NM or LM and NM were further selected; of this number, 1,036 probes with a gene symbol were further selected (without redundancy of gene symbols). Gene ontology (GO) analysis was performed using the Database for Annotation, Visualization, and Integrated Discovery (DAVID) version 6.7 (https://david.ncifcrf.gov/). From the lists of probes ranked by fold-change values, the top 1,500 gene symbols were selected from up- and downregulated genes for each LM and LMS sample and subjected to GO analysis.

2.6. Genome-Wide DNA Methylation Analysis. Genomic DNA (1.5 μg) was bisulfite converted using the EpiTect Plus DNA Bisulfite Kit (Qiagen). After determining the concentration of bisulfite-treated DNA, 300 ng of bisulfite DNA from each sample was subjected to Illumina Infinium HumanMethylation450 BeadChip analysis according to the manufacturer's standard protocol (Illumina). The array slides were scanned on an iScan system (Illumina). The scanned image data were processed using GenomeStudio Methylation Analysis Module version 1.9.0 with background subtraction and control normalization options. Methylation levels for each of over 480,000 CpG sites were calculated using a β value (= intensity of the methylated allele/[intensity of the unmethylated allele + intensity of the methylated allele + 100]), ranging from 0 (completely unmethylated) to 1 (completely methylated).

Of the 485,577 probes, probes with a detection P value of >0.05 or blank β value were excluded from further analyses. GenomeStudio was used to draw boxplots and scatter plots and to perform hierarchical clustering analysis (complete linkage with Euclidean distance). The hierarchical clustering analyses for the β values of subsets of hypermethylated probes were performed using Heatmap2 with default parameters. The difference in β values between the two samples was defined as delta beta ($\Delta\beta$), and $\Delta\beta > 0.2$ and $\Delta\beta < -0.2$ were regarded as hyper- and hypomethylated, respectively, in this study. Differentially methylated regions between two groups of samples were extracted using Illumina Methylation Analyzer (IMA), an R package for analyzing site-level and region-level methylation changes between the two groups [12]. The BED-formatted lists of hyper- and hypomethylated regions were compiled for each of the six gene feature groups (TSS1500, TSS200, 5′UTR, first exon, gene body, and 3′UTR) by binning two or more probes found in the same gene feature group of the same gene as one region and analyzed one by one using the GREAT annotation website (http://bejerano.stanford.edu/great/public/html/) [13] with the default parameters of the "single nearest gene" mode.

2.7. Combined Bisulfite Restriction (COBRA) Analysis for LINE1. Bisulfite PCR for LINE1 elements were conducted as described previously [14]. The PCR primers used were 5′-TTGAGTTGTGGTGGGTTTATTTAG-3′ and 5′-TCATCTCACTAAAAAATACCAAACA-3′. The thermal cycling conditions were 25 cycles of 95°C for 30 seconds (s), 50°C for 30 s, and 72°C for 30 s, with an initial step of 95°C for 5 minutes (min) and a final step of 72°C for 2 min. PCR products (413 bp) were purified using the illustra GFX 96 PCR Purification Kit (GE Healthcare) and digested with *Hinf*I. The digestion DNA products were analyzed using BioAnalyzer 2100 (Agilent).

2.8. Data Deposition. DNA methylation and gene expression array data used in publication have been deposited in NCBI's

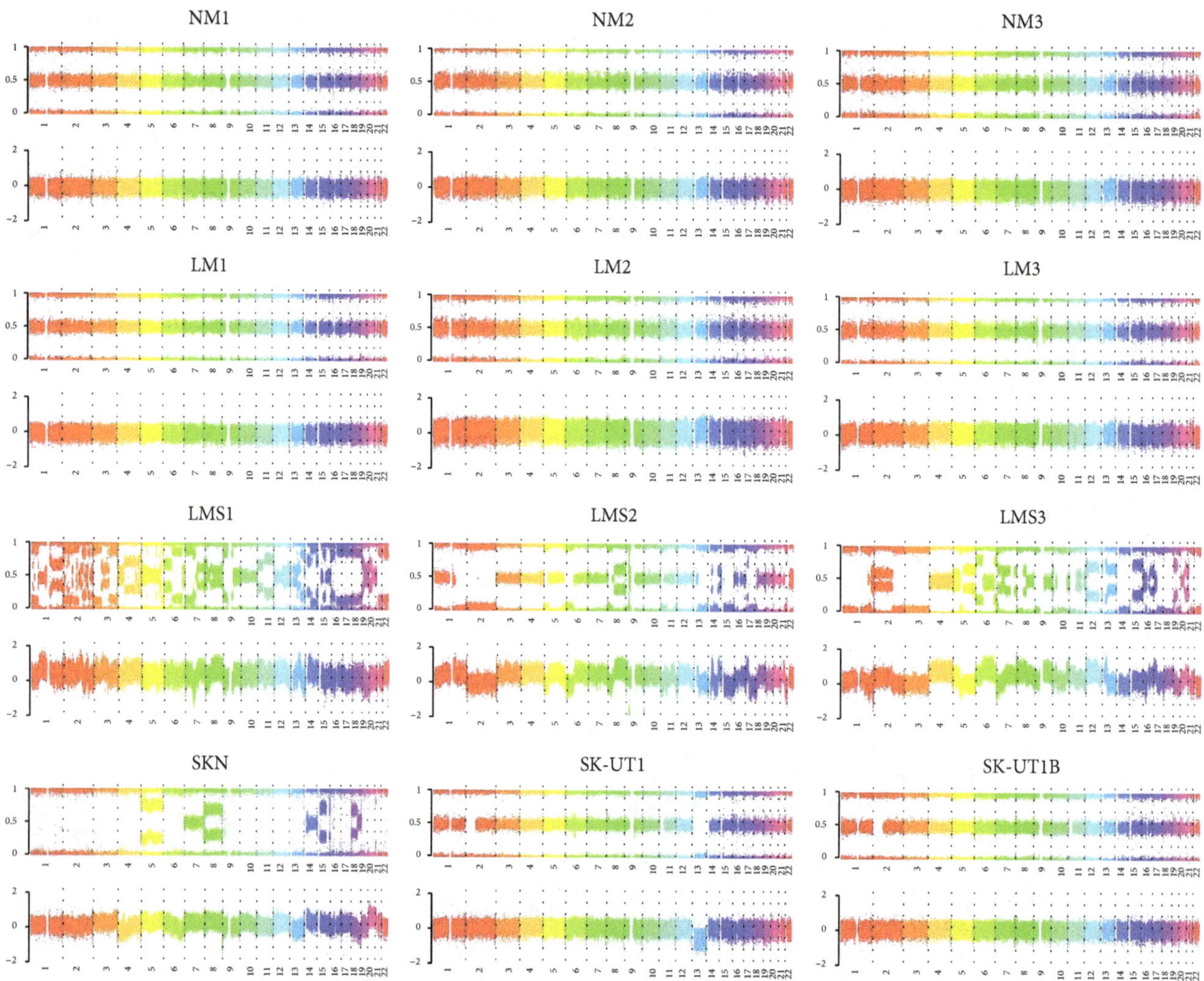

FIGURE 1: Chromosomal constitutions of normal metrium tissues (NM), leiomyoma (LM), and leiomyosarcoma (LMS) cases, and LMS-derived cell lines determined by SNP-array analysis. BAF (upper) and LRR (lower) are shown for 22 autosomal chromosomes of each of the 12 samples. The data ranges shown are 0 to 1 for BAF and −2 to 2 for LRR.

Gene Expression Omnibu (http://www.ncbi.nlm.nih.gov/geo/) and are accessible through GEO Series accession number GSE68312.

3. Results and Discussion

3.1. Extensive Chromosomal Abnormalities Specific to Leiomyosarcoma. We assessed the extent of chromosomal copy number alterations in NM, LM, and LMS samples and LMS-derived cell lines using SNP BeadChip arrays carrying probes for approximately 300,000 SNPs. This array platform uses log R ratio (LRR) and B allele frequency (BAF) as metrics to detect copy number changes. Although microarray-based comparative genomic hybridization (array-CGH) has been previously used to assess the chromosomal abnormalities of uterine LMS [15, 16], this is the first study to apply a SNP-array platform to analyze the genomic structural alterations of LMS together with LM. SNP-array platforms are advantageous over the array-CGH method in that the platforms can detect copy neutral loss of heterozygosity and mosaics in addition to copy number alterations. LMS samples showed highly disturbed LRR and BAF distributions compared to NM and LM samples, suggesting extensive numerical and structural changes as well as a highly mosaic constitution of chromosomes (Figure 1).

To estimate the extent of chromosomal aberrations for each sample, we used two copy number variation (CNV) calling tools, the CNV partition plug-in V3.0.7.0 (Illumina) and the R-GADA package [11]. We initially used the CNV partition, which detected copy neutral loss of heterozygosity (CN-LOH) accurately but failed to call gains and losses under mosaic chromosomal constitution. Therefore, we subsequently used R-GADA, which better detected gains and losses at chromosomally mosaic regions. We regarded the sum of the ratio of the copy number altering changes (gain and loss) detected by R-GADA and that of copy neutral changes (CN-LOH) detected by CNV partition as the approximate ratio of chromosomal abnormalities in this study. Consistent with the appearance of their LRR and BAF plots (Figure 1), LMS samples were highly chromosomally abnormal (66.7–89.5%) (Supplementary Material, Table S1, in Supplementary Material available online at http://dx.doi.org/10.1155/2015/412068). Compared to the LRR patterns of the LMS samples, those of the LMS-derived cell lines (SKN, SK-UT1, and SK-UT1B) were less complex, indicating that these cell lines are composed of cells with a single type or limited types of chromosomal constitution(s), which is likely due to a selection for cells capable of rapid and infinite cell division. LM samples were found to contain no or limited ratios of chromosomal abnormalities (0.7 to 8.7%). The numerical and structural abnormalities across almost all chromosomes are the genomic features specific to LMS, at least among the samples examined in this study, suggesting the possible use of CNV profiles as diagnostic information for LMS.

We found that the *CDKN2A* locus was homozygously deleted in LMS2 and SKN (Figure 2). The p16 protein, encoded by the *CDKN2A* gene, plays a critical role in the regulation of the G1 cell cycle phase by inhibiting cyclin D and RB proteins and is known to be inactivated in many types of carcinomas and sarcomas [17]. A study of 77 LMS cases in soft tissues other than the uterus showed that decreased p16 expression correlates with promoter methylation of the *CDKN2A* gene and poor prognoses in patients [18]. Consistent with a previous study reporting the homozygous deletion of the *CDKN2A* locus in uterine LMS [19], our data further confirms the involvement of the functional loss of p16 during the development of uterine LMS.

Somatic mutations in the *FH* gene (encoding fumarate hydratase) [20] and in the *MED12* gene (encoding mediator complex subunit 12) [21] have been identified in 1.3% of sporadic and 70% of unselected uterine LMs, respectively. Approximately 40% to 50% of LMs are reported to contain cytogenetic rearrangements, such as those involving 12q15 or 6p21 and 7q deletions [22]. Furthermore, complex chromosomal rearrangements involving 7q, *COL4A5-COL4A6*, *HMGA2*, and *RAD51B* loci have been reported to be observed in a subset of LMs [23]. Therefore, not only mutations in specific genes but also chromosomal abnormalities are likely involved in genetic causes of LM and should be further explored. The accumulation of CNV profiles of unusual variants of LM (such as mitotically active cases) is urgently needed.

3.2. Gene Expression Signatures and Candidate Expression Markers Distinguishing LMS from LM. We obtained gene expression profiles of NM, LM, and LMS samples together with those of LMS cell lines and found that hierarchical clustering for a subset of differentially expressed genes (1,036 genes selected as described in Section 2) and the PCA for the entire dataset reliably distinguished LMS samples (and LMS cell lines) from NM and LM samples (Figures 3(a) and 3(b)), as shown previously [24]. To search for candidate expression markers distinguishing NM, LM, and LMS, we selected probes whose signal intensities are high in one (or two) of the three types and are low (below the background level) in the other types. Using flag (present/absent call) and normalized log 2 intensity of ">6" as filters (Supplementary Material, Table S2), four NM/LM-specific, four NM-specific, one LM-specific, and 45 LMS-specific genes were selected (Figure 3(c) and Supplementary Material, Table S3). The selected LMS-specific genes were found to contain many genes known to encode a key cell cycle-related protein (such as *TICRR* [25] and *KIF4A* [26]) and to be involved in the cell cycle progression of cancerous cells (such as *CDCA2* [27] and *MELK* [28]). The 45 LMS-specific genes contain a number of critical cell cycle regulators and transcription factors that were not identified as genes overexpressed in LMS in a previous expression array study [24]. Therefore, the expression array dataset in this study provides additional information that facilitates understanding of the cancer biology of LMS. Although these candidate markers need to be validated in larger numbers of samples for their specificity, it is likely possible to establish a quantitative RT-PCR-based diagnostic method to distinguish LMS and LM using a combination of highly specific markers, for example, the *PGR* gene (encoding progesterone receptor) silenced in LMS and one of the LMS-specific cell cycle-related genes.

We counted the numbers of differentially expressed genes, upregulated (>2.0-fold) or downregulated (<0.5-fold), in three each of LM and LMS samples compared to the average of three NM samples (Supplementary Material, Figure S1). Although the numbers of upregulated and downregulated genes in six samples were similar, ranging from 5,999 to 8,932 and from 3,473 to 6,155, respectively (Supplementary Material, Figure S1), the numbers of probes commonly up- or downregulated among three samples differed significantly. In the three LMS samples, 20.4% and 22.1% of probes were commonly up- and downregulated, respectively, whereas only 2.9% and 4.7% were commonly up- and downregulated among the three LM samples (Supplementary Material, Figure S1), indicating that the contents of differentially expressed genes were similar among LMS samples but diverse among LM samples.

We performed GO analysis (see Section 2) to elucidate functional features of differentially expressed genes in LM and LMS samples compared to NM tissues. The results for the GOTERM_BP_FAT category (BP, biological process) were summarized in Figure 3(d) (full results are provided in Supplementary Material, Table S4). Commonly in all three LMS samples, genes related to the "cell cycle phase" and "cell adhesion" were statistically significantly enriched among up- and downregulated genes, respectively. In contrast, enrichment of GO terms differed across the three LM samples. Statistically significant (Benjamini's corrected P value < 0.05) enrichment of GO terms among upregulated genes was observed only in LM2 ("chromosome segregation"). Although the GO terms enriched among downregulated genes were very similar between LM1 and LM2 ("regulation of cell motion"), those in LM3 were totally different ("translation"). The observed downregulation of translation-related genes including many ribosomal protein genes and translation initiation/elongation factor genes was considered to be associated with the administration of the gonadotrophin-releasing hormone analogue to the patient of LM3 (Table 1).

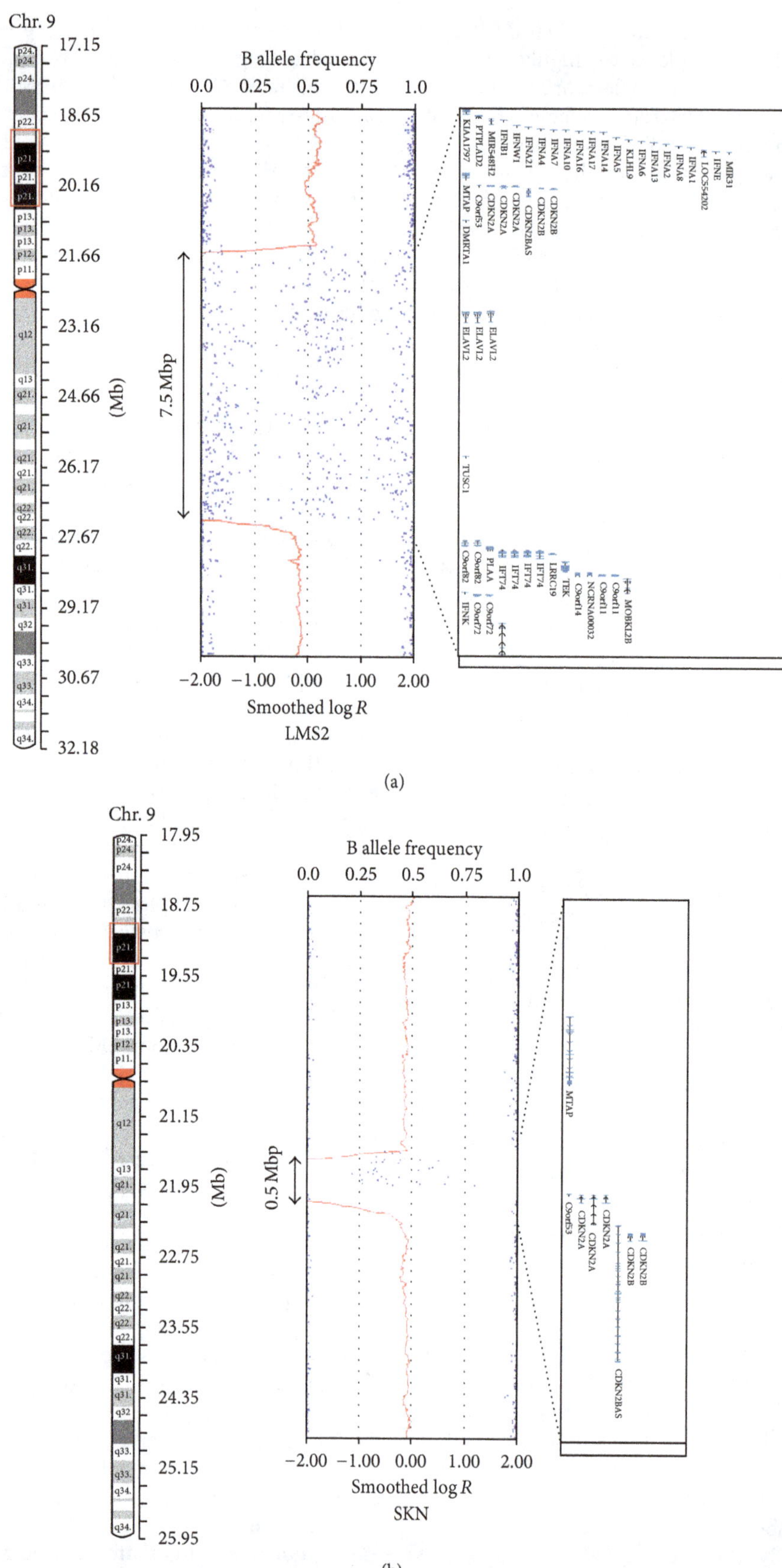

FIGURE 2: Homozygous deletions involving the *CDKN2A* and *CDKN2B* genes at chromosome 9p21.3 detected in LMS2 and SKN. A 7.5 Mb region (Chr9: 20,908,374–28,420,020, hg19) and a 0.5 Mb region (Chr9: 21,695,893-22,195,820, hg19) were found to be homozygously deleted in LMS2 (a) and in SKN (b), respectively.

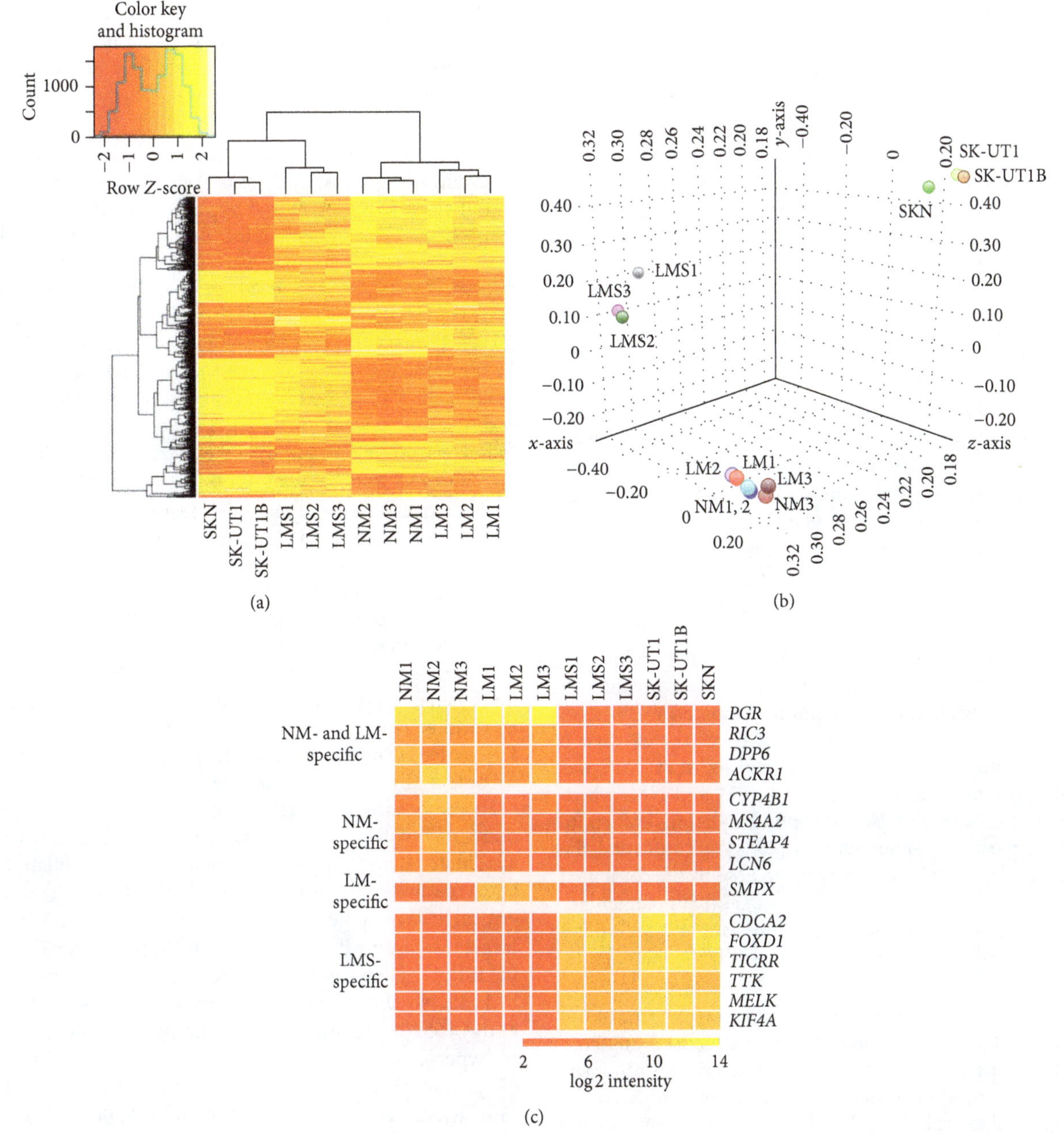

	Upregulated (fold-change >2.0) Term	*P* value	Downregulated (fold-change <0.5) Term	*P* value		Upegulated (fold-change >2.0) Term	*P* value	Downregulated (fold-change <0.5) Term	*P* value
LM1	Cytoskeleton-dependent intracellular transport	7.8*E* − 05	Regulation of cell motion	4.8*E* − 10	LMS1	Cell cycle phase	4.4*E* − 36	Cell adhesion	1.5*E* − 13
	Wnt receptor signaling pathway	2.9*E* − 04	Angiogenesis	4.3*E* − 10		M phase	4.8*E* − 35	Biological adhesion	1.6*E* − 13
	Cell cycle process	2.3*E* − 04	Regulation of cell migration	1.4*E* − 09		Cell cycle process	3.3*E* − 32	Muscle system process	1.1*E* − 09
LM2	Chromosome segregation	2.1*E* − 09	Regulation of cell motion	2.3*E* − 11	LMS2	Cell cycle phase	5.5*E* − 36	Response to wounding	6.3*E* − 12
	Organelle fission	9.2*E* − 08	Regulation of locomotion	8.8*E* − 10		M phase	2.5*E* − 34	Cell adhesion	3.8*E* − 11
	Cell cycle	2.8*E* − 07	Regulation of cell migration	6.8*E* − 10		Organelle fission	5.4*E* − 34	Biological adhesion	4.2*E* − 11
LM3	Cell-cell signaling	5.9*E* − 05	Translation	7.4*E* − 16	LMS3	Cell cycle phase	8.0*E* − 42	Blood vessel morphogenesis	6.9*E* − 08
	Neuron differentiation	1.4*E* − 04	Translational elongation	8.0*E* − 11		M phase	3.4*E* − 39	Muscle organ development	6.9*E* − 08
	Neuron development	1.9*E* − 04	Ubiquitin-dependent protein catabolic process	4.8*E* − 10		Cell cycle process	6.5*E* − 37	Blood vessel development (cell adhesion)	7.0*E* − 08 1.3*E* − 06 (9th)

(d)

FIGURE 3: Transcriptome analysis for NM, LM, LMS, and LMS-derived cell lines. (a) Hierarchical clustering analysis for the normalized log 2-transformed intensities of the 1,036 differentially expressed genes using Heatmap2. (b) Three-dimensional visualization of PCA for the entire probe set. (c) Candidate expression markers. Of the 45 LMS-specific genes selected, only six, whose log 2 intensities in LMS and LMS-derived cell lines are >9, are shown (full genes are shown in Supplementary Material, Table S3). (d) GO analysis for up- and downregulated genes in each of the LM and LMS samples. The top three GO terms of biological process and their *P* values are shown in black when the corresponding Benjamini's corrected *P* value was <0.05 or are otherwise shown in grey.

Taken together, our annotations for the gene expression profiles of LM and LMS confirmed that these benign and malignant tumors can be distinguished by transcriptomic features as well as specific expression markers. However, as the three LM samples examined showed considerable variations in the contents of differentially expressed genes, data should be interpreted with caution. This also highlights the need for a dataset with a larger number of LM cases that can be used to define and classify the gene expression variations among the spectrum of LM cases.

3.3. Characterization of Genome-Wide DNA Methylation Profiles of LMS. We obtained genome-wide DNA methylation profiles of NM, LM, and LMS samples and LMS-derived cell lines and used β values (DNA methylation levels) of 471,511 probes that passed quality control procedures (Figure 4(a)) for subsequent analyses. It should be noted that this is the first study describing the genome-wide DNA methylation profiles of LMS and LMS-derived cell lines. In a hierarchical clustering analysis, four groups (three histological types and the group of cell lines) were branched into different clusters (Figure 4(b)), clearly indicating that genome-wide DNA methylation datasets can distinguish NM, LM, and LMS. Boxplot representation (Figure 4(c)) of β values for all 471,511 probes revealed that the medians of β values in LMS samples were apparently lower compared to those of NM and LM. Scatter plots (Figure 4(d)) of the average β values for the same probe set also showed that LMS was globally hypomethylated compared to LM and NM, which is consistent with the global hypomethylation known to occur in most malignant tumors [29]. We confirmed the hypomethylation of LINE1 elements in LMS by the combined bisulfite restriction analysis (Figure 4(e) and Supplementary Material, Figure S2). These results demonstrate that LM and LMS can be distinguished by their global DNA methylation levels.

Since the genome-wide DNA methylation patterns of LM have been described previously [30], we focused on those of LMS in this study. To explore genomic features of hyper- and hypomethylation observed in LMS, we compared the average β values of LMS and NM samples in six gene feature categories, namely, intergenic, TSS1500 (200 bp to 1500 bp upstream from a transcription start site (TSS)), TSS200 (within 200 bp upstream from a TSS), 5′UTR (untranslated region) and the first exon, gene body, and 3′UTR (Figures 4(f)–4(k) and Table 2). The extent of hypomethylation was striking in the intergenic, TSS1500, gene body, and 3′UTR categories (29.0%, 14.4%, 15.8%, and 14.4%, resp.) (Figures 4(f), 4(g), 4(j), and 4(k)) but less striking in the TSS200 and 5′UTR/first-exon categories (7.2% and 10.0%) (Figures 4(h) and 4(i)). The extent of hypermethylation was consistently lower than that of hypomethylation in all six categories and tended to be lower in the TSS and its vicinities (2.1% to 3.2%) compared to other categories (3.9% to 4.5%). CpG sites within CpG islands (CGIs), the majority of which are unmethylated, were found to be more frequently hypermethylated (4.5%) than those outside of CGIs (2.5% in open sea) and to be much less frequently hypomethylated (4.6%) than those outside CGIs (16.7% in shores and shelves, and 28.1% in open sea) (Figures 4(l)–4(n) and Table 2). These results demonstrate that TSS and/or CGI regions tended to be resistant to genome-wide demethylation and were partly methylated *de novo*, during tumorigenesis.

When averages of the β values were compared between LMS and NM groups, 17,037 (3.6%) and 80,549 (17.1%) probes were hyper- ($\Delta\beta > 0.2$) and hypomethylated ($\Delta\beta < -0.2$), respectively. We subjected the same dataset to the IMA [12]: 1,151 and 6,095 genes were found to host hyper- and hypomethylated regions in at least one of the six gene feature groups of TSS1500, TSS200, 5′UTR, first exon, gene body, and 3′UTR (Figure 4(a) and Supplementary Material, Table S5). In the same analyses conducted for LM compared to NM, 14,053 (3.0%) and 9,510 (2.0%) probes were found to be hyper- and hypomethylated (Table 2), and 869 and 770 genes were found to host hyper- and hypomethylated regions in at least one of the six gene feature groups (data not shown).

We assessed the functional features of differentially methylated regions in LMS by GO analysis using the GREAT annotation website [13] as described in Section 2. We observed that hypermethylated regions were highly significantly enriched with homeobox and *PCDH* (protocadherin) genes (Supplementary Material, Table S5 and Figure S3). Polycomb group (PcG) target genes including many homeobox genes are known to be abnormally hypermethylated in various cancers [31]. Hypermethylation of the subset of PcG genes encoding developmental regulators is considered to potentially contribute to the stem-like state of cancer [32]. Protocadherin proteins contain extracellular cadherin domains involved in cell adhesion and are suggested to be candidate tumor suppressors because they modulate regulatory pathways (such as canonical Wnt signaling) that are critical in development and disease [33, 34]. Among 1,893 PcG target (SUZ12-positive) genes identified previously (Table S8 in [35]), 197 genes (10.4%) were found to be hypermethylated in LMS. Notably, 37 out of 197 genes were hypermethylated at the TSS200 region, which was found to be most resistant to hypermethylation (Figure 4(h)). Likewise, we identified 29 protocadherin genes to be hypermethylated in LMS, 15 of which were hypermethylated at TSS200. Hierarchical clustering of DNA methylation values of the aforementioned 37 PcG target genes and 15 protocadherin genes distinguished NM, LM, and LMS (Figure 5(a)).

A whole-genome bisulfite sequencing study has revealed that large blocks (up to several Mb) of hypomethylation were observed for more than half of the genome in colon cancers and that this feature was common in other solid tumors [36]. In the GO analysis, we observed that hypomethylated regions in LMS were frequently enriched with gene clusters such as olfactory receptor genes, kallikrein-related peptidase (*KLK*) genes, keratin-associated protein genes, and serine protease genes (Supplementary Material, Table S6 and Figure S4). These gene clusters were found to be located within genomic regions that were identified as hypomethylation blocks in colon cancers [36]. Taken together, the annotations for differentially methylated regions in LMS compared to NM demonstrate that LMS exhibits epigenomic features such as

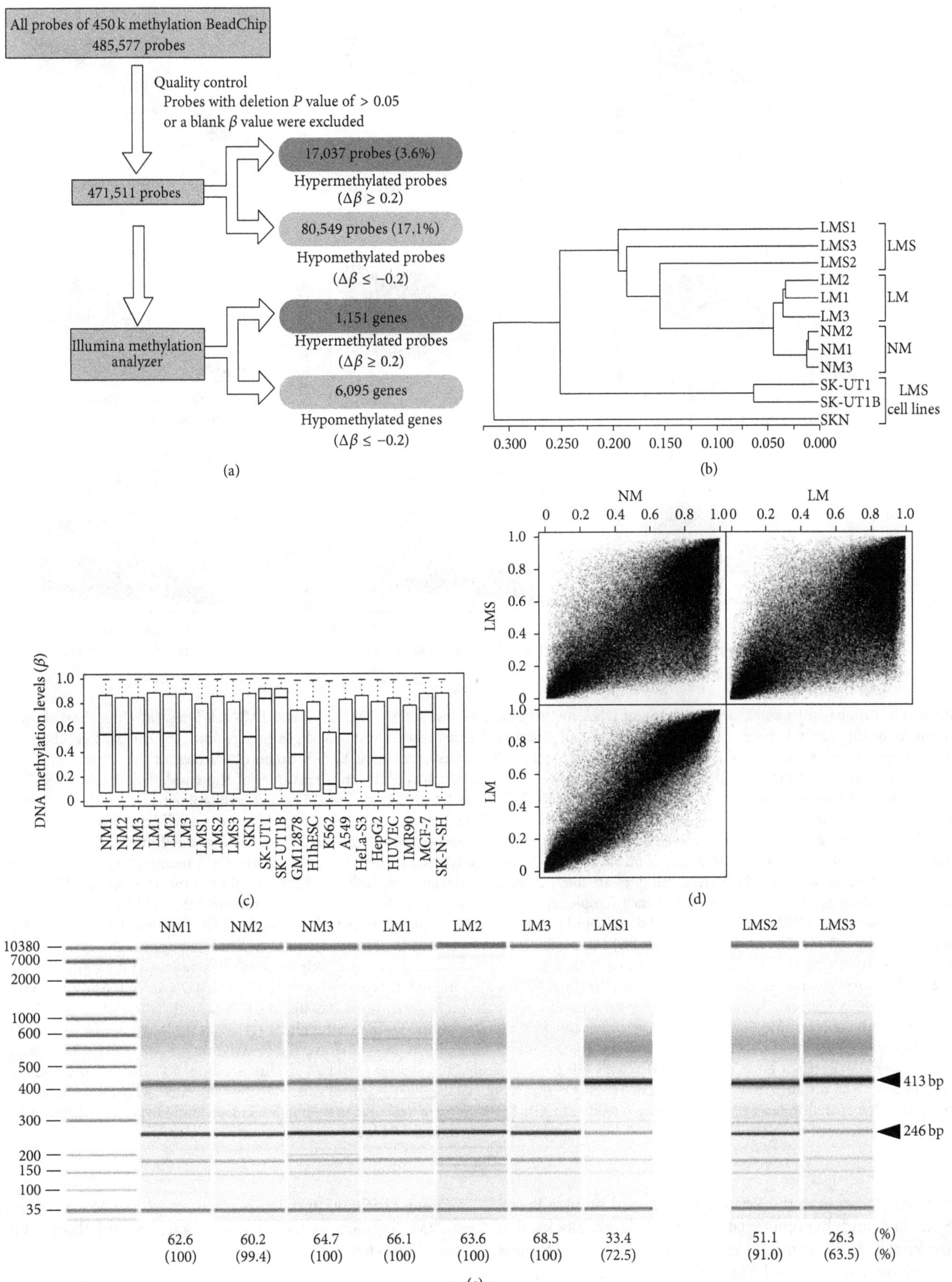

FIGURE 4: Continued.

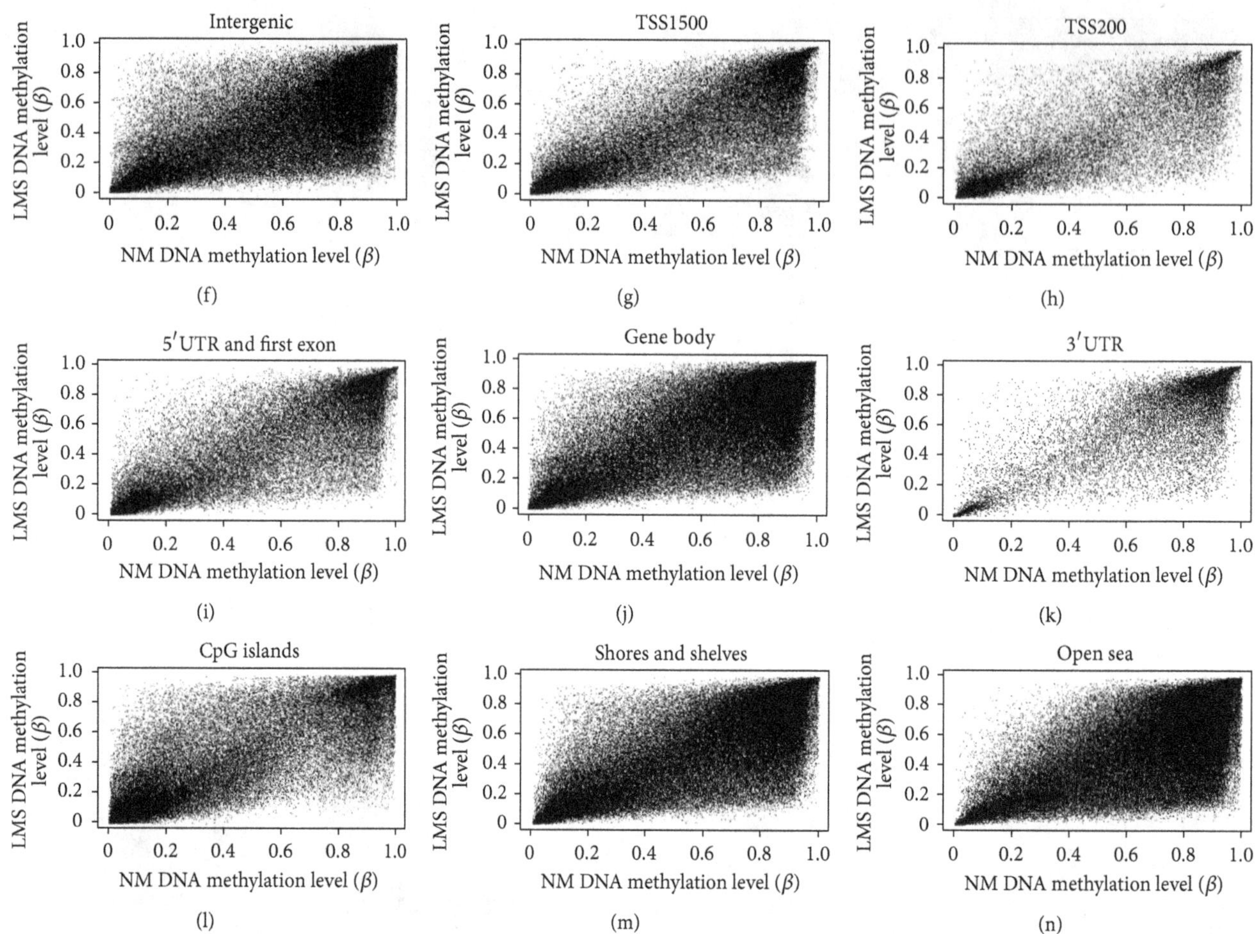

FIGURE 4: Comparisons and characterization of DNA methylation profiles of NM, LM, LMS, and LMS cell lines. (a) Flow chart showing results of quality control procedures and the extraction of differentially methylated probes and genomic regions. (b) Hierarchical clustering of 12 samples using β values of 471,511 probes that passed the data QC procedures (see (a)). (c) Boxplots of β values for the 471,511 probes that passed QC procedures for 12 samples analyzed in this study, as well as boxplots of the entire β values of HumanMethylation450 BeadChip data for ten cell lines obtained from the ENCODE DNA Methylation Track (http://hgdownload.cse.ucsc.edu/goldenPath/hg19/encodeDCC/wgEncodeHaibMethyl450/). Whereas LMS tissues exhibited global hypomethylation tendencies, LMS-derived cell lines did not. To assess whether observed global methylation levels (normal or hyper) are specific to LMS-derived cell lines, we examined those of six cancer cell lines (K562, A549, HeLa-S3, HepG2, MCF-7, and SK-N-SH) and confirmed their highly various levels. The DNA methylation profiles of these cancer cell lines as well as LMS-derived cell lines are likely extensively deviated from those of their origin (a cancerous tissue). (d) Scatter (x-y) plots showing the average β values of each sample for the 471,511 probes (NM versus LM, NM versus LMS, and LM versus LMS). (e) COBRA assays for LINE1 methylation. 413-bp and 246-bp bands represent uncut (unmethylated) and cut (methylated) bands upon *Hinf*I digestion, respectively. The methylation index (%) was calculated as (the intensity of the cut band/246)/((the intensity of the cut band/246) + (the intensity of the uncut band/413)) and shown at the bottom. The measured methylation index was corrected using the standard curve (Supplementary Material, Figure S2) obtained with the methylated and unmethylated control bisulfite-converted DNAs (EpiTect PCR Control DNA Set #59695, Qiagen). The corrected methylation levels (%) are shown in parentheses. Though the LINE1 methylation levels of LM were similar to those of NM, LMS samples showed lower levels of LINE1 methylation. (f)–(k) Scatter plots of β values (LMS average (y-axis) versus NM average (x-axis)) in the six gene feature groups. (l)–(n) Scatter plots of β values (LMS average (y-axis) versus NM average (x-axis)) of three subgroups in relation to CpG islands (CGIs): CGIs (l), CGI shores and shelves (within 4 kb distance from a CGI) (m), and non-CGI regions (over 4 kb distance from a CGI, open sea) (n). CpG sites within CGIs, the majority of which are unmethylated, were found to be more frequently hypermethylated (4.5%) than those outside of CGIs (2.5% in open sea) and to be much less frequently hypomethylated (4.6%) than those outside of CGIs (16.7% in shores and shelves, and 28.1% in open sea) (Table 2).

hypermethylation at the PcG target gene and protocadherin gene loci and hypomethylation within large blocks that are known to be common among malignant solid tumors (Supplementary Material, Figure S4).

We also assessed the relation between changes in the gene expression and the DNA methylation at gene promoter regions (TSS1500 and TSS200) observed in LMS compared to NM (Supplementary Material, Figure S5) and observed no correlation between them.

3.4. Selection of Candidate Methylation Markers to Distinguish LMS from LM. As an attempt to identify candidate DNA

TABLE 2: Numbers of differentially methylated CpG sites in LM and LMS compared to normal metrium (NM) tissues.

Feature	# of CpG probes	Leiomyoma (LM)		Leiomyosarcoma (LMS)	
		Hypermethylated ($\Delta\beta > 0.2$)	Hypomethylated ($\Delta\beta < -0.2$)	Hypermethylated ($\Delta\beta > 0.2$)	Hypomethylated ($\Delta\beta < -0.2$)
Gene feature groups					
Intergenic	115,382	4,910 (4.3%)	2,776 (2.4%)	4,533 (3.9%)	33,513 (29.0%)
TSS1500	67,542	1,841 (2.7%)	1,059 (1.6%)	1,614 (2.4%)	9,741 (14.4%)
TSS200	50,513	877 (1.7%)	415 (0.8%)	1,043 (2.1%)	3,625 (7.2%)
5′UTR and 1st exon	63,745	1,504 (2.4%)	913 (1.4%)	2,025 (3.2%)	6,383 (10.0%)
Gene body	157,160	4,539 (2.9%)	3,894 (2.5%)	7,072 (4.5%)	24,809 (15.8%)
3′UTR	17,170	382 (2.2%)	453 (2.6%)	750 (4.4%)	2,478 (14.4%)
Total	**471,512**	**14,053 (3.0%)**	**9,510 (2.0%)**	**17,037 (3.6%)**	**80,549 (17.1%)**
Relation to CGI					
CGI	145,443	3,848 (2.6%)	884 (0.6%)	6,541 (4.5%)	6,612 (4.5%)
Shore and shelf	156,254	5,230 (3.3%)	2,960 (1.9%)	6,180 (4.0%)	26,231 (16.8%)
Open sea*	169,815	4,975 (2.9%)	5,666 (3.3%)	4,316 (2.5%)	47,706 (28.1%)
Total	**471,512**	**14,053 (3.0%)**	**9,510 (2.0%)**	**17,037 (3.6%)**	**80,549 (17.1%)**

*Outside of island, shore, and shelf.

$\Delta\beta$ of LM: average of the β values of three LM samples − average of the β values of three NM samples.

$\Delta\beta$ of LMS: average of the β values of three LMS samples − average of the β values of three NM samples.

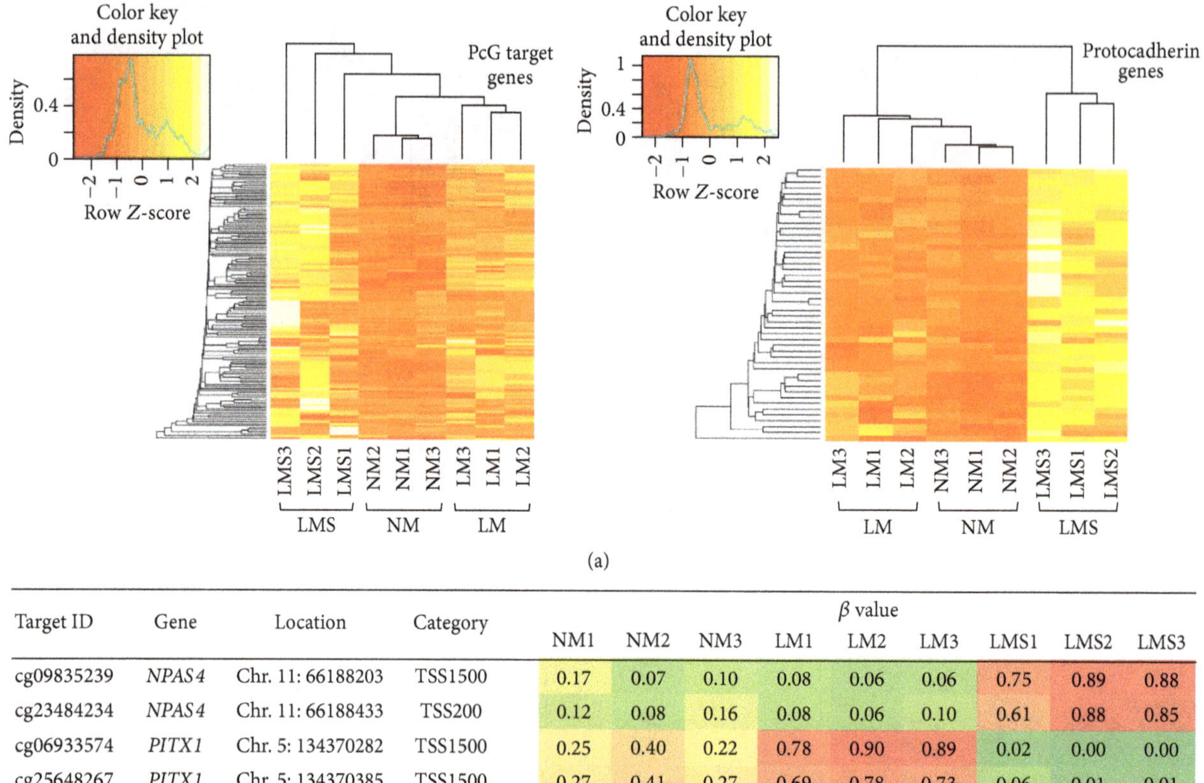

(a)

Target ID	Gene	Location	Category	β value								
				NM1	NM2	NM3	LM1	LM2	LM3	LMS1	LMS2	LMS3
cg09835239	*NPAS4*	Chr. 11: 66188203	TSS1500	0.17	0.07	0.10	0.08	0.06	0.06	0.75	0.89	0.88
cg23484234	*NPAS4*	Chr. 11: 66188433	TSS200	0.12	0.08	0.16	0.08	0.06	0.10	0.61	0.88	0.85
cg06933574	*PITX1*	Chr. 5: 134370282	TSS1500	0.25	0.40	0.22	0.78	0.90	0.89	0.02	0.00	0.00
cg25648267	*PITX1*	Chr. 5: 134370385	TSS1500	0.27	0.41	0.27	0.69	0.78	0.73	0.06	0.01	0.01

0 0.5 1

(b)

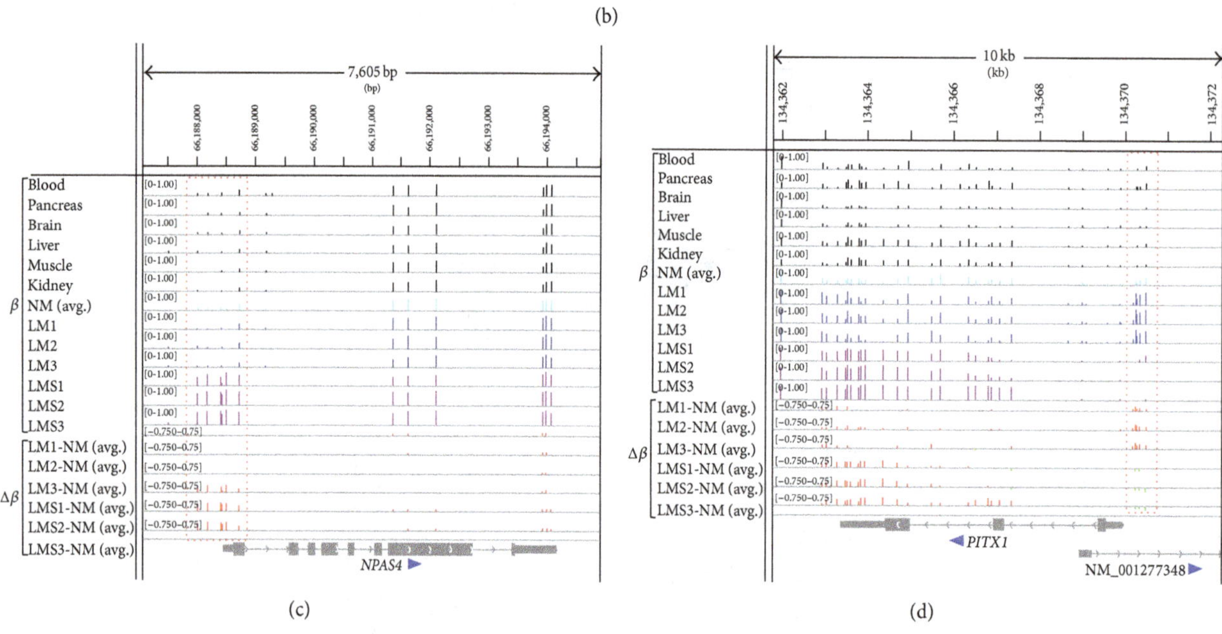

(c) (d)

FIGURE 5: Candidate methylation markers to distinguish LM and LMS. (a) Clustering analyses of TSS200 probes at 37 PcG target gene loci (left) and 15 protocadherin gene loci (right) hypermethylated ($\Delta\beta > 0.2$) in LMS compared to NM. The standard deviations of β values of 133 CpG probes (at 37 PcG target loci) ranged from 0.01 to 0.38 (median 0.22). The standard deviations of β values of 47 CpG probes (at 15 protocadherin genes) ranged from 0.06 to 0.31 (median 0.22). β values and Z-scores of those 133 and 47 CpG probes in NM, LM, and LMS samples are shown in Supplementary Material, Table S7. (b) Four selected promoter CpG sites whose methylation levels were strikingly different between LMS and LM. (c) and (d) DNA methylation profiles at *NPAS4* and *PITX1* loci. Methylation β values (data range: 0 to 1) and $\Delta\beta$ values (data range: −0.75 to 0.75) are shown as vertical bars using the Integrative Genomics Viewer. The colors of vertical bars for β values are as follows: black for six normal tissues (blood, pancreas, brain, liver, muscle, and kidney), light blue for the average of three NM samples ("NM(avg.)"), blue for LM samples, and purple for LMS samples. Positive and negative $\Delta\beta$ values for each of the LM and LMS samples (compared to NM(avg.)) are indicated by red and green vertical bars, respectively. The promoter region containing the probes shown in (b) is boxed by red dashed lines. Exon-intron structure and transcriptional orientation of the gene(s) are shown at the bottom.

methylation marker loci to reliably distinguish LMS and LM, we selected 69 probes whose methylation levels were strikingly different between LMS and LM using β value > 0.6 in all three samples in one group and β value < 0.1 in all three samples in the other group as filter conditions (data not shown; 69 probes consisted of 13 probes and 56 probes hypermethylated in LMS and LM, resp.). Among the 69 probes, 38 probes were mapped to 31 gene loci (the remaining 31 probes were located intergenically). These 38 probes were further selected using the following conditions: two or more probes were mapped within the TSS1500/TSS200 categories of one gene. As a result, the promoter regions of *NPAS4* and *PITX1* genes were selected as examples of candidate methylation marker loci (Figures 5(b)–5(d)). It should be noted that different candidates can be selected by changing filter conditions. The promoter region of the *NPAS4* gene (encoding the neuronal PAS domain Protein 4) was nearly unmethylated in normal tissues and LM samples but highly methylated only in LMS samples (Figure 5(c)). The promoter region of the *PITX1* gene (encoding the paired-like homeodomain 1 protein) was highly methylated only in LM samples but not in normal tissues and LMS samples (Figure 5(d)).

3.5. Feasibility of Developing Molecular Diagnostic Tests to Distinguish LMS from LM. We successfully identified omics features as well as candidate biomarkers that can distinguish LMS from LM. The array-based methods used in this study require only a few hundred nanograms of genomic DNA or total RNA. Therefore, omics profiles can be obtained for limited amounts of specimens such as those collected by transcervical needle biopsy. There is also the option to introduce next-generation sequencing-based methods, which require even smaller amounts of starting materials. Recently, a method to capture sarcoma cells circulating in peripheral blood has been developed [37]. Combining such a method with LMS-specific markers or omics signatures identified in this study will open up the possibility to develop a preoperative and noninvasive diagnostic test to distinguish LM and LMS.

4. Conclusions

We have demonstrated that omics profiles clearly distinguish typical uterine LMS and LM and represent reservoirs for molecular markers highly specific to LMS. While the numbers of the samples assessed were limited in this study, the array platforms adopted and the data analysis methods established in this study are directly applicable to a larger number of samples. In clinical settings, there is an urgent need for gynecologic oncologists to establish reliable methodologies that distinguish the intermediate grades of tumors, such as uterine smooth muscle tumors of uncertain malignant potential and atypical LM, from LMS. By obtaining omics profiles for such intermediate grades of tumors, it could be plausible to screen for good molecular markers for these tumors using the dataset in this study as a reference. The omics profiling methods and the dataset described in this study could help to develop preoperative and noninvasive diagnostic tests for LMS.

Acknowledgments

This study was supported by a grant from the Ministry of Health, Labour and Welfare of Japan (H26-Nambyo-Ippan-082) to Kenichiro Hata and a grant from the National Center for Child Health and Development (NCCHD) of Japan (24-3) to Kazuhiko Nakabayashi. The authors are grateful to Hiromi Kamura for her technical assistance. The paper was proofread and edited by Emma Barber of the Department of Education for Clinical Research, NCCHD.

References

[1] E. D'Angelo and J. Prat, "Uterine sarcomas: a review," *Gynecologic Oncology*, vol. 116, no. 1, pp. 131–139, 2010.

[2] S. E. Brooks, M. Zhan, T. Cote, and C. R. Baquet, "Surveillance, epidemiology, and end results analysis of 2677 cases of uterine sarcoma 1989–1999," *Gynecologic Oncology*, vol. 93, no. 1, pp. 204–208, 2004.

[3] R. L. Giuntoli II, D. S. Metzinger, C. S. DiMarco et al., "Retrospective review of 208 patients with leiomyosarcoma of the uterus: prognostic indicators, surgical management, and adjuvant therapy," *Gynecologic Oncology*, vol. 89, no. 3, pp. 460–469, 2003.

[4] E. A. Pritts, D. J. Vanness, J. S. Berek et al., "The prevalence of occult leiomyosarcoma at surgery for presumed uterine fibroids: a meta-analysis," *Gynecological Surgery*, vol. 12, no. 3, pp. 165–177, 2015.

[5] V. M. Abeler, O. Røyne, S. Thoresen et al., "Uterine sarcomas in Norway. A histopathological and prognostic survey of a total population from 1970 to 2000 including 419 patients," *Histopathology*, vol. 54, pp. 355–364, 1970.

[6] E. A. Vucic, K. L. Thu, K. Robison et al., "Translating cancer 'omics' to improved outcomes," *Genome Research*, vol. 22, no. 2, pp. 188–195, 2012.

[7] H. Ueno, H. Okita, S. Akimoto et al., "DNA methylation profile distinguishes clear cell sarcoma of the kidney from other pediatric renal tumors," *PLoS ONE*, vol. 8, no. 4, Article ID e62233, 2013.

[8] W. Zhang, Y. Liu, N. Sun et al., "Integrating genomic, epigenomic, and transcriptomic features reveals modular signatures underlying poor prognosis in ovarian cancer," *Cell Reports*, vol. 4, no. 3, pp. 542–553, 2013.

[9] M. Buyse and S. Michiels, "Omics-based clinical trial designs," *Current Opinion in Oncology*, vol. 25, no. 3, pp. 289–295, 2013.

[10] M. L. Hensley, B. A. Barrette, K. Baumann et al., "Gynecologic Cancer InterGroup (GCIG) consensus review: uterine and ovarian leiomyosarcomas," *International Journal of Gynecological Cancer*, vol. 24, no. 9, pp. S61–S66, 2014.

[11] R. Pique-Regi, A. Cáceres, and J. R. González, "R-Gada: A fast and flexible pipeline for copy number analysis in association studies," *BMC Bioinformatics*, vol. 11, article 380, 2010.

[12] D. Wang, L. Yan, Q. Hu et al., "IMA: an R package for high-throughput analysis of Illumina's 450K Infinium methylation data," *Bioinformatics*, vol. 28, no. 5, pp. 729–730, 2012.

[13] C. Y. McLean, D. Bristor, M. Hiller et al., "GREAT improves functional interpretation of cis-regulatory regions," *Nature Biotechnology*, vol. 28, no. 5, pp. 495–501, 2010.

[14] A. S. Yang, M. R. H. Estécio, K. Doshi, Y. Kondo, E. H. Tajara, and J.-P. J. Issa, "A simple method for estimating global DNA methylation using bisulfite PCR of repetitive DNA elements," *Nucleic Acids Research*, vol. 32, article e38, 2004.

[15] M. Raish, M. Khurshid, M. A. Ansari et al., "Analysis of molecular cytogenetic alterations in uterine leiomyosarcoma by array-based comparative genomic hybridization," *Journal of Cancer Research and Clinical Oncology*, vol. 138, no. 7, pp. 1173–1186, 2012.

[16] S. Croce, A. Ribeiro, C. Brulard et al., "Uterine smooth muscle tumor analysis by comparative genomic hybridization: a useful diagnostic tool in challenging lesions," *Modern Pathology*, vol. 28, no. 7, pp. 1001–1010, 2015.

[17] S. Negrini, V. G. Gorgoulis, and T. D. Halazonetis, "Genomic instability—an evolving hallmark of cancer," *Nature Reviews Molecular Cell Biology*, vol. 11, no. 3, pp. 220–228, 2010.

[18] K.-I. Kawaguchi, Y. Oda, T. Saito et al., "Mechanisms of inactivation of the p16INK4a gene in leiomyosarcoma of soft tissue: decreased p16 expression correlates with promoter methylation and poor prognosis," *Journal of Pathology*, vol. 201, no. 3, pp. 487–495, 2003.

[19] Y.-L. Zhai, T. Nikaido, A. Orii, A. Horiuchi, T. Toki, and S. Fujii, "Frequent occurrence of loss of heterozygosity among tumor suppressor genes in uterine leiomyosarcoma," *Gynecologic Oncology*, vol. 75, no. 3, pp. 453–459, 1999.

[20] R. Lehtonen, M. Kiuru, S. Vanharanta et al., "Biallelic inactivation of *Fumarate hydratase* (FH) occurs in nonsyndromic uterine leiomyomas but is rare in other tumors," *The American Journal of Pathology*, vol. 164, no. 1, pp. 17–22, 2004.

[21] N. Mäkinen, M. Mehine, J. Tolvanen et al., "MED12, the mediator complex subunit 12 gene, is mutated at high frequency in uterine leiomyomas," *Science*, vol. 334, no. 6053, pp. 252–255, 2011.

[22] A. A. Sandberg, "Updates on the cytogenetics and molecular genetics of bone and soft tissue tumors: leiomyoma," *Cancer Genetics and Cytogenetics*, vol. 158, no. 1, pp. 1–26, 2005.

[23] M. Mehine, E. Kaasinen, N. Mäkinen et al., "Characterization of uterine leiomyomas by whole-genome sequencing," *The New England Journal of Medicine*, vol. 369, no. 1, pp. 43–53, 2013.

[24] K. M. Skubitz and A. P. N. Skubitz, "Differential gene expression in leiomyosarcoma," *Cancer*, vol. 98, no. 5, pp. 1029–1038, 2003.

[25] C. G. Sansam, D. Goins, J. C. Siefert, E. A. Clowdus, and C. L. Sansam, "Cyclin-dependent kinase regulates the length of S phase through TICRR/TRESLIN phosphorylation," *Genes & Development*, vol. 29, no. 5, pp. 555–566, 2015.

[26] M. Mazumdar, S. Sundareshan, and T. Misteli, "Human chromokinesin KIF4A functions in chromosome condensation and segregation," *Journal of Cell Biology*, vol. 166, no. 5, pp. 613–620, 2004.

[27] F. Uchida, K. Uzawa, A. Kasamatsu et al., "Overexpression of CDCA2 in human squamous cell carcinoma: correlation with prevention of G1 phase arrest and apoptosis," *PLoS ONE*, vol. 8, no. 2, Article ID e56381, 2013.

[28] L. W. Hebbard, J. Maurer, A. Miller et al., "Maternal embryonic leucine zipper kinase is upregulated and required in mammary tumor-initiating cells in vivo," *Cancer Research*, vol. 70, no. 21, pp. 8863–8873, 2010.

[29] C. de Smet and A. Loriot, "DNA hypomethylation in cancer: epigenetic scars of a neoplastic journey," *Epigenetics*, vol. 5, no. 3, pp. 206–213, 2010.

[30] R. Maekawa, S. Sato, Y. Yamagata et al., "Genome-wide DNA methylation analysis reveals a potential mechanism for the pathogenesis and development of uterine leiomyomas," *PLoS ONE*, vol. 8, no. 6, Article ID e66632, 2013.

[31] D. J. Weisenberger, "Characterizing DNA methylation alterations from The Cancer Genome Atlas," *Journal of Clinical Investigation*, vol. 124, no. 1, pp. 17–23, 2014.

[32] H. Easwaran, S. E. Johnstone, L. Van Neste et al., "A DNA hypermethylation module for the stem/progenitor cell signature of cancer," *Genome Research*, vol. 22, no. 5, pp. 837–849, 2012.

[33] Q. Wu and T. Maniatis, "A striking organization of a large family of human neural cadherin-like cell adhesion genes," *Cell*, vol. 97, no. 6, pp. 779–790, 1999.

[34] A. R. Dallosso, B. Øster, A. Greenhough et al., "Long-range epigenetic silencing of chromosome 5q31 protocadherins is involved in early and late stages of colorectal tumorigenesis through modulation of oncogenic pathways," *Oncogene*, vol. 31, no. 40, pp. 4409–4419, 2012.

[35] T. I. Lee, R. G. Jenner, L. A. Boyer et al., "Control of developmental regulators by Polycomb in human embryonic stem cells," *Cell*, vol. 125, no. 2, pp. 301–313, 2006.

[36] K. D. Hansen, W. Timp, H. C. Bravo et al., "Increased methylation variation in epigenetic domains across cancer types," *Nature Genetics*, vol. 43, no. 8, pp. 768–775, 2011.

[37] A. Satelli, A. Mitra, J. J. Cutrera et al., "Universal marker and detection tool for human sarcoma circulating tumor cells," *Cancer Research*, vol. 74, no. 6, pp. 1645–1650, 2014.

15

Intra-Articular Synovial Sarcomas: Incidence and Differentiating Features from Localized Pigmented Villonodular Synovitis

D. Nordemar,[1] J. Öberg,[2] O. Brosjö,[3] and M. Skorpil[4,5]

[1] *Department of Radiology, Capio S:t Göran Hospital, S:t Göransplan 1, 112 81 Stockholm, Sweden*
[2] *Department of Medical Physics, Karolinska University Hospital, Karolinska Vägen 1, 171 76 Solna, Sweden*
[3] *Department of Orthopaedics, Karolinska University Hospital, Karolinska Vägen 1, 171 76 Solna, Sweden*
[4] *Department of Radiology, Karolinska University Hospital, Karolinska Vägen 1, 171 76 Solna, Sweden*
[5] *Department of Molecular Medicine and Surgery, Karolinska Institute, Solnavägen 1, 171 77 Solna, Sweden*

Correspondence should be addressed to M. Skorpil; mikael.skorpil@ki.se

Academic Editor: Akira Kawai

Purpose. To determine the incidence of intra-articular synovial sarcomas and investigate if any radiological variables can differentiate them from localized (unifocal) pigmented villonodular synovitis (PVNS) and if multivariate data analysis could be used as a complementary clinical tool. *Methods.* Magnetic resonance images and radiographs of 7 cases of intra-articular synovial sarcomas and 14 cases of localized PVNS were blindedly reviewed. Variables analyzed were size, extra-articular growth, tumor border, blooming, calcification, contrast media enhancement, effusion, bowl of grapes sign, triple signal intensity sign, synovial low signal intensity, synovitis, age, and gender. Univariate and multivariate data analysis, the method of partial least squares-discriminant analysis (PLS-DA), were used. Register data on all synovial sarcomas were extracted for comparison. *Results.* The incidence of intra-articular synovial sarcomas was 3%. PLS-DA showed that age, effusion, size, and gender were the most important factors for discrimination between sarcomas and localized PVNS. No sarcomas were misclassified as PVNS with PLS-DA, while some PVNS were misclassified as sarcomas. *Conclusions.* The most important variables in differentiating intra-articular sarcomas from localized PVNS were age, effusion, size, and gender. Multivariate data analysis can be helpful as additive information to avoid a biopsy, if the tumor is classified as most likely being PVNS.

1. Introduction

Magnetic resonance imaging (MRI) is the method of choice when examining soft tissue tumors [1, 2]. Some benign tumors, such as lipomas and hemangiomas, can be safely diagnosed using MRI without the need of a biopsy [1, 3, 4]. Intra-articular sarcomas however pose a diagnostic problem, since they have similar MRI features to benign localized (unifocal) pigmented villonodular synovitis (PVNS) [5–9]. Since asymptomatic localized PVNS does not require surgical intervention, avoiding unnecessary biopsies of the much more common localized PVNS, without missing sarcomas, would be valuable. Localized PVNS is a benign neoplastic process representing approximately 6% of all PVNS and can, if the lesion is symptomatic, be removed arthroscopically with a negligible risk of recurrence [9, 10]. Sarcomas on the other hand are intermediate or high-grade malignant tumors with a high potential for metastases. Extensive surgery is required, sometimes ending in amputation [8]. Synovial sarcomas have the highest incidence among intra-articular sarcomas [11]. The term "synovial" is a misnomer, as the tumor does not origin from synovia. It merely reflects the histopathological similarities to developing synovial tissue [5]. No radiological distinguishing features have been established to differentiate intra-articular synovial sarcomas from benign tumors and in the literature there are only case reports or reviews of case reports [5, 6, 12–16]. In this study we reviewed 7 patients with intra-articular synovial sarcomas, which is a comparatively large material of these rare tumors. These were blindly reviewed together with localized PVNS to evaluate if any variables would be useful for differentiation. We also investigated if multivariate data analysis could add differential diagnostic information. Finally, data from the Scandinavian Sarcoma Group (SSG) on synovial sarcomas were compared to the intra-articular synovial sarcomas.

2. Materials and Methods

2.1. Patients and Register Data. Within the SSG 7 cases (6 males and 1 female) of intra-articular synovial sarcomas have been recorded between the years 2000 and 2013, all having MRI examinations. The mean age was 21 years (range 9–35 years). Six were located in the knee joint and 1 in the elbow joint. All 7 cases had chronic pain and pain on movement. One patient had symptoms for 5 months and the other 6 for at least 1 year. All diagnoses were histopathologically confirmed by pathologists subspecialized in sarcomas, based on histological appearance in combination with immunohistochemistry. Four cases were also tested and found to be positive for the translocation between chromosome X and chromosome 18 (SYT-SSX), which is specific for synovial sarcomas [14]. Three synovial sarcomas were monophasic and four were biphasic. Four patients were treated by operation and chemotherapy, one patient had operation and radiotherapy, one patient had only operation, and one patient refused operation but was treated with both chemotherapy and radiotherapy. No metastases were found at presentation. One patient had a recurrence and died 2.5 years after diagnosis, while 6 patients are disease-free.

For comparison, 14 MRI examinations of patients with localized (unifocal) PVNS (5 males and 9 females) diagnosed at a Sarcoma Center were included. Mean age was 42 years (range 15–70 years). Seven cases had histopathological specimens and all were diagnosed by pathologists subspecialized in sarcomas and soft tissue pathology. The other 7 were not operated on, but all were followed up clinically for up to 3 years with no signs of progression.

A senior radiologist with more than 30 years of experience in bone and soft tissue tumors, blinded to the diagnoses and clinical data, reviewed all 21 MRI examinations with regard to variables chosen from previous studies [5, 17, 18]: largest diameter (size), extra-articular growth, tumor border (well-defined or infiltrative), bowl of grapes sign, triple signal intensity sign, blooming (magnetic susceptibility artifact seen on gradient echo sequences (GRE)), calcification on radiographs, and contrast media enhancement [8, 18]. The amount of effusion ("small" refers to normal amounts of fluid, "large" refers to the bursa suprapatellaris or elbow joint being clearly distended with fluid, and "moderate" refers to being in-between small and large), low signal intensity in the synovia (suggesting hemosiderin), and synovitis (general synovial contrast enhancement and/or "rice bodies") were also investigated. MRI sequences differed since most cases were referred.

Data on soft tissue sarcomas were extracted from the SSG Central Register, where data on all sarcoma patients in Scandinavia from 1979 and forward are recorded. Up until July 2014, a total of 9327 soft tissue sarcomas were registered. 334 of them lacked some relevant information and were therefore excluded. A total of 446 cases of synovial sarcomas (Table 1) were diagnosed between 1986 and 2013, which amounts to 5% of all soft tissue sarcomas in the register. Mean age at diagnosis was 39 years (range 6–86 years). The male : female ratio was 1 : 1. Between 2000 and 2013 a total of 226 synovial sarcomas were diagnosed. During this period approximately 3% of the synovial sarcomas were intra-articular (7/226). In addition to the 7 synovial sarcomas, there was one case of an intra-articular chondrosarcoma and one case of an intra-articular liposarcoma in the SSG Register between 2000 and 2013.

Table 1: Data on all synovial sarcomas from the SSG Central Register.

	Mean (SD)
Age (years)	38.8 (19.2)
Size (cm)	7.3 (4.9)
Male : female ratio	1 : 1
Metastasis at primary diagnosis	8.3%
Disease-free survival at latest follow-up	54%
Disease-free survival versus age*	
≤20 years of age (68/83)	82%
>20 years of age (157/331)	47%
Disease-free survival versus tumor size**	
≤5 cm (131/175)	75%
>5 cm (95/240)	40%
Disease-free survival versus age and tumor size	
≤20 years of age and ≤5 cm (40/41)	98%
>20 years of age and >5 cm (58/179)	32%
Patients with metastasis at primary diagnosis	Mean (SD)
Size (cm)	10.6 (4.8)

*32 cases had missing data regarding age. **31 cases had missing data regarding tumor size.

2.2. Statistics. For univariate data analysis Kruskal-Wallis 1-way ANOVA and Fisher's exact test were used. Bonferroni correction was subsequently used. Phi was used for covariation analysis. $p < 0.05$ was chosen as the significance level.

For multivariate data analysis the method partial least squares-discriminant analysis (PLS-DA) was used (SIMCA; Umetrics AB, Umea, Sweden). PLS-DA relates data matrices to each other by a linear multivariate model. Before performing PLS-DA, data are mean-centered and scaled to unit variance. A Y-matrix is formed, encoding class membership by a set of "dummy" variables (e.g., group one = 0 and group two = 1). PLS-DA then relates the X-matrix, containing the observed data, and Y to each other by a linear multivariate model. The aim of PLS-DA is to create a predictive model that, using linear combinations of the variables, best separates groups within the data. The prediction parameter, Q^2, provides an estimate of the predictive power of a principal component. For the models built in this study Q^2 needs to

Table 2: Univariate data analysis.

	PVNS Mean (range)	Sarcoma Mean (range)	p value
Size (cm)	2.5 (1.5–5)	4.6 (2–9)	0.059
Age (years)	41 (15–70)	21 (9–35)	0.012*
	Number of patients/total#	Number of patients/total#	
Gender (male)	5/14	6/7	0.063
Extra-articular growth	0/14	1/7	0.33
Blooming	1/5	1/2	1.0
Calcification	0/7	2/2	0.028*
Effusion			0.016*
Small	6/14	7/7	
Moderate	5/14	0/7	
Large	3/14	0/7	
Low signal intensity in synovia	2/14	0/7	0.53
Synovitis	4/14	0/7	0.25

Total# refers to all patients with available information. *Significant prior to Bonferroni correction.

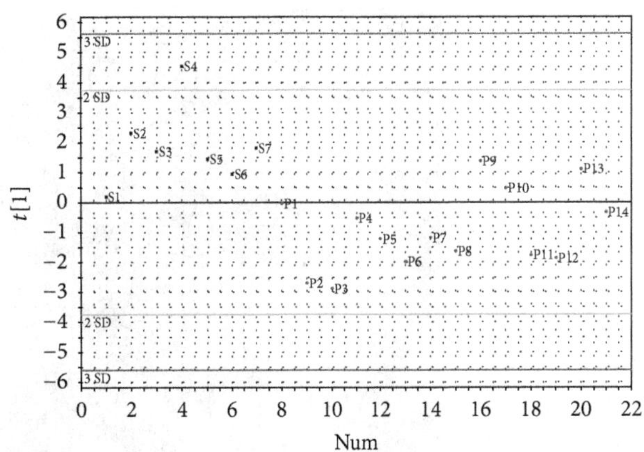

Figure 1: One-dimensional PLS-DA score plot showing the separation of the two groups. The color of each dot represents the actual diagnosis of that case, where black corresponds to sarcoma and red to localized PVNS. Green and red horizontal lines correspond to two or three standard deviations (SD) of the t_1 vector.

Table 3: Variable influence on projection (VIP) parameters for the variables in the model.

Age	1.32
Effusion	1.32
Size	1.22
Gender (F)	1.16
Gender (M)	1.16
Synovitis (Y)	0.84
Synovitis (N)	0.84
Extra-articular growth (Y)	0.78
Extra-articular growth (N)	0.78
Low signal intensity in synovia (Y)	0.56
Low signal intensity in synovia (N)	0.56

be larger than 0.05. PLS-DA gives one or more vectors of scores (t), which summarizes all the variables entering the analysis. A score plot can be seen as a window in the X-space, displaying the observations (i.e., patients) as situated on the projection planes. The variable influence on projection (VIP) parameters reflect the importance of terms in the model with respect to both Y and X. Terms with large VIP, larger than 1, are the most relevant for explaining Y. Effusion was treated as a quantitative variable ranging from 1 (small) to 3 (large).

When analyzing SSG-data on all synovial sarcomas, receiver operating characteristics (ROC) analysis was used to find the best cut-off values for age and tumor size as prognostic factors.

3. Results

All patients with available MRI sequences had the same results for well-defined borders (all), bowl of grapes sign (none), triple signal intensity sign (none), and contrast enhancement (all), and these variables were excluded in the final analysis. Covariation was tested for size and calcification in the intra-articular sarcomas and was not significant (p = 0.06).

3.1. Univariate Data Analysis. Data for localized PVNS and intra-articular sarcomas are shown in Table 2. No variables were significant after Bonferroni correction.

3.2. Multivariate Data Analysis. Calcification and blooming were excluded in the multivariate data analysis due to the number of cases with missing radiographs (12 cases) or missing GRE sequences (14 cases). PLS-DA gave a one-component model. R^2X, the variance in X explained by the model, was 0.33. R^2Y, the variance in Y explained by the model, was 0.51. Q^2 was 0.43. Figure 1 shows the score plot of the significant component (t_1) of the PLS-DA model. Figures 2 and 3 show two sarcomas with different t_1 values: one with a high t_1 and one with more indeterminate t_1. Figure 4 shows localized PVNS with large amounts of effusion.

The VIP of the PLS-DA in Figure 1 is shown in Table 3. VIPs are sorted in descending order of importance and it can be concluded that the variables age, effusion, size, and gender were the most important variables for the separation.

3.3. ROC Analysis. Most important prognostic factors on all synovial sarcomas were age ≤ 20 years and size ≤ 5 cm. 82% of patients aged ≤ 20 and 75% of patients with a tumor ≤ 5 cm had disease-free survival at latest follow-up.

4. Discussion

Using multivariate data analysis, the most important variables to differentiate intra-articular synovial sarcomas from localized PVNS were size, effusion, age, and gender. With univariate analysis no variables were significant after Bonferroni correction.

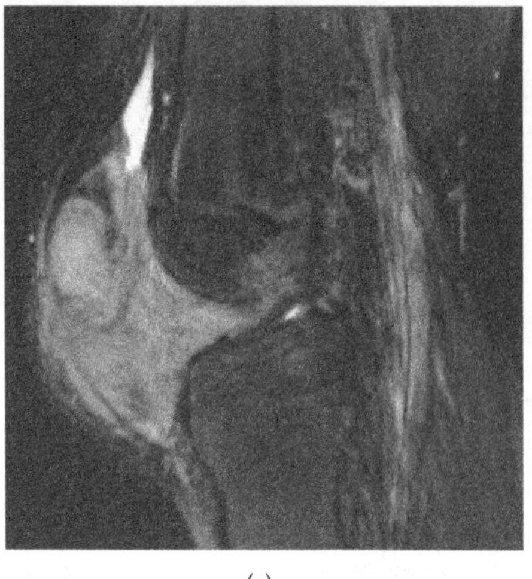

(a)

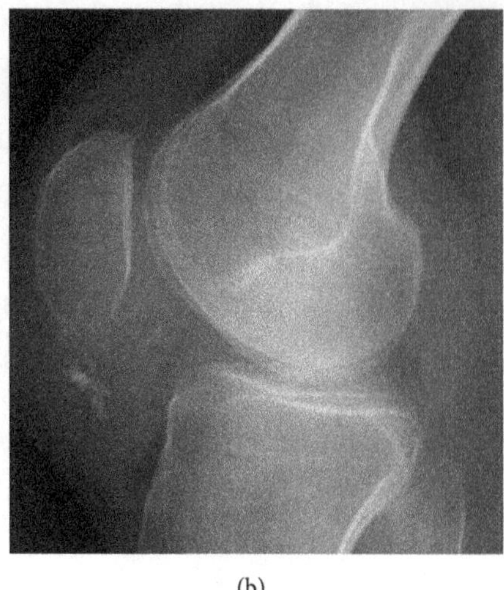

(b)

FIGURE 2: 17-year-old boy with a large sarcoma in Hoffa's fat pad (case #S4). (a) Sagittal fat-saturated T2-weighted MR image shows the tumor growing extra-articularly and invading the patella. (b) Lateral radiograph shows intratumoral calcifications.

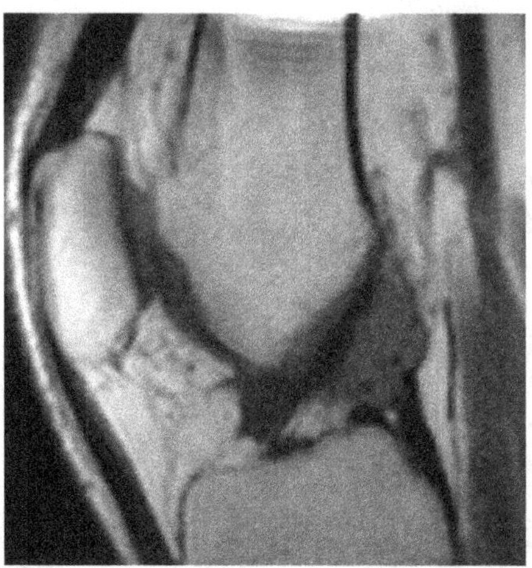

FIGURE 3: 34-year-old man with a small sarcoma at the cruciate ligaments (case #S6). Sagittal T1-weighted MR image.

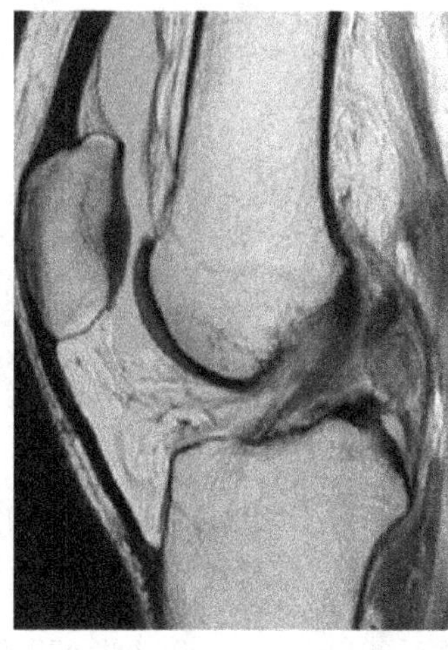

FIGURE 4: 24-year-old female with localized PVNS at the posterior cruciate ligament (case #P5). Bursa suprapatellaris is clearly distended with fluid. Sagittal proton density-weighted MR image.

Differentiating intra-articular synovial sarcomas from benign tumors is difficult and no certain radiological features have been established. The most challenging differential diagnosis is localized PVNS [5, 6, 10, 12–16]. Using multivariate data analysis this study showed that the most important variables for differentiation were size, effusion, age, and gender. PVNS had a size of 1–4 cm in a study by Murphey et al., although larger localized PVNS have been found [9, 10]. In our material all but one localized PVNS were ≤3 cm; that is, larger tumors should raise suspicion of a sarcoma. Importantly, however, intra-articular synovial sarcomas can be small [5]. Interestingly, moderate and large amounts of effusion were only found in PVNS. According to a study by Huang et al. on PVNS 8 out of 21 had effusion [10]. In previous reports of intra-articular synovial sarcomas a mean age of approximately 34 years has been presented, with only one patient being >50 years old [5]. The oldest sarcoma patient in our data was 35 years old. According to Murphey et al. PVNS is most common in the 3rd to 5th decades of life [9]. Since the male : female ratio is 1 : 1 in extra-articular synovial sarcomas, it was surprising that 6/7 intra-articular sarcoma patients were males. Friedman et al. have presented similar gender data on intra-articular synovial sarcomas with more than 70% of patients being males [5, 19]. However, the reason remains unclear. In synovial sarcomas chromosome X involves a *SYT-SSX* fusion gene, a very specific chromosomal translocation between chromosome X and chromosome 18 (t(X; 18)), which thereby could be subject to some gender difference [14].

Calcification and blooming were excluded in the multivariate data analysis due to several cases with missing radiographs or GRE sequences. Nevertheless, calcification is an important variable. Approximately 30% of synovial sarcomas have calcifications, while calcifications are not present in PVNS [6, 9]. In our material only 2 sarcomas had radiographs performed, but both had calcifications. This emphasizes the value of radiographs for differentiating intra-articular tumors. In our material only 7 patients had a GRE sequence performed, with 1/5 localized PVNS having "blooming" and 1/2 sarcomas also having "blooming." Thus, it could be questioned if GRE sequence is of value in localized intra-articular tumors. Extra-articular growth was not found to be significant in our study. However, it was only seen in one case (Figure 2), which was a sarcoma. In this study we also evaluated low signal intensity in the synovia (suggesting hemosiderin) and synovitis (contrast enhancement and/or "rice bodies"), but none of them was significant. For the following variables the results were identical for both groups, well-defined border, bowl of grapes sign, triple signal intensity sign, and contrast enhancement, which therefore ought to be of no clinical use. Although evaluated in other studies, we choose not to test for lobulation or bone invasion. In our experience, lobulation is too subjective for evaluation, and without radiographs or computed tomography bone invasion is difficult to differentiate from pressure erosions, which can be seen in PVNS [8].

No sarcoma was misclassified as PVNS in the multivariate data analysis, while some PVNS were misclassified as sarcomas. Since sensitivity is more important than specificity for malignant tumors, this is useful in a clinical setting. A biopsy would be indicated when the multivariate data analysis suggests a sarcoma, while a biopsy could be avoided when the tumor is classified as most likely being a localized PVNS. However, one sarcoma was close to being misclassified as a PVNS. In clinical practice, when an unknown intra-articular tumor needs to be differentiated between a sarcoma and localized PVNS, it should be tested against the model and inserted to the PLS-DA t_1 score plot. The further it is from the zero line, the stronger the suggestion is for either sarcoma or PVNS. This information will be regarded as additive to the radiologist's own judgement.

Extra-articular synovial sarcomas in the SSG Register had a higher mean age and larger mean size at diagnosis than intra-articular synovial sarcomas. This could be due to intra-articular tumors presenting with earlier symptoms. The incidence of synovial sarcoma arising in a joint has been unknown but believed to be low [6]. According to our data the incidence of intra-articular synovial sarcomas is 3% of all synovial sarcomas. The overall disease-free survival for intra-articular synovial sarcomas was 86% and for all synovial sarcomas 54%. For all synovial sarcomas in the SSG Register the disease-free survival was 98% in patients with tumor size ≤ 5 cm and age ≤ 20 years, compared to 32% in the group with size > 5 cm and age > 20 years. The only patient with intra-articular sarcoma in our study that did not survive had a tumor size of 3 cm.

There are some limitations to this study. Because of the rareness of the tumor, the material is small and the statistical analysis must be interpreted with care. However, we believe that the multivariate data analysis gives valuable clinical guidance. The database used only exists in our Sarcoma Center at this point, although an international database could be created. An advantage of using and expanding the database is that this could further improve the PLS-DA model in separating the tumors. We chose to include only localized PVNS as differential diagnosis, since other diagnoses rarely cause a problem. Multifocal PVNS is easily differentiated from a sarcoma, while hemangiomas and synovial osteochondromatosis also have a specific appearance [5, 6, 11]. Other sarcomas can exist intra-articularly but are even rarer. In 7 cases of localized PVNS there was no histopathological specimen, but all these patients are followed up at the Sarcoma Center with no suspicion of a sarcoma. In localized PVNS with no symptoms an operation is not advocated.

In conclusion, size, effusion, age, gender, and calcification are most useful for differentiation between sarcomas and localized PVNS. Sarcomas tend to be larger, have a small effusion, and be calcified, and the patients are younger and of male gender. To detect calcifications we recommend using radiographs as a complement to MRI. Although univariate analysis can be helpful, it is problematic in knowing how to best combine variables or which ones to rely upon. To overcome this a new approach was used, multivariate data analysis, which can be used as additive information to the radiologist. A biopsy could be avoided if it predicts that the tumor most likely is a localized PVNS.

References

[1] E. A. Walker, M. E. Fenton, J. S. Salesky, and M. D. Murphey, "Magnetic resonance imaging of benign soft tissue neoplasms in adults," *Radiologic Clinics of North America*, vol. 49, no. 6, pp. 1197–1217, 2011.

[2] ESMO/European Sarcoma Network Working Group, "Soft tissue and visceral sarcomas: ESMO Clinical Practice Guidelines for diagnosis, treatment and follow-up," *Annals of Oncology*, vol. 25, supplement 3, pp. iii102–iii112, 2014.

[3] H. Einarsdottir, V. Söderlund, O. Larson, G. Jenner, and H. C. F. Bauer, "MR imaging of lipoma and liposarcoma," *Acta Radiologica*, vol. 40, no. 1, pp. 64–68, 1999.

[4] M. D. Murphey, J. F. Carroll, D. J. Flemming, T. L. Pope, F. H. Gannon, and M. J. Kransdorf, "From the archives of the AFIP: benign musculoskeletal lipomatous lesions," *Radiographics*, vol. 24, no. 5, pp. 1433–1466, 2004.

[5] M. V. Friedman, M. Kyriakos, M. J. Matava, D. J. McDonald, J. W. Jennings, and D. E. Wessell, "Intra-articular synovial sarcoma," *Skeletal Radiology*, vol. 42, no. 6, pp. 859–867, 2013.

[6] L. T. Bui-Mansfield and S. D. O'Brien, "Magnetic resonance appearance of intra-articular synovial sarcoma: case reports and review of the literature," *Journal of Computer Assisted Tomography*, vol. 32, no. 4, pp. 640–644, 2008.

[7] M. F. Blacksin, J. R. Siegel, J. Benevenia, and S. C. Aisner, "Synovial sarcoma: frequency of nonaggressive MR characteristics," *Journal of Computer Assisted Tomography*, vol. 21, no. 5, pp. 785–789, 1997.

[8] M. D. Murphey, M. S. Gibson, B. T. Jennings, A. M. Crespo-Rodríguez, J. Fanburg-Smith, and D. A. Gajewski, "Imaging of synovial sarcoma with radiologic-pathologic correlation," *Radiographics*, vol. 26, no. 5, pp. 1543–1565, 2006.

[9] M. D. Murphey, J. H. Rhee, R. B. Lewis, J. C. Fanburg-Smith,

D. J. Flemming, and E. A. Walker, "From the archives of the AFIP pigmented villonodular synovitis: radiologic-pathologic correlation," *Radiographics*, vol. 28, no. 5, pp. 1493–1518, 2009.

[10] G.-S. Huang, C.-H. Lee, W. P. Chan, C.-Y. Chen, J. S. Yu, and D. Resnick, "Localized nodular synovitis of the knee: MR imaging appearance and clinical correlates in 21 patients," *American Journal of Roentgenology*, vol. 181, no. 2, pp. 539–543, 2003.

[11] C. Helpert, A. M. Davies, N. Evans, and R. J. Grimer, "Differential diagnosis of tumours and tumour-like lesions of the infrapatellar (Hoffa's) fat pad: pictorial review with an emphasis on MR imaging," *European Radiology*, vol. 14, no. 12, pp. 2337–2346, 2004.

[12] S. D. Gresswell, A. A. Corsini, L. H. Balsamo, and E. F. Miles, "Intra-articular synovial sarcoma treated with a transfemoral amputation: a case report and review of the literature," *Military Medicine*, vol. 178, no. 8, pp. e956–e962, 2013.

[13] T. Ishida, T. Iijima, S. Moriyama, C. Nakamura, T. Kitagawa, and R. Machinami, "Intra-articular calcifying synovial sarcoma mimicking synovial chondromatosis," *Skeletal Radiology*, vol. 25, no. 8, pp. 766–769, 1996.

[14] H. Kimura, N. Yamamoto, H. Nishida et al., "Synovial sarcoma in knee joint, mimicking low-grade sarcoma confirmed by molecular detection of SYT gene split," *Anticancer Research*, vol. 34, no. 6, pp. 3105–3111, 2014.

[15] H. A. Mann, A. Hilton, N. J. Goddard, M. A. Smith, B. Holloway, and C. A. Lee, "Synovial sarcoma mimicking haemophilic pseudotumour," *Sarcoma*, vol. 2006, Article ID 27212, 3 pages, 2006.

[16] Y. Namba, A. Kawai, N. Naito, Y. Morimoto, S. Hanakawa, and H. Inoue, "Intraarticular synovial sarcoma confirmed by SYT-SSX fusion transcript," *Clinical Orthopaedics and Related Research*, no. 395, pp. 221–226, 2002.

[17] A. Daniel, E. Ullah, S. Wahab, and V. Kumar, "Relevance of MRI in prediction of malignancy of musculoskeletal system—a prospective evaluation," *BMC Musculoskeletal Disorders*, vol. 10, no. 1, article 125, 2009.

[18] B. C. Jones, M. Sundaram, and M. J. Kransdorf, "Synovial sarcoma: MR imaging findings in 34 patients," *American Journal of Roentgenology*, vol. 161, no. 4, pp. 827–830, 1993.

[19] M. J. Kransdorf, "Malignant soft-tissue tumors in a large referral population: distribution of diagnoses by age, sex, and location," *American Journal of Roentgenology*, vol. 164, no. 1, pp. 129–134, 1995.

16

Can Orthopedic Oncologists Predict Functional Outcome in Patients with Sarcoma after Limb Salvage Surgery in the Lower Limb?

Sjoerd Kolk,[1] Kevin Cox,[2] Vivian Weerdesteyn,[1,3] Gerjon Hannink,[2] Jos Bramer,[4] Sander Dijkstra,[5] Paul Jutte,[6] Joris Ploegmakers,[6] Michiel van de Sande,[5] Hendrik Schreuder,[7] Nico Verdonschot,[2,8] and Ingrid van der Geest[7]

[1] *Department of Rehabilitation, Radboud Institute for Health Sciences, Radboud University Medical Center, P.O. Box 9101, 6500 HB Nijmegen, The Netherlands*
[2] *Orthopaedic Research Laboratory, Radboud Institute for Health Sciences, Radboud University Medical Center, P.O. Box 9101, 6500 HB Nijmegen, The Netherlands*
[3] *Sint Maartenskliniek Research, P.O. Box 9011, 6500 GM Nijmegen, The Netherlands*
[4] *Department of Orthopaedic Surgery, Amsterdam University Medical Centre, P.O. Box 22660, 1100 DD Amsterdam, The Netherlands*
[5] *Department of Orthopaedic Surgery, Leiden University Medical Centre, P.O. Box 9600, 2300 RC Leiden, The Netherlands*
[6] *Department of Orthopaedic Surgery, Groningen University Medical Centre, P.O. Box 30001, 9700 RB Groningen, The Netherlands*
[7] *Department of Orthopaedic Surgery, Radboud Institute for Health Sciences, Radboud University Medical Center, P.O. Box 9101, 6500 HB Nijmegen, The Netherlands*
[8] *Laboratory for Biomechanical Engineering, Faculty of Engineering Technology, University of Twente, P.O. Box 217, 7500 AE Enschede, The Netherlands*

Correspondence should be addressed to Ingrid van der Geest; ingrid.vandergeest@radboudumc.nl

Academic Editor: Peter C. Ferguson

Accurate predictions of functional outcome after limb salvage surgery (LSS) in the lower limb are important for several reasons, including informing the patient preoperatively and, in some cases, deciding between amputation and LSS. This study aimed to elucidate the correlation between surgeon-predicted and patient-reported functional outcome of LSS in the Netherlands. Twenty-three patients (between six months and ten years after surgery) and five independent orthopedic oncologists completed the Toronto Extremity Salvage Score (TESS) and the RAND-36 physical functioning subscale (RAND-36 PFS). The orthopedic oncologists made their predictions based on case descriptions (including MRI scans) that reflected the preoperative status. The correlation between patient-reported and surgeon-predicted functional outcome was "very poor" to "poor" on both scores (r^2 values ranged from 0.014 to 0.354). Patient-reported functional outcome was generally underestimated, by 8.7% on the TESS and 8.3% on the RAND-36 PFS. The most difficult and least difficult tasks on the RAND-36 PFS were also the most difficult and least difficult to predict, respectively. Most questions had a "poor" intersurgeon agreement. It was difficult to accurately predict the patient-reported functional outcome of LSS. Surgeons' ability to predict functional scores can be improved the most by focusing on accurately predicting more demanding tasks.

1. Introduction

Limb salvage surgery (LSS) rather than amputation is the operation of choice in 70–85% of all malignant bone and soft tissue lower limb sarcomas [1, 2]. Since the oncological results for amputation and LSS in the surgical treatment of sarcomas are comparable [3, 4], the decision to perform an amputation or LSS is based on the tumor size, the tumor location, patient preferences, the expected risk of complications and multiple reoperations, and the expected functional outcome [3]. If it is surgically possible, LSS is generally the preferred treatment, unless a poor functional outcome is expected. It has been shown that the functional outcome of LSS is superior to amputation, with the exception of below-knee amputation, which yields a similar function as limb salvage [5]. The expected functional outcome of patients after LSS is thus an important part of the preoperative decision making process for the surgical treatment.

Several known predictors of functional outcome include tumor size, location, grade, bone resection, muscle involvement, use of radiotherapy, and motor nerve sacrifice [6]. The functional outcome is predicted by the surgeon based on these parameters combined with his/her clinical experience. However, to the best of our knowledge, there are no reports about how well surgeons are able to actually predict functional outcome after LSS. Insight into the level of accuracy of these predictions is important for several reasons. First, accurate predictions of functional outcome are highly relevant in informing the patient preoperatively about the expected final functional outcome. Second, in some cases, the predictions are helpful in deciding between amputation or LSS. Third, information about the correlation between predicted functional outcome and patient-reported functional outcome provides valuable information for surgeons in training.

In this study, (1) we aimed to establish whether orthopedic oncologists can accurately predict patient-reported functional outcome of LSS in the treatment of sarcoma in the lower limb in a selected group of patients. (2) We also examined whether there was a tendency to over- or underestimate patient-reported functional outcome. Additionally, (3) we sought to identify which items on the functional outcome scores were least difficult and which were most difficult to predict, and whether the surgeons agreed amongst themselves (interrater reliability) in their predictions.

2. Materials and Methods

2.1. Patients. We selected patients who had undergone a LSS for a sarcoma in the lower limb from a database of orthopedic oncologic patients at the Department of Orthopedic Surgery of the Radboud University Medical Center (RUMC), Nijmegen, The Netherlands. The database contained 216 patients who had undergone LSS or amputation for any type of tumor in the hip or knee region. We selected patients using the following inclusion criteria: follow-up at least six months after the surgery (before July 1, 2012) for patients without adjuvant treatment and at least twelve months for patients with adjuvant treatment, a maximum follow-up of ten years (after February 1, 2003), and age between 18–70 years, and preoperative MRI scans had to be available. The follow-up of at least six months was chosen because functional scores tend to plateau within that time frame [6, 7]. We excluded patients who had a bone tumor with an intact cortical bone, as almost no functional deficits were expected to occur in those patients. Patients who had suffered local recurrence or complications that required reoperation in the last six months before the study were excluded. A flow chart of the patient selection is shown in Figure 1. Twenty-four patients were eligible for inclusion in the study, of whom 23 were successfully contacted. All 23 patients were included in the study. The study procedures were approved by the Local Ethical Committee of the RUMC. Written informed consent was obtained from all participants.

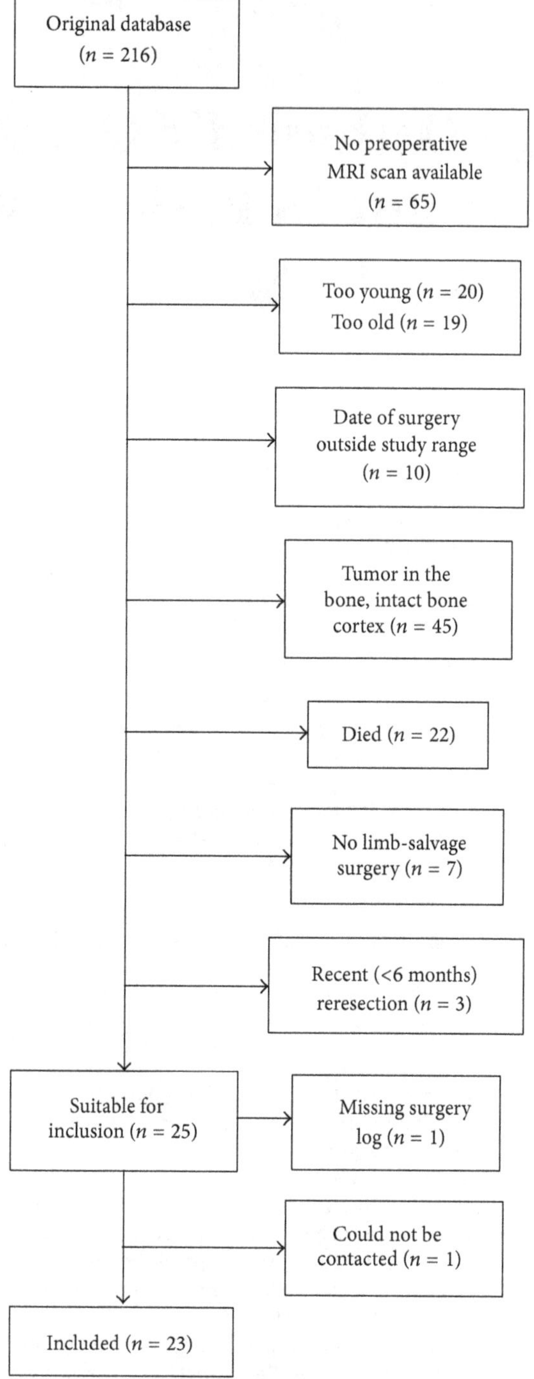

Figure 1: Flow chart of patient selection. Some patients fitted into multiple exclusion criteria (e.g., "no preoperative MRI scan available" and "too old"); in such cases, the patient was counted as belonging to the first of those exclusion criteria.

2.2. Materials. To evaluate the functional outcome, we used the Toronto Extremity Salvage Score (TESS) for the lower extremity and the RAND-36 physical functioning subscale (RAND-36 PFS). The TESS is a patient-reported questionnaire that has been specifically designed to measure the physical functional status of patients after limb-salvage surgery [7]. It contains 30 questions, and the final score ranges from 0% to 100%, 100% being the highest achievable score. The RAND-36 PFS is intended to measure physical functioning in any patient cohort [8, 9], which makes it more general than the TESS. Like the TESS, the RAND-36 PFS also is a patient-reported questionnaire. The RAND-36 PFS consists of ten questions, and the final score ranges from 0% to 100%, 100% being the highest achievable score. The RAND-36 PFS is identical to the SF-36 PFS. In addition to the TESS and RAND-36 PFS, we also used the RAND-36 pain subscale to examine postoperative pain levels. The RAND-36 pain subscale contains two questions; one regarding the amount of pain and one regarding the hindrance experienced due to pain when performing everyday activities in the previous four weeks [8, 9]. The final score ranges from 0% to 100%, where 100% represents no pain. We did not employ the Musculoskeletal Tumor Society score [10], as that score is not patient-reported and includes the domains of pain and emotional acceptance, which would have been impossible to predict solely on the basis of case descriptions.

A case description of each patient was made, which reflected the preoperative status of the patient. It contained the patient's age, sex, body mass index (BMI), tumor diagnosis, diagnostic MRI scans, a description of the performed surgical procedure for tumor resection and reconstruction, whether the patient had received adjuvant pre- or postoperative chemo- or radiotherapy, and whether there were any complications from the surgery (a case example is shown in Figure 2). The information did not include follow-up time. If a reresection had been performed, the preoperative MRI scans from before the primary resection surgery were provided, rather than those made after the local recurrence. The case descriptions were distributed through a central electronic platform. Whenever bone was removed, it was replaced by tumor prosthesis and/or an allograft.

2.3. Study Procedures. The patients were interviewed about their current functional status in a structured telephone call (done by KC, an independent researcher who was not a medical doctor), consisting of the TESS, the RAND-36 PFS, and the RAND-36 pain subscale. Five independent orthopedic oncologists (JB, PD, PJ, JP, and MvdS), working in one of the other three Dutch orthopedic oncologic referral centers (other than the RUMC) participated in the study. They were asked to give a prediction of the total TESS score (one percentage for the total functional status of the patient without addressing all separate items) and a prediction of the ten individual items of the RAND-36 PFS, based on the case descriptions. They had never been involved in the treatment of the patients and were unaware of their patient-reported functional outcome. All orthopedic oncologists were experienced and specialized in orthopedic oncology. They were familiar with the employed functional scales and were provided with a copy of the TESS questionnaire for reference.

2.4. Outcome Measures and Statistical Analyses. Descriptive statistics were calculated and stated as mean ± standard deviation. We compared the patient-reported and surgeon-predicted TESS and RAND-36 PFS scores in three ways.

First, Pearson correlations were calculated between the patients' reported scores and individual surgeon predicted scores, as well as for the average scores of all the surgeons combined. The squared correlation coefficient, r^2, (coefficient of determination), represents the variation in the values of the patient-reported outcome that can be explained by variations in the value of the surgeon-predicted outcome [11]. An r^2-value of 0.75–1.00 was interpreted as a "very good" prediction, 0.50–0.74 as "good," 0.25–0.49 as "poor," and 0-0.24 as "very poor." The r^2-values were considered the primary outcome measure.

Second, the mean differences and 95% confidence intervals (95% CI) between the patient-reported scores on the TESS and RAND-36 PFS and the surgeon-predicted scores were calculated to reveal whether the predictions had a bias towards being too optimistic or pessimistic.

Third, the agreement between patient-reported and the median surgeon-predicted answers to the separate questions of the RAND-36 PFS were examined using percent agreement and Gwet's agreement coefficient (AC1). Compared with Cohen's Kappa [12, 13], Gwet's AC1 has a more stable interrater reliability and is less affected by prevalence and marginal probability [14]. This allowed us to identify which questions were the least difficult and most difficult to predict. The intersurgeon agreement on each separate question was also calculated, using percent agreement and Gwet's AC1. To calculate the intersurgeon agreement on the TESS, we used the intraclass correlation coefficient (ICC; absolute single measure/absolute agreement). Agreement coefficients below 0.40 were considered to represent a "poor" agreement; between 0.40 and 0.59 "fair"; between 0.60 and 0.74 "good"; and between 0.75 and 1.00 "excellent," analogous to commonly used guidelines for interexaminer agreement [15].

The associations between each separate variable (age, sex, BMI, pain, and time since surgery) and patient-reported TESS and RAND-36 were examined using univariate regression analyses to examine whether they were associated with the functional outcome scores.

Matlab R2011a (The Mathworks, Natick, MA, USA) and R version 3.0.2. [16] were used for the statistical analyses.

3. Results

3.1. Patients. The characteristics of all 23 patients are listed in Table 1. The age at the time of surgery was 39.9 ± 18.8 years and the time after surgery was 47 ± 27 months. All patients were ambulatory and able to at least walk short distances without a walking aid. Two patients (cases 10 and 21) had undergone a reresection; this was mentioned in the case file. All other patients had not suffered from local recurrence

Case 7: ♂ 37 years
BMI: 23,74 (83 kg/1 m87[2])
Indication:
Malignant fibrous hystiocytoma
left distal femur, pretreated with chemotherapy.
An incision biopsy has been done on the left
anterolateral side.

Surgical treatment:
Reconstruction Extra-articular distal femur
resection and reconstruction with tumour
prosthesis.

Preoperative MRI:
Top row: transversal (T1-FS)
Middle row: transversal (T1)
Bottom row: sagittal (T1)

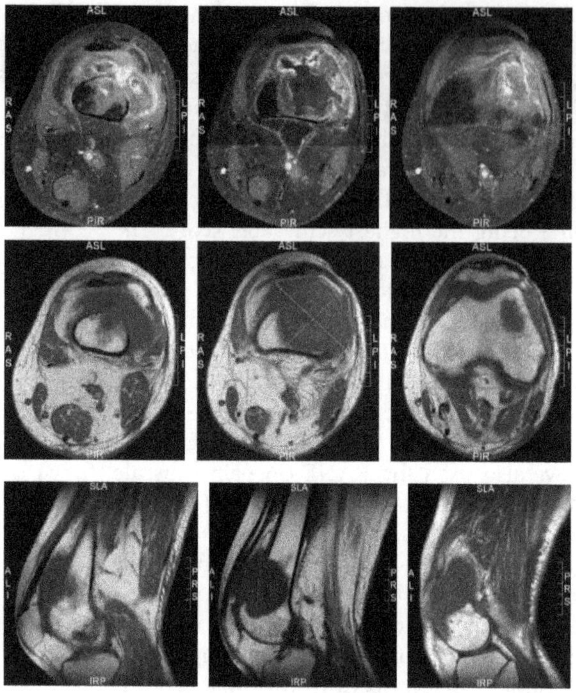

FIGURE 2: Example case as given to the orthopedic oncologists. This is patient 7 in Table 1.

or complications that required follow-up surgery. The mean patient-reported scores were TESS 87.0 ± 12.1, RAND-36 PFS 73.3 ± 18.7, and RAND-36 pain subscale 85.5 ± 24.7.

3.2. Surgeon Predictions—TESS. The surgeon-predicted scores and their correlations with the patient-reported scores of all five surgeons and the average predictions of all surgeons on the TESS are shown in Figure 3 and in Table 2. The correlations with the patient-reported scores were "very poor" for all surgeons, with the best correlation for surgeon 2 ($r^2 = 0.185$). The TESS was underestimated for most patient cases (Figure 3); the mean underestimation ranged from 1.5 to 22.6 percentage points (Table 2). The correlations with the patient-reported TESS formed by averaging all five surgeons' predictions were "very poor" ($r^2 = 0.159$) and underestimated patient-reported functional outcome by 8.7 (95% CI: 3.62–13.7) percentage points. The intersurgeon agreement on the TESS was "poor" with an ICC of 0.29 (95% CI: 0.10–0.53).

3.3. Surgeon Predictions—RAND-36 PFS. The surgeon-predicted RAND-36 PFS scores and their correlations with the patient-reported scores are shown in Figure 4 and in Table 2. The correlations to the patient-reported scores were either "very poor" (surgeons 1, 4, and 5) or "poor" (surgeons 2 and 3). Surgeon 3's predictions had the highest correlation with the patient-reported scores ($r^2 = 0.354$). The patient-reported RAND-36 PFS score was underestimated by all surgeons, except for surgeon 2 (5.4 percentage points overestimation) (Table 2). The average correlations with the patient-reported scores were "poor" ($r^2 = 0.255$) and underestimated patient-reported functional outcome by 8.3 (95% CI: 0.64–16.0) percentage points.

In the analysis of the individual questions that make up the RAND-36 PFS, "*Climbing several flights of stairs*" and "*Walking more than a mile*" were the most difficult items to predict, with "poor" agreement coefficients (AC1) of 0.15 and 0.19, respectively, between surgeon-predicted and patient-reported scores (Table 3). "*Walking one block*" and "*Bathing or dressing yourself*" were the least difficult items to predict, with "excellent" agreement coefficients of 0.81 and 0.76, respectively, between surgeon-predicted and patient-reported scores. Similar to the overall RAND-36 PFS scores, most of its separate questions were underestimated; only two questions were overestimated ("*Bending, kneeling, or stooping*" and "*Lift-ing or carrying groceries*").

On most questions of the RAND-36 PFS, the intersurgeon agreement coefficient was "poor," but there was a "fair" agreement on "*Bathing or dressing yourself*" and "*Moderate activities*" and a "good" agreement on "*Vigorous activities*" and "*Walking one block*" (Table 3).

3.4. Other Potential Predictors. No correlations were found between the TESS or RAND-36 PFS and any of the potential predicting factors (Table 4).

4. Discussion

This national survey aimed to investigate how well orthopedic oncologists are able to predict the patient-reported functional outcome of patients that had undergone LSS in the lower limb. We found "very poor" to "poor" correlations between patient-reported outcomes and surgeon-predicted outcomes

TABLE 1: Patient characteristics, indication, tumor location, surgical treatment, adjuvant therapy, and functional scores.

Pat. number	Gender, age (y)	BMI (kg/m^2)	Indication	Tumor location	Side	Surgical treatment	Adjuvant therapy	Time post-OR (months)	TESS score	RAND-36 phys. func.	RAND-36 pain
1	M, 50	26.0	Paget's osteosarcoma	Distal femur	Left	Extra-articular distal femur resection including part of the quadriceps muscle. Reconstruction with tumor prosthesis and biceps femoris tendon transposition for quadriceps reconstruction	Pre- and postoperative chemotherapy	67	79.6	65.0	89.8
2	M, 36	21.4	Clear cell chondrosarcoma	Proximal femur	Right	Proximal femur resection, including the greater trochanter Reconstruction with tumor prosthesis		28	89.2	70.0	67.3
3	V, 44	28.3	Myxoid liposarcoma next to the medial femoral epicondyle	Distal femur	Left	Soft tissue tumor resection, including the medial collateral ligament Reconstruction of the pes anserinus		75	98.3	100.0	100.0
4	V, 63	25.2	Sarcoma not otherwise specified tibial tuberosity	Proximal tibia	Left	Proximal tibia resection Reconstruction with allograft and tumor prosthesis. Soft tissue closure with gastrocnemius transfer and split skin graft		62	95	75.0	100.0
5	V, 60	25.4	Liposarcoma	Medial thigh	Left	Resection soft-tissue tumor		21	88.8	80.0	100.0
6	V, 66	25.2	Parosteal osteosarcoma	Distal femur	Right	Distal femur resection Reconstruction with tumor prosthesis		12	98.3	70.0	100.0
7	M, 37	23.7	Sarcoma not otherwise specified	Distal femur	Left	Extra-articular distal femur resection and reconstruction with tumor prosthesis	Pre- and postoperative chemotherapy	65	92.9	90.0	100.0
8	V, 60	24.1	Soft tissue sarcoma adductor muscles compartment	Medial thigh	Right	En block resection	Preoperative chemotherapy	14	93.1	90.0	100.0
9	V, 41	34.3	Chondrosarcoma grade 2	Proximal tibia	Left	Proximal tibia resection Reconstruction with tumor prosthesis		10	83.3	75.0	100.0
10	M, 47	28.7	Soft tissue sarcoma; previous incomplete resection	Thigh	Right	Reresection		105	96.7	85.0	79.6
11	M, 15	19.2	Osseous lipoma like liposarcoma	Proximal femur	Right	Proximal femur resection (osteotomy at 250 mm) and reconstruction with tumor prosthesis	Preoperative chemo- and radiotherapy	46	82.8	60.0	79.6

TABLE 1: Continued.

Pat. number	Gender, age (y)	BMI (kg/m^2)	Indication	Tumor location	Side	Surgical treatment	Adjuvant therapy	Time post-OR (months)	TESS score	RAND-36 phys. func.	RAND-36 pain
12	V, 16	24.5	Osteosarcoma	Tibia shaft	Right	Segment resection tibia shaft, saving tibia epiphysis Reconstruction with allograft, intramedullary pen, cement, and plate osteosynthesis	Pre- and postoperative chemotherapy	30	92.5	75.0	100.0
13	V, 15	26.9	Osteosarcoma	Distal femur	Right	Distal femur resection (235 mm), reconstruction with tumor prosthesis	Pre- and postoperative chemotherapy	79	72.4	25.0	100.0
14	V, 65	25.9	Osteosarcoma	Distal femur	Left	Distal femur resection, reconstruction with tumor prosthesis		55	79.8	60.0	0.0
15	V, 39	24.9	Synovial sarcoma between proximal fibula and tibia	Proximal fibula	Left	Proximal fibula resection, including lateral cortex of tibia Reconstruction with plate and cement.		40	93.1	80.0	100.0
16	M, 59	25.8	Chondrosarcoma grade 2	Distal femur	Left	Distal femur resection, reconstruction with tumor prosthesis		7	52.9	50.0	79.6
17	V, 59	23.8	Soft tissue sarcoma not otherwise specified	Dorsal thigh	Right	Resection soft tissue tumor	Postoperative radiotherapy	51	60.8	45.0	100.0
18	M, 15	26.6	Telangiectatic osteosarcoma	Distal femur	Left	Distal femur resection, reconstruction with tumor prosthesis	Pre- and postoperative chemotherapy	84	83.6	65.0	57.1
19	M, 21	24.2	Osteosarcoma	Distal femur	Left	Distal femur resection, reconstruction with tumor prosthesis	Pre- and postoperative chemotherapy	12	83.9	55.0	44.9
20	V, 30	21.7	Myxoid liposarcoma	Rectus femoris	Left	Resection soft tissue sarcoma		45	100.0	100.0	100.0
21	V, 49	26.8	Liposarcoma, previous incomplete resection	Anterolateral thigh	Right	Reresection (last part vastus lateralis anteromedial and distal)	Postoperative radiotherapy	50	95.8	90.0	69.4
22	M, 17	22.6	Osteosarcoma	Lateral femoral epicondyles	Right	Distal femur resection, reconstruction with tumor prosthesis	Pre- and postoperative chemotherapy	50	87.5	85.0	100.0
23	M, 14	21.5	Ewing's sarcoma	Diaphysis femur	Right	Segment resection right femur Reconstruction with allograft, intramedullary nail, and plate osteosynthesis	Pre- and postoperative chemotherapy	77	100.0	100.0	100.0

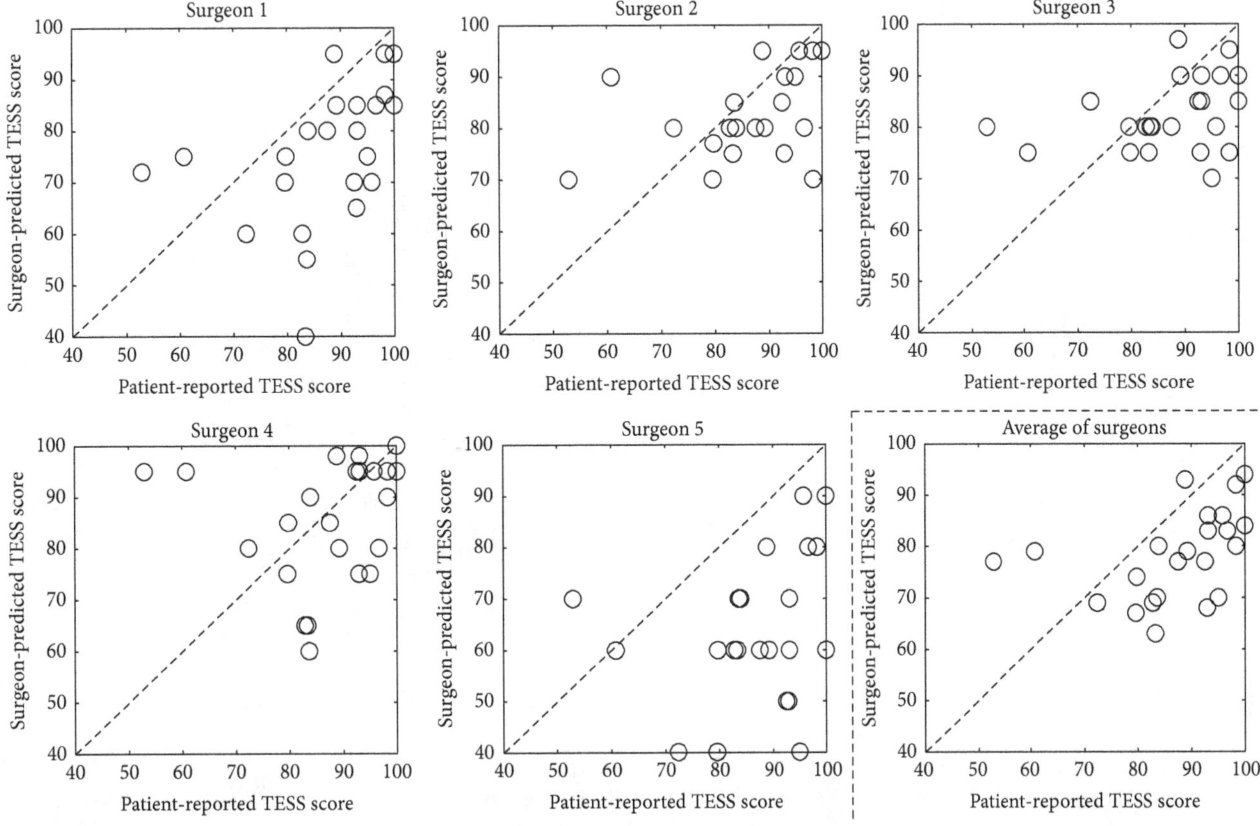

FIGURE 3: Scatter plots of patient-reported outcome and orthopedic tumor surgeon predictions on the Toronto Extremity Salvage Scale (TESS). The dashed lines indicate a hypothetical perfect correlation; if a patient case lies above or below this line, the functional outcome was overestimated or underestimated, respectively.

TABLE 2: Patient-reported and surgeon-predicted mean TESS and RAND-36 PFS scores and coefficients of determination for TESS and RAND-36 PFS scores.

	TESS		RAND-36 PFS	
	Mean score[a]	r^2	Mean score[a]	r^2
Patient-reported	87.0 (12.1)		73.3 (18.7)	
Surgeon 1	75.6 (13.6)	0.167	50.9 (20.3)	0.142
Surgeon 2	83.6 (8.6)	0.185	78.7 (15.5)	0.336
Surgeon 3	82.5 (7.1)	0.096	70.2 (17.9)	0.354
Surgeon 4	85.5 (11.9)	0.014	72.2 (18.7)	0.081
Surgeon 5	64.3 (14.7)	0.088	52.8 (26.8)	0.118
Average of surgeons	78.3 (8.7)	0.159	65.0 (16.6)	0.255

[a]Scores are reported as mean (SD).

on both the TESS and the RAND-36 PFS. The orthopedic oncologists tended to underestimate patient-reported functional outcome on both scales. The most difficult tasks on the RAND-36 PFS were also the most difficult to predict, whereas, for the least difficult tasks, it was easy to predict that these could be performed without substantial limitations by nearly all patients. The intersurgeon agreement on the RAND-36 PFS questions was mostly "poor" but was "good" for some of the most and least demanding tasks. None of the potentially predicting factors were related to the primary outcome measures.

Our results indicate that it was difficult for the participating orthopedic oncologists to accurately predict the patient-reported functional outcome of limb salvage surgery. On the TESS, for instance, the coefficients of determination (r^2) between patient-reported and surgeon-predicted outcomes were lower than 0.20, indicating that less than 20% of the variance in TESS could be explained by the predictions made by the orthopedic oncologists. We did not expect such a poor predictive ability, considering the experience level of the orthopedic oncologists with limb salvage surgery. Several aspects may underlie this seemingly rather poor predictive ability.

First, each limb salvage patient presents a unique case in terms of anatomical involvement. Even in patients with the same type of tumor at a similar location, for instance, the distal femur, final functional results can differ to a large extent. In part, this depends on the amount and precise location of soft tissue involvement, which may have been difficult to see from the limited set of MRI images in the case files. Moreover, patients are unique in terms of adaptive capacity. The adaptation of the patient to the new anatomical and sensorimotor situation plays a large role in the recovery of function [17]. The amount of adaptive capacity may have been

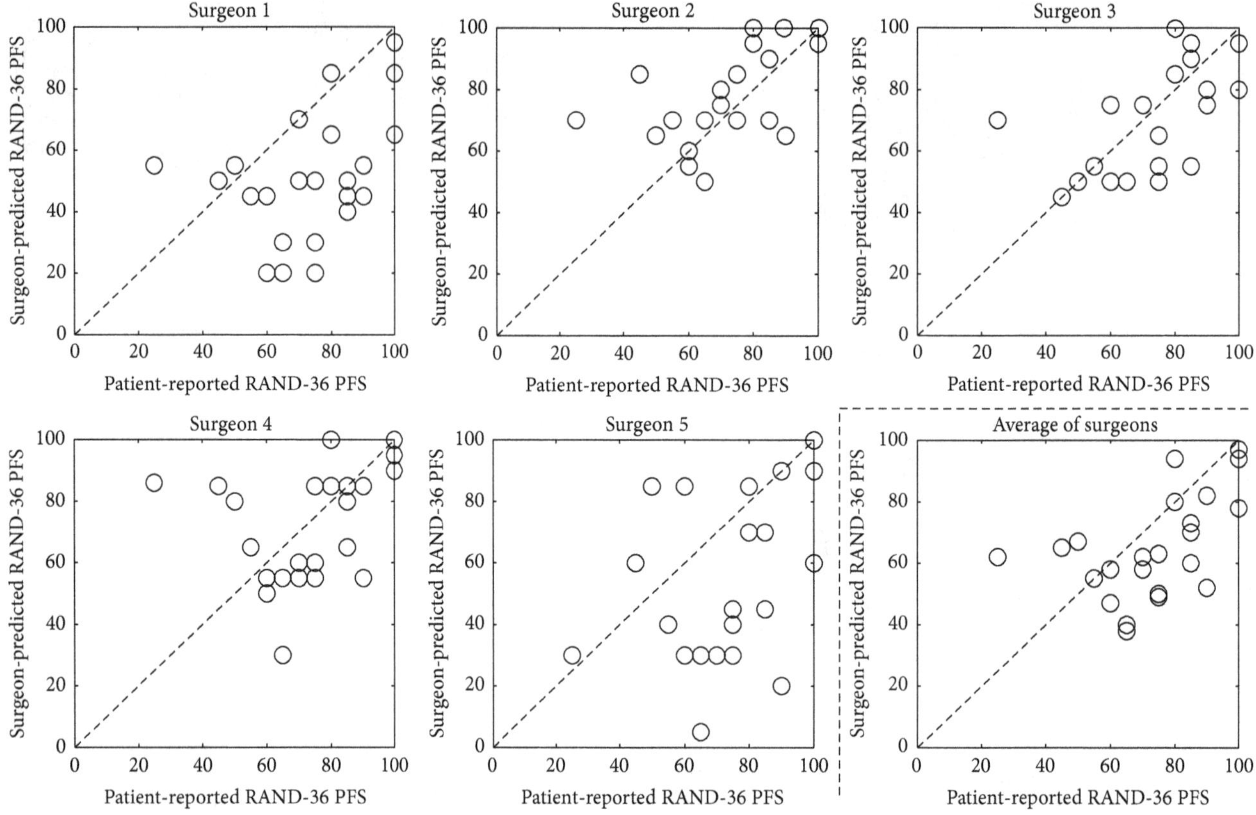

FIGURE 4: Scatter plots of patient-reported outcome and orthopedic tumor surgeon predictions on the RAND-36 physical functioning subscale (RAND-36 PFS). The dashed lines indicate a hypothetical perfect correlation; if a patient case lies above or below this line, the functional outcome was overestimated or underestimated, respectively.

hard or impossible to estimate by the orthopedic oncologists from the case files. Second, we measured functional outcome with questionnaires, which are inherently subjective. Thus, the patients' own perception of functioning may have played a large role in the functional outcome score. It might be that functional outcome measured by objective means, such as, for example, gait analysis, more closely reflects the orthopedic oncologists' predictions. Third, in the case files, we mimicked as well as possible the information typically available preoperatively to the surgeon in a clinical setting, but the study design did not permit the independent surgeons to review the medical history of the patients nor perform a physical examination before the surgery. As such, predictions of patient-reported functional outcome in a "real" clinical setting (e.g., including a physical examination) might be more accurate than those made in this study. Fourth, patients who had a bone tumor with an intact cortical bone were not included; the patient-reported functional outcome in those patients would potentially have been less difficult to predict than that in the patients with larger tumors.

The poor predictive ability raises the question of which other factors determine functional outcome in limb saving surgery and to what degree. Davis et al. showed that large tumor size, deep lesions, high grade tumor, use of radiotherapy, bone resection, and motor nerve sacrifice are significantly related to increased disability on the TESS [6]. In their study, those combined parameters were able to predict 20% of the variance in TESS score. This is in the same order of magnitude as the presently reported results, indicating that the surgeons were unable to "add" predictive value on top of the given parameters in the case files. The rehabilitation protocol may also have an effect on functional outcome; Shehadeh et al. showed that adherence to a strict rehabilitation protocol after limb salvage surgery led to a relatively high level of functional outcome compared with other studies [18]. If we interpret our findings concurrent with those of Davis et al. and Shehadeh et al., it appears that still a large percentage of functional outcome cannot be predicted by the surgeon nor by anatomical and surgery or adjuvant therapy-related factors nor by rehabilitation protocols. Other factors that may play a significant role in the patient-reported functional outcome include the preoperative physical and mental state of the patient. For example, a patient who is highly motivated and athletic may recover to a far higher level of functioning than one who is less motivated and leads a sedentary lifestyle. From this perspective, one may intuitively expect a correlation between patient-reported functional outcome and age or BMI, but we did not find this (Table 4). Further studies are required to clarify the role each factor plays in patient-reported functional outcome after limb salvage surgery.

TABLE 3: Analysis of separate questions on the RAND-36 physical functioning subscale.

	Patient-reported score			Surgeon-predicted score			Patients versus median surgeon				Intersurgeon agreement	
	"Yes, limited a lot"	"Yes, limited a little"	"No, not limited at all"	"Yes, limited a lot"	"Yes, limited a little"	"No, not limited at all"	Percent agreement	Percent of cases underestimated	Percent of cases overestimated	AC1	Percent agreement	AC1
Vigorous activities	14	6	3	14	8	1	60.9%	26.1%	13.0%	0.47	70.0%	0.60
Moderate activities	0	7	16	0	16	7	60.9%	39.1%	0%	0.48	66.5%	0.55
Lifting or carrying groceries	2	7	14	0	9	14	65.2%	13.0%	21.7%	0.53	50.4%	0.32
Climbing several flights of stairs	2	10	11	4	16	3	39.1%	47.8%	13.0%	0.15	44.3%	0.20
Climbing one flight of stairs	1	4	18	0	9	14	52.2%	30.4%	17.4%	0.39	52.2%	0.35
Bending, kneeling, or stooping	6	13	4	0	16	7	52.2%	4.3%	43.5%	0.35	49.1%	0.28
Walking more than a mile	5	6	12	1	17	5	43.4%	34.8%	21.7%	0.19	54.3%	0.36
Walking several blocks	1	4	18	0	10	13	52.2%	34.8%	13.0%	0.38	50.9%	0.33
Walking one block	1	1	21	0	2	21	82.6%	8.7%	8.7%	0.81	67.8%	0.61
Bathing or dressing yourself	0	1	22	0	4	19	78.3%	17.4%	4.3%	0.76	60.0%	0.50

TABLE 4: Coefficients of determination between patient characteristics and functional outcomes (TESS and RAND-36 physical functioning subscale).

	TESS r^2	RAND-36 PFS r^2
Age	0.011	0.001
Sex	0.024	0.001
Body mass index	0.008	0.003
Pain (RAND-36 pain subscale)	0.042	0.079
Time since surgery	0.036	0.015

The orthopedic oncologists tended to underestimate patient-reported functional outcome on both the TESS and the RAND-36 PFS. Thus, it appears that the patients adapted to the new anatomical and functional situation better than the surgeons predicted. It is possible that this is due to some surgeons being used to picturing a somewhat more pessimistic scenario to their patients so that the actual achieved functional result exceeds the patients' expectations. However, we specifically instructed the surgeons to provide their most accurate predictions of patient-reported functional outcome, rather than to provide predictions that they would share with patients. As for clinical relevance, we did not set a specific threshold, but the underestimation of patient-reported functional outcome on both the TESS and the RAND-36 PFS was rather consistent, as demonstrated by the 95% confidence intervals that did not pass through zero.

Interestingly, we found that the "*Walking one block*" question was the least difficult to predict, whereas the "*Walking more than a mile*" question was one of the most difficult questions to predict (only "*Climbing several flights of stairs*" was more difficult to predict). It appears that the ultimate level of function that is reached in patients is hard to predict, whereas it is easier to predict lower levels of function. Thus, surgeons' ability to predict functional scores can be improved the most by focusing on accurately predicting more demanding tasks. Additional improvement might be gained by analyzing the prediction for the "*Bending, kneeling, or stooping*" question. If the prediction for this question did not match with the patient-reported outcome, it was mostly overestimated (43.5% of cases). This overestimation breaks with the general trend to underestimate patient-reported functional outcome and indicates that bending the knees is more difficult to do for patients than the median surgeon predicted.

The intersurgeon agreement on most RAND-36 PFS questions was "poor," indicating that there was a high intersurgeon variability in the predictions to the questions. Notable exceptions were "*Walking one block*" and "*Vigorous activities*," with "good" intersurgeon agreement. The prior arguably is the least difficult activity on the scale, whereas the latter represents the most demanding activities on the scale (including running, heavy lifting, and strenuous sports). However, this does not imply that there was also a high agreement with the patient-reported outcome; "*Vigorous activities*" had only a "fair" agreement with the patient-reported score. "*Walking one block*," on the other hand, was the only question that had both an "excellent" agreement with the patient-reported score as well as a "good" intersurgeon agreement. This might be due to the surgeons' familiarity with predicting this basic level of functional outcome or because being able to walk at least short distances is considered one of the criteria for attempting limb salvage surgery, and most patients indeed achieved that goal.

This study has some limitations. First, the surgeons only predicted the total TESS score, instead of predicting each of the 30 questions that comprise the score. This was done because some questions were already present in the much shorter RAND-36 PFS, and to reduce the time it would take the surgeons to predict the 23 cases. Second, we used a translated version of the TESS which has not been validated in Dutch. However, as the TESS is the gold standard assessment tool after limb salvage surgery, we decided to use it [19]. The RAND-36 PFS has been validated in Dutch [8, 9], and its results showed the same trend in the comparisons as the translated TESS. Third, we found a wide range of patient-reported functional outcome scores, including in patients that had undergone similar surgery. Of course, each case is unique, but the perception of effort required to perform the activities in the questionnaires and the interpretation of the questions can vary between patients. Measuring actual functional outcome (e.g., in a movement laboratory or by observing patients in their home setting) could yield more knowledge of actual functioning, eliminate the subjectivity inherent in questionnaires, and establish the construct validity of the employed functional scoring systems. Fourth, the surgeons predicted the functional outcome based on a case description without being allowed to review the medical history of the patients or perform a physical examination. The time since surgery was also not provided, which might have negatively affected the predictions. This, however, does not explain the large differences found between predicted and patient-reported functional outcome nor does it explain the differences in predictions between surgeons. Furthermore, there was no correlation between the patient-reported functional scores and the time since surgery (Table 4).

5. Conclusions

It was difficult for the participating orthopedic oncologists to accurately predict the patient-reported functional outcome of limb salvage surgery. Patient-reported functional outcome tended to recover to a higher level than the surgeons predicted. The ultimate level of function that the patients reached was hard to predict, whereas it was easier to predict lower levels of function. Thus, surgeons' ability to predict functional scores can be improved the most by focusing on accurately predicting more demanding tasks. Intersurgeon agreement to most questions was "poor," indicating the high variability in the surgeons' predictions, and, possibly, treatment decisions. The poor predicting ability warrants research into objective tools to assist orthopedic oncologists in the decision making process. Such tools could include, for instance, computational musculoskeletal models that prospectively calculate whether enough muscle strength remains to perform activities of daily living.

Acknowledgment

The authors gratefully acknowledge financial support by the European Commission (Grant FP7-ICT-247860) for the TLEM*safe* project (http://www.tlemsafe.eu/).

References

[1] R. P. H. Veth, R. van Hoesel, M. Pruszczynski, J. Hoogenhout, B. Schreuder, and T. Wobbes, "Limb salvage in musculoskeletal oncology," *The Lancet Oncology*, vol. 4, no. 6, pp. 343–350, 2003.

[2] M. C. Gebhardt, "What's new in musculoskeletal oncology," *Journal of Bone and Joint Surgery A*, vol. 84, no. 4, pp. 694–701, 2002.

[3] M. A. Ghert, A. Abudu, N. Driver et al., "The indications for and the prognostic significance of amputation as the primary surgical procedure for localized soft tissue sarcoma of the extremity," *Annals of Surgical Oncology*, vol. 12, no. 1, pp. 10–17, 2005.

[4] R. Niimi, A. Matsumine, K. Kusuzaki et al., "Usefulness of limb salvage surgery for bone and soft tissue sarcomas of the distal lower leg," *Journal of Cancer Research and Clinical Oncology*, vol. 134, no. 10, pp. 1087–1095, 2008.

[5] L. H. Aksnes, H. C. F. Bauer, N. L. Jebsen et al., "Limb-sparing surgery preserves more function than amputation," *Journal of Bone and Joint Surgery B*, vol. 90, no. 6, pp. 786–794, 2008.

[6] A. M. Davis, S. A. M. Sennik, J. S. Griffin et al., "Predictors of functional outcomes following limb salvage surgery for lower-extremity soft tissue sarcoma," *Journal of Surgical Oncolog*, vol. 73, no. 4, pp. 206–211, 2000.

[7] A. M. Davis, J. G. Wright, J. I. Williams, C. Bombardier, A. Griffin, and R. S. Bell, "Development of a measure of physical function for patients with bone and soft tissue sarcoma," *Quality of Life Research*, vol. 5, no. 5, pp. 508–516, 1996.

[8] K. I. VanderZee, R. Sanderman, J. W. Heyink, and H. de Haes, "Psychometric qualities of the RAND 36-item health survey 1.0: a multidimensional measure of general health status," *International Journal of Behavioral Medicine*, vol. 3, no. 2, pp. 104–122, 1996.

[9] K. I. van der Zee and R. Sanderman, "Het meten van de algemene gezondheidstoestand met de RAND-36, een handleiding. Tweede herziene druk," UMCG/Rijksuniversiteit Groningen, Research Institute SHARE, 2012.

[10] W. F. Enneking, W. Dunham, M. C. Gebhardt, M. Malawar, and D. J. Pritchard, "A system for the functional evaluation of reconstructive procedures after surgical treatment of tumors of the musculoskeletal system," *Clinical Orthopaedics and Related Research*, no. 286, pp. 241–246, 1993.

[11] R. Taylor, "Interpretation of the correlation coefficient: a basic review," *Journal of Diagnostic Medical Sonography*, vol. 6, no. 1, pp. 35–39, 1990.

[12] J. Cohen, "A coefficient of agreement for nominal scales," *Educational and Psychological Measurement*, vol. 20, no. 1, pp. 37–46, 1960.

[13] J. Cohen, "Weighted kappa: nominal scale agreement provision for scaled disagreement or partial credit," *Psychological Bulletin*, vol. 70, no. 4, pp. 213–220, 1968.

[14] N. Wongpakaran, T. Wongpakaran, D. Wedding, and K. L. Gwet, "A comparison of Cohen's Kappa and Gwet's AC1 when calculating inter-rater reliability coefficients: a study conducted with personality disorder samples," *BMC Medical Research Methodology*, vol. 13, no. 1, article 61, 2013.

[15] D. V. Cicchetti, "Guidelines, criteria, and rules of thumb for evaluating normed and standardized assessment instruments in psychology," *Psychological Assessment*, vol. 6, no. 4, pp. 284–290, 1994.

[16] R Core Team, "R: a language and environment for statistical computing," R Foundation for Statistical Computing, 2014, http://www.R-project.org/.

[17] E. De Visser, T. Mulder, H. W. B. Schreuder, R. P. H. Veth, and J. Duysens, "Gait and electromyographic analysis of patients recovering after limb-saving surgery," *Clinical Biomechanics*, vol. 15, no. 8, pp. 592–599, 2000.

[18] A. Shehadeh, M. El Dahleh, A. Salem et al., "Standardization of rehabilitation after limb salvage surgery for sarcomas improves patients' outcome," *Hematology/Oncology and Stem Cell Therapy*, vol. 6, no. 3-4, pp. 105–111, 2013.

[19] M. Clayer, S. Doyle, N. Sangha, and R. Grimer, "The toronto extremity salvage score in unoperated controls: an age, gender, and country comparison," *Sarcoma*, vol. 2012, Article ID 717213, 5 pages, 2012.

miR-125b and miR-100 are Predictive Biomarkers of Response to Induction Chemotherapy in Osteosarcoma

Daisuke Kubota,[1,2] Nobuyoshi Kosaka,[3] Tomohiro Fujiwara,[3] Akihiko Yoshida,[4] Yasuhito Arai,[5] Zhiwei Qiao,[1] Fumitaka Takeshita,[6] Takahiro Ochiya,[3] Akira Kawai,[5] and Tadashi Kondo[1]

[1]*Division of Rare Cancer Research, National Cancer Center Research Institute, 5-1-1 Tsukiji, Chuo-ku, Tokyo 104-0045, Japan*
[2]*Division of Musculoskeletal Oncology, National Cancer Center Hospital, 5-1-1 Tsukiji, Chuo-ku, Tokyo 104-0045, Japan*
[3]*Division of Molecular and Cellular Medicine, National Cancer Center Research Institute, 5-1-1 Tsukiji, Chuo-ku, Tokyo 104-0045, Japan*
[4]*Pathology and Clinical Laboratory Division, National Cancer Center Hospital, 5-1-1 Tsukiji, Chuo-ku, Tokyo 104-0045, Japan*
[5]*Division of Cancer Genomics, National Cancer Center Research Institute, 5-1-1 Tsukiji, Chuo-ku, Tokyo 104-0045, Japan*
[6]*Department of Functional Analysis, National Cancer Center Research Institute, 5-1-1 Tsukiji, Chuo-ku, Tokyo 104-0045, Japan*

Correspondence should be addressed to Tadashi Kondo; proteomebioinformatics@gmail.com

Academic Editor: Valerae O. Lewis

Osteosarcoma is the most common primary malignancy in bone. Patients who respond poorly to induction chemotherapy are at higher risk of adverse prognosis. The molecular basis for such poor prognosis remains unclear. We investigated miRNA expression in eight open biopsy samples to identify miRNAs predictive of response to induction chemotherapy and thus maybe used for risk stratification therapy. The samples were obtained from four patients with inferior necrosis (Huvos I/II) and four patients with superior necrosis (Huvos III/IV) following induction chemotherapy. We found six miRNAs, including miR-125b and miR-100, that were differentially expressed > 2-fold ($p < 0.05$) in patients who respond poorly to treatment. The association between poor prognosis and the abundance of miR-125b and miR-100 was confirmed by quantitative reverse transcriptase-polymerase chain reaction in 20 additional osteosarcoma patients. Accordingly, overexpression of miR-125b and miR-100 in three osteosarcoma cell lines enhanced cell proliferation, invasiveness, and resistance to chemotherapeutic drugs such as methotrexate, doxorubicin, and cisplatin. In addition, overexpression of miR-125b blocked the ability of these chemotherapy agents to induce apoptosis. As open biopsy is routinely performed to diagnose osteosarcoma, levels of miR-125b and miR-100 in these samples may be used as basis for risk stratification therapy.

1. Introduction

Osteosarcoma is the most common primary malignancy in bone and a leading cause of cancer death among children and adolescents [1, 2]. Cure rates of 15–20% were achieved in the 1970s by surgery alone in patients with localized osteosarcoma. These rates dramatically improved to as high as 80% following the introduction of higher-dose and multiagent chemotherapy regimens and induction chemotherapy [3, 4]. Induction chemotherapy downstages tumors and facilitates complete resection by inhibiting micrometastatic tumors and decreasing tumor vascularity. Response to induction chemotherapy is histologically evaluated according to the Huvos grading system [5], which is based on the degree of tumor necrosis in surgically resected tissues. Patients with ≥90% tumor necrosis after induction chemotherapy are considered good responders, and all others are deemed to be poor responders [2]. It is noteworthy that histological response to induction chemotherapy is the most reliable prognostic factor, aside from metastasis at time of diagnosis [6–15].

Therefore, prediction of response to induction chemotherapy could potentially be used to determine the most appropriate treatment regimen [16].

Although Huvos grading is widely used, it is obtained after chemotherapy and is thus not predictive. On the other hand, clinically useful predictive biomarkers have not been identified, even though osteosarcoma has been extensively characterized. This has prevented effective stratification of patients according to risk of drug resistance and may prevent further innovations in treatment. Therefore, it is imperative to understand the molecular basis of chemoresistance to develop more effective therapies.

Osteosarcoma is genetically heterogeneous among patients, across tumors, and within tumors [17, 18]. Indeed, osteosarcoma karyotypes indicate numerous numerical and structural changes [19]. Therefore, a comprehensive omics approach to survey molecular events at multiple levels may identify novel molecular mechanisms underlying resistance to treatments. Given the complex mechanisms that can contribute to chemoresistance, significant biological insights may yet be uncovered.

Previously, we investigated the proteomic profiles of open biopsy samples obtained from osteosarcoma patients before chemotherapy and identified peroxiredoxin 2 (PRDX2) as a novel predictive biomarker with response to induction chemotherapy with ifosfamide, doxorubicin, and cisplatin [20]. Subsequently, we found PRDX2 to be also predictive of the response to induction chemotherapy with different combinations of drugs, and we characterized its functional significance [21]. As open biopsy is routinely performed to diagnose osteosarcoma, predictive biomarkers that can be measured in samples collected during this procedure may prove to be useful in clinical settings.

microRNAs (miRNAs) are small, noncoding RNA 21–25 nucleotides in length that control growth, development, and differentiation by regulating gene expression posttranscriptionally. The human genome encodes more than 1,000 miRNAs [22] that regulate thousands of human genes [23, 24]. In osteosarcoma, global expression of miRNAs has been examined in relation to onset [25, 26], progression [27, 28], response to treatments [29, 30], and prognosis [31]. However, the clinical significance of these miRNAs has not been definitively established.

In this study, we explored the possibility that expression of miRNAs may have a utility in predicting responsiveness to neoadjuvant chemotherapy in osteosarcoma patients. We analyzed miRNA expression in frozen tissue samples obtained before induction chemotherapy. We found that abundant expression of miR-125b and miR-100 was significantly associated with poor response to chemotherapy. We validated this result using qRT-PCR in an independent sample set and verified the functional significance of these miRNAs by *in vitro* assays.

2. Material and Methods

2.1. Patients and Clinical Information. Frozen clinical specimens, collected by open biopsy before chemotherapy, were retrieved from the National Cancer Center Hospital, Japan. The samples were obtained from eight patients (Table 1) who were diagnosed between 2009 and 2011 and treated according to the standard treatment protocol with methotrexate, doxorubicin, and cisplatin, which are considered key drugs [32]. Response to preoperative chemotherapy was histologically assessed by a pathologist according to the Huvos grading system [2]; when less than 10% tumor cells were found to be viable, the patients were defined as responders, and if not, they were considered as nonresponders (chemoresistant). Samples were snap-frozen in liquid nitrogen at the time of collection and stored at −80°C.

An independent cohort of 20 patients (Table 2) was used to validate results by qRT-PCR, using formalin-fixed paraffin-embedded specimens also collected by open biopsy before chemotherapy. These patients were diagnosed between 1990 and 2008. Nine patients were chemoresistant, and 11 were chemosensitive. All patients were monitored from 0.5 to 11.1 years, with mean 7.7 years. Seven patients have been continuously disease-free, seven died of the disease, and six were living with osteosarcoma.

Written informed consent was obtained from all patients, and the study was approved by the ethics committee of the National Cancer Center.

2.2. RNA Extraction and miRNA and mRNA Array. Frozen tissues were powdered under liquid nitrogen using Multi-beads shocker (Yasui Kikai, Osaka, Japan). Total RNA was then extracted using miRNeasy Mini Kit (Qiagen, Venlo, Netherlands). Formalin-fixed paraffin-embedded samples were sectioned at 10 μm, and total RNA was extracted from several of such slices using the miRNeasy FFPE Kit (Qiagen).

miRNA expression profiles of frozen samples were obtained by hybridizing total RNA to the Agilent human miRNA Microarray V3 (021827, 8 × 15 K, v12.0, Agilent Technologies, Santa Clara, CA), following the manufacturer's instructions. Hybridized microarrays were scanned with a DNA microarray scanner (Agilent G2565BA) with default protocols and settings. miRNA expression was analyzed in GeneSpring GX software (Agilent Technologies). miRNAs were considered differentially expressed when expression increased or decreased > 1.5-fold, with $p < 0.05$ in an unpaired t-test.

mRNA expression profiles of osteosarcoma cells were obtained by hybridizing total RNA to SurePrint G3 Human GE microarray (8 × 60 K, Ver3.0, Agilent Technologies, Santa Clara, CA), following the manufacturer's instructions. The DNA microarray data were analyzed by Bioconductor agilp package (http://bioconductor.org/packages/agilp/). The probes were selected, when their intensity was considerably (more than 1.5-fold change) different between two samples.

2.3. Validation of miR-100 and miR-125b in Independent Samples. miR-100 and miR-125b were amplified by quantitative real-time reverse transcriptase-polymerase chain reaction (qRT-PCR) from formalin-fixed paraffin-embedded samples. First, cDNA was synthesized from 10 ng total RNA using TaqMan MicroRNA hsa-miR-100 and hsa-miR-125b (Applied Biosystems) and TaqMan MicroRNA Reverse Transcription

Table 1: Clinical and pathological data of osteosarcoma patients for global miRNA expression study.

Case number	Gender	Age	Location	Histologic type	Neoadjuvant chemotherapy	Viable cells (%)[A]
Case 1	Female	11	Tibia	Osteoblastic	MTX + DOX + CDDP	0%
Case 2	Male	18	Tibia	Osteoblastic	MTX + DOX + CDDP	9%
Case 3	Male	15	Tibia	Osteoblastic	MTX + DOX + CDDP	0%
Case 4	Female	13	Femur	Osteoblastic	MTX + DOX + CDDP	0%
Case 5	Female	10	Femur	Osteoblastic	MTX + DOX + CDDP	70%
Case 6	Male	25	Tibia	Osteoblastic	MTX + DOX + CDDP	40%
Case 7	Male	12	Femur	Osteoblastic	MTX + DOX + CDDP	20%
Case 8	Female	16	Femur	Osteoblastic	MTX + DOX + CDDP	22%

A: probability of viable cells was pathologically evaluated by surgical specimen.

Table 2: Clinical and pathological data of osteosarcoma patients for validation study.

Case number	Gender	Age	Location	Histologic type	Neoadjuvant chemotherapy	Viable cells (%)[A]	Prognosis[C]
Number 1	Male	19	Tibia	Osteoblastic	MTX + DOX + CDDP	0–10%	NED
Number 2	Female	9	Femur	Osteoblastic	MTX + DOX + CDDP	0%	CDF
Number 3	Female	9	Tibia	Chondroblastic	MTX + DOX + CDDP	0–10%	DOD
Number 4	Female	14	Femur	Osteoblastic	MTX + DOX + CDDP	0	CDF
Number 5	Female	15	Femur	Osteoblastic	MTX + DOX + CDDP	0–10%	DOD
Number 6	Female	9	Tibia	Osteoblastic	MTX + DOX + CDDP	0%	NED
Number 7	Male	17	Femur	Osteoblastic	MTX + DOX + CDDP	0–10%	CDF
Number 8	Female	17	Tibia	Osteoblastic	MTX + DOX + CDDP	1%	CDF
Number 9	Female	11	Femur	Chondroblastic	MTX + DOX + CDDP	7%	CDF
Number 10	Male	13	Femur	Osteoblastic	MTX + DOX + CDDP	0–10%	DOD
Number 11	Male	16	Femur	Chondroblastic	MTX + DOX + CDDP	0–10%	DOD
Number 12	Female	13	Tibia	Osteoblastic	MTX + DOX + CDDP	60–70%	DOD
Number 13	Male	22	Femur	Osteoblastic	MTX + DOX + CDDP	30%	DOD
Number 14	Male	18	Femur	Osteoblastic	MTX + DOX + CDDP	60–70%	NED
Number 15	Male	14	Tibia	Osteoblastic	MTX + DOX + CDDP	50–60%	CDF
Number 16	Male	13	Femur	Osteoblastic	MTX + DOX + CDDP	30–40%	AWD
Number 17	Male	9	Femur	Chondroblastic	MTX + DOX + CDDP	30–40%	NED
Number 18	Female	10	Femur	Chondroblastic	MTX + DOX + CDDP	70%	CDF
Number 19	Male	17	Ilium	Fibroblastic	MTX + DOX + CDDP	Clinically poor[B]	DOD
Number 20	Male	15	Tibia	Osteoblastic	MTX + DOX + CDDP	50–60%	NED

A: Probability of viable cells was pathologically evaluated by surgical specimen. B: patients with disease progression in diagnostic imaging by computed tomography and magnetic resource imaging. C: CDF: continuously disease-free, DOD: died of disease, NED: no evidence of disease, and AWD: alive with disease.

Kit (Applied Biosystems). Target miRNAs were amplified over 45 cycles of denaturation at 95°C for 10 sec, annealing at 60°C for 10 sec, and extension at 65°C for 10 sec, following initial denaturation at 95°C for 10 min. PCR was performed in triplicate in 96-well plates using the 7300 Real-Time PCR System (Applied Biosystems), and miRNA expression was normalized to small nuclear RNA RNU6B (Applied Biosystems).

2.4. Cell Culture and Transfection. Differentially expressed miRNAs were functionally characterized in osteosarcoma cell lines MNNG-HOS, 143B, and MG63, American Type Culture Collection. Briefly, cells were cultured at 37°C in a humidified 5% CO_2 chamber using DMEM supplemented with 10% fetal bovine serum, 1 mmol/L sodium pyruvate, nonessential amino acids, and 2 mmol/L glutamine. Cells were then transfected with 25 nM negative control miRNA (Cosmo Bio, Tokyo, Japan), miR-100 (Bonac Corporation, Fukuoka, Japan), and miR-125 (Bonac Corporation, Fukuoka, Japan) using DharmaFECT transfection reagents (Thermo Scientific, Tokyo, Japan), following the manufacturer's protocol.

2.5. Cell Proliferation Assay. Cell proliferation was measured using a standard MTS assay. In brief, cells were seeded at 3×10^3 cells/well in a 96-well plate containing 100 μL culture medium, grown overnight, and transfected with miRNAs as described or incubated in conditioned medium. The media in transfected cells were replaced with fresh medium A 24 h after transfection. Cell viability was determined 3 d thereafter by Cell Counting Kit-8 (Dojindo, Kumamoto, Japan) according to the manufacturer's protocol. In this assay, WST-8 is reduced by dehydrogenase activity in viable cells to yield a formazan dye, which is soluble in tissue culture media, and assayed by absorbance at 450 nm [33]. The amount of formazan dye was produced in directly proportional to the number of viable cells. Three wells were examined for each treatment, and experiments were independently repeated three times. Results are reported as mean ± SD. Statistical significance was tested by t-test.

2.6. Cell Invasion Assay. Cell invasion was evaluated using the BD BioCoat™ Invasion Chamber (BD Bioscience), following the manufacturer's protocol. In brief, cells transfected with miR-125b or miR-100 for 24 h were seeded onto the membrane in the upper chamber of the transwell at 5×10^5 cells in 500 μL serum-free medium. The medium in the lower chamber contained 10% fetal calf serum as source of chemoattractants. Cells that passed through the Matrigel-coated membrane were stained with Diff-Quick (Sysmex, Kobe, Japan) and counted. Experiments were performed three times independently, and statistical significance was determined by t-test.

2.7. Apoptosis Assay. Cells were transfected as described with 25 nM negative control miRNA, miR-100, and miR-125b and treated 24 h thereafter with methotrexate for 72 h, doxorubicin for 48 h, and cisplatin for 48 h. Proteins were extracted, and expression of apoptosis-associated proteins was measured by western blotting.

2.8. Protein Extraction and Western Blotting. Frozen tissues were powdered under liquid nitrogen with the Multi-beads shocker and resuspended in 6 mol/L urea, 2 mol/L thiourea, 3% CHAPS, and 1% Triton X-100. The supernatant was then cleared by centrifugation at 15,000 rpm for 30 min. Cultured cells were washed with PBS, fixed with 10% TCA for 30 min, and lysed in the same buffer for 30 min. The supernatant was collected after centrifugation for 30 min.

Proteins were separated on SDS-polyacrylamide gels and transferred to a nitrocellulose membrane (Bio-Rad). After blocking for 1 h in Tris-buffered saline and Tween 20 (TBS-T) supplemented with 5% nonfat milk, membranes were incubated overnight at 4°C with primary antibodies against Bakl (monoclonal, 1:250, MBL), PARP (1:1000, BD), Caspase-3 (1:1000, BD), Caspase-9 (1:1000, MBL), Caspase-2 (1:1000, BD), BMF (polyclonal, 1:1000, MBL), PUMA (monoclonal, 1:1000, BD), Bcl-2 (monoclonal, 1:500, BD), PP2A-catalytic α (1:1000, BD), MCL-1 (1:1000, BD), and β-actin (1:1000, BD). Membranes were then extensively washed with TBS-T and labeled with horseradish peroxidase-conjugated secondary anti-mouse (1:1000, GE) or anti-rabbit IgG (1:2000, GE). After additional washes with TBS-T, antigen-antibody complexes were visualized with ECL-Prime Kit (GE).

2.9. Transfection of miRNA to Osteosarcoma Cells Followed by Global Gene Expression Analysis. For preparation of RNA samples, MG63 cells were transfected with 25 nM negative control miRNA, miR-100, and miR-125 using DharmaFECT transfection reagents. Cells were harvested at 72 hours after transfection. mRNA expression profiles of miRNA transfected cells were obtained for the global mRNA expression study using DNA microarray as mentioned above.

3. Results

We analyzed global miRNA expression in eight frozen diagnostic open biopsy specimens. Clinical and pathological data are summarized in Table 1. The tumors included in the miRNA expression study were histologically osteoblastic and originated from either the femur or the tibia. Since a previous study has suggested there was a significant correlation between response to chemotherapy and histology [34], we aimed to omit the histological bias in our study by using samples with similar histological and anatomical backgrounds. Patients who had less than 10% viable tumor cells after chemotherapy were considered good responders, and all others were deemed to be poor responders according to the Huvos grading system. Expression profiling identified six miRNAs expressed at significantly different levels ($p < 0.05$) between good responders and poor responders (Figure 1(a), Supplementary Table 1 in Supplementary Material available online at http://dx.doi.org/10.1155/2016/1390571). Of these, the miRNAs 483-3p, 100, 124, 125b, and 127-3p were expressed more abundantly in poor responders, while miR-887 expression was suppressed. Clinical or pathological factors were not obviously correlated with differential expression. To confirm results, these miRNAs were amplified by qRT-PCR from the same eight samples. This assay confirmed significantly different ($p < 0.05$) expression of miR-125b and miR-100 in poor responders (Figures 1(b) and 1(c)) but not of miRNAs 124, 127-3p, 483-3p, and 887 (Figures 1(d)–1(g)). Nevertheless, expression levels measured by qRT-PCR show the same general trends as microarray data.

To investigate these observations further, we measured miRNA expression by qRT-PCR in 20 formalin-fixed paraffin-embedded open biopsy samples of primary osteosarcoma (Supplementary Table 2). The tumor tissues used for validation purposes were heterogeneous; they included osteoblastic, chondroblastic, or fibroblastic tumors, and their site of origin included the tibia, the femur, or the ilium. By exploring such heterogeneous tumor samples, we aimed to demonstrate the versatility of these miRs in predicting responsiveness to neoadjuvant chemotherapy. We also found miR-125b and miR-100 to be expressed at significantly higher levels ($p < 0.05$) in poor responders (Figures 2(a) and 2(b)). The receiver operating characteristic curve had areas under the curves 0.909 and 0.899 for miR-125b and miR-100, respectively ($p < 0.05$, Figures 2(c) and 2(d)).

In light of these results, we characterized the functional significance of miR-125b and miR-100 overexpression in osteosarcoma cells. In cell proliferation assays, we observed miR-125b and miR-100 to significantly enhance growth in MNNG/HOS, 143B, and MG63 (Figures 3(a)–3(c)). Moreover, we found that miR-125b promoted cell invasiveness in MNNG/HOS and 143B, while miR-100 enhanced cell invasiveness in all three cell lines (Figures 4(a) and 4(b)). These observations suggested that overexpression of miR-125b and miR-100 had significant effects on tumorigenicity.

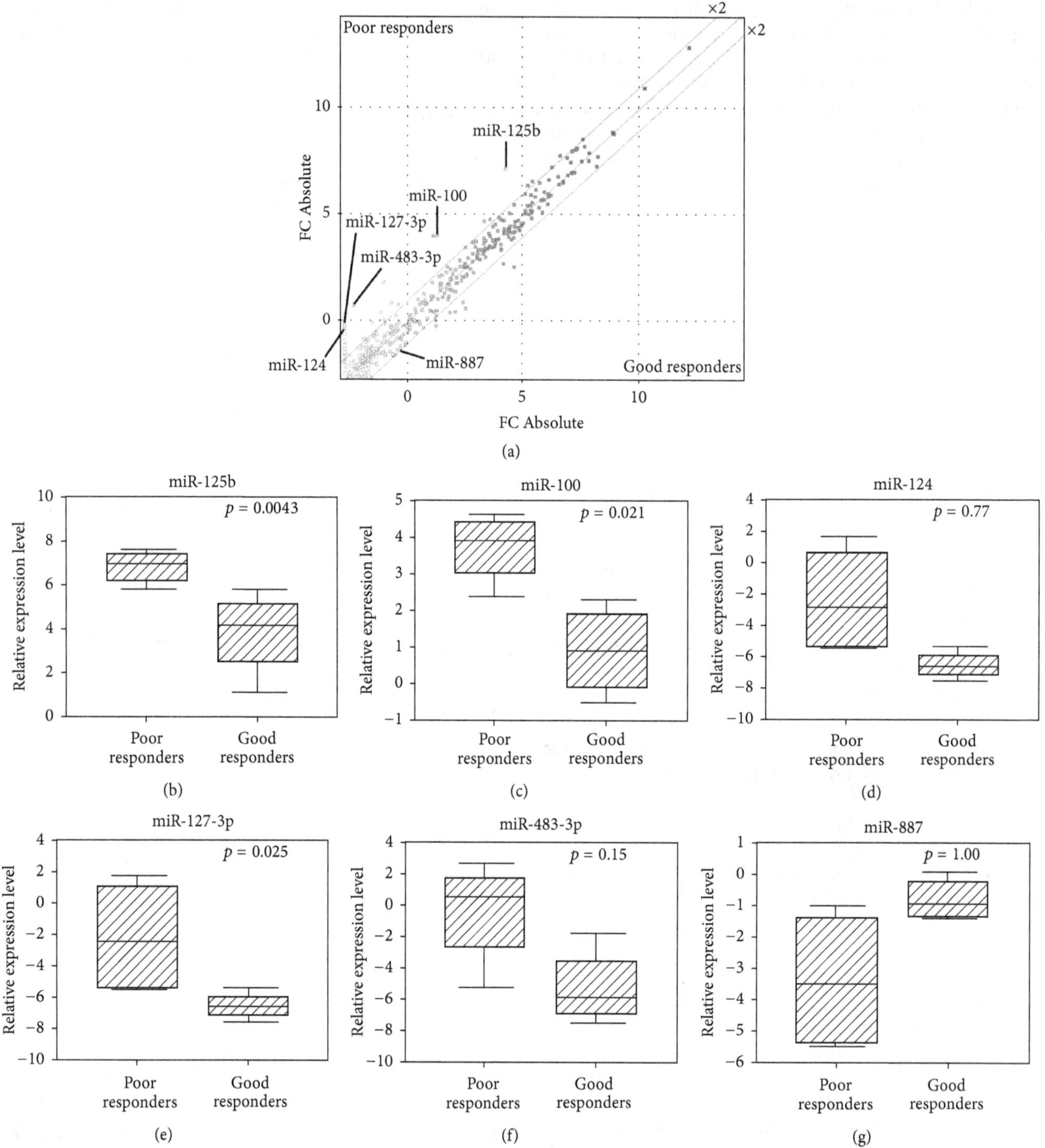

FIGURE 1: Expression of six miRNAs was significantly different between poor and good responders, as measured by microarray analysis of open biopsy samples (a). qRT-PCR (b–g) of these six miRNAs confirmed that miRNA-125b (b) and miR-100 (c) were expressed at significantly higher levels in chemoresistant patients.

We investigated the impact of miR-125b and miR-100 on the effectiveness of chemotherapy drugs. Overexpression of miR-125b significantly blocked the cytotoxic effects of methotrexate, doxorubicin, and cisplatin in all cells (Supplementary Figure 1, Supplementary Table 3). miR-100 also blocked cytotoxicity, except that of doxorubicin in MNNG/HOS cells (Supplementary Figure 1, Supplementary Table 3). Subsequently, we focused on miR-125b because of its ability to block all chemotherapy drugs in all cells examined.

We hypothesized that the known ability of miR-125b to inhibit apoptosis drives tumor progression and resistance to chemotherapy. Indeed, we found that overexpression of miR-125b markedly reduced the expression of apoptosis proteins, including p53, Caspase-2, MCL-1, PUMA, and PP2A catalytic

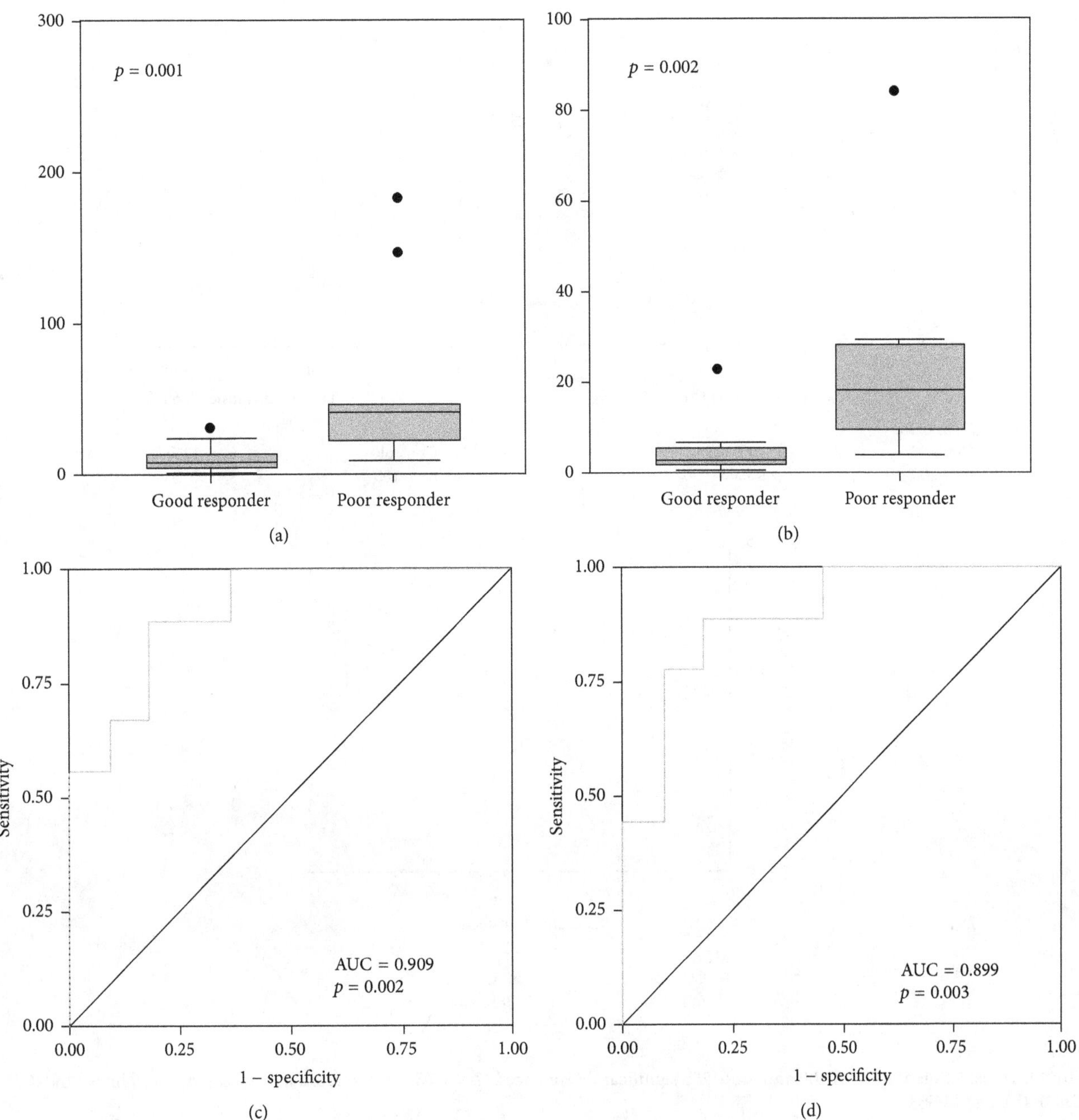

FIGURE 2: In an independent cohort of patients, expression of miR-125b (a) and miR-100 (b) was higher in patients resistant induction chemotherapy. miR-125b (c) and miR-100 (d) showed significant sensitivity and specificity in receiver operating curves, with area under the curve 0.909 and 0.899, respectively. The black circles represent the patients' data.

α (Supplementary Figure 2(A)). We also found that miR-125b blocked the ability of methotrexate, doxorubicin, and cisplatin to induce expression of Bakl and cleaved PARP (Supplementary Figure 2(B)). On the other hand, overexpression of miR-100 resulted in reduced expression of CTDSPL and Rb (Supplementary Figure 2(C)). These results are consistent with our hypothesis that miR-125b may contribute to drug resistance by inhibiting apoptosis.

To explore the effects of miR-100 and miR-125b, we examined the global expression of mRNA after transfecting miR-100 or miR-125b. The transfection of miR-100 and miR-125b induced the differential expression of 35 and 88 genes, respectively (Supplementary Tables 4 and 5). The 16 mRNAs were commonly up- or downregulated by transfection of miR-100 and miR-125b (Table 3).

4. Discussion

As osteosarcoma patients have significantly favorable prognosis when they respond well to neoadjuvant treatments, molecular biomarkers predictive of this response may be useful to determine the appropriate course of treatment.

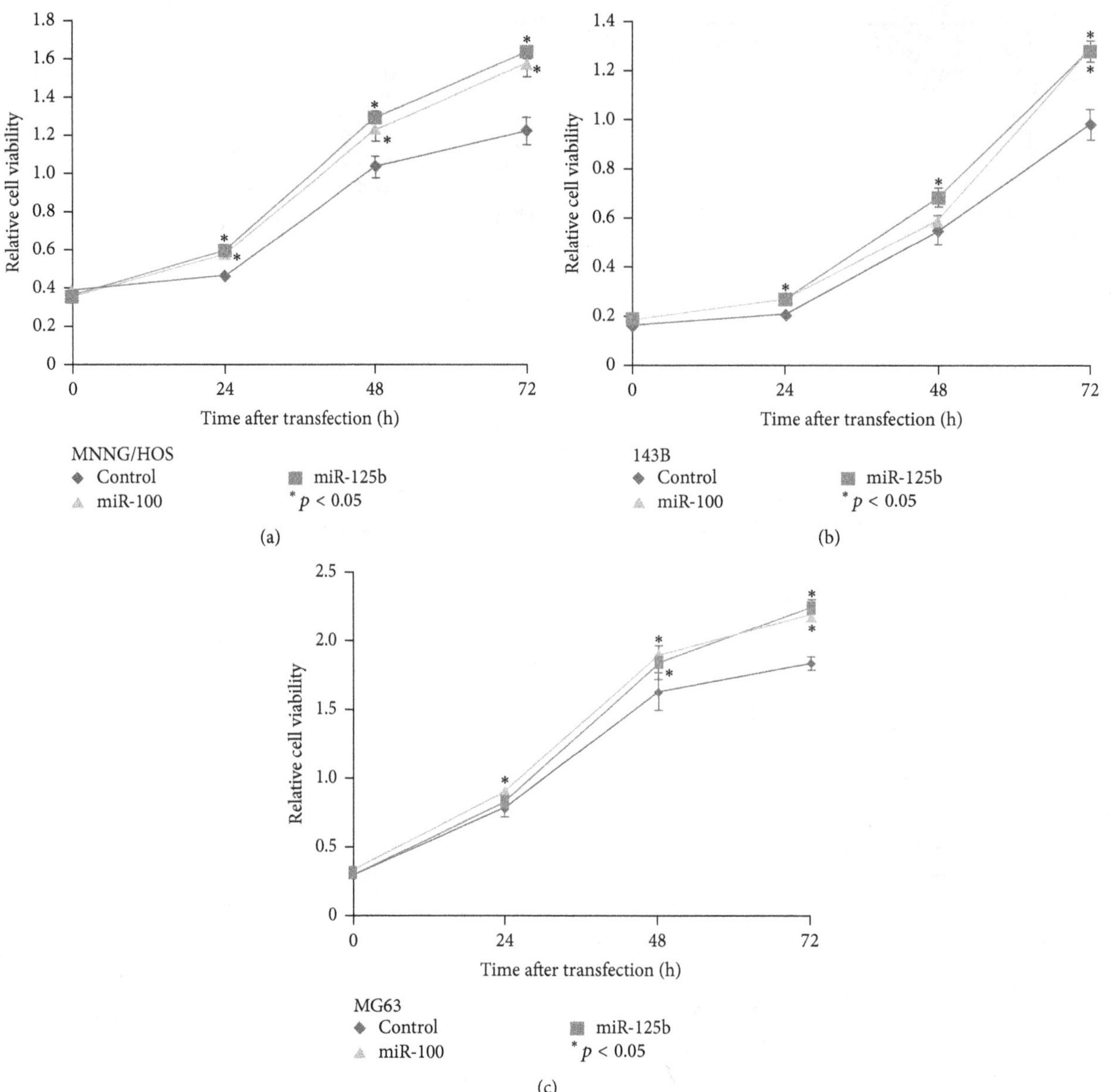

FIGURE 3: Transfection of miRNA-100 and miR-125b significantly enhanced ($p < 0.05$) proliferation in osteosarcoma cell lines MNNG/HOS (a), 143B (b), and MG63 (c).

Several of such biomarkers have been reported, including P-glycoprotein [15] and PRDX2, which was associated with resistance to neoadjuvant treatments in two independent studies [20, 21]. In contrast, Borys et al. [35] reported that p16 was correlated with a therapeutic response. Although these studies concerning miR-100 and miR-125b appear promising, there is insufficient evidence to support their practical use. Extensive validation studies will be required to establish the predictive utility of these biomarkers prior to application in the clinic.

We now report that abundant expression of miR-100 and miR-125b in osteosarcoma tissues prior to treatment is predictive of a poor response to neoadjuvant chemotherapy. Notably, expression of miR-100 and miR-125b was found to be lower in osteosarcoma tissues than in adjacent healthy tissues [36, 37]. As we examined expression of these miRNAs only in tumor tissues, it might be informative to investigate whether expression in adjacent tissues is correlated in some way with clinical and pathological parameters. The superiority of miR-100 and miR-125b over other previously reported predictive biomarkers should be noted. The area under the ROC curve for PRDX2 has been reported to be 0.90 ($p = 0.015$) [20, 21]. The predictive performances of miR-100 and miR-125b noted here (areas under the ROC curve of approximately 0.9 in each case) are equivalent to that of PRDX2. However, the expression of PRDX2 was measured by western blotting, a methodology that cannot be easily automated. In contrast, the expression levels of miR-100 and miR-125b were measured

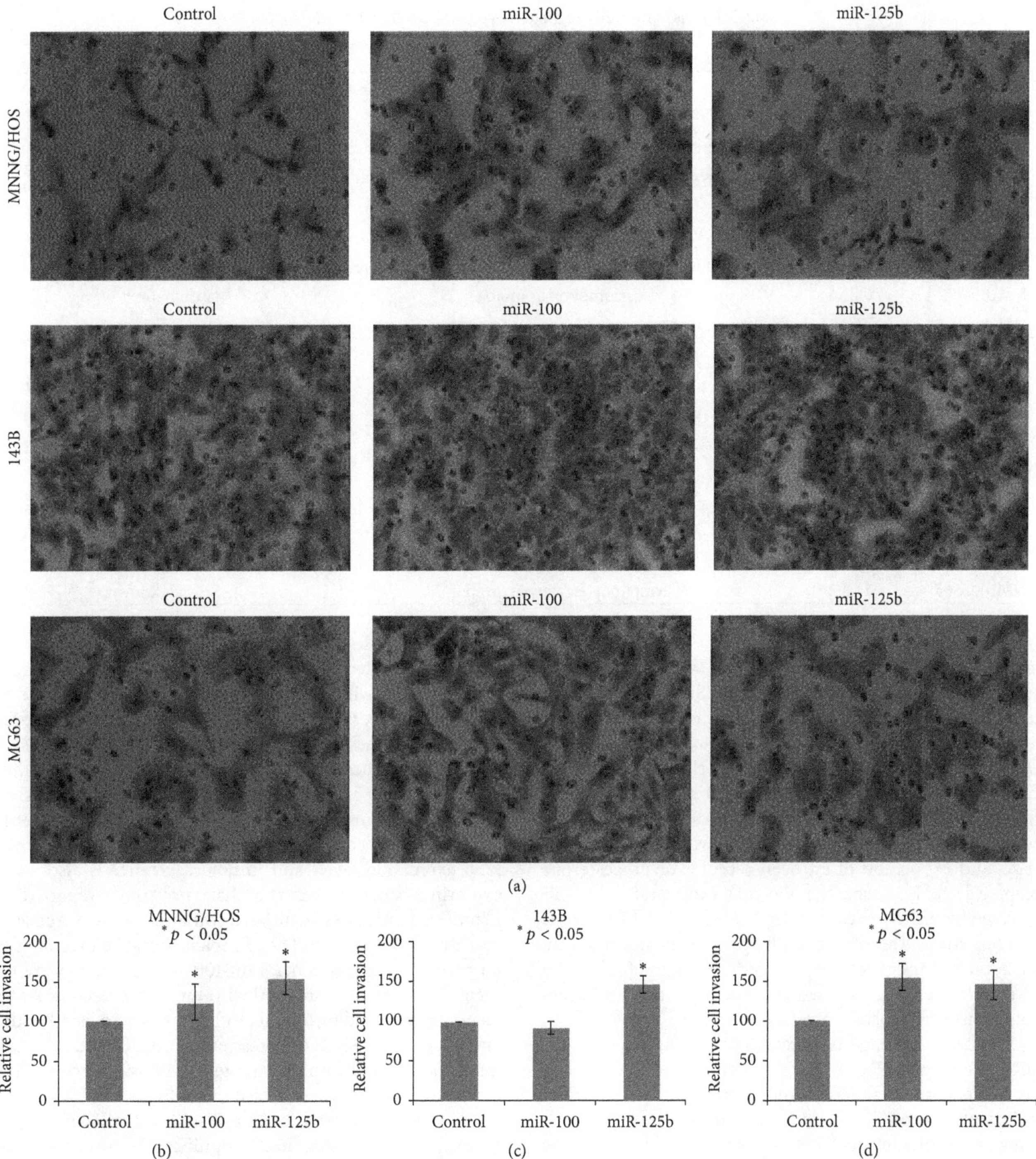

FIGURE 4: Transfection of miR-100 and miR-125b enhanced cell invasiveness in MNNG/HOS (a), 143B (b), and MG63 (c) osteosarcoma cell lines.

by qRT-PCR, which can be easily automated. The practical utility of miR-100 and miR-125b should therefore be further explored.

The reported effects of miR-100 and miR-125b on proliferation of osteosarcoma cells are controversial. Huang et al. [36] demonstrated that miR-100 suppresses proliferation of Saos-2 and MG63 cells, an effect reversed by antisense RNA against miR-100. In contrast, we found miR-100 as well as miR-125b to stimulate proliferation in MNNB/HOS, 143B, and MG63 cells (Figure 3). A possible explanation for this discrepancy is the use of different assays to measure cell proliferation [33]. As osteosarcoma is a heterogeneous malignancy, in order to establish the molecular mechanisms of chemoresistance we may need to explore a range of osteosarcoma cell lines.

We found the mRNAs expression which was commonly upregulated by the transfection of miR-100 and miR-125b.

TABLE 3: Genes commonly regulated by miRNA-100 and miRNA-125b.

Accession number	Symbol	Gene title	Biological function
Upregulated genes			
NM_006868	RAB31	RAB31, member RAS oncogene family	Nucleotide binding
NM_012241	SIRT5	Sirtuin (silent mating type information regulation 2 homolog) 5	NAD+ ADP-ribosyltransferase activity
NM_001142864	PIEZO1	Piezo-type mechanosensitive ion channel component 1	Cation channel activity
NM_002383	MAZ	MYC-associated zinc finger protein	Metal ion binding
NM_004997	MYBPH	Myosin binding protein H	Structural constituent of muscle
NM_000261	MYOC	Myocilin, trabecular meshwork inducible glucocorticoid response	Structural molecule activity
NM_014292	CBX6	Chromobox homolog 6	Chromatin binding
NM_145267	C6orf57	Chromosome 6 open reading frame 57	Unknown
Downregulated genes			
NM_000576	IL1B	Interleukin 1, beta	Cytokine activity
NM_014510	PCLO	piccolo (presynaptic cytomatrix protein)	Calcium ion binding
NM_001017402	LAMB3	Laminin, beta 3	Structural molecule activity
NM_004864	GDF15	Growth differentiation factor 15	Cytokine activity
NM_000379	XDH	Xanthine dehydrogenase	Nucleotide binding
NM_182507	KRT80	Keratin 80	Structural molecule activity
NM_213602	SIGLEC15	Sialic acid binding Ig-like lectin 15	Unknown
NM_005565	LCP2	Lymphocyte cytosolic protein 2	Unknown

Among them, the expression of sirtuin (silent mating type information regulation 2 homolog 5, SIRT5) was previously associated with the resistance against the *in vitro* and *in vivo* treatments with cis-diamminedichloroplatinum, 5-fluorouracil, or bleomycin in non-small cell lung cancer [38]. The aberrant regulation of SIRT5 was reported in various types of malignancies. For example, in breast cancer, the expression of SIRT5 had significant relation with tumor location, grade, and expression of estrogen receptor or progesterone receptor [39]. However, the aberrant expression of SIRT5 regulated by miRNAs was not implicated with osteosarcoma until our study. The sirtuin family genes play an important role in the carcinogenesis and cancer progression [40], and it is worth challenging to investigate the regulation and functions of sirtuins in osteosarcomas.

Our next challenge is to establish the clinical utility of miR-100 and miR-125b. As the number of cases in this study was limited, more validation studies may be required before clinical application. Prediction of a poor response to neoadjuvant chemotherapy may prevent the use of time-consuming but ultimately ineffective treatments and thereby prevent patients from experiencing unnecessary side effects. Unfortunately, there are no alternative therapeutic strategies. Nevertheless, immediate surgical resection due to a predicted risk of chemoresistance may improve clinical outcomes for some patients. Identification of chemoresistant patients may also justify their inclusion in clinical trials of novel anticancer agents. Finally, we may be able to identify new therapeutic targets by characterizing the molecular basis of the correlation between miR-100 and miR-125b expression and response to neoadjuvant chemotherapy.

The global expression of miRNAs and especially the expression level of miR-100 and miR-125b in metastatic tumors is intriguing. Recently, Berlanga et al. compared primary osteosarcomas with lung metastatic osteosarcomas and identified twenty-six miRNAs with significantly different expression between the two [41]. Although miR-100 and miR-125b were not identified in their study, it is worth examining their expression in paired primary and metastatic tumor tissues in patients having different responses to chemotherapeutic treatment. The correlation between the miR-100 and miR-125b expression levels and tumor recurrence is also worth exploring. Sanchez-Diaz et al. have previously reported the identity of miRNAs associated with tumor recurrence in pediatric osteosarcoma [42]. Probably because they focused on pediatric osteosarcoma, miR-100 and miR-125b were not identified as being associated with tumor recurrence. As the response to neoadjuvant chemotherapy is associated with a favorable prognosis, the expression of miR-100 and miR-125b may be associated with poor prognosis in osteosarcoma. This hypothesis should be addressed in a future study.

In summary, expression of miR-100 and miR-125b in pretreatment of osteosarcoma is significantly correlated with poor chemotherapy response and is a promising biomarker to guide treatment decisions.

Disclosure

Present address of Daisuke Kubota is Department of Orthopaedic Surgery, Juntendo University School of Medicine, Tokyo, Japan. Present address of Nobuyoshi Kosaka is Department of Zoology, University of Oxford, Oxford, UK. Present address of Tomohiro Fujiwara is Department of Orthopaedic Surgery, Okayama University Graduate School of Medicine, Dentistry, and Pharmaceutical Sciences, Okayama, Japan.

Acknowledgments

This research was supported by Practical Research for Innovative Cancer Control (15ck0106089h0002 and 15ck0106089h0003) from Japan Agency for Medical Research and Development, by the National Cancer Center Development Fund (26-A-3), and by Grant-in-Aid for Scientific Research 25871161.

References

[1] C. P. Gibbs, K. Weber, and M. T. Scarborough, "Malignant bone tumors," *Journal of Bone and Joint Surgery—Series A*, vol. 83, no. 11, pp. 1728–1745, 2001.

[2] P. A. Meyers and R. Gorlick, "Osteosarcoma," *The Pediatric Clinics of North America*, vol. 44, no. 4, pp. 973–989, 1997.

[3] A. J. Provisor, L. J. Ettinger, J. B. Nachman et al., "Treatment of nonmetastatic osteosarcoma of the extremity with preoperative and postoperative chemotherapy: a report from the Children's Cancer Group," *Journal of Clinical Oncology*, vol. 15, no. 1, pp. 76–84, 1997.

[4] G. Rosen, "Preoperative (neoadjuvant) chemotherapy for osteogenic sarcoma: a ten year experience," *Orthopedics*, vol. 8, no. 5, pp. 659–664, 1985.

[5] G. Rosen, R. C. Marcove, A. G. Huvos et al., "Primary osteogenic sarcoma: eight-year experience with adjuvant chemotherapy," *Journal of Cancer Research and Clinical Oncology*, vol. 106, no. 1, pp. 55–67, 1983.

[6] G. Rosen, B. Caparros, S. Groshen et al., "Primary osteogenic sarcoma of the femur: a model for the use of preoperative chemotherapy in high risk malignant tumors," *Cancer Investigation*, vol. 2, no. 3, pp. 181–192, 1984.

[7] G. Bacci, M. Avella, D. P. A. Brach et al., "Neoadjuvant chemotherapy for osteosarcoma of the extremities. Good response of the primary tumor after preoperative chemotherapy with high-dose methotrexate followed by cisplatinum and adriamycin. Preliminary results," *Chemioterapia*, vol. 7, no. 2, pp. 138–142, 1988.

[8] K. Winkler, G. Beron, G. Delling et al., "Neoadjuvant chemotherapy of osteosarcoma: results of a randomized cooperative trial (COSS-82) with salvage chemotherapy based on histological tumor response," *Journal of Clinical Oncology*, vol. 6, no. 2, pp. 329–337, 1988.

[9] A. M. Davis, R. S. Bell, and P. J. Goodwin, "Prognostic factors in osteosarcoma: a critical review," *Journal of Clinical Oncology*, vol. 12, no. 2, pp. 423–431, 1994.

[10] S. Weeden, R. J. Grimer, S. R. Cannon, A. H. M. Taminiau, and B. M. Uscinska, "The effect of local recurrence on survival in resected osteosarcoma," *European Journal of Cancer*, vol. 37, no. 1, pp. 39–46, 2001.

[11] G. Bacci, A. Longhi, M. Versari, M. Mercuri, A. Briccoli, and P. Picci, "Prognostic factors for osteosarcoma of the extremity treated with neoadjuvant chemotherapy: 15-year experience in 789 patients treated at a single institution," *Cancer*, vol. 106, no. 5, pp. 1154–1161, 2006.

[12] S. S. Bielack, B. Kempf-Bielack, G. Delling et al., "Prognostic factors in high-grade osteosarcoma of the extremities or trunk. An analysis of 1702 patients treated on Cooperative Osteosarcoma Study Group protocols," *Journal of Clinical Oncology*, vol. 20, no. 3, pp. 776–790, 2002.

[13] D. B. Glasser, J. M. Lane, A. G. Huvos, R. C. Marcove, and G. Rosen, "Survival, prognosis, and therapeutic response in osteogenic sarcoma. The memorial hospital experience," *Cancer*, vol. 69, no. 3, pp. 698–708, 1992.

[14] T. Akatsuka, T. Wada, Y. Kokai et al., "ErbB2 expression is correlated with increased survival of patients with osteosarcoma," *Cancer*, vol. 94, no. 5, pp. 1397–1404, 2002.

[15] N. Baldini, K. Scotlandi, G. Barbanti-Bròdano et al., "Expression of P-glycoprotein in high-grade osteosarcomas in relation to clinical outcome," *The New England Journal of Medicine*, vol. 333, no. 21, pp. 1380–1385, 1995.

[16] G. Rosen, B. Caparros, A. G. Huvos et al., "Preoperative chemotherapy for osteogenic sarcoma: *selection of postoperative adjuvant chemotherapy based on the response of the primary tumor to preoperative chemotherapy*," *Cancer*, vol. 49, no. 6, pp. 1221–1230, 1982.

[17] M. J. Klein and G. P. Siegal, "Osteosarcoma: anatomic and histologic variants," *American Journal of Clinical Pathology*, vol. 125, no. 4, pp. 555–581, 2006.

[18] M. L. Kuijjer, P. C. W. Hogendoorn, and A.-M. Cleton-Jansen, "Genome-wide analyses on high-grade osteosarcoma: making sense of a genomically most unstable tumor," *International Journal of Cancer*, vol. 133, no. 11, pp. 2512–2521, 2013.

[19] A. K. Boehm, J. R. Neff, J. A. Squire, J. Bayani, M. Nelson, and J. A. Bridge, "Cytogenetic findings in 36 osteosarcoma specimens and a review of the literature," *Pediatric Pathology and Molecular Medicine*, vol. 19, no. 5, pp. 359–376, 2000.

[20] K. Kikuta, N. Tochigi, S. Saito et al., "Peroxiredoxin 2 as a chemotherapy responsiveness biomarker candidate in osteosarcoma revealed by proteomics," *Proteomics—Clinical Applications*, vol. 4, no. 5, pp. 560–567, 2010.

[21] D. Kubota, K. Mukaihara, A. Yoshida, H. Tsuda, A. Kawai, and T. Kondo, "Proteomics study of open biopsy samples identifies peroxiredoxin 2 as a predictive biomarker of response to induction chemotherapy in osteosarcoma," *Journal of Proteomics*, vol. 91, pp. 393–404, 2013.

[22] D. P. Bartel, "MicroRNAs: genomics, biogenesis, mechanism, and function," *Cell*, vol. 116, no. 2, pp. 281–297, 2004.

[23] B. P. Lewis, C. B. Burge, and D. P. Bartel, "Conserved seed pairing, often flanked by adenosines, indicates that thousands of human genes are microRNA targets," *Cell*, vol. 120, no. 1, pp. 15–20, 2005.

[24] L. P. Lim, N. C. Lau, P. Garrett-Engele et al., "Microarray analysis shows that some microRNAs downregulate large numbers of target mRNAs," *Nature*, vol. 433, no. 7027, pp. 769–773, 2005.

[25] R. R. Lulla, F. F. Costa, J. M. Bischof et al., "Identification of differentially expressed microRNAs in osteosarcoma," *Sarcoma*, vol. 2011, Article ID 732690, 6 pages, 2011.

[26] G. Maire, J. W. Martin, M. Yoshimoto, S. Chilton-MacNeill, M. Zielenska, and J. A. Squire, "Analysis of miRNA-gene expression-genomic profiles reveals complex mechanisms of microRNA deregulation in osteosarcoma," *Cancer Genetics*, vol. 204, no. 3, pp. 138–146, 2011.

[27] E. Kobayashi, R. Satow, M. Ono et al., "MicroRNA expression and functional profiles of osteosarcoma," *Oncology*, vol. 86, no. 2, pp. 94–103, 2014.

[28] K. B. Jones, Z. Salah, S. Del Mare et al., "miRNA signatures associate with pathogenesis and progression of osteosarcoma," *Cancer Research*, vol. 72, no. 7, pp. 1865–1877, 2012.

[29] M. B. Mintz, R. Sowers, K. M. Brown et al., "An expression signature classifies chemotherapy-resistant pediatric osteosarcoma," *Cancer Research*, vol. 65, no. 5, pp. 1748–1754, 2005.

[30] A. Gougelet, D. Pissaloux, A. Besse et al., "Micro-RNA profiles in osteosarcoma as a predictive tool for ifosfamide response," *International Journal of Cancer*, vol. 129, no. 3, pp. 680–690, 2011.

[31] A. D. Kelly, B. Haibe-Kains, K. A. Janeway et al., "MicroRNA paraffin-based studies in osteosarcoma reveal reproducible independent prognostic profiles at 14q32," *Genome Medicine*, vol. 5, no. 1, article 2, 2013.

[32] Y. Iwamoto, K. Tanaka, K. Isu et al., "Multiinstitutional phase II study of neoadjuvant chemotherapy for osteosarcoma (NECO study) in Japan: NECO-93J and NECO-95J," *Journal of Orthopaedic Science*, vol. 14, no. 4, pp. 397–404, 2009.

[33] M. Ishiyama, Y. Miyazono, K. Sasamoto, Y. Ohkura, and K. Ueno, "A highly water-soluble disulfonated tetrazolium salt as a chromogenic indicator for NADH as well as cell viability," *Talanta*, vol. 44, no. 7, pp. 1299–1305, 1997.

[34] G. Bacci, S. Ferrari, N. Delepine et al., "Predictive factors of histologic response to primary chemotherapy in osteosarcoma of the extremity: study of 272 patients preoperatively treated with high-dose methotrexate, doxorubicin, and cisplatin," *Journal of Clinical Oncology*, vol. 16, no. 2, pp. 658–663, 1998.

[35] D. Borys, R. J. Canter, B. Hoch et al., "P16 expression predicts necrotic response among patients with osteosarcoma receiving neoadjuvant chemotherapy," *Human Pathology*, vol. 43, no. 11, pp. 1948–1954, 2012.

[36] J. Huang, K. Gao, J. Lin, and Q. Wang, "MicroRNA-100 inhibits osteosarcoma cell proliferation by targeting Cyr61," *Tumor Biology*, vol. 35, no. 2, pp. 1095–1100, 2014.

[37] L.-H. Liu, H. Li, J.-P. Li et al., "miR-125b suppresses the proliferation and migration of osteosarcoma cells through down-regulation of STAT3," *Biochemical and Biophysical Research Communications*, vol. 416, no. 1-2, pp. 31–38, 2011.

[38] W. Lu, Y. Zuo, Y. Feng, and M. Zhang, "SIRT5 facilitates cancer cell growth and drug resistance in non-small cell lung cancer," *Tumor Biology*, vol. 35, no. 11, pp. 10699–10705, 2014.

[39] M. Igci, M. E. Kalender, E. Borazan et al., "High-throughput screening of Sirtuin family of genes in breast cancer," *Gene*, vol. 586, no. 1, pp. 123–128, 2016.

[40] J. George and N. Ahmad, "Mitochondrial sirtuins in cancer: emerging roles and therapeutic potential," *Cancer Research*, vol. 76, no. 9, pp. 2500–2506, 2016.

[41] P. Berlanga, L. Muñoz, M. Piqueras et al., "miR-200c and phospho-AKT as prognostic factors and mediators of osteosarcoma progression and lung metastasis," *Molecular Oncology*, vol. 10, no. 7, pp. 1043–1053, 2016.

[42] P. C. Sanchez-Diaz, T.-H. Hsiao, Y. Zou et al., "In silico functional analyses and discovery of survival-associated microRNA signatures in pediatric osteosarcoma," *Oncoscience*, vol. 1, no. 9, pp. 599–608, 2014.

18

Early Evidence of Cardiotoxicity and Tumor Response in Patients with Sarcomas after High Cumulative Dose Doxorubicin given as a Continuous Infusion

Raymundo A. Quintana,[1] Jose Banchs,[1] Ridhi Gupta,[2] Heather Y. Lin,[1] Sean D. Raj,[3] Anthony Conley,[3] Vinod Ravi,[3] Dejka Araujo,[3] Robert S. Benjamin,[3] Shreyaskumar Patel,[3] Saroj Vadhan-Raj,[3] and Neeta Somaiah[3]

[1]*Department of Cardiology, University of Texas MD Anderson Cancer Center, 1515 Holcombe Blvd., Unit 1451, Houston, TX 77030, USA*
[2]*Division of Hematology/Oncology, Department of Medicine, Medical University of South Carolina, Charleston, SC 29425, USA*
[3]*Department of Sarcoma Medical Oncology, University of Texas MD Anderson Cancer Center, 1515 Holcombe Boulevard, Unit 450, Houston, TX 77030, USA*

Correspondence should be addressed to Raymundo A. Quintana; raquint@emory.edu

Academic Editor: Fritz C. Eilber

Background. Despite the dose-dependent response rate of sarcomas to doxorubicin, clinicians limit its cumulative dose due to cardiotoxicity. This study evaluates early evidence of cardiotoxicity in patients treated with high-dose doxorubicin given as a continuous infusion. *Methods.* Data was collected on patients who received 90 mg/m^2 doxorubicin as a continuous infusion and 10 gm/m^2 ifosfamide for up to 6 cycles as part of a phase II study. Cardiotoxicity was assessed with serial echocardiograms or multigated acquisition scans and serum brain natriuretic peptide and troponin levels. Tumor responses were determined by serial radiographic imaging per RECIST. *Result.* Out of the 48 patients enrolled, no patient developed heart failure symptoms; however, 4 out of the 38 (10%) patients with serial left ventricular ejection fraction assessments developed subclinical cardiotoxicity (asymptomatic drop in LVEF ≥ 10%). Twenty-three patients received all six 72-hour cycles of doxorubicin with a mean cumulative dose of 540 mg/m^2. Among these patients, 4% ($n = 1$) developed subclinical cardiotoxicity. In the advanced disease group ($n = 39$), patients with a complete or partial response received a higher mean cumulative dose than those with stable disease ($p < 0.033$). *Conclusions.* Doxorubicin cardiotoxicity can be limited by administering doxorubicin as a continuous infusion, allowing higher cumulative dosing to maximize efficacy.

1. Introduction

Sarcomas account for 1% of all malignancies in adults worldwide. These rare tumors originate from mesenchymal cells in different areas of the body. Since the 1970s, doxorubicin (an anthracycline) has been shown to prolong survival in patients with advanced sarcomas [1, 2]. The response to doxorubicin is dose-dependent, with doses above 60 mg/m^2 considered to be effective in sarcomas [3]. However, the most important limiting factor in the use of doxorubicin is the adverse effect of cardiotoxicity [4]. Anthracycline-induced cardiotoxicity is currently defined as the development of signs or symptoms consistent with heart failure or an asymptomatic decrease in baseline left ventricular ejection fraction (LVEF) ≥ 10% to a level < 50% [5–7]. Prior studies have shown that using a higher cumulative anthracycline dose when administered as a bolus infusion increases the risk of cardiotoxicity in children and adults [8, 9]. In one of these studies, 36% of patients ($n = 10$) developed a ≥10% decline in LVEF and 28% ($n = 8$) of them received a cumulative dose ≥ 400 mg/m^2 [10]. Therefore, most clinicians limit the cumulative dose to 400–450 mg/m^2, considered a lifetime maximum in some institutions, to prevent cardiotoxicity regardless of continued therapeutic response. However, it is well documented in studies that cardiotoxicity can be reduced significantly by administration of dexrazoxane, a cardioprotective agent, prior to bolus infusion or by continuous infusion of anthracycline, since anthracycline-induced cardiotoxicity is a peak-dose effect [11–16]. More recently, studies have shown that a brain natriuretic peptide (BNP) level > 100 ng/dl and a troponin I level ≥ 0.08 ng/ml are good predictors of anthracycline-induced cardiotoxicity [17–23]. Herein we report the results of the phase II clinical trial DM00-435, where early doxorubicin-induced cardiotoxicity was assessed by measuring serial LVEF and levels of troponin I and BNP in sarcoma patients receiving high-dose doxorubicin as a continuous infusion and ifosfamide for up to 6 cycles.

2. Materials and Methods

From August 2001 to October 2002, forty-eight adult patients enrolled in the phase II clinical trial DM00-435 at MD Anderson Cancer Center who had newly diagnosed high-grade sarcomas, with either advanced disease (American Joint Committee on Cancer Staging system stages IIC, III, or IV) or localized disease with high risk of relapse, were evaluated. All patients received front-line chemotherapy with doxorubicin 90 mg/m^2 and ifosfamide 10 g/m^2 every 3 weeks for up to 6 cycles. Doxorubicin was given as a continuous infusion over 72 hours (30 mg/m^2 over 24 hours × 3 days). Patients were excluded from the study if they had (1) leiomyosarcoma of gastrointestinal origin; (2) structural heart disease or cardiomyopathy; (3) prior radiation therapy; or (4) prior chemotherapy.

2.1. Systolic Function Determination. Every patient in our study underwent either a transthoracic echocardiogram (TTE) or a multigated acquisition (MUGA) scan at baseline, midstudy, and end of study. All transthoracic echocardiograms were obtained using the same Vivid 7 or E9 [General Electrics (GE) Healthcare, Milwaukee, WI] ultrasound machine and interpreted by a single reader. Patient's LVEF was calculated from the apical four- and two-chamber views using the biplane method of disks (modified Simpson biplane method). MUGA scans were obtained using the GE Infinia camera with low-energy high-resolution collimator in 180 degrees' configuration (H mode). The GE R-wave trigger was used to gate the acquisition. Patient's red blood cells were labeled with technetium-99m (Ultratag® RBC kit). The LVEF was calculated with data collected from three standard views: anterior, best septal left anterior oblique (45 degrees), and left lateral (70–90 degrees). Some patients underwent additional TTEs and MUGA scans during the follow-up period as part of their future treatment protocols.

2.2. Cardiotoxicity. In our study, cardiotoxicity was defined as the development of signs or symptoms consistent with heart failure or an asymptomatic decrease in LVEF ≥ 10% from baseline to a level less than 50% by either TTE or MUGA scan.

2.3. Biomarkers. Serum BNP and troponin I measurements were performed at baseline, midstudy, and end of study in all patients. A commercial, multibiomarker panel (Biosite Triage Profiler, Biosite Incorporated®, 9975 Summers Ridge Road, San Diego, CA 92121, USA) was used to quantify BNP and troponin I levels.

2.4. Tumor Response Assessment. In patients with advanced disease, we assessed tumor response by computed tomography or magnetic resonance imaging every two chemotherapy cycles according to the Response Evaluation Criteria In Solid Tumors (RECIST) [24, 25]. Treatment responses were classified as follows: (1) complete response (CR): disappearance of all target lesions; (2) partial response (PR): 30% decrease in the sum of the longest diameter of all target lesions; (3) disease progression (PD): 20% increase or more in the sum of the longest diameter of all target lesions; or (4) stable disease (SD): changes in the size of target lesions that do not meet above criteria.

2.5. Statistical Analysis. Descriptive statistics such as frequency distribution, mean (±standard deviation), and median (range) were used to summarize patients demographic, tumor characteristic, and cardiac function parameters including LVEF, troponin I, and BNP. Spearman correlation coefficient was used to assess the correlation between the changes of ejection fraction or BNP from baseline to midstudy or end of study with doxorubicin cumulative dose. Chi-square test or Fisher's exact test was used to test differences in categorical variables. Wilcoxon rank-sum test or Kruskal-Wallis test was used to detect differences in continuous variables between groups.

3. Results

A total of 48 patients with diverse sarcoma histologies were evaluated for doxorubicin-induced cardiotoxicity and tumor response. Male-to-female ratio was 1 : 1 with a median age of 38.9 years. The clinical features of the studied patients are listed in Table 1. Left ventricular ejection fraction assessments at both baseline and end of study were available for only 38 patients (79%). Twenty-three patients (48%) received six full 72-hour cycles of doxorubicin with a mean cumulative dose of approximately 540 mg/m^2, and all of these patients had LVEF assessments at baseline and end of study. Midstudy LVEF assessments when done did not differ from end-of-study LVEF and were not always done at the same point in time. The mean number of cycles received among the 48 patients was 4.85 (mean cumulative dose of 433.85 mg/m^2 and median cumulative dose of 502 mg/m^2). Fifteen patients (31%) had their infusion duration reduced from 72 to 48 hours due to development of mucositis. Thirty-nine patients (81%) had advanced disease and were evaluable for tumor response. The remaining nine patients (19%) had early disease with high risk of relapse and received doxorubicin as an adjuvant therapy; thus, their response was not evaluable.

None of the patients experienced any clinical signs of cardiotoxicity during the study or during the available follow-up period of 3.7 years (range, 1 month–10.4 years). All pre- and postchemotherapy LVEF measurements were within

TABLE 1: Patient and treatment characteristics.

Features	n	Percent
Gender		
Female	24	50.00
Male	24	50.00
Tumor histology		
Liposarcoma	9	18.75
Synovial sarcoma	9	18.75
Unclassified sarcoma	9	18.75
Leiomyosarcoma	7	14.58
Osteosarcoma	5	10.42
Ewing's sarcoma/primary neuroectodermal tumor	4	8.33
Angiosarcoma	1	2.08
Desmoplastic small round cell tumor	1	2.08
Chondrosarcoma	1	2.08
Malignant phyllodes tumor	1	2.08
Rhabdomyosarcoma	1	2.08
Location of primary tumors		
Upper limbs	4	8.33
Lower limbs	8	16.67
Nonextremities	36	75.00
High-grade sarcoma stage		
Early disease with high risk of relapse	9	18.75
Advanced disease	39	81.25
Metastatic at diagnosis		
Yes	14	29.17
No	34	70.83
LVEF assessments at both baseline and end of study		
Yes	38	79.17
No	10	20.83
Doxorubicin infusion cycles duration		
72 hours	33	68.75
72/48 hours	15	31.25

normal limits (LVEF $\geq$ 50%). Out of the 38 patients with LVEF assessments at baseline and end of study, only 4 (10%) developed subclinical cardiotoxicity, that is, a drop in LVEF of ≥10% (range, 10–15%). Their clinical characteristics are summarized in Table 2. Interestingly, these 4 patients received a lower mean cumulative dose of doxorubicin than those who did not experience a drop in their LVEF ($p = 0.04$, Table 3). The follow-up period for these 4 patients was 1 year (2 patients) and 4 years (2 patients), during which no clinical heart failure symptoms were noted. All 23 patients that received 6 cycles of doxorubicin over 72 hours were among those evaluated with LVEF assessments at baseline and end of study. Among them, only one patient (4%) developed subclinical cardiotoxicity. Troponin and BNP levels were available in 44 patients at baseline, 48 at midstudy, and 29 at end of study. None of the patients had serum troponin levels $\geq$ 0.05 ng/ml or BNP levels $\geq$ 100 pg/ml. Analysis of baseline to end-of-study BNP values showed that none of the patients had a BNP increase > 10 ng/dl. Three out of the four patients who experienced a drop in their LVEF $\geq$ 10% demonstrated a BNP increase $\leq$ 10 ng/dl. Nonetheless, the difference was not statistically significant ($p = 1.0$). No statistically significant correlation was found between changes from baseline to end-of-study LVEF (Spearman correlation coefficient, Rho = 0.23, p-value = 0.16) or BNP levels (Rho = −0.23, p-value = 0.25) and cumulative doxorubicin dose.

Out of the 39 patients (81%) evaluable for tumor response, a complete response was observed in 1 patient (3%), a partial response was seen in 20 patients (51%), stable disease was found in 16 patients (41%), and disease progression was seen in 2 patients (5%). Patients with a complete or partial response received a higher mean cumulative dose than those with stable disease ($p < 0.033$, Table 4).

4. Discussion

Cardiotoxicity is a well-known side effect related to the peak dose of doxorubicin. Standard dosing is usually 75 mg/m^2 per cycle routinely maxed at 6 cycles irrespective of clinical benefit (widely accepted lifetime cumulative doxorubicin dose of 450 mg/m^2). Continuous infusion (over 72 hours) and dexrazoxane administered prior to bolus infusion are well-known cardioprotective mechanisms employed to mitigate this risk. Our study shows that patients receiving a continuous infusion of high-dose doxorubicin (90 mg/m^2 per cycle for up to a total of 6 cycles) with a median cumulative dose around 500 mg/m^2 (majority getting a total of 540 mg/m^2) did not experience any significant early evidence of cardiotoxicity (based on LVEF, BNP, and troponin I assessment) or clinical heart failure during the available follow-up period of 3.7 years (range, 1 month to 10.4 years). This is in contrast to bolus administration; in a 28-patient study using bolus infusion led to cardiotoxicity in 7%, 21%, and 36% of patients after 200 mg/m^2, 400 mg/m^2, and 500 mg/m^2 of doxorubicin, respectively [10]. In the case of cardiotoxicity during treatment, discontinuation of doxorubicin usually results in improvement of LVEF over time. Echocardiogram monitoring is recommended in all patients at baseline and after 4–6 cycles in high-risk patients, to detect asymptomatic contractile dysfunction that may progress to symptomatic disease with continued therapy [10, 26]. In our study, in the 29 patients who had end-of-study troponin I or BNP levels (including 3 of the 4 patients who had a subclinical decline in LVEF), no significant changes were noted. Although different studies have reported a strong association between BNP levels > 100 ng/dl or a troponin I level $\geq$ 0.08 ng/ml and early anthracycline-induced cardiotoxicity [17–23], recent evidence suggests that newer assays such as ultrasensitive troponin I or N-Terminal Pro-BNP are more sensitive and should be incorporated in any future studies [24, 25].

While therapy discontinuation may reverse acute systolic dysfunction, there is data to suggest that early evidence of cardiotoxicity correlates with the development of future

TABLE 2: Clinical characteristics of 4 patients who developed subclinical cardiotoxicity.

Age (years)	Mean cumulative dose (mg/m^2)	Number of chemotherapy cycles	Baseline LVEF (%)	Baseline troponin I levels (ng/ml)	Midstudy troponin I levels (ng/ml)	End-study troponin I (ng/ml)	Baseline BNP (ng/dl)	Midstudy BNP (ng/dl)	End-study BNP (ng/dl)	Tumor response
45	405	6	65	<0.05	<0.05	<0.05	4.9	4.9	11.7	Neoadjuvant
44	360	4	77	<0.05	<0.05	NA	6.6	4.9	NA	Neoadjuvant
32	525	6	66	<0.05	<0.05	<0.05	4.9	4.9	4.9	Stable disease
53	450	5	68	<0.05	<0.05	<0.05	4.9	4.9	4.9	Stable disease

TABLE 3: Associations between mean doxorubicin cumulative dose and changes in LVEF and BNP.

Variables	Level	n	Cumulative dose Mean cumulative dose (mg/m^2)	Max dose (mg/m^2)	Median cumulative dose (mg/m^2)	p value
LVEF drop from baseline to end of study	<10%	34	490	540	540	0.040
	>10%	4	435	525	428	
BNP increase from baseline to end of study	<10%	21	521	540	540	0.551
	>10%	5	504	540	540	

TABLE 4: Doxorubicin mean cumulative dose and tumor response.

Variable	Tumor response	n	Mean cumulative dose (mg/m^2)	Min dose (mg/m^2)	Max dose (mg/m^2)	Median cumulative dose (mg/m^2)	p value
Doxorubicin mean cumulative dose	Complete response	1	540	540	540	540	0.033
	Partial response	20	490	270	540	540	
	Stable disease	16	416	180	540	450	

LVEF impairment; therefore, long-term cardiac follow-up should be considered on an individual basis in these patients.

In our study, patients with CR/PR received higher cumulative dose of doxorubicin. This could be because those with progression stopped therapy sooner, but since only two patients had PD, it suggests that patients who managed to get all cycles of therapy had a higher likelihood of CR/PR. We also found that the 4 patients with subclinical cardiotoxicity received a significant lower mean cumulative dose of doxorubicin. This was probably a result of earlier discontinuation due to unacceptable toxicities or earlier discontinuation upon noting the lower LVEF on midstudy assessment.

Multiple alternate approaches have been evaluated to avoid anthracycline-induced cardiotoxicity, such as structural modifications (epirubicin and mitoxantrone) and liposomal encapsulation of the anthracycline molecule but these have not been able to match the established efficacy of doxorubicin as the standard backbone for sarcoma regimens [27–31]. Currently aldoxorubicin, a tumor-targeted doxorubicin conjugate (doxorubicin attached to an acid sensitive liker and N-ε-maleimidocaproic acid hydrazide for preferential tumor uptake), is in clinical trial testing and might offer an alternative in the future with lower cardiotoxicity and higher dose administration. For now, using continuous infusion or dexrazoxane prior to bolus infusion of doxorubicin can allow clinicians to cautiously continue doxorubicin (with frequent LVEF monitoring) beyond the cumulative dose of 450 mg/m^2, in patients with continued benefit and good tolerance. Since this could potentially open up surgical options for previously unresectable disease and there are limited treatment options for most sarcoma patients, cardioprotection is critical with doxorubicin. Concerns have been raised about the possibility of decreased treatment efficacy when using dexrazoxane with bolus doxorubicin, though a head-to-head study comparing the efficacy with continuous infusion doxorubicin has not been conducted in adults.

Although our study supports the cardioprotective effects of doxorubicin administration as a continuous infusion, high cumulative doses of doxorubicin, especially when given ifosfamide, are not completely devoid of other acute toxicities. In our study, almost one-third of patients (31%) developed mucositis, warranting a decrease in doxorubicin infusion duration to 48 hours, and other expected toxicities, which lead to a subsequent lowering of the dose or discontinuation of therapy. While myelosuppression is a peak-dose-dependent toxicity, mucositis is linked to the duration of exposure/infusion. Patients must be assessed after each cycle to make adjustments in the regimen if needed based on the severity and duration of the acute toxicities, with a higher threshold for acute self-limiting toxicities in the setting of curative therapy. In this study, the median age was 38.9 years (range 19–65), whereas in previous studies of standard dose doxorubicin (75 mg/m^2) and ifosfamide (10 g/m^2) the median was 45–48 years [32, 33]. Given the potential for high acute toxicity with this combination, younger patients with fewer comorbidities were probably preferentially enrolled and it is important to note that this high-dose regimen would not be recommended for patients above 65 years.

5. Conclusion

In patients with aggressive sarcomas susceptible to doxorubicin, cardiotoxicity can be limited by administering doxorubicin as a continuous infusion over 72 hours per cycle, allowing higher cumulative dosing to maximize efficacy. Physicians should tailor treatment strategies based on the goals of therapy (curative versus palliative), baseline cardiac function, and overall risks when deciding the dose and number of cycles of doxorubicin to administer.

References

[1] R. S. Benjamin, P. H. Wiernik, and N. R. Bachur, "Adriamycin: A new effective agent in the therapy of disseminated sarcomas," *Medical and Pediatric Oncology*, vol. 1, no. 1, pp. 63–76, 1975.

[2] R. M. O'Bryan, J. K. Luce, R. W. Talley, J. A. Gottlieb, L. H. Baker, and G. Bonadonna, "Phase II evaluation of adriamycin in human neoplasia," *Cancer*, vol. 32, no. 1, pp. 1–8, 1973.

[3] R. M. O'Bryan, L. H. Baker, J. E. Gottlieb et al., "Dose response evaluation of adriamycin in human neoplasia," *Cancer*, vol. 39, no. 5, pp. 1940–1948, 1977.

[4] D. D. von Hoff, M. W. Layard, P. Basa et al., "Risk factors for doxorubicin-induced congestive heart failure," *Annals of Internal Medicine*, vol. 91, no. 5, pp. 710–717, 1979.

[5] I. Mitani, D. Jain, T. M. Joska, B. Burtness, and B. L. Zaret, "Doxorubicin cardiotoxicity: prevention of congestive heart failure with serial cardiac function monitoring with equilibrium radinuclide angiocardiography in the current era," *Journal of Nuclear Cardiology*, vol. 10, no. 2, pp. 132–139, 2003.

[6] R. Altena, P. J. Perik, D. J. van Veldhuisen, E. G. de Vries, and J. A. Gietema, "Cardiovascular toxicity caused by cancer treatment: strategies for early detection," *The Lancet Oncology*, vol. 10, no. 4, pp. 391–399, 2009.

[7] R. G. Schwartz, W. B. McKenzie, J. Alexander et al., "Congestive heart failure and left ventricular dysfunction complicating doxorubicin therapy. Seven-year experience using serial radionuclide angiocardiography," *The American Journal of Medicine*, vol. 82, no. 6, pp. 1109–1118, 1987.

[8] M. A. Grenier and S. E. Lipshultz, "Epidemiology of anthracycline cardiotoxicity in children and adults," *Seminars in Oncology*, vol. 25, no. 4, pp. 72–85, 1998.

[9] J. P. Krischer, S. Epstein, D. D. Cuthbertson, A. M. Goorin, M. L. Epstein, and S. E. Lipshultz, "Clinical cardiotoxicity following anthracycline treatment for childhood cancer: The Pediatric Oncology Group experience," *Journal of Clinical Oncology*, vol. 15, no. 4, pp. 1544–1552, 1997.

[10] T. Nousiainen, E. Jantunen, E. Vanninen, and J. Hartikainen, "Early decline in left ventricular ejection fraction predicts doxorubicin cardiotoxicity in lymphoma patients," *British Journal of Cancer*, vol. 86, no. 11, pp. 1697–1700, 2002.

[11] S. S. Legha, R. S. Benjamin, B. Mackay et al., "Reduction of doxorubicin cardiotoxicity by prolonged continuous intravenous infusion," *Annals of Internal Medicine*, vol. 96, no. 2, pp. 133–139, 1982.

[12] E. S. Casper, J. J. Gaynor, S. I. Hajdu et al., "A prospective randomized trial of adjuvant chemotherapy with bolus versus continuous infusion of doxorubicin in patients with high-grade extremity soft tissue sarcoma and an analysis of prognostic factors," *Cancer*, vol. 68, no. 6, pp. 1221–1229, 1991.

[13] G. N. Hortobagyi, H. Yap, S. W. Kau et al., "A Comparative Study of Doxorubicin and Epirubicin in Patients with Metastatic Breast Cancer," *American Journal of Clinical Oncology*, vol. 12, no. 1, pp. 57–62, 1989.

[14] J. Shapira, M. Gotfried, M. Lishner, and M. Ravid, "Reduced cardiotoxicity of doxorubicin by a 6-hour infusion regimen. A prospective randomized evaluation," *Cancer*, vol. 65, no. 4, pp. 870–873, 1990.

[15] M. Zalupski, B. Metch, S. Balcerzak et al., "Phase III comparison of doxorubicin and dacarbazine given by bolus versus infusion in patients with soft-tissue sarcomas: A southwest oncology group study," *Journal of the National Cancer Institute*, vol. 83, no. 13, pp. 926–932, 1991.

[16] E. C. Van Dalen, H. J. H. Van Der Pal, H. N. Caron, and L. C. M. Kremer, "Different dosage schedules for reducing cardiotoxicity in cancer patients receiving anthracycline chemotherapy," *Cochrane Database of Systematic Reviews*, no. 4, Article ID CD005008, 2009.

[17] M.-F. Pichon, F. Cvitkovic, K. Hacene et al., "Drug-induced cardiotoxicity studied by longitudinal B-type natriuretic peptide assays and radionuclide ventriculography," *In Vivo*, vol. 19, no. 3, pp. 567–576, 2005.

[18] H. Okumura, K. Iuchi, T. Yoshida et al., "Brain natriuretic peptide is a predictor of anthracycline-induced cardiotoxicity," *Acta Haematologica*, vol. 104, no. 4, pp. 158–163, 2000.

[19] W. J. Reagan, M. York, B. Berridge, E. Schultze, D. Walker, and S. Pettit, "Comparison of Cardiac Troponin I and T, Including the Evaluation of an Ultrasensitive Assay, as Indicators of Doxorubicin-induced Cardiotoxicity," *Toxicologic Pathology*, vol. 41, no. 8, pp. 1146–1158, 2013.

[20] J. P. Bertinchant, A. Polge, J. M. Juan et al., "Evaluation of cardiac troponin I and T levels as markers of myocardial damage in doxorubicin-induced cardiomyopathy rats, and their relationship with echocardiographic and histological findings," *Clinica Chimica Acta*, vol. 329, no. 1-2, pp. 39–51, 2003.

[21] D. Cardinale, M. T. Sandri, A. Colombo et al., "Prognostic value of troponin I in cardiac risk stratification of cancer patients undergoing high-dose chemotherapy," *Circulation*, vol. 109, no. 22, pp. 2749–2754, 2004.

[22] D. Cardinale, M. T. Sandri, A. Martinoni et al., "Left ventricular dysfunction predicted by early troponin I release after high-dose chemotherapy," *Journal of the American College of Cardiology*, vol. 36, no. 2, pp. 517–522, 2000.

[23] D. Cardinale, M. T. Sandri, A. Martinoni et al., "Myocardial injury revealed by plasma troponin I in breast cancer treated with high-dose chemotherapy," *Annals of Oncology*, vol. 13, no. 5, pp. 710–715, 2002.

[24] B. Ky, M. Putt, H. Sawaya et al., "Early increases in multiple biomarkers predict subsequent cardiotoxicity in patients with breast cancer treated with doxorubicin, taxanes, and trastuzumab," *Journal of the American College of Cardiology*, vol. 63, no. 8, pp. 809–816, 2014.

[25] T. Cil, A. M. Kaplan, A. Altintas, A. M. Akin, S. Alan, and A. Isikdogan, "Use of N-terminal pro-brain natriuretic peptide to assess left ventricular function after adjuvant doxorubicin

therapy in early breast cancer patients: A prospective series," *Clinical Drug Investigation*, vol. 29, no. 2, pp. 131–137, 2009.

[26] P. Therasse, S. G. Arbuck, E. A. Eisenhauer et al., "New guidelines to evaluate the response to treatment in solid tumors. European Organization for Research and Treatment of Cancer, National Cancer Institute of the United States, National Cancer Institute of Canada ," *Journal of the National Cancer Institute*, vol. 92, no. 3, pp. 205–216, 2000.

[27] E. A. Eisenhauer, P. Therasse, J. Bogaerts et al., "New response evaluation criteria in solid tumours: revised RECIST guideline (version 1.1)," *European Journal of Cancer*, vol. 45, no. 2, pp. 228–247, 2009.

[28] M. T. Meinardi, D. J. Van Veldhuisen, J. A. Gietema et al., "Prospective evaluation of early cardiac damage induced by epirubicin-containing adjuvant chemotherapy and locoregional radiotherapy in breast cancer patients," *Journal of Clinical Oncology*, vol. 19, no. 10, pp. 2746–2753, 2001.

[29] M. Ryberg, D. Nielsen, T. Skovsgaard, J. Hansen, B. V. Jensen, and P. Dombernowsky, "Epirubicin cardiotoxicity: An analysis of 469 patients with metastatic breast cancer," *Journal of Clinical Oncology*, vol. 16, no. 11, pp. 3502–3508, 1998.

[30] J. A. Neidhart, D. Gochnour, R. Roach, D. Hoth, and D. Young, "A comparison of mitoxantrone and doxorubicin in breast cancer," *Journal of Clinical Oncology*, vol. 4, no. 5, pp. 672–677, 1986.

[31] L. A. Smith, V. R. Cornelius, C. J. Plummer et al., "Cardiotoxicity of anthracycline agents for the treatment of cancer: systematic review and meta-analysis of randomised controlled trials," *BMC Cancer*, vol. 10, article 337, 2010.

[32] A. M. Young, T. Dhillon, and M. Bower, "Cardiotoxicity after liposomal anthracyclines," *Lancet Oncology*, vol. 5, no. 11, p. 654, 2004.

[33] A. A. Gabizon, O. Lyass, G. J. Berry, and M. Wildgust, "Cardiac safety of pegylated liposomal doxorubicin (Doxil®/Caelyx®) demonstrated by endomyocardial biopsy in patients with advanced malignancies," *Cancer Investigation*, vol. 22, no. 5, pp. 663–669, 2004.

19

When do Orthopaedic Oncologists Consider the Implantation of Expandable Prostheses in Bone Sarcoma Patients?

Magdalena M. Gilg,[1] **Christine Wibmer**,[1] **Marko Bergovec**,[1] **Robert J. Grimer**,[2] **and Andreas Leithner**[1]

[1]*Department of Orthopaedic Surgery and Traumatology, Medical University of Graz, Graz, Austria*
[2]*Royal Orthopaedic Hospital NHS Foundation Trust, Birmingham, UK*

Correspondence should be addressed to Magdalena M. Gilg; magdalena.gilg@medunigraz.at

Academic Editor: Dae-Geun Jeon

Introduction. Indications discussed for the implantation of expandable prostheses in bone sarcoma patients are unclear. This survey aimed to analyse common practice with this implant type in orthopaedic oncology. *Methods.* A web-based survey was sent to 98 orthopaedic oncology surgeons. Factors reported in literature to influence the decision on the implantation of a growing prosthesis were covered in individual questions and three case scenarios. *Results.* The completion rate of the survey was 45% ($n = 44$). Twenty-seven of 44 surgeons (61%) had implanted between 1 and 15 expandable prostheses within three years. The minimum median patient age was 6.5 years, and 3–5 cm of predicted growth deficit was the minimum before implanting a growing prosthesis. One-third of surgeons do not use growth calculation methods. Two out of three surgeons would rather not implant a growing prosthesis in children with metastatic disease. *Conclusions.* Our survey confirmed the literature with 3-4 cm as the minimum estimated growth deficit. The minimum age for the implantation of a growing prosthesis is approx. 6.6 years, and therefore the patients are younger than those reported in previous publications. One-quarter of orthopaedic surgeons do not use growing prostheses at all. It remains unclear whether growing prostheses are indicated in patients with metastatic disease.

1. Introduction

Paediatric bone sarcoma frequently arises in the meta-diaphyseal regions of the distal femur or the proximal tibia. Wide resection can include the growth plate, and there will be a leg-length discrepancy by skeletal maturity. In the past, amputations in the very young patients or multiple revision surgeries were performed to address the leg-length discrepancy [1].

In 1976, the first expandable prostheses (synonyms: extendible or growing prostheses) were introduced, allowing minimally invasive lengthening via a small skin incision [2]. Still, general anaesthetics and surgical interventions were required, which ultimately increased the risk of infection and the loss of prosthesis [3], so that noninvasively expandable prostheses are now considered to be the gold standard in paediatric limb-salvage surgery [4]. Different types of noninvasive lengthening mechanisms are currently available and can be applied in an outpatient setting [1, 2, 5, 6].

To implant a growing prosthesis, at least 3-4 cm of growth has to be expected for the child until skeletal maturity [7–9]. Furthermore, expandable prostheses require a minimal resection length between 123 and 170 mm depending on the prosthesis type and a sufficient bone diameter, limiting its use in very young children [6, 10]. There is no consensus on the minimum age for the implantation of a growing prosthesis [4, 6, 8, 10, 11].

Our survey aimed to clarify the indications for implantation of a growing prosthesis in bone sarcoma patients by conducting a survey among experts in orthopaedic oncology. Furthermore, we aimed to identify alternative methods other than expandable prostheses to compensate for limb-length inequality.

2. Materials and Methods

A ten-minute web-based survey (Question Pro©) was distributed via email to 98 active orthopaedic surgeons of the European Musculo-Skeletal Oncology Society (EMSOS) (Supplementary Materials (available here)). Nonorthopaedic members were not invited to participate in the survey. Participants who stated via email that they are retired or do not operate on children were excluded from the survey (2 surgeons). Forty-four invited orthopaedic surgeons from thirteen European countries responded to the survey (participation rate 45%), and the completion rate was 93%.

The questionnaire consisted of 15 items on 3 pages including case-specific questions. The first three survey questions asked about participants' personal experience with expandable prostheses, including years in practice, previous experience in orthopaedic oncology, and experience with the implantation of growing prostheses over the last three years. Questions 4–10 were based on relevant factors reported in literature (minimum age, minimum predicted growth, metastatic disease, and "dummy prostheses," i.e., a growing prosthesis implanted without a motor immediately after wide resection, with implantation of the motor at a later stage). Questions 11 and 12 asked for other methods to maintain limb-length equality including epiphysiodesis. Finally, to check consistency, there were three case scenarios based on osteosarcoma patients aged 6.5, 8, and 10.5 years. For all three case scenarios, bone sarcomas were located in the distal femur and tumour extent was depicted. Total femur length as well as required minimal resection lengths of different types of growing prostheses was provided for each case. In addition to multiple choice answers, survey participants could provide information on their own surgical technique in a separate comment field. None of the cases involved skip metastasis, metastatic disease, intra-articular tumour infiltration, or pathological fracture.

The survey was constructed according to the "Checklist for Reporting Results of Internet E-Surveys (CHERRIES)" [12]. Before the survey was distributed, three specialists in orthopaedic oncology tested it for usability and technical functionality as well as comprehensibility. The survey was accessible only via email invitation with password protection, and unique visitors were identified by IP address. Survey visitors who did not start the questionnaire were excluded. All surveys were completed within a normal time frame. Duplicate database entries having the same user ID were eliminated before analysis, and the most complete entry was kept for analysis.

Statistical analysis was conducted with Microsoft Excel (Excel Version 2010). Categorical variables are presented as absolute and relative frequencies and numerical variables as means and ranges.

3. Results

Regarding personal experience, about one-half of the participants have been in practice for more than 20 years and two out of three orthopaedic surgeons dedicated more than 50% of their working time to musculoskeletal oncology.

Table 1: Participants' characteristics.

Years in practice	n	%
0–5	2	5
6–10	3	7
11–15	14	32
16–20	3	7
>20	22	50
Percentage of practice dedicated to musculoskeletal oncology	n	%
0–25	3	7
26–50	7	16
51–75	8	19
76–100	25	58
Number of growing prostheses implanted over the last 3 years	n	%
0	13	30
1–5	14	32
6–15	13	30
16–25	1	2
26–35	1	2
>35	2	5

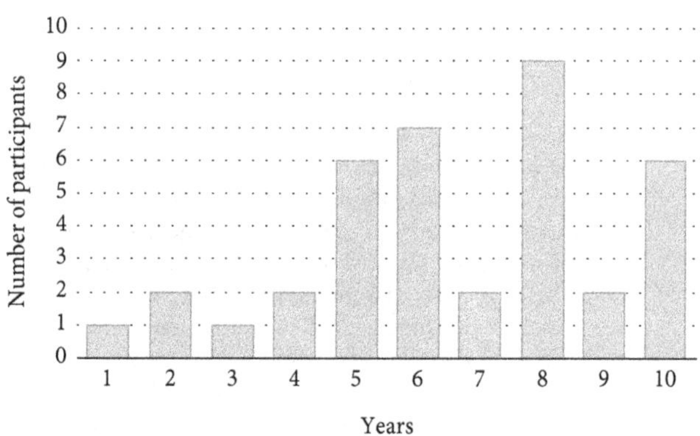

Figure 1: Minimum ages at the time of implantation.

Twenty-seven of 44 surgeons (61%) had implanted between 1 and 15 expandable prostheses within the last three years, whereas about 30% ($n = 13$) of survey participants had not implanted any (Table 1).

The answers concerning factors influencing the decision for or against a growing prosthesis revealed a median minimum age of 6.5 years (range, 1–10) (Figure 1). The minimum predicted growth was given as 3–5 cm by a majority of participants ($n = 26$, 59%). To calculate the growth potential, one specific method is used by 45% (18/40), multiple methods by 20% (8/40), and none by 35% (14/40) of surgeons (Figure 2). In detail, Paley's multiplier method [13] is most frequently applied (9/40, 23%), followed by bone age estimation (8/40, 20%) and growth charts (6/40, 15%). About one-third of surgeons (12/39, 31%) would consider the implantation of an expandable prosthesis despite the presence of metastatic disease. The use of dummy prostheses is supported by 21% (8/38) of surgeons.

As alternative surgical option, about one-half of orthopaedic surgeons (20/43, 47%) would lengthen by callus distraction, either with intramedullary nailing devices or with Ilizarov technique. Additionally, 40% (17/42) of

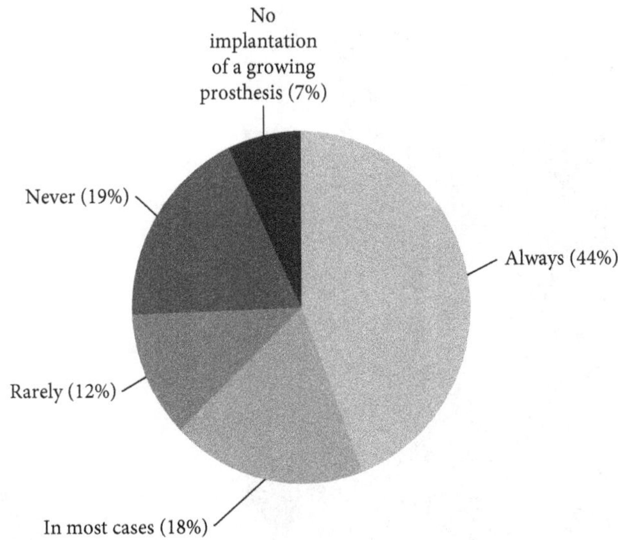

FIGURE 2: Growth prediction methods used by the survey participants (multiple answers possible).

participants often or always consider epiphysiodesis as an option to guide growth.

All three case scenarios were based on patients prior to the pubertal growth spurt (Figure 3). In line with the answers given in the survey questions, the implantation rate of a growing prosthesis increased from 53% ($n = 23/43$) for Case A to 76% ($n = 32/42$) and 83% ($n = 34/41$) for Cases B and C. Amputation was not considered by any of the respondents in any of the three case scenarios. Approximately one-quarter of surgeons (26%, $n = 11/43$) would use other surgical options for Case A, 14% ($n = 6/42$) for Case B, and 12% ($n = 5/41$) for Case C (Table 2).

4. Discussion

The use of expandable prostheses is one possible reconstruction method for children in whom limb-salvage surgery is feasible and sarcoma resection will result in significant leg-length discrepancy, and the literature fails to define the circumstances under which these prostheses are indicated. This survey aimed to identify expert opinions and consensus factors.

In our study population of experienced orthopaedic oncologists, 3-4 cm was confirmed as the minimum of estimated growth deficit prior to the implantation of an expandable device. The median minimum age for this surgical procedure was 6.5 (range 2–10) years. Apart from that, answers for specific factors were quite heterogeneous for the remaining questions. Demographics of survey participants, including years in practice and percentage of time dedicated to orthopaedic oncology, were representative of an expert population. It is unclear why one-third of participating surgeons do not consider the implantation of a growing prosthesis. Apart from individual surgical preferences, nonmedical reasons like the availability of implants in some countries and other socioeconomic reasons might influence the use of expandable prostheses.

We looked at factors influencing the surgical indication for a growing prosthesis that have been described in the literature, including age, expected growth deficit, growth prediction methods, metastatic disease, and alternative treatment options to compensate for leg-length discrepancy [1, 6–10]. Age has been described as a limiting factor since enough bone stock has to be available, and the minimum resection length varies between 123 and 170 mm for the implantation of a growing prosthesis. Furthermore, the younger the patient at first implantation, the more revision surgeries will be needed to overcome the maximum expansion capacities of implants. Our survey results depict a younger patient age than reported previously. Schinhan et al. [9] and Weisstein et al. [14] recommend growing prostheses in patients older than 8 years, whereas Yoshida et al. [15] suggest 10 years and older in their review articles. Staals et al. [8] reported using expandable prostheses in the 7- to 10-year age group. Apart from that, there are only descriptive data from single-centre analyses, with minimum ages between 5.5 and 8.2 years [11, 16, 17]. These studies did not include an outcome analysis correlating age at implantation with the amount of lengthening and the number of complications, and age recommendations do not differentiate between genders. As to age limits, there are neither validated recommendations nor an expert consensus.

It is important to predict growth accurately since 3-4 cm of remaining growth is seen as an indication for a growing prosthesis [7–9]. This calculation can be quite challenging, especially in children who undergo polychemotherapy, and to date there is no clear preference for a particular method [18]. In our survey, surgeons favoured Paley's multiplier method, bone age estimation, and growth charts. Interestingly, about one-third of survey participants do not conduct growth estimation prior to the implantation of an expandable implant. Baumgart and Lenze [7] emphasized the importance of a reliable method to calculate for growth potential and recommend Paley's multiplier method. Grimer et al. [1] use growth charts and bone age estimation with hand radiographs to obtain prospective data. Neither literature nor our survey results provide conclusive information as to which method is best applicable to this particular patient group.

Opinions as to whether expandable implants should be considered in patients with metastatic disease were divisive, though a majority would rather not use them with metastatic disease. The literature offers only minimal information, apart from Schinhan et al. [9], who see metastases at the time of implantation as a contraindication, but it must be taken into account that only 10–20% of patients have macroscopic evidence of metastatic disease, whereas 80–90% of patients with osteosarcoma are assumed to have micrometastatic disease at initial diagnosis [19].

Since this made it difficult to decide which patients would have a favourable prognosis at the time of implantation, some centres began to use dummy prostheses. The costly motor is implanted only later since response to chemotherapy cannot be predicted before surgery. It must also be considered here that chemotherapy reduces the growth velocity and most relapses occur within 2-3 years

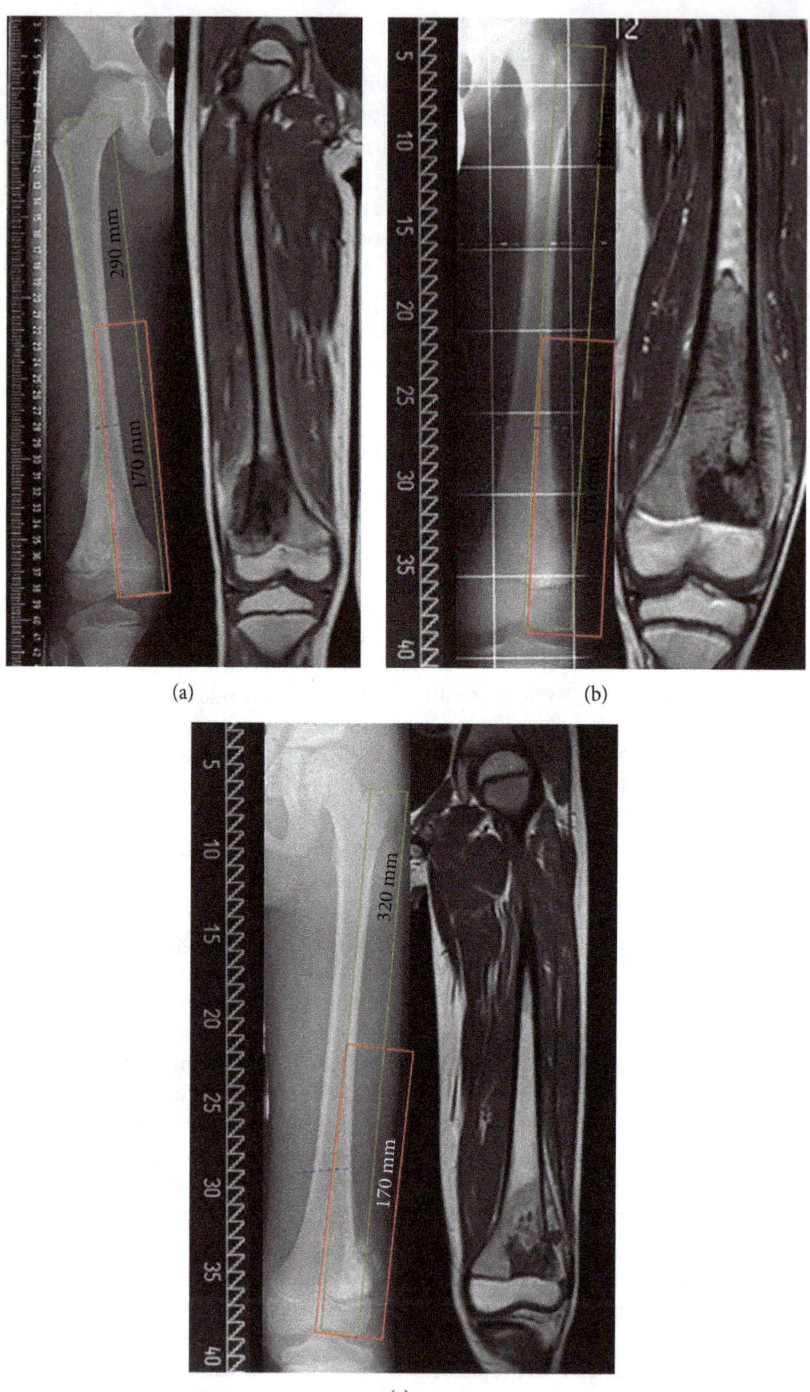

(a) (b) (c)

Figure 3: X-ray and MRI showing three case scenarios including specific answers for treatment options. None of the cases involved skip metastasis, metastatic disease, intra-articular tumour infiltration, or pathological fracture. (a) Male, 6.5 years at initial diagnosis, osteosarcoma of distal femur, and femur length (greater trochanter to eminentia intercondylaris) is 290 mm. (b) Female, 8.0 years at initial diagnosis, osteosarcoma of distal femur, and femur length (greater trochanter to eminentia intercondylaris) is 340 mm. (c) Male, 10.5 years at initial diagnosis, osteosarcoma of distal femur, and femur length (greater trochanter to eminentia intercondylaris) is 320 mm.

following initial diagnosis. There is no peer-reviewed literature on this practice, but our survey results showed that a considerable number of surgeons do use dummy prostheses.

The use of growing prostheses is only one possibility to compensate for leg-length discrepancy. In the case scenarios, we could see that the younger the patients were, the more cautious the participants were in opting for an expandable prosthesis. Instead, participants proposed biological reconstruction, temporary spacer, or callus distraction techniques. Our survey does not explain why one-third of

TABLE 2: Case scenarios A–C and possible alternative treatment options.

Case scenario	Expandable prosthesis	Amputation	Rotationplasty	Conventional tumour prosthesis	Other techniques	
Case A	53%	0%	16%	5%	26%	Allograft reconstruction (4), spacer techniques (2), callus distraction by intramedullary nailing devices (2), Canadell's epiphyseal distraction (1), "Pamplona technique" (1), decision according to family (1)
Case B	76%	0%	7%	3%	14%	Allograft reconstruction (3), spacer techniques (1), callus distraction by intramedullary nailing devices (1), Canadell's epiphyseal distraction (1)
Case C	83%	0%	0%	5%	12%	Allograft reconstruction (3), intraepiphyseal distraction and allograft reconstruction (1), Canadell's epiphyseal distraction (1)

surgeons do not consider expandable implants. In any case, alternative treatment option for paediatric sarcoma patients has to be discussed, since the currently available noninvasive expandable prostheses are still associated with complications, such as prosthetic joint infection or mechanical failure [4, 8]. Endoprosthetic devices are, however, in a phase of intensive and continuing development, and long-term outcome data are awaited with great interest.

5. Conclusions

Extendable implants were constructed to compensate for the limb-length discrepancy following metaepiphyseal sarcoma resection. At least 3-4 cm of leg-length discrepancy should be expected before a growing prosthesis is considered. Otherwise, there is no consensus on surgical indications among orthopaedic oncologists. Our survey showed that the opinions of experts in orthopaedic oncology from a wide geographic range are quite divergent that it would be a matter of some priority to work toward a consensus on the use of expandable prostheses in paediatric bone sarcoma patients.

References

[1] R. J. Grimer, M. Belthur, S. R. Carter, R. M. Tillman, and P. Cool, "Extendible replacements of the proximal tibia for bone tumours," *Journal of Bone and Joint Surgery-British Volume*, vol. 82, no. 12, pp. 255–260, 2000.

[2] R. Abed and R. Grimer, "Surgical modalities in the treatment of bone sarcoma in children," *Cancer Treatment Reviews*, vol. 36, no. 4, pp. 342–347, 2010.

[3] A. Abudu, R. Grimer, R. Tillman, and S. Carter, "The use of prostheses in skeletally immature patients," *Orthopedic Clinics of North America*, vol. 37, no. 1, pp. 75–84, 2006.

[4] N. Hwang, R. J. Grimer, S. R. Carter, R. M. Tillman, A. Abudu, and L. M. Jeys, "Early results of a non-invasive extendible prosthesis for limb-salvage surgery in children with bone tumours," *Bone & Joint Journal*, vol. 94-B, no. 2, pp. 265–269, 2012.

[5] M. D. Neel, R. M. Wilkins, B. N. Rao, and C. M. Kelly, "Early multicenter experience with a noninvasive expandable prosthesis," *Clinical Orthopaedics and Related Research*, vol. 415, pp. 72–81, 2003.

[6] C. A. Cipriano, I. S. Gruzinova, R. M. Frank, S. Gitelis, and W. W. Virkus, "Frequent complications and severe bone loss associated with the Repiphysis expandable distal femoral prosthesis," *Clinical Orthopaedics and Related Research*, vol. 473, no. 3, pp. 831–838, 2015.

[7] R. Baumgart and U. Lenze, "Expandable endoprostheses in malignant bone tumors in children: indications and limitations," *Recent Results in Cancer Research*, vol. 179, pp. 59–73, 2009.

[8] E. L. Staals, M. Colangeli, N. Ali, J. M. Casanova, D. M. Donati, and M. Manfrini, "Are complications associated with the Repiphysis expandable distal femoral prosthesis acceptable for its continued use?," *Clinical Orthopaedics and Related Research*, vol. 473, no. 9, pp. 3003–3013, 2015.

[9] M. Schinhan, P. Funovics, M. Dominkus, and R. Windhager, "Growing prostheses for reconstruction of lower limb defects in children," *Operative Orthopädie und Traumatologie*, vol. 24, no. 3, pp. 235–245, 2012.

[10] L. M. Nystrom and J. A. Morcuende, "Expanding endoprosthesis for pediatric musculoskeletal malignancy: current concepts and results," *Iowa Orthopaedic Journal*, vol. 30, pp. 141–149, 2010.

[11] S. Saghieh, M. R. Abboud, S. A. Muwakkit, R. Saab, B. Rao, and R. Haidar, "Seven-year experience of using Repiphysis expandable prosthesis in children with bone tumors," *Pediatric Blood & Cancer*, vol. 55, no. 3, pp. 457–463, 2010.

[12] G. Eysenbach, "Improving the quality of web surveys: the Checklist for Reporting Results of Internet E-Surveys (CHERRIES)," *Journal of Medical Internet Research*, vol. 6, no. 3, p. e34, 2004.

[13] J. Paley, J. Talor, A. Levin, A. Bhave, D. Paley, and J. E. Herzenberg, "The multiplier method for prediction of

adult height," *Journal of Pediatric Orthopaedics*, vol. 24, no. 6, pp. 732–737, 2004.

[14] J. S. Weisstein, R. E. Goldsby, and R. J. O'Donnell, "Oncologic approaches to pediatric limb preservation," *Journal of the American Academy of Orthopaedic Surgeons*, vol. 13, no. 8, pp. 544–554, 2005.

[15] Y. Yoshida, S. Osaka, and Y. Tokuhashi, "Experience with extendable prostheses for malignant bone tumors in children," *Journal of the Formosan Medical Association*, vol. 110, no. 11, pp. 711–715, 2011.

[16] P. Ruggieri, A. F. Mavrogenis, E. Pala, M. Romantini, M. Manfrini, and M. Mercuri, "Outcome of expandable prostheses in children," *Journal of Pediatric Orthopaedics*, vol. 33, no. 3, pp. 244–253, 2013.

[17] K. K. Ness, M. D. Neel, S. C. Kaste et al., "A comparison of function after limb salvage with non-invasive expandable or modular prostheses in children," *European Journal of Cancer*, vol. 50, no. 18, pp. 3212–3220, 2014.

[18] M. M. Gilg, C. Wibmer, D. Andreou et al., "Paley's multiplier method does not accurately predict adult height in children with bone sarcoma," *Clinical Orthopaedics and Related Research*, vol. 472, no. 8, pp. 2506–2513, 2014.

[19] A. Luetke, P. A. Meyers, I. Lewis, and H. Juergens, "Osteosarcoma treatment-where do we stand? A state of the art review," *Cancer Treatment Reviews*, vol. 40, no. 4, pp. 523–532, 2014.

20

HIV-1 Evolutionary Patterns Associated with Metastatic Kaposi's Sarcoma during AIDS

Susanna L. Lamers,[1] Rebecca Rose,[1] David J. Nolan,[2] Gary B. Fogel,[3] Andrew E. Barbier,[1] Marco Salemi,[2] and Michael S. McGrath[4]

[1] *Bioinfoexperts, LLC, 718 Bayou Lane, Thibodaux, LA 70302, USA*
[2] *Department of Pathology and Laboratory Medicine, University of Florida, 2055 Mowry Road, Gainesville, FL 32610, USA*
[3] *Natural Selection, Inc., 5910 Pacific Center Blvd., 6480 Weathers Place, San Diego, CA 92121, USA*
[4] *The AIDS and Cancer Specimen Resource, University of California at San Francisco and the Department of Laboratory Medicine, Pathology, and Medicine, University of California at San Francisco, 1001 Poterero Ave, Bldg 3, Rm 207, UCSF Box 1317, San Francisco, CA 94110, USA*

Correspondence should be addressed to Michael S. McGrath; mike.mcgrath@ucsf.edu

Academic Editor: C. Verhoef

Kaposi's sarcoma (KS) in HIV-infected individuals can have a wide range of clinical outcomes, from indolent skin tumors to a life-threatening visceral cancer. KS tumors contain endothelial-related cells and inflammatory cells that may be HIV-infected. In this study we tested if HIV evolutionary patterns distinguish KS tumor relatedness and progression. Multisite autopsies from participants who died from HIV-AIDS with KS prior to the availability of antiretroviral therapy were identified at the AIDS and Cancer Specimen Resource (ACSR). Two patients (KS1 and KS2) died predominantly from non-KS-associated disease and KS3 died due to aggressive and metastatic KS within one month of diagnosis. Skin and visceral tumor and nontumor autopsy tissues were obtained ($n = 12$). Single genome sequencing was used to amplify HIV RNA and DNA, which was present in all tumors. Independent HIV tumor clades in phylogenies differentiated KS1 and KS2 from KS3, whose sequences were interrelated by both phylogeny and selection. HIV compartmentalization was confirmed in KS1 and KS2 tumors; however, in KS3, no compartmentalization was observed among sampled tissues. While the sample size is small, the HIV evolutionary patterns observed in all patients suggest an interplay between tumor cells and HIV-infected cells which provides a selective advantage and could promote KS progression.

1. Introduction

Prior to the human immunodeficiency virus (HIV) epidemic, Kaposi's sarcoma (KS) was considered a very rare disease, found primarily in Mediterranean countries and in organ transplant recipients [1]. Although Human Herpes Virus 8 (HHV8) is the etiological cause of KS [2], most HHV8$^+$ individuals do not develop KS. Early in the HIV epidemic, KS was so frequently diagnosed that it was considered an AIDS-defining illness [3–5]. Prior to the mid-1990s and the use of combined antiretroviral therapy (cART), HIV$^+$ patients had a 40% lifetime risk of developing KS [6]. Although combined antiretroviral therapy (cART) has undeniably reduced KS-associated mortality among HIV-infected patients [7–9], the statistical impact is unclear due to differing clinical definitions and cART adherence problems [10, 11]. Furthermore, KS is still one of the most common cancers among HIV$^+$ patients [12] despite cART-improved CD4$^+$ T-cell counts, low viral loads, and reduced risk of opportunistic infections [13–16]. KS is particularly problematic in resource-poor settings where cART and chemotherapy are limited [6, 17–19]; however, even in resource-rich settings, full remission of KS using cART and chemotherapy occurs in less than 50% of HIV$^+$ patients with disseminated disease [20].

KS lesions can be solitary, localized, or disseminated, but the relationship among tumors in a single individual is largely unknown. While many KS lesions are cutaneous and indolent, tumors can occur in the oral cavity, lymph nodes, and viscera, which can result in fatal complications due to interference with normal body function. The growth of lesions can be very slow or explosively fast. The KS defining cell-type is a spindle cell (SC) [21, 22] that expresses markers of both endothelial and macrophage lineages [23]. KS tumors are polyclonal, positive for the presence of HHV8 virus, which infects the tumor-associated B-cells and SCs [23], and highly vascularized, giving them a distinguishing purple color. Inflammatory lymphocytes and monocytes/macrophages populate and enrich the KS tumor environment for tumor growth through production of a variety of cytokines [23]. These immune cells are all potential targets for HIV; however, to our knowledge, only one study assessed KS tumors for the presence of HIV using an early hybridization technique [24]. SCs can be cultured from PBMCs of patients with KS, suggesting that circulating SCs may lead to the appearance of multiple KS lesions [23].

HIV has the potential to infect and evolve in many anatomical tissues, including tumors [25–27]. Previously, we showed that the viral populations in lymphoma tumors were distinct from HIV in healthy tissues [25]. Here, our goal was to characterize HIV populations in KS tumors to determine whether HIV evolution could be used to track tumor relatedness and progression in native KS uncomplicated by the use of cART. We obtained tumor and nontumor tissues sampled *post mortem* from the AIDS and Cancer Specimen Resource (ACSR) from three HIV^+/KS^+ patients who died from aggressive AIDS, and we generated HIV *env-nef* sequences using single genome sequencing (SGS) to characterize viral evolutionary patterns.

2. Materials and Methods

2.1. Patients and Biomaterial. The three male patients included in this study were diagnosed with HIV infection and died with advanced AIDS without receiving cART (Table 1). 100 mg of frozen autopsy tumor and nontumor tissues was obtained through the ACSR (http://acsr.ucsf.edu/). Tissues were classified as tumor or nontumor by histological examination. The ACSR is a National Cancer Institute-funded tissue-banking program that obtains tissues from patients after appropriate consent and releases tissues to investigators following approval of the proposed study and deidentification of samples and clinical histories. The ACSR is recognized by the Office of Biorepositories and Biospecimen Research at the National Institutes of Health as being HIPAA compliant and in accordance with the ethical standards of the Declaration of Helsinki. Additionally, all material was obtained under approval from the University of California at San Francisco Committee on Human Research.

2.2. RNA/DNA Extractions. Total RNA and genomic DNA were isolated separately from each tissue section (30–50 ng) using AllPrep DNA/RNA Mini Kit (Qiagen #80204). Tissues were homogenized just prior to extraction in Buffer RLT Plus (lysis buffer) using a TissueRupter rotor-stator homogenizer (Qiagen #9001271) with a fresh sterile disposable probe (Qiagen #990890) for each sample. Manufacturer's guidelines were followed, with the exception of two 50 μL final elutions using RNase-free water during the RNA isolation. The 100 μL final volume of RNA generated was concentrated using RNeasyMinElute Cleanup Kit (Qiagen #74204). RNA and DNA extractions, cDNA synthesis, and first-round PCR setup were conducted in a restricted-access, amplicon-free room with separate air handling and laboratory equipment where no amplified PCR products or recombinant cloned plasmids were allowed, and work surfaces and equipment were thoroughly cleaned before and after use with Eliminase® (Decon Labs, Inc.). cDNA was synthesized using SuperScript® III First-Strand Synthesis System (Invitrogen Life Technologies #18080-051) using the provided Oligo$(dT)_{20}$ primer according to manufacturer's recommendations. RNA was incubated at 65°C for 5 minutes with deoxynucleoside triphosphates (0.5 mM) and 5 μM Oligo$(dT)_{20}$ and then cooled quickly to 4°C. First-Strand cDNA Synthesis was performed in a 40 μL reaction volume containing 1x reverse transcription buffer (10 mM Tris-HCl [pH 8.4], 25 mMKCl), 5 mM $MgCl_2$, 10 mM dithiothreitol, 2 U/μL of RNase-OUT™ (RNase inhibitor), and 10 U/μL SuperScript III RT. The reaction was heated to 50°C for 50 minutes, followed by 85°C for 5 minutes. The reaction was cooled to 37°C and 0.1 U/μL of *E. coli* RNase H was added, followed by a 20-minute incubation. cDNA was stored at −20°C.

2.3. Sequencing Protocol. A modified single genome sequencing protocol was used to amplify linked HIV *env* and *nef* sequences [28]. cDNA and genomic DNA were serially diluted until an average of 30% or less of the nested PCR reactions were positive. During the first-round PCR, diluted cDNA or genomic DNA was amplified in 25 μL reactions containing 1x Platinum® Blue PCR SuperMix (Invitrogen Life Technologies) and 0.2 μM of each primer: EF2, 5′-ACAGTCTATTATGGGGTRCC-3′ and NR1, 5′-AGCTCCCAGGCTCAGATCT-3′ (6333–6352 bp and 9558–9576 bp of HIV HXB2, resp.) with the following cycling parameters: initial denaturation 95°C for 5 minutes, followed by 35 cycles of denaturing at 94°C for 1 minute, annealing at 58°C for 1 minute, and extension at 72°C for 4 minutes, with a final extension time of 10 minutes at 72°C. A second round of gp120 PCR consisted of 1 μL of the first-round PCR added to a 24 μL second-round reaction consisting of 1x Platinum Blue PCR SuperMix (Invitrogen Life Technologies) and 0.2 μM of each primer: EF3, 5′ CATAATGTTTGGGCCACACA-3′ and ER2, 5′-CACCACTCTTCTYTTTGCC-3′ (6420–6439 bp and 7724–7742 bp of HIV HXB2, resp.) with the following cycling parameters: initial denaturation 95°C for 5 minutes, followed by 35 cycles of denaturation at 94°C for 1 minute, annealing at 58°C for 1 minute, and extension at 72°C for 2 minutes, with a final extension time of 10 minutes at 72°C. This second-round PCR generated a 1.3 Kb product, nearly covering the entire *env* gp120 gene. Second-round *env* gp120 PCR products were visualized on 1% agarose gels stained with ethidium bromide, and reactions containing a single 1.3 Kb product were considered positive and selected

TABLE 1: Patient clinical history.

Patient	Age[1]	Major comorbidities[2]	KS location	Time since KS diagnosis (months)	Length of HIV infection (years)	Anatomical location of biopsy	Concentration (ng/μL)		Number of *env* sequences		Number of *nef* sequences	
							RNA	DNA	RNA	DNA	RNA	DNA
KS1	34	Lymphoma, MAC, PCP, cytomegalovirus	Skin, pleura, lungs, trachea, lymph node, liver, adrenal glands	Unknown	7	KS skin	144	154	22	8	24	9
						KS lymph node	168	276	13	21	14	21
						Lymph node	120	12.1	37	22	35	26
						Kidney	>200	8.18	5	0	9	0
KS2	31	BCBL	Skin, pleura, lungs, esophagus, small bowel	~5	Unknown	KS skin	165	44	14	10	18	12
						KS small bowel	192	9.84	4	0	5	0
						Liver	191	8.42	0	0	0	0
						Spleen	190	13.9	23	1	31	2
KS3	28	Aggressive KS	Skin, pleura, lungs, trachea, esophagus, small bowel, colon, rectum, iliac lymph nodes, mesenteric lymph nodes, para-aortic lymph nodes, paratracheal lymph nodes	~1	9	KS skin	49	51	6	2	2	6
						KS small bowel	164	39.4	16	25	14	24
						Liver	161	33.4	14	5	15	5
						Stomach	78.2	40.2	24	8	20	8

[1]Age in years; [2]MAC: *Mycobacterium avium* complex; PCP: *Pneumocystis pneumonia*; BCBL: body cavity based lymphoma.

for sequencing. Subsequently, the first-round reactions that corresponded to positive second-round gp120 PCRs were then used to amplify the *nef* gene sequence. Second-round *nef* PCR consisted of 1 μL of the first-round PCR added to a 24 μL second-round reaction consisting of 1x Platinum Blue PCR SuperMix (Invitrogen Life Technologies) and 0.2 μM of each primer: NF1, 5′-TTAGGCAGGGATAYTCACC-3′ and NR2, 5′-ATCTGAGGGCTCGCCACT-3′ (8347–8365 bp and 9488–9505 of HIV HXB2, resp.) with the following cycling parameters: initial denaturation 95°C for 5 minutes, followed by 35 cycles of denaturation at 94°C for 1 minute, annealing at 58°C for 1 minute, and extension at 72°C for 2 minutes, with a final extension at 72°C for 10 minutes. Second-round *nef* PCRs were visualized on 1% agarose gels stained with ethidium bromide, and reactions containing single 1.1 Kb products were considered positive and selected for sequencing. The primers were designed using Primer3 (http://bioinfo.ut.ee/primer3-0.4.0/) and by observing regions of conservation in alignments of published HIV subtype B sequences downloaded from Los Alamos HIV Sequence Database (http://www.hiv.lanl.gov/). Sequencing was performed on an Applied Biosystems 3730xl DNA Analyzer (Life Technologies) at the University of Florida Interdisciplinary Center for Biotechnology Research (UF ICBR). All sequences were assembled and aligned with the Geneious R7 software package (Biomatters http://www.geneious.com/) followed by a manual optimization of regions containing insertions and deletions. Sequence data has been submitted to GenBank (Accession numbers KU709129–KU709831).

2.4. Sequence Analysis. Env and *nef* alignments were generated using ClustalW [29] in MEGA5 [30] with further optimization performed by hand. Due to a large number of insertions and deletions that are typically problematic to align, regions with substantial insertions and deletions in *env* V1, V2, and V4 domains were removed. An initial maximum-likelihood phylogeny was inferred using sequences from all patients for both genes to ensure no cross-contamination. Pairwise distance analysis within and between RNA and DNA tissue sequence populations over time was assessed in MEGA5 [30] using the Tamura-Nei molecular model (identified using Model-Selection) with standard error estimated by 1000 bootstrap replicates. The Kruskal-Wallis test was used to determine significance between the mean pairwise distances in different anatomical tissues. Individual maximum-likelihood phylogenies were inferred for each patient under a GTR model of nucleotide evolution and gamma distributed rate variation among sites (+G) using PhyML [31]. Statistical support was assessed with 200 bootstrap replicates. The Slatkin-Maddison test [32] was used to determine compartmentalization between sequences derived from different tissues, and significance was assessed using 1,000 replicates of tip randomization, implemented in HYPHY v.1.0 [33]. The fast, unconstrained Bayesian approximations for inferring selection (FUBAR) model, implemented in Data Monkey (http://datamonkey.org/), were used to identify amino acid sites under selection in sequences derived from different tissues for each individual. Sites with posterior probability >0.9 of an increased (diversifying) or decreased (purifying) rate of nonsynonymous relative to synonymous substitutions were considered to have experienced a significant level of selective pressure. Selected sites were numbered according to the molecular HIV clone HXB2 (GenBank Accession #AF358141).

3. Results

3.1. Clinical Characteristics of the Patient Cohort. All patients (KS1–KS3) had CD4 counts <50 cells/mm^3 at death and were diagnosed with KS only months prior to death (Table 1). KS1 lived with HIV infection for seven years. He was hospitalized due to *Mycobacterium avium* complex, *Pneumocystis pneumonia,* and wasting syndrome eleven months prior to death. Five months prior to death, medical notes indicate multiple AIDS-like symptoms; however, KS was not specified. At autopsy, numerous infections were identified throughout his body, including disseminated KS, which either had not been previously reported or had originated closer to death. KS2's clinical history is similar to that of KS1 in having multiple infections; however, this patient had an initial KS diagnosis five months prior to death. Also, this patient was diagnosed with an aggressive body cavity based lymphoma (BCBL) four months prior to death that was treated with chemotherapy. BCBL may be related to primary effusion lymphoma which is typically caused by HHV8, the Kaposi sarcoma herpes virus. KS3 had a nine-year history of HIV infection with reoccurring upper respiratory tract infections. He was diagnosed with KS one month prior to death. His KS lesions became rapidly disseminated on the skin and internally, which lead directly to his death due to respiratory distress.

3.2. HIV RNA and DNA Was Successfully Sequenced from All KS Tumors. Viral sequences were obtained from RNA in 13/14 tissues and from DNA in 12/14 tissues (Table 1). A preliminary maximum-likelihood (ML) phylogenetic tree of all sequences confirmed a distinct population of HIV sequences for each patient, indicating no laboratory cross-contamination.

3.3. KS Tumors Can Contain Distinct HIV Isolates. ML phylogenies were inferred for *env* and *nef* sequence populations for all three patients. In the KS1 *env* phylogeny, four distinct and well-supported clades (A–D) were apparent that contained the majority of tumor-derived sequences (Figure 1). The relatively long internal branches leading to each clade indicate considerable divergence from the rest of the viral population. The majority of lymph node tumor sequences (19/34) were within two distinct clades (A, D). The majority of skin tumor sequences (20/32) were also located in two different distinct clades (B-C). One of these (B) contained both DNA and RNA sequences, while the other (C) was comprised exclusively of RNA skin tumor sequences. Most of the terminal branches leading directly to skin tumor-derived sequences were very short, while those leading to the lymph node tumor-derived sequences were considerably longer and showed more branching within the clade. The

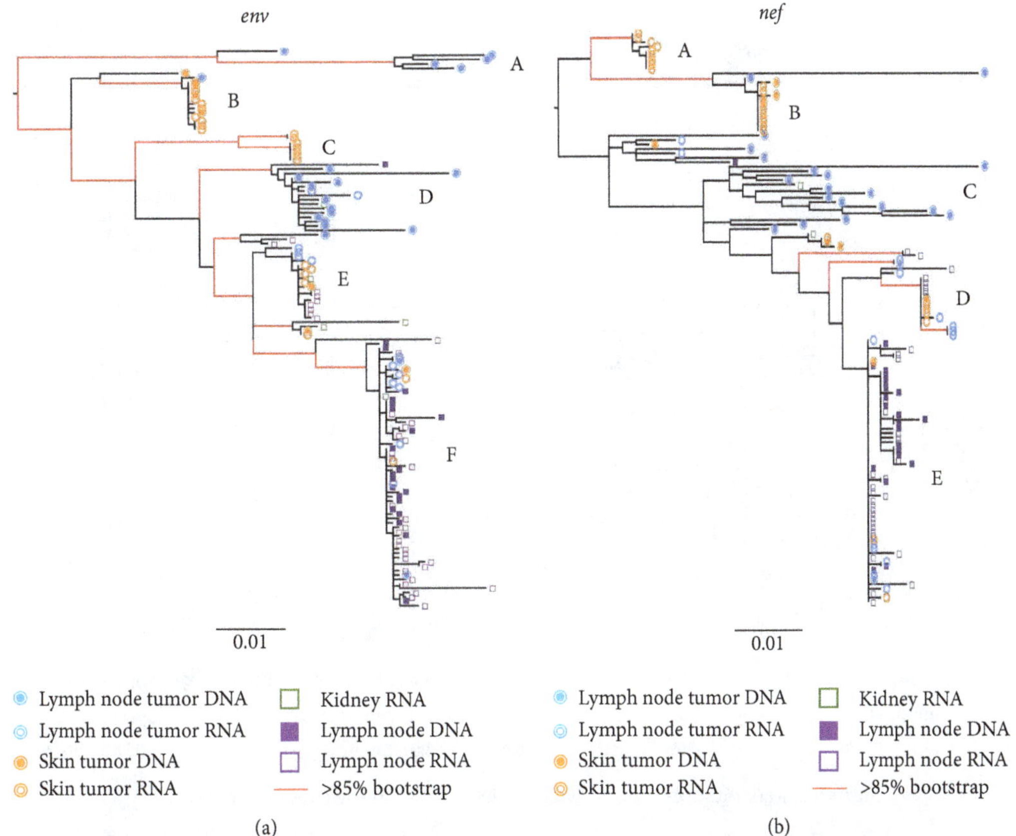

FIGURE 1: Maximum-likelihood phylogenies for KS1. Phylogenies were inferred for each patient using *env* (a) and *nef* (b) sequence alignments. Tips are labeled with symbols corresponding to the tissue of origin for each sequence. Branches with red lines indicate bootstrap values >85/200. Branches are scaled in substitutions/site according to the scale under each tree. Clades labeled A–F are discussed in the text.

remaining lymph node and skin tumor RNA and DNA sequences were located in highly mixed clades (E-F). The *nef* phylogeny for KS1 had similar branching patterns, with even more pronounced diversity in one lymph node tumor clade (C). Similarly, all skin tumor-derived sequences except one clustered together in a distinct and well-supported clade in KS2 for both *env* and *nef* (A) (Figure 2). Small bowel tumor-derived RNA sequences were interspersed with the nontumor spleen-derived sequences in both genes; however, few bowel-derived sequences were obtained ($n = 9$). Branches in the nontumor clade showed considerable structure in both genes, consistent with a continuously diversifying virus population. In the *nef* phylogeny, two distinct clades were evident within the mixed clade, which was not present in the *env* tree. In contrast, for KS3, all tumor- and nontumor-derived sequences were largely interspersed in both *env* and *nef* phylogenies (Figure 3). Three well-supported clades were present in both genes (A–C). Interestingly, this patient was diagnosed with advanced and aggressive tumorigenesis less than one month prior to death.

3.4. KS-Associated Virus Is Compartmentalized in Tumors in KS1 and KS2 but Not in KS3. When pairwise distances were calculated for sequences derived from each tumor and nontumor tissue, only one significant difference was observed ($p < 0.001$) (KS1 lymph node tumor *nef* versus nontumor *nef* sequences). Viral populations were significantly compartmentalized within each of the two tumors and normal tissues for both env and nef in KS1 and KS2 ($p < 0.001$). On the other hand, gene flow among the three sites was found in both genes in KS3 (*env*: $p = 0.021$; *nef*: $p = 0.171$). Viral populations from combined tumor locations were again significantly compartmentalized compared with nontumor populations in *env* and *nef* in KS1 and KS2, as well as in *nef* for KS3 ($p < 0.001$).

3.5. Positively and Negatively Selected Codons Were Fewer and Tissue-Specific in KS1 and KS2 in Contrast to KS3 (Tables 2 and 3). The proportion of codons under selection in *env* did not significantly vary between positively and negatively selected sites overall or within any single subject. However, the number of positions under either selective pressure was significantly higher in KS3 than in KS1 and KS2 ($p < 0.01$). In *nef*, a significantly higher number of negatively selected codons over positively selected codons were observed in all patients ($p < 0.01$). Codons under selection were tissue-specific in both KS1 and KS2, with only one being shared between two tissues in KS2. In contrast, in KS3 *env* sequence populations, all shared positively and negatively selected codons in tumor tissues were also identified within nontumor

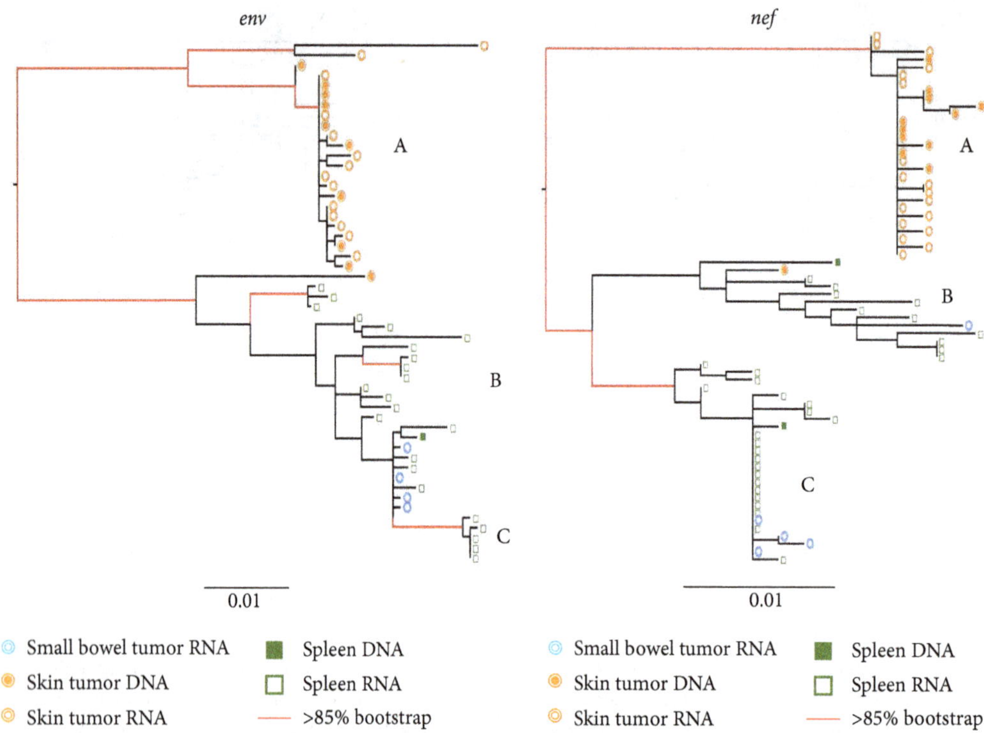

FIGURE 2: Maximum-likelihood phylogenies for KS2. See legend under Figure 1.

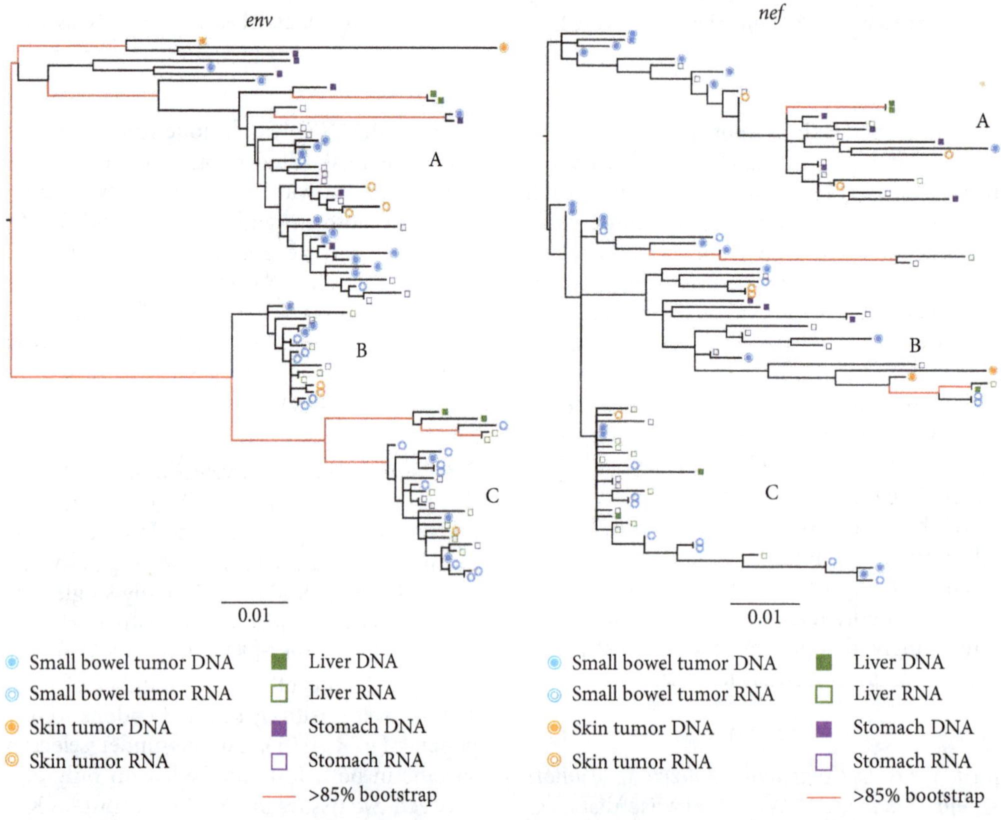

FIGURE 3: Maximum-likelihood phylogenies for KS3. See legend under Figure 1.

TABLE 2: Number (and percent) of codons under positive or negative selection in tumor and nontumor sites in *env* sequence populations.

Patient	Tissue	# positively selected sites (%)	Codon position of shared positively selected sites	# negatively selected sites	Codon position of shared negatively selected sites
KS1 (359)	Skin tumor	7 (1.9)	None	7 (1.9)	na
	Lymph node tumor	1 (0.3)	None	7 (1.9)	122
	Nontumor	None	None	8 (2.2)	122
KS2 (394)	Skin tumor	8 (2.0)	464	5 (1.2)	150
	Small bowel tumor	None	None	None	None
	Nontumor	5 (1.2)	373	4 (1.0)	150
KS3 (373)	Skin tumor	3 (0.8)	464	6 (1.6)	207, 247
	Small bowel tumor	10 (2.6)	183, 336, 396	16 (4.2)	103, 118, 207, 228, 238, 246, 254, 276, 374, 408, 415, 445
	Nontumor	11 (2.9)	143, 167, 183, 336, 454	21 (5.6)	103, 118, 207, 228, 238, 246, 254, 276, 374, 408, 415, 445

TABLE 3: Number (and percent) of codons under positive or negative selection in tumor and nontumor sites in *nef* sequence populations.

Patient	Tissue	# positively selected sites	Codon position of shared positively selected sites	# negatively selected sites	Codon position of shared negatively selected sites
KS1 (207)	Skin tumor	0	None	3 (1.5)	188
	Lymph node tumor	4 (1.9)	None	18 (8.7)	8, 37, 188
	Nontumor	1 (0.5)	None	4 (1.9)	8, 37, 188
KS2 (205)	Skin tumor	1 (0.5)	190	0	None
	Small bowel tumor	1 (0.5)	190	4 (2.0)	81
	Nontumor	2 (1.0)	190	5 (2.4)	81
KS3 (207)	Skin tumor	1 (0.5)	None	7 (3.4)	30, 65, 147, 151, 191, 195
	Small bowel tumor	1 (0.5)	None	14 (6.8)	4, 30, 63, 65, 111, 129, 151, 164, 191, 195
	Nontumor	1 (0.5)	None	21 (10.1)	4, 63, 111, 129, 147, 151, 164, 191, 195

sequences; similarly, in KS3 *nef* sequence populations, all shared selected codons from tumors were identified in nontumor tissues except codon positions 31 and 67.

4. Discussion

In this study we examined if HIV evolutionary patterns could differentiate metastatic KS in patients untreated with cART. We analyzed HIV *env* and *nef* sequences from tumor and nontumor anatomical sites from three subjects who died with KS. Medical records indicated that subjects KS1 and KS2 had a slower KS progression than subject KS3; however, all patients had visceral KS, indicating an advanced cancer at death from AIDS. HIV RNA and/or DNA was amplified from all tumors in the study, demonstrating that, similar to a previous study [25], cancer tissues contain substantial amounts of HIV. Furthermore, HIV sequence populations from most tissues had similar genetic distances, indicating no constraints to HIV evolution in any of the tissue environments examined.

HIV from tumor sites in KS1 and KS2 was compartmentalized relative to the nontumor virus, with limited gene flow between compartments; however, subpopulations of virus were also present within tumors. Additionally, codon selection analysis demonstrated that, at the protein level, KS1 and KS2 had sequence populations evolving under independent selective pressures in different tumor/nontumor sites. In contrast, the patient who died from highly aggressive KS (KS3) showed remarkably different patterns. Here the virus in tumor and nontumor tissue was completely interspersed with a non-tissue-specific viral population structure. These findings could result from a number of scenarios, including the following: (1) subpopulations of virus in tumor could result from recent viral migration from another, unsampled anatomical location; (2) the viral population in the tumors is evolving independently due to a physical barrier restricting gene flow; (3) the viral populations in the tumors are evolving in response to local selective pressures; (4) viral sequences in one or more sites could represent archival virus that was reactivated because of the cancer growth. The first scenario is untestable here; however, we are conducting additional studies with more tumor and nontumor tissues from other KS patients, including KS derived from patients on cART with no detectable plasma viral load. While the second scenario is possible, unlike the brain in which viral flow is impeded by the blood-brain barrier, KS tumors are highly vascularized which would in theory provide ample opportunity for migration. Furthermore, a small number of tumor viruses were found in nontumor tissues, also suggesting a lack of physical barrier. In considering the third and fourth scenario, we did find that codon positions were under varied selective pressures in the tumors from KS1 and KS2 when compared to nontumor tissues (as expected from the phylogeny). For KS3, most, but not all, selected codons were shared among tissues; however, this patient had widely metastatic KS at the time of death. Therefore, it is possible that tumor-compartmentalized HIV populations could have existed in this patient prior to the rapid outgrowth and spread of the cancer, perhaps represented by one of the distinct subpopulations.

Reactivation and clonal expansion of viral populations could be consistent with the large clades of identical or nearly identical tumor-associated virus in KS1 and KS2 phylogenies and with the separation of DNA and RNA derived sequences into different clades within tumors of KS1. This hypothesis could be investigated further by identifying the infected cells types within each tumor. Furthermore, identifying the insertion sites within the host genome in these tumors could help understand if HIV-infected cells in tumors are physically migrating to other tumor sites. A recent HIV integration site study showed that one mechanism of HIV persistence within T-cells is related to clonal expansion [34]. Interestingly, the authors also found that insertion sites were enriched for genes involved in cell growth [34], suggesting that the insertion sites themselves may promote tumorigenesis. Studies within cancer and AIDS dementia tissue macrophages performed in our lab showed that major HIV integration sites in tissue-associated macrophages (TAMs) were related to cellular activation including those just upstream of the *c-fes* oncogene, which could contribute to clonal expansion [35–38]. This is consistent with a sequential pathogenesis model in which the insertion site of the virus promotes persistent cellular activation, clonal expansion, and migration of HIV^+ from the tumor to nontumor sites [36].

The patients studied here were all cART-naïve; however, KS remains a substantial comorbidity even for patients undergoing cART. For some patients, rapid progression of KS occurs under cART even with an undetectable viral load [39]. These cases are frequently classified as related to immune reconstitution inflammatory syndrome (IRIS) [19, 39, 40], a well-studied phenomenon of resurgence of underlying pathologies during cART [41–46]. IRIS-related worsening of coinfections typically occurs within the first 6 months of therapy, is associated with localized tissue inflammation and low CD4 counts, and is most often observed in limited-resource settings [41, 47]. Although T-cell restoration and activation have been suggested as causing KS progression in these patients, no direct link has been demonstrated [47]. Innate immune dysfunction (e.g., macrophage-activation) has also been offered as an explanation for progressive KS during cART, whereby the interaction of restored T-cell populations with existing activated macrophages leads to increased IRIS [19].

5. Conclusions

Kaposi's sarcoma (KS) is a major cancer that still occurs in HIV positive patients despite immune-restorative combined antiretroviral therapy (cART). In this study we isolated HIV from tumor and nontumor tissue sites from patients who died with KS which had metastasized to the viscera (KS1–KS3). KS1 and KS2 died from other AIDS-associated complications, whereas KS3 died directly due to a highly aggressive KS that metastasized to lungs and caused death within 1 month of initial KS diagnosis. We compared the HIV sequences among patient's tissue sites and found that KS1 and KS2 had unique HIV in tumors compared to nontumor sites, whereas HIV was freely migrating among all tissues in KS3. While the study is based on a very small sample size, the results suggest that an HIV-associated mechanism may promote the metastatic process in aggressive KS. It is also important to note that it is unclear how the other AIDS-associated cancers may have impacted the study (e.g., lymphoma in KS1 and BCBL in KS2). Continued studies of the evolutionary patterns within and among KS tumors could help in understanding the mechanisms of metastasis as well as describing an additional HIV reservoir during cART. Evolutionary studies of HIV in tumor tissues are sorely lacking, and further investigation could provide additional clarity into the mechanisms of HIV-associated cancers.

Disclosure

The funders had no role in study design, data collection and interpretation, or the decision to submit the work for publication.

Competing Interests

The authors declare that they have no competing interests.

Authors' Contributions

Susanna L. Lamers and Rebecca Rose contributed equally to this work.

Acknowledgments

This work was supported by the U.S. National Institutes of Health under Grants NIMH R01-MH100984 and NCI ACSR UM1-CA181255-03 to Michael S. McGrath and Grants P50-GM103297 and R01-NS063897 to Marco Salemi. Additional support was provided by Navidea Biopharmaceuticals, Inc.

References

[1] P. Cook-Mozaffari, R. Newton, V. Beral, and D. P. Burkitt, "The geographical distribution of Kaposi's sarcoma and of

lymphomas in Africa before the AIDS epidemic," *British Journal of Cancer*, vol. 78, no. 11, pp. 1521–1528, 1998.

[2] Y. Chang, E. Cesarman, M. S. Pessin et al., "Identification of herpesvirus-like DNA sequences in AIDS-associated Kaposi's sarcoma," *Science*, vol. 266, no. 5192, pp. 1865–1869, 1994.

[3] http://www.cdc.gov/mmwr/preview/mmwrhtml/rr5710a2.htm.

[4] A. Stewart, S. Chan Carusone, K. To, N. Schaefer-Mcdaniel, M. Halman, and R. Grimes, "Causes of death in HIV patients and the evolution of an AIDS hospice: 1988–2008," *AIDS Research and Treatment*, vol. 2012, Article ID 390406, 7 pages, 2012.

[5] R. Rothenberg, M. Woelfel, R. Stoneburner, J. Milberg, R. Parker, and B. Truman, "Survival with the acquired immunodeficiency syndrome. Experience with 5833 cases in New York City," *The New England Journal of Medicine*, vol. 317, no. 21, pp. 1297–1302, 1987.

[6] J. H. Campbell, A. C. Hearps, G. E. Martin, K. C. Williams, and S. M. Crowe, "The importance of monocytes and macrophages in HIV pathogenesis,treatment,and cure," *AIDS*, vol. 28, no. 15, pp. 2175–2187, 2014.

[7] M. A. Eltom, A. Jemal, S. M. Mbulaiteye, S. S. Devesa, and R. J. Biggar, "Trends in Kaposi's sarcoma and non-Hodgkin's lymphoma incidence in the United States from 1973 through 1998," *Journal of the National Cancer Institute*, vol. 94, no. 16, pp. 1204–1210, 2002.

[8] A. M. Cattelan, M. L. Calabrò, P. Gasperini et al., "Acquired immunodeficiency syndrome-related Kaposi's sarcoma regression after highly active antiretroviral therapy: biologic correlates of clinical outcome," *Journal of the National Cancer Institute. Monographs*, no. 28, pp. 44–49, 2001.

[9] G. Di Lorenzo, P. A. Konstantinopoulos, L. Pantanowitz, R. Di Trolio, S. De Placido, and B. J. Dezube, "Management of AIDS-related Kaposi's sarcoma," *The Lancet Oncology*, vol. 8, no. 2, pp. 167–176, 2007.

[10] A. S. Semeere, N. Busakhala, and J. N. Martin, "Impact of antiretroviral therapy on the incidence of Kaposi's sarcoma in resource-rich and resource-limited settings," *Current Opinion in Oncology*, vol. 24, no. 5, pp. 522–530, 2012.

[11] S. E. Krown, "Highly active antiretroviral therapy in AIDS-associated Kaposi's sarcoma: implications for the design of therapeutic trials in patients with advanced, symptomatic Kaposi's sarcoma," *Journal of Clinical Oncology*, vol. 22, no. 3, pp. 399–402, 2004.

[12] E. L. Yanik, K. Tamburro, J. J. Eron, B. Damania, S. Napravnik, and D. P. Dittmer, "Recent cancer incidence trends in an observational clinical cohort of HIV-infected patients in the US, 2000 to 2011," *Infectious Agents and Cancer*, vol. 8, no. 1, article no. 18, 2013.

[13] D. Serraino, A. De Paoli, A. Zucchetto et al., "The impact of Kaposi sarcoma and non-Hodgkin lymphoma on mortality of people with AIDS in the highly active antiretroviral therapies era," *Cancer Epidemiology*, vol. 34, no. 3, pp. 257–261, 2010.

[14] L. Martín-Carbonero, R. Palacios, E. Valencia et al., "Long-term prognosis of HIV-infected patients with Kaposi sarcoma treated with pegylated liposomal doxorubicin," *Clinical Infectious Diseases*, vol. 47, no. 3, pp. 410–417, 2008.

[15] M. Bower, J. Weir, N. Francis et al., "The effect of HAART in 254 consecutive patients with AIDS-related Kaposi's sarcoma," *AIDS*, vol. 23, no. 13, pp. 1701–1706, 2009.

[16] S. E. Krown, J. Y. Lee, and D. P. Dittmer, "More on HIV-associated Kaposi's sarcoma," *The New England Journal of Medicine*, vol. 358, no. 5, pp. 535–536, 2008.

[17] A. Jemal, F. Bray, M. M. Center, J. Ferlay, E. Ward, and D. Forman, "Global cancer statistics," *CA—A Cancer Journal for Clinicians*, vol. 61, no. 2, pp. 69–90, 2011.

[18] E. A. Mesri, E. Cesarman, and C. Boshoff, "Kaposi's sarcoma and its associated herpesvirus," *Nature Reviews Cancer*, vol. 10, no. 10, pp. 707–719, 2010.

[19] E. Letang, J. J. Lewis, M. Bower et al., "Immune reconstitution inflammatory syndrome associated with Kaposi sarcoma: higher incidence and mortality in Africa than in the UK," *AIDS*, vol. 27, no. 10, pp. 1603–1613, 2013.

[20] H. Q. Nguyen, A. S. Magaret, M. M. Kitahata, S. E. Van Rompaey, A. Wald, and C. Casper, "Persistent Kaposi sarcoma in the era of highly active antiretroviral therapy: characterizing the predictors of clinical response," *AIDS*, vol. 22, no. 8, pp. 937–945, 2008.

[21] S. Uccini, S. Scarpino, F. Ballarini et al., "In situ study of chemokine and chemokine-receptor expression in Kaposi sarcoma," *The American Journal of Dermatopathology*, vol. 25, no. 5, pp. 377–383, 2003.

[22] N. Dupin and P. A. Grange, "Looking for the target cell of Kaposi's sarcoma-associated herpesvirus," *The Journal of Investigative Dermatology*, vol. 126, no. 3, pp. 545–547, 2006.

[23] B. Ensoli, C. Sgadari, G. Barillari, M. C. Sirianni, M. Stürzl, and P. Monini, "Biology of Kaposi's sarcoma," *European Journal of Cancer*, vol. 37, no. 10, pp. 1251–1269, 2001.

[24] P. Delli Bovi, E. Donti, D. M. Knowles II et al., "Presence of chromosomal abnormalities and lack of AIDS retrovirus DNA sequences in AIDS-associated Kaposi's sarcoma," *Cancer Research*, vol. 46, no. 12, part 1, pp. 6333–6338, 1986.

[25] M. Salemi, S. L. Lamers, L. C. Huysentruyt et al., "Distinct patterns of HIV-1 evolution within metastatic tissues in patients with non-hodgkins Lymphoma," *PLoS ONE*, vol. 4, no. 12, Article ID e8153, 2009.

[26] S. L. Lamers, M. Salemi, D. C. Galligan et al., "Human immunodeficiency virus-1 evolutionary patterns associated with pathogenic processes in the brain," *Journal of NeuroVirology*, vol. 16, no. 3, pp. 230–241, 2010.

[27] S. L. Lamers, M. Salemi, D. C. Galligan et al., "Extensive HIV-1 intra-host recombination is common in tissues with abnormal histopathology," *PLoS ONE*, vol. 4, no. 3, Article ID e5065, 2009.

[28] S. Palmer, M. Kearney, F. Maldarelli et al., "Multiple, linked human immunodeficiency virus type 1 drug resistance mutations in treatment-experienced patients are missed by standard genotype analysis," *Journal of Clinical Microbiology*, vol. 43, no. 1, pp. 406–413, 2005.

[29] J. D. Thompson, T. J. Gibson, F. Plewniak, F. Jeanmougin, and D. G. Higgins, "The CLUSTAL_X windows interface: flexible strategies for multiple sequence alignment aided by quality analysis tools," *Nucleic Acids Research*, vol. 25, no. 24, pp. 4876–4882, 1997.

[30] K. Tamura, D. Peterson, N. Peterson, G. Stecher, M. Nei, and S. Kumar, "MEGA5: molecular evolutionary genetics analysis using maximum likelihood, evolutionary distance, and maximum parsimony methods," *Molecular Biology and Evolution*, vol. 28, no. 10, pp. 2731–2739, 2011.

[31] S. Guindon, F. Delsuc, J.-F. Dufayard, and O. Gascuel, "Estimating maximum likelihood phylogenies with PhyML," *Methods in Molecular Biology*, vol. 537, pp. 113–137, 2009.

[32] M. Slatkin and W. P. Maddison, "A cladistic measure of gene flow inferred from the phylogenies of alleles," *Genetics*, vol. 123, no. 3, pp. 603–613, 1989.

[33] D. W. Huang, B. T. Sherman, and R. A. Lempicki, "Bioinformatics enrichment tools: paths toward the comprehensive functional analysis of large gene lists," *Nucleic Acids Research*, vol. 37, no. 1, pp. 1–13, 2009.

[34] F. Maldarelli, X. Wu, L. Su et al., "Specific HIV integration sites are linked to clonal expansion and persistence of infected cells," *Science*, vol. 345, no. 6193, pp. 179–183, 2014.

[35] B. Shiramizu, B. Herndier, H. Abby, and M. S. McGrath, "Clonal HIV is present in a wide variety of HIV-associated malignancies and cell separation studies map the clone to tumor-associated macrophages," *Journal of Acquired Immune Deficiency Syndromes & Human Retrovirology*, vol. 14, no. 4, article A50, 1997.

[36] M. S. McGrath, B. T. Shiramizu, and B. G. Herndier, "Identification of a clonal form of HIV in early Kaposi's sarcoma: evidence for a novel model of ontogenesis, 'sequential neoplasia,'" *Journal of Acquired Immune Deficiency Syndromes and Human Retrovirology*, vol. 8, no. 4, pp. 379–385, 1995.

[37] B. Shiramizu, B. G. Herndier, and M. S. McGrath, "Identification of a common clonal human immunodeficiency virus integration site in human immunodeficiency virus-associated lymphomas," *Cancer Research*, vol. 54, no. 8, pp. 2069–2072, 1994.

[38] K. D. Mack, X. Jin, S. Yu et al., "HIV insertions within and proximal to host cell genes are a common finding in tissues containing high levels of HIV DNA and macrophage-associated p24 antigen expression," *Journal of Acquired Immune Deficiency Syndromes*, vol. 33, no. 3, pp. 308–320, 2003.

[39] R. S. Leidner and D. M. Aboulafia, "Recrudescent Kaposi's sarcoma after initiation of HAART: a manifestation of immune reconstitution syndrome," *AIDS Patient Care and STDs*, vol. 19, no. 10, pp. 635–644, 2005.

[40] E. Letang, J. M. Almeida, J. M. Miró et al., "Predictors of immune reconstitution inflammatory syndrome-associated with kaposi sarcoma in mozambique: a prospective study," *Journal of Acquired Immune Deficiency Syndromes*, vol. 53, no. 5, pp. 589–597, 2010.

[41] M. Müller, S. Wandel, R. Colebunders, S. Attia, H. Furrer, and M. Egger, "Immune reconstitution inflammatory syndrome in patients starting antiretroviral therapy for HIV infection: a systematic review and meta-analysis," *The Lancet Infectious Diseases*, vol. 10, no. 4, pp. 251–261, 2010.

[42] S. A. Shelburne and R. J. Hamill, "The immune reconstitution inflammatory syndrome," *AIDS Reviews*, vol. 5, no. 2, pp. 67–79, 2003.

[43] S. A. Shelburne III, R. J. Hamill, M. C. Rodriguez-Barradas et al., "Immune reconstitution inflammatory syndrome: emergence of a unique syndrome during highly active antiretroviral therapy," *Medicine*, vol. 81, no. 3, pp. 213–227, 2002.

[44] M. A. French, P. Price, and S. F. Stone, "Immune restoration disease after antiretroviral therapy," *AIDS*, vol. 18, no. 12, pp. 1615–1627, 2004.

[45] S. F. Stone, P. Price, and M. A. French, "Immune restoration disease: a consequence of dysregulated immune responses after HAART," *Current HIV Research*, vol. 2, no. 3, pp. 235–242, 2004.

[46] P. Price, N. Mathiot, R. Krueger, S. Stone, N. M. Keane, and M. A. French, "Immune dysfunction and immune restoration disease in HIV patients given highly active antiretroviral therapy," *Journal of Clinical Virology*, vol. 22, no. 3, pp. 279–287, 2001.

[47] N. F. Walker, N. F. Walker, N. F. Walker et al., "Immune reconstitution inflammatory syndrome in HIV-infected patients," *HIV/AIDS - Research and Palliative Care*, vol. 7, pp. 49–64, 2015.

Predictors of Wound Complications following Radiation and Surgical Resection of Soft Tissue Sarcomas

Drake G. LeBrun,[1] David M. Guttmann,[2] Jacob E. Shabason,[2] William P. Levin,[2] Stephen J. Kovach,[3] and Kristy L. Weber[4]

[1] *Perelman School of Medicine, University of Pennsylvania, Jordan Medical Education Center, 3400 Civic Center Blvd., Philadelphia, PA 19104, USA*
[2] *Department of Radiation Oncology, Perelman School of Medicine, University of Pennsylvania, 3400 Civic Center Boulevard, TRC 2 West, Philadelphia, PA 19104, USA*
[3] *Department of Plastic Surgery, Perelman School of Medicine, University of Pennsylvania, 3400 Civic Center Boulevard, 7th Floor South Pavilion, Philadelphia, PA 19104, USA*
[4] *Department of Orthopaedic Surgery, Perelman School of Medicine, University of Pennsylvania, 3400 Civic Center Boulevard, 10-179 South Pavilion, Philadelphia, PA 19104, USA*

Correspondence should be addressed to Kristy L. Weber; kristy.weber@uphs.upenn.edu

Academic Editor: Peter C. Ferguson

Wound complications represent a major source of morbidity in patients undergoing radiation therapy (RT) and surgical resection of soft tissue sarcomas (STS). We investigated whether factors related to RT, surgery, patient comorbidities, and tumor histopathology predict the development of wound complications. An observational study of patients who underwent STS resection and RT was performed. The primary outcome was the occurrence of any wound complication up to four months postoperatively. Significant predictors of wound complications were identified using multivariable logistic regression. Sixty-five patients representing 67 cases of STS were identified. Median age was 59 years (range 22–90) and 34 (52%) patients were female. The rates of major wound complications and any wound complications were 21% and 33%, respectively. After adjusting for radiation timing, diabetes (OR 9.6; 95% CI 1.4–64.8; $P = 0.02$), grade ≥2 radiation dermatitis (OR 4.8; 95% CI 1.2–19.2; $P = 0.03$), and the use of 3D conformal RT (OR 4.6; 95% CI 1.1–20.0; $P = 0.04$) were associated with an increased risk of any wound complication on multivariable analysis. These data suggest that radiation dermatitis and radiation modality are predictors of wound complications in patients with STS.

1. Introduction

The current standard of care for local control of disease in patients with soft tissue sarcoma (STS) of the extremities and trunk where an adequate margin cannot be obtained with resection alone is surgical resection combined with radiation therapy (RT). The use of RT is also preferred in patients with deep, high-grade, large tumors regardless of the ability to achieve adequate margins. However, multiple studies have demonstrated overall wound complication rates ranging from 22 to 35% when radiation was given in combination with surgery [1–4], with even higher rates seen when individual limbs were assessed. In fact, a large randomized control trial found a wound complication rate of 45% in patients with STS of the thigh [4].

Wound complications are treatable with good long-term functional status, yet they can be sources of substantial morbidity in patients with STS. Major wound complications encompass a broad array of wounds including those that require reoperation, an invasive procedure without general or regional anesthesia, readmission for wound management, or prolonged deep packing or dressing changes [4]. In contrast, minor wound complications—those that necessitate clinical follow-up but do not fit within the scope of major wound complications—are also clinically important though not as frequently reported in the literature. To reduce the risk of wound complications, it has been standard practice at sarcoma centers to perform soft tissue reconstruction with the use of rotational or free flaps to bring viable muscle or fasciocutaneous tissues to the defect left after tumor resection. Despite these efforts, wound complications remain a significant problem in this population.

Although RT is known to increase the risk of wound complications, there is limited available data on radiation-related factors other than radiation timing that may be predictive of wound complications in the setting of RT and surgical resection of STS. In addition, further work is needed to refine our understanding of baseline demographic factors that may predispose patients to wound complications. We therefore sought to identify predictors of wound complications in this population with a specific focus on radiation-related parameters that have not been extensively studied in the literature. We hypothesized that factors associated with radiation technique would be correlated with the development of wound complications after adjusting for established clinical risk factors.

2. Materials and Methods

2.1. Patient Population. After obtaining approval from our Institutional Review Board, we identified all patients who had primary resection or reresection of biopsy-proven STS at our institution between August 2013 and November 2016. Patients were excluded from analysis if they underwent resection for regionally recurrent disease, were less than 18 years old, did not undergo RT, or had retroperitoneal tumors. All surgical resections were performed at one institution. Use of muscle, fasciocutaneous, and/or skin grafts was anticipated preoperatively with surgical planning between an orthopaedic oncologist and a plastic surgeon. Indications included a substantial skin or soft tissue defect that could not be closed primarily or a need for vascularized tissue over exposed bone, joint, or neurovascular structures. Radiation was delivered at our institution or at outside institutions. For the six patients who underwent RT at outside institutions, radiation reports were obtained from the patient's primary radiation oncologist. These reports included all relevant radiation parameters including modality and the presence of acute skin toxicities. If any parameters were missing or unclear, these were confirmed via contact with the patient's radiation oncologist. Generally, patients with intermediate- or high-grade tumors or tumors larger than 5 cm underwent RT. All patients are followed routinely in the clinic and there was no loss to follow-up over the study period.

2.2. Data Collection. Patient, tumor, and treatment-related data were collected by retrospective review of the medical record. Patient data included patient age, sex, obesity (defined as BMI ≥ 30), diabetes status, and smoking history. Diabetes status included both Type I and Type II diabetes mellitus.

Tumor data included resected specimen size, tumor size, tumor depth relative to the fascia, and tumor location. Resected specimen size and tumor size were defined by the maximal cross-sectional diameters of the total resected specimen and tumor, respectively, as indicated in the pathology report. Tumor depth was defined as either deep or superficial relative to the fascia. Tumors that were both deep and superficial to the fascia with subcutaneous extension were considered superficial for the purposes of data analysis.

Treatment-related data included history of chemotherapy, type of wound closure, radiation timing (pre- versus postoperative), radiation modality, grade of radiation dermatitis, use of radiation boost, use of radiation bolus, planning target volume (PTV), and cumulative radiation dose. Radiation dermatitis was a dichotomous variable (grade <2 versus grade $\geq$2) determined by the radiation oncologist's summary report and based on the 2010 National Cancer Institute Common Terminology Criteria for Adverse Events [5]. Radiation boost is defined as the escalation of the total radiation dose prescription to a subvolume of the initial treatment region believed to be at higher risk for local recurrence. Radiation bolus is the use of tissue equivalent material placed over the treatment region to increase dose deposition in more superficial structures such as skin. PTV is the total volume of tissue targeted to receive the prescription dose of radiation.

2.3. Outcomes. Major and minor wound complications were assessed up to four months postoperatively. Major wound complications were defined according to the National Cancer Institute of Canada trial as a reoperation for wound repair, an invasive procedure for wound management without regional or general anesthesia, hospital readmission for nonoperative wound management, or prolonged deep packing or dressing changes for 120 days or longer [4]. Minor wound complications were defined as any other surgical wounds that did not meet criteria for a major wound. These included wounds requiring in-office debridement or oral antibiotics. A prespecified composite outcome "any wound" was defined as the development of either a major or minor wound complication. The time interval between surgery and first identification of a wound complication was also recorded.

2.4. Statistical Analysis. Descriptive statistics were used to summarize demographic, histopathologic, and treatment characteristics of the study population. Fisher's exact test and the Wilcoxon rank-sum test were used to determine whether categorical and continuous characteristics were associated with the development of wound complications, respectively. Due to the limited number of events in this dataset, a parsimonious model was desired to avoid model overfitting. A backward selection strategy was used with a threshold to enter $P < 0.2$ to screen weak prognostic covariates from the multivariable model. Variables were retained in the multivariable model if Wald tests yielded a P value of <0.05. Generalized estimating equations (GEE) were used to adjust for correlated exposures and outcomes among individuals with multiple observations in the sample [6]. Collinearity was assessed by calculating variance inflation factors and the final model was evaluated for two-way interactions. Model goodness-of-fit was assessed via the Hosmer-Lemeshow test. Discrimination—the ability of our model to assign higher probabilities of wound complications to those with true wound complications compared to those without—was assessed via the C-statistic, also known as the area under

TABLE 1: Patient and tumor characteristics.

Characteristic	Major wound complication			Any wound complication		
	Yes	No	P	Yes	No	P
Sex			0.95			0.55
Female	7 (50%)	27 (51%)		10 (45%)	24 (53%)	
Male	7 (50%)	26 (49%)		12 (55%)	21 (47%)	
Age	62.2 (19.5)	57.0 (16.3)	**0.19**	62.8 (17.7)	55.7 (16.3)	**0.08**
Obese (BMI ≥ 30)			0.75			**0.08**
Yes	5 (36%)	16 (30%)		10 (45%)	11 (24%)	
No	9 (64%)	37 (70%)		12 (55%)	34 (76%)	
Diabetes mellitus			**0.05**			**0.01**
Yes	4 (29%)	4 (8%)		6 (27%)	2 (4%)	
No	10 (71%)	49 (92%)		16 (73%)	43 (96%)	
Tobacco use			0.69			0.65
Current or past smoker	5 (36%)	22 (42%)		14 (64%)	26 (58%)	
Never smoker	9 (64%)	31 (58%)		8 (36%)	19 (42%)	
Tumor location			1.0			0.24
Upper extremity	2 (14%)	8 (15%)		5 (23%)	5 (11%)	
Lower extremity	12 (86%)	42 (79%)		17 (77%)	37 (82%)	
Trunk	0 (0%)	3 (6%)		0 (0%)	3 (7%)	
Tumor location in extremity			0.74			0.77
Proximal	11 (79%)	36 (68%)		17 (77%)	30 (67%)	
Distal	3 (21%)	14 (26%)		5 (23%)	12 (27%)	
Trunk	0 (0%)	3 (6%)		0 (0%)	3 (6%)	
Tumor depth relative to fascia			0.83			**0.09**
Deep	8 (57%)	32 (60%)		10 (45%)	30 (67%)	
Superficial	6 (43%)	21 (40%)		12 (55%)	15 (33%)	
*Resected specimen size (cm)**	13.0 (13.7)	11.9 (13.1)	0.65	12.9 (8.7)	13.3 (6.4)	0.31
*Tumor size (cm)**	11.1 (9.6)	7.9 (4.7)	0.60	10.1 (7.6)	7.8 (5.0)	0.49

*Continuous variables are reported as mean (SD). Categorical variables are reported as N (%). Total count values may not sum to 67 due to missing data. Bolded P values correspond to covariates that met a level of significance of $P < 0.2$ for inclusion in the multivariable model. BMI: body mass index. cm: centimeter.

the receiver operating curve [7]. Fewer than 5% of observations were missing for any variable included in the regression analysis. For all analyses, two-sided tests were used with a level of significance of $\alpha \leq 0.05$. All analyses were performed using STATA 14.0 (StataCorp, College Station, TX, USA).

3. Results

Patient and tumor characteristics are summarized in Table 1. A total of 65 patients met inclusion criteria for the study. Two patients had separate resections and radiation treatments in the setting of metastatic disease and were each considered as two distinct cases for the purposes of this study for a total of 67 cases. The median age of patients was 59 years (range 24–90 years) and 34 (52%) of patients were female.

Treatment characteristics are summarized in Table 2. Among preoperative RT patients, resection occurred a median of 28 days (range 18–49 days) after completion of RT. Surgery for patients who underwent reresection occurred between 25 and 162 days after their primary resection at an outside hospital. All patients underwent limb-salvage resection, and all patients were alive at the 120-day cutoff to assess wound complications. With a median postoperative follow-up of 20.7 months, 60 patients (92%) were alive at the time of the study analysis.

A summary of wound types is shown in Table 3. Among all cases, 14 (21%) major wound complications were noted within four months of surgery. An additional 8 (12%) minor wound complications were noted; thus, a total of 22 cases (33%) experienced *any* wound complication. Wounds were first documented a median of 30 days postoperatively (range 11 to 100 days).

On univariate analysis, only diabetes was associated with the development of a major wound complication ($P = 0.05$). Diabetes ($P = 0.01$), skin graft and/or vascularized flap reconstruction ($P = 0.01$), grade ≥2 radiation dermatitis ($P = 0.02$), and 3D conformal RT relative to intensity-modulated radiation therapy (IMRT) or proton therapy ($P = 0.008$) were associated with an increased risk of any wound complication.

Among patients undergoing preoperative RT, 7 of 13 (54%) with grade >2 radiation dermatitis developed any wound complications compared to 11 of 43 (26%) without high-grade radiation dermatitis. Although there was evidence of an association among this subgroup, it did not meet statistical significance (OR 3.39; 95% CI 0.94–12.30; $P = 0.06$). Among patients undergoing postoperative RT, 3

TABLE 2: Treatment characteristics.

Characteristic	Major wound complication			Any wound complication		
	Yes	No	*P*	Yes	No	*P*
Resection type			1.0			0.76
Primary resection	11 (79%)	43 (81%)		17 (77%)	37 (82%)	
Reresection	3 (21%)	10 (19%)		5 (23%)	8 (18%)	
Wound closure			**0.19**			**0.01**
Primary	6 (43%)	33 (62%)		8 (36%)	31 (69%)	
Skin graft and/or vascularized flap reconstruction	8 (57%)	20 (38%)		14 (64%)	14 (31%)	
Preoperative chemotherapy			1.0			0.48
Yes	4 (29%)	15 (28%)		5 (23%)	14 (31%)	
No	10 (71%)	38 (72%)		17 (77%)	31 (69%)	
Institution providing radiation therapy			0.6			0.39
Our institution	12 (86%)	49 (92%)		19 (87%)	42 (93%)	
Other	2 (14%)	4 (8%)		3 (13%)	3 (7%)	
Radiation modality			0.74			**0.008**
3D conformal	4 (29%)	13 (25%)		10 (45%)	7 (16%)	
IMRT	10 (71%)	30 (57%)		12 (55%)	28 (62%)	
Proton therapy	0 (0%)	10 (18%)		0 (0)	10 (22%)	
Radiation timing			0.43			0.72
Preoperative	11 (79%)	46 (87%)		18 (82%)	39 (87%)	
Postoperative	3 (21%)	7 (13%)		4 (18%)	6 (13%)	
Use of radiation boost			1.0			1.0
Yes	1 (8%)	5 (10%)		2 (10%)	4 (9%)	
No	12 (92%)	46 (90%)		19 (90%)	39 (91%)	
Use of radiation bolus			0.5			**0.16**
Yes	5 (36%)	12 (24%)		8 (38%)	9 (21%)	
No	9 (64%)	37 (76%)		13 (62%)	33 (79%)	
Grade ≥2 radiation dermatitis			0.51			**0.02**
Yes	5 (36%)	13 (25%)		10 (45%)	8 (19%)	
No	9 (64%)	38 (75%)		12 (55%)	35 (81%)	
*Cumulative radiation dose (gy)**	5027 (410)	5015 (296)	0.85	5021 (323)	5016 (323)	0.34
*Radiation planning target volume (cc)**	1646 (1526)	1314 (1663)	**0.12**	1747 (2382)	1206 (1092)	0.53

*Continuous variables are reported as mean (SD). Categorical variables are reported as *N* (%). Total count values may not sum to 67 due to missing data. Bolded *P* values correspond to covariates that met a level of significance of $P < 0.2$ for inclusion in the multivariable model. IMRT: intensity-modulated radiation therapy. gy: gray. cc: cubic centimeters.

TABLE 3: Wound complications in study sample.

Wound type	*N* (%)
Major wounds	*14 (21%)*
Reoperation	12
Nonsurgical readmission	1
Prolonged deep packing	1
Minor wounds	*8 (12%)*
In-office debridement	5
Oral antibiotics	2
Hyperbaric oxygen	1
Any wounds	*22 (33%)*

of 5 (60%) with grade >2 radiation dermatitis developed any wound complications compared to 1 of 4 (25%) with grade <2 radiation dermatitis (OR 4.50; 95% CI 0.25–80.57; $P = 0.31$).

No patients who underwent proton therapy ($n = 10$) developed wound complications. When proton therapy was excluded, the use of 3D conformal RT was still associated with more wound complications relative to IMRT ($P = 0.04$). Tumor depth did not significantly affect any wound development, with any wounds seen in 25% of those with deep tumors and 45% of those with superficial tumors ($P = 0.09$).

In the multivariable model, diabetes remained associated with an increased risk of major wounds (OR 5.10; 95% CI 1.07–24.29; $P = 0.04$). For any wounds (Table 4), diabetes (OR 9.58; 95% CI 1.42–64.83; $P = 0.02$) and grade ≥2 radiation dermatitis (OR 4.82; 95% CI 1.20–19.21; $P = 0.03$) remained associated with an increased risk of wound complications. The use of 3D conformal RT was also found to be significantly associated with an increased risk of wound complications relative to IMRT or proton radiation (OR 4.55; 95% CI 1.09–20.0; $P = 0.04$). Radiation timing was included in the multivariable logistic regression model to account for known

TABLE 4: Multivariable analysis of predictors for any wound complications.

Predictors	Adjusted OR (95% CI)	P
Diabetes versus no diabetes	9.58 (1.42–64.83)	0.02
Grade ≥2 versus grade <2 radiation dermatitis	4.82 (1.20–19.21)	0.03
3D conformal RT versus IMRT or proton radiation	4.55 (1.09–20.0)	0.04

OR: odds ratio; CI: confidence interval; IMRT: intensity-modulated radiation therapy.

differential risk associated with pre- versus postoperative RT; however, it was not associated with wound complications in either model. The C-statistic was 0.80 suggesting good ability of the model to discriminate between individuals who did and did not experience any wound complication. The Hosmer-Lemeshow test demonstrated adequate goodness-of-fit. No collinearity was detected and no significant interactions were identified.

4. Discussion

In this single-center observational study of 67 cases of STS of the extremity and trunk that underwent surgical resection and RT, we found that 3D conformal RT was associated with a greater risk of wound complications relative to more conformal modalities such as IMRT or proton therapy. Moreover, we found that grade ≥2 radiation dermatitis was associated with an increased risk of wound complications, a finding that has not been identified in other studies.

Radiation therapy is an integral component of limb-sparing treatment for most patients with STS and allows marked improvement in local control compared to surgical resection alone [8]. However, the addition of RT is not without risks. Wound complications are a source of considerable morbidity for these patients. Although much of the existing literature has focused on major wound complications, we sought to expand this definition given the occurrence of other wound complications that are clinically important but not accounted for in previous studies [4]. In doing so, we sought to more precisely establish the risk factors associated with the development of major wound complications and any wound complications, with an expanded focus on radiation parameters and outcomes.

To our knowledge, this exploratory study is the second to show that the use of 3D conformal RT was associated with a greater risk of wound complications relative to more conformal modalities such as IMRT or proton therapy. Our findings are consistent with a recent study by Saeed et al. [9] that demonstrated a decreased risk of postoperative wound complications (OR 0.4, $P = 0.02$) among patients undergoing IMRT compared to patients who underwent 3D conformal RT for STS. Otherwise, a 2013 study showed that the rate of wound complications using IMRT was lower than that of the landmark NCI study that used 3D conformal radiation but failed to meet statistical significance [10]. A recent prospective phase II trial assessed the use of image-guided RT with reduced volumes, with all patients undergoing preoperative RT and 75% receiving IMRT [11]. This study demonstrated a similar acute wound complication rate (36.6%) to the National Cancer Institute of Canada trial with a lower rate of late toxicities. Importantly, these studies had larger sample sizes and were better powered than the current study [10, 11]. Results of the prospective phase II trial Preoperative Radiotherapy for Sarcomas of the Extremities with Intensity-Modulation, Image-Guidance, and Small Safety-Margins (PREMISS) are awaited to clarify whether IMRT can reduce wound complications in this population [12].

There is a pressing need for additional studies to corroborate the recent findings by Saeed and colleagues [9]. Our study addresses that need by providing further evidence to support the association between radiation modality and wound complications. Compared to 3D conformal RT, IMRT and proton radiation permit more conformal targeting of complicated volumes, sparing normal tissue from excess dose and decreasing associated toxicity [13]. 3D conformal radiation techniques may deliver a higher dose to a larger volume of the skin and subcutaneous tissues, placing the patient at higher risk for wound breakdown. This may be the basis for the observed association between 3D conformal radiation and wound complications. In contrast, IMRT limits the high dose radiation volume more tightly to the tumor by using multiple beam angles of varying fluency to deliver dose to the target. Proton therapy even better spares normal tissue due to the physical properties of protons that cause them to deposit all their energy in the target tissue and completely spare dose distally. This is distinct from traditional photon radiation in which there is always "exit" dose along the beam path. In this study, the small size precluded a reliable statistical comparison between IMRT versus proton therapy or proton therapy versus 3D conformal RT. Although our study was not designed to assess outcomes associated with proton therapy alone, no patients who underwent proton therapy developed wound complications, highlighting an area for further inquiry. From a practical perspective, it is not infrequent that insurance companies deny the use of IMRT or proton therapy for treatment of patients with soft tissue sarcomas, citing no evidence to justify its increased cost. The data in this manuscript may be helpful in obtaining authorization for these advanced treatments, as the risk of wound complications is reduced.

This study is also the first to identify grade ≥2 radiation dermatitis as an independent predictor of wound complications in the setting of STS. It is unclear if there is a direct causal relationship between radiation dermatitis and surgical wound complications or if the development of radiation dermatitis is a surrogate marker for a patient who is biologically more susceptible to radiation injury. Radiation incites an active inflammatory response in irradiated tissue, which is associated with poor wound healing. The observed association between brisk radiation skin reaction and wound complications in this cohort likely results from a larger biological effect of the radiation in the tissues of those patients who experienced worse dermatitis based on both technical (e.g., choice of radiation modality) and patient factors (e.g., diabetes). It is also possible that the soft tissues in these patients were predisposed to complications or poor cutaneous healing due to unstudied patient factors such as inadequate nutrition.

Our results confirm the importance of diabetes in the development of wound complications, a finding that has been demonstrated in other studies assessing wound complication risk in patients undergoing resection and RT for STS [14–16]. When treating patients with STS and comorbid diabetes, clinicians should consider strategies to lower the risk of wound complications such as communicating with the patient's primary care physician at the time of diagnosis to optimize diabetes control and monitoring fasting glucose levels over the course of preoperative RT. Although we did not routinely check hemoglobin A1c preoperatively, this is another strategy to stratify patients by their degree of chronic hyperglycemia.

There are important limitations to this study. The study is retrospective and therefore subject to selection bias. Although we attempted to control for any measured confounding with multivariable analysis, unmeasured factors not accounted for in the data set may bias the estimates of wound complication risk. For example, we do not know why certain patients received IMRT or proton therapy and others did not. In addition, the study is underpowered to detect all relevant risk factors for wound complications in multimodality therapy for STS. This may explain why some previously identified risk factors did not meet statistical significance in our study, including smoking history, obesity, specimen size, and preoperative radiation [4, 14–17]. Other known risk factors such as vascular involvement of the tumor and tumor volume were not assessed in our study [18, 19]. Baldini and colleagues found that tumor depth, defined as tumor distance less than 3 mm from the skin surface, was associated with wound complications after radiation [15]. Our study defined tumor depth relative to the fascia, considering deep tumors with superficial extension as superficial given the need to manage these superficial tumors to remove the subcutaneous margin, and found no association between tumor depth and wound complications. When these tumors were considered deep, the results of the analysis did not significantly change.

5. Conclusions

In this study, the use of IMRT or proton therapy was associated with a decreased risk of wound complications relative to the use of 3D conformal RT after adjusting for radiation timing. These data suggest that utilizing IMRT or proton therapy in place of 3D conformal RT could reduce the incidence of wound complications in patients with STS. Moreover, this study suggests that grade ≥ 2 radiation dermatitis is associated with an increased risk of wounds, highlighting a previously undescribed predictor of postoperative wound complications. Additional studies are needed to corroborate and elucidate these findings.

References

[1] C. P. Cannon, M. T. Ballo, G. K. Zagars et al., "Complications of combined modality treatment of primary lower extremity soft-tissue sarcomas," *Cancer*, vol. 107, no. 10, pp. 2455–2461, 2006.

[2] W. W. Virkus, A. Mollabashy, J. D. Reith, R. A. Zlotecki, B. H. Berrey, and M. T. Scarborough, "Preoperative radiotherapy in the treatment of soft tissue sarcomas," *Clinical Orthopaedics and Related Research*, no. 397, pp. 177–189, 2002.

[3] J. F. Tseng, M. T. Ballo, H. N. Langstein et al., "The effect of preoperative radiotherapy and reconstructive surgery on wound complications after resection of extremity soft-tissue sarcomas," *Annals of Surgical Oncology*, vol. 13, no. 9, pp. 1209–1215, 2006.

[4] B. O'Sullivan, A. M. Davis, R. Turcotte et al., "Preoperative versus postoperative radiotherapy in soft-tissue sarcoma of the limbs: a randomised trial," *The Lancet*, vol. 359, no. 9325, pp. 2235–2241, 2002.

[5] NCI (2010) Common Terminology Criteria for Adverse Events (CTCAE) Version 4.03.

[6] J. A. Hanley, A. Negassa, M. D. D. Edwardes, and J. E. Forrester, "Statistical analysis of correlated data using generalized estimating equations: an orientation," *American Journal of Epidemiology*, vol. 157, no. 4, pp. 364–375, 2003.

[7] P. Royston, K. G. M. Moons, D. G. Altman, and Y. Vergouwe, "Prognosis and prognostic research: Developing a prognostic model," *BMJ (Online)*, vol. 338, no. 7707, pp. 1373–1377, 2009.

[8] J. C. Yang, A. E. Chang, A. R. Baker et al., "Randomized prospective study of the benefit of adjuvant radiation therapy in the treatment of soft tissue sarcomas of the extremity," *Journal of Clinical Oncology*, vol. 16, no. 1, pp. 197–203, 1998.

[9] H. Saeed, C. Johnstone, D. M. King et al., "The impact of 3D conformal radiotherapy versus intensity-modulated radiotherapy on post-operative wound complications in soft tissue sarcomas of the extremity and chest-wall," *Journal of Radiation Oncology*, vol. 5, no. 4, pp. 389–394, 2016.

[10] B. O'Sullivan, A. M. Griffin, C. I. Dickie et al., "Phase 2 study of preoperative image-guided intensity-modulated radiation therapy to reduce wound and combined modality morbidities in lower extremity soft tissue sarcoma," *Cancer*, vol. 119, no. 10, pp. 1878–1884, 2013.

[11] D. Wang, Q. Zhang, B. L. Eisenberg et al., "Significant reduction of late toxicities in patients with extremity sarcoma treated with image-guided radiation therapy to a reduced target volume: Results of radiation therapy oncology group RTOG-0630 trial," *Journal of Clinical Oncology*, vol. 33, no. 20, pp. 2231–2238, 2015.

[12] B. Röper, C. Heinrich, V. Kehl et al., "Study of preoperative radiotherapy for sarcomas of the extremities with intensity-modulation, image-guidance and small safety-margins (PREMISS)," *BMC Cancer*, vol. 15, pp. 1–8, 2015.

[13] L. Hong, K. M. Alektiar, M. Hunt, E. Venkatraman, and S. A. Leibel, "Intensity-modulated radiotherapy for soft tissue sarcoma of the thigh," *International Journal of Radiation Oncology Biology Physics*, vol. 59, no. 3, pp. 752–759, 2004.

[14] J. Moore, M. Isler, J. Barry, and S. Mottard, "Major wound complication risk factors following soft tissue sarcoma resection," *European Journal of Surgical Oncology*, vol. 40, no. 12, pp. 1671–1676, 2014.

[15] E. H. Baldini, M. R. Lapidus, Q. Wang et al., "Predictors for major wound complications following preoperative radiotherapy and surgery for soft-tissue sarcoma of the extremities and trunk: importance of tumor proximity to skin surface," *Annals of Surgical Oncology*, vol. 20, no. 5, pp. 1494–1499, 2013.

[16] B. Kim, Y.-L. E. Chen, D. G. Kirsch et al., "An effective preoperative three-dimensional radiotherapy target volume for extremity soft tissue sarcoma and the effect of margin width on local control," *International Journal of Radiation Oncology Biology Physics*, vol. 77, no. 3, pp. 843–850, 2010.

[17] D. S. Geller, F. J. Hornicek, H. J. Mankin, and K. A. Raskin, "Soft tissue sarcoma resection volume associated with wound-healing complications," *Clinical Orthopaedics and Related Research*, no. 459, pp. 182–185, 2007.

[18] M. Ziegele, D. M. King, and M. Bedi, "Tumor volume is a better predictor of post-operative wound complications compared to tumor size in soft tissue sarcomas of the proximal lower extremity," *Clinical Sarcoma Research*, vol. 6, pp. 1–9, 2016.

[19] A. Schwartz, A. Rebecca, A. Smith et al., "Risk factors for significant wound complications following wide resection of extremity soft tissue sarcomas," *Clinical Orthopaedics and Related Research*, vol. 471, no. 11, pp. 3612–3617, 2013.

The Volume-Outcome Relationship in Retroperitoneal Soft Tissue Sarcoma: Evidence of Improved Short- and Long-Term Outcomes at High-Volume Institutions

Sanjay P. Bagaria,[1] Matthew Neville,[2] Richard J. Gray,[3] Emmanuel Gabriel,[1] Jonathan B. Ashman,[4] Steven Attia,[5] and Nabil Wasif[3,6]

[1]*Department of Surgery, Section of Surgical Oncology, Mayo Clinic, Jacksonville, FL, USA*
[2]*Department of Biostatistics, Mayo Clinic, Scottsdale, AZ, USA*
[3]*Department of Surgery, Section of Surgical Oncology, Mayo Clinic, Phoenix, AZ, USA*
[4]*Department of Radiation Oncology, Mayo Clinic, Phoenix, AZ, USA*
[5]*Division of Hematology/Oncology, Mayo Clinic, Jacksonville, FL, USA*
[6]*Robert D. and Patricia E. Kern Center for the Science of Health Care Delivery, Surgical Outcomes Division, Mayo Clinic, Phoenix, AZ, USA*

Correspondence should be addressed to Sanjay P. Bagaria; bagaria.sanjay@mayo.edu

Academic Editor: C. Verhoef

Background. We sought to study the association between RPS case volume and outcomes. Although a relationship has been demonstrated between case volume and patient outcomes in some cancers, such a relationship has not been established for retroperitoneal sarcomas (RPSs). *Study Design.* The National Cancer Database (NCDB) was queried for patients undergoing treatment for primary RPS diagnosed between 2004 and 2013. Mean annual patient volume for RPS resection was calculated for all hospitals and divided into low volume (<5 cases/year), medium volume (5–10 cases/year), and high volume (>10 cases/year). Risk-adjusted regression analyses were performed to identify predictors of 30-day surgical mortality, *R*0 margin status, and overall survival (OS). *Results.* Our study population consisted of 5,407 patients with a median age of 61 years, of whom 47% were male and 3,803 (70%) underwent surgical resection. Absolute 30-day surgical mortality and *R*0 margin rate following surgery for low-, medium-, and high-volume institutions were 2.4%, 1.3%, and 0.5% ($p = 0.027$) and 68%, 65%, and 82%, ($p < 0.001$), respectively. Five-year overall survival rates for low, medium, and high-volume institutions were 56%, 57%, and 66%, respectively ($p < 0.001$). Patients treated at low-volume institutions had a significantly higher risk of 30-day mortality (adjusted OR = 4.66, 95% CI 2.26–9.63) and long-term mortality (adjusted HR = 1.56, 95% CI 1.16–2.11) compared to high-volume institutions. *Conclusion.* We demonstrate the existence of a hospital sarcoma service line volume-oncologic outcome relationship for RPS at the national level and provide benchmark data for cancer care delivery systems and policy makers.

1. Introduction

Retroperitoneal sarcomas (RPSs) are rare tumors that account for 15–20% of all soft tissue sarcomas. The majority of cases present with localized disease, and therefore, surgical resection is the mainstay of treatment. Extirpations are complex procedures that often require removal of adjacent organs and dissection along critical structures, and as a result, they can be associated with significant morbidity. Furthermore, the efficacy of surgery depends on the ability to achieve negative margins, which requires multidisciplinary preoperative and intraoperative expertise in radiology, pathology, and surgical subspecialties.

Hospital surgical volume is a well-studied measure associated with improved outcomes in multiple tumor subtypes [1–4]. In particular, such a relationship has been reported for complex surgical oncologic procedures such as colectomy, nephrectomy, and pancreatectomy, all of which are commonly performed for RPS [5–7]. As a result, centralization of complex surgical oncologic procedures to high-volume centers has been advocated [1, 2, 4]. The premise is that high-volume centers have the experience and expertise to perform these complex procedures in an optimal manner with correspondingly superior outcomes compared to low-volume centers.

Such a volume-outcome association has not been demonstrated at the national level for RPS, likely due to the rarity of the disease. Nevertheless, due to the multispecialty expertise required to optimally treat these tumors, an association may exist. Our hypothesis is that high-volume centers treating primary RPS have a lower 30-day postoperative mortality, higher margin negative resection rate, and improved overall survival compared to low-volume centers.

2. Methods

2.1. Data Source. Data from the National Cancer Database (NCDB) were used to conduct this study. The NCDB, a joint program of the Commission on Cancer (CoC) of the American College of Surgeons (ACoS) and the American Cancer Society (ACS), is a nationwide database for more than 1,500 commission-accredited cancer programs in the United States and Puerto Rico. Approximately 70% of all newly diagnosed cases of cancer in the United States are captured at the institutional level and reported to the NCDB. Variables in the database cover demographics, socioeconomic status, tumor stage, treatment received, and hospital characteristics. NCDB data contain no protected health information; hence, this study was exempt from formal IRB review.

2.2. Inclusion/Exclusion Criteria. Patients diagnosed with RPS from 2004 to 2013 were identified from the NCDB and constituted our study population (note that patients with extraabdominal sarcoma and gastrointestinal stromal tumors were not included). This time period was chosen to ensure up-to-date coding in the NCDB for the variables of interest for this study and to provide at least 5 years of follow-up for survival analyses.

Two patient cohorts were created. The first comprised all patients diagnosed with RPS irrespective of whether they underwent surgery or not. This group included all stages and represents the institutional experience with RPS. We believe this group better represents any association between volume and long-term survival as it captures multidisciplinary care. The second cohort is a subset of this group comprising only of patients who underwent curative intent surgery. This group was defined to study the association between surgical volume and short-term outcomes. NCDB surgical codes distinguish between curative intent surgery and procedures such as open biopsies. For this surgery-only group, patients with metastatic disease and those not undergoing curative intent surgery were excluded. For both groups, only patients who had all treatment (surgery, radiation therapy, and/or chemotherapy) at the reporting hospital were included in order to provide valid volume-outcome comparisons.

2.3. Outcome, Exposure, and Independent Variables. The exposure variable was the hospital volume status. Primary outcome variables were overall survival (OS), surgical margins, and 30-day surgical mortality. Surgical margins were defined as negative ($R0$) or positive ($R1/R2$). Independent variables included age, sex, race, insurance status, education, modified Charlson score, primary tumor site, pathologic tumor size, grade, histology, radiation therapy, and chemotherapy. Tumor histology was grouped into clinically significant categories by using ICD codes. Tumor grade was divided into GX (unknown), G1 (well differentiated), G2 (moderately differentiated), and G3 (poorly or undifferentiated).

2.4. Hospital Volume Calculations. Average annual volume/hospital of curative intent surgery for RPS was calculated by dividing the total number of surgical resections performed at a hospital by the number of years that data were reported to the NCDB. A histogram of average annual volume/hospital was then plotted, and volume cutoffs were chosen to divide our patient cohorts into three groups: low volume (<5 cases/year), medium volume (5–10 cases/year), and high volume (>10 cases/year) to ensure volume groups with adequate number of patients to enable robust statistical analyses. For analyses involving the all cases cohort, the same volume cutoffs were used to ensure comparability.

2.5. Statistical Analyses. Bivariate analyses were initially performed to identify demographic, tumor, and treatment differences between different volume categories using the chi-square test or analysis of variance. Logistic regression analyses were used to model the margin negative resection and 30-day mortality following surgery, and adjusted odds ratios (OR) and 95% confidence intervals (CI) were reported. OS was estimated by the Kaplan–Meier method, and the comparison in the survival curves between different surgical volumes was assessed by the log rank test. Cox regression analyses were used to model overall survival, and adjusted hazard ratios (HR) and 95% CIs were reported. Patients who died within 30 days of surgery were excluded from survival analyses. A p value of <0.05 was set as our threshold for statistical significance. The analysis was performed using SAS 9.4 and R 3.3.0.

3. Results

3.1. Demographics. We identified 5,407 patients with primary RPS who comprised our primary study population (Table 1). The median age was 61 years, and 53% were female. The mean tumor size was 18.5 cm (median = 15.5 cm), and a plurality of tumors were well differentiated (36%). Approximately 76% of patients underwent surgery, 26% received radiation therapy, and 17% received systemic therapy. There were 3,807 patients who underwent surgical resection for curative intent of primary RPS (Table 2) excluding stage-4 cancers. The median age was 62 years, and 53% were female. The median tumor size was 16.8 cm. Most tumors were well differentiated (36%).

Table 1: Patient characteristics: all patients.

	High volume ($N = 563$)	Medium volume ($N = 373$)	Low volume ($N = 4471$)	Total ($N = 5407$)	p value
Age at diagnosis					0.0085
Mean (SD)	59.6 (14.3)	58.5 (14.4)	60.7 (14.2)	60.4 (14.2)	
Median	60.0	59.0	62.0	61.0	
Q1, Q3	51.0, 70.0	50.0, 68.0	52.0, 71.0	52.0, 71.0	
Range	(19.0–90.0)	(18.0–88.0)	(18.0–90.0)	(18.0–90.0)	
Sex					0.0001
Male	304 (54.0%)	193 (51.7%)	2028 (45.4%)	2525 (46.7%)	
Female	259 (46.0%)	180 (48.3%)	2443 (54.6%)	2882 (53.3%)	
Race					0.0010
Black	34 (6.0%)	30 (8.0%)	500 (11.2%)	564 (10.4%)	
Other	29 (5.2%)	26 (7.0%)	271 (6.1%)	326 (6.0%)	
White	500 (88.8%)	317 (85.0%)	3700 (82.8%)	4517 (83.5%)	
Charlson–Deyo score					0.0047
0	472 (83.8%)	307 (82.3%)	3500 (78.3%)	4279 (79.1%)	
1	79 (14.0%)	52 (13.9%)	755 (16.9%)	886 (16.4%)	
2	12 (2.1%)	14 (3.8%)	216 (4.8%)	242 (4.5%)	
Year of diagnosis					0.37
2004	49 (8.7%)	20 (5.4%)	353 (7.9%)	422 (7.8%)	
2005	41 (7.3%)	25 (6.7%)	392 (8.8%)	458 (8.5%)	
2006	56 (9.9%)	37 (9.9%)	404 (9.0%)	497 (9.2%)	
2007	56 (9.9%)	38 (10.2%)	422 (9.4%)	516 (9.5%)	
2008	66 (11.7%)	37 (9.9%)	453 (10.1%)	556 (10.3%)	
2009	64 (11.4%)	34 (9.1%)	452 (10.1%)	550 (10.2%)	
2010	51 (9.1%)	38 (10.2%)	479 (10.7%)	568 (10.5%)	
2011	68 (12.1%)	48 (12.9%)	522 (11.7%)	638 (11.8%)	
2012	59 (10.5%)	59 (15.8%)	508 (11.4%)	626 (11.6%)	
2013	53 (9.4%)	37 (9.9%)	486 (10.9%)	576 (10.7%)	
Facility type					<0.0001
Missing	48	39	364	451	
Community cancer program	0 (0.0%)	1 (0.3%)	230 (5.6%)	231 (4.7%)	
Comprehensive community cancer program	0 (0.0%)	0 (0.0%)	1428 (34.8%)	1428 (28.8%)	
Academic/research program	515 (100.0%)	283 (84.7%)	2023 (49.3%)	2821 (56.9%)	
Integrated network cancer program	0 (0.0%)	50 (15.0%)	426 (10.4%)	476 (9.6%)	
Primary payor					<0.0001
Not insured	7 (1.2%)	10 (2.7%)	181 (4.0%)	198 (3.7%)	
Private insurance	243 (43.2%)	195 (52.3%)	2127 (47.6%)	2565 (47.4%)	
Medicaid	17 (3.0%)	25 (6.7%)	271 (6.1%)	313 (5.8%)	
Medicare	168 (29.8%)	131 (35.1%)	1774 (39.7%)	2073 (38.3%)	
Other government	5 (0.9%)	1 (0.3%)	61 (1.4%)	67 (1.2%)	
Insurance status unknown	123 (21.8%)	11 (2.9%)	57 (1.3%)	191 (3.5%)	
Median income quartiles					0.0078
Missing	36	10	159	205	
<$30,000	36 (6.8%)	41 (11.3%)	547 (12.7%)	624 (12.0%)	
$30,000–$35,999	98 (18.6%)	67 (18.5%)	716 (16.6%)	881 (16.9%)	
$36,000–$45,999	139 (26.4%)	101 (27.8%)	1124 (26.1%)	1364 (26.2%)	
$46,000+	254 (48.2%)	154 (42.4%)	1925 (44.6%)	2333 (44.8%)	
No high school degree (%)					<0.0001
Missing	36	10	159	205	
≥29%	58 (11.0%)	33 (9.1%)	681 (15.8%)	772 (14.8%)	
20–28.9%	96 (18.2%)	91 (25.1%)	961 (22.3%)	1148 (22.1%)	
14–19.9%	125 (23.7%)	96 (26.4%)	994 (23.1%)	1215 (23.4%)	
<14%	248 (47.1%)	143 (39.4%)	1676 (38.9%)	2067 (39.7%)	
Distance to treating center (miles)					<0.0001
Mean (SD)	223.5 (389.7)	68.2 (119.1)	39.5 (136.1)	60.6 (187.7)	
Median	75.9	38.4	12.4	15.4	
Q1, Q3	22.4, 242.7	15.0, 89.8	5.1, 33.5	5.8, 46.2	
Range	(1.0–4040.1)	(1.0–1495.6)	(1.0–4710.1)	(1.0–4710.1)	

Table 1: Continued.

	High volume ($N=563$)	Medium volume ($N=373$)	Low volume ($N=4471$)	Total ($N=5407$)	p value
Histologic subtype					<0.0001
Dedifferentiated liposarcoma	160 (28.4%)	81 (21.7%)	755 (16.9%)	996 (18.4%)	
Fibrosarcoma	10 (1.8%)	5 (1.3%)	67 (1.5%)	82 (1.5%)	
Leiomyosarcoma	98 (17.4%)	88 (23.6%)	1069 (23.9%)	1255 (23.2%)	
Liposarcoma	188 (33.4%)	98 (26.3%)	1468 (32.8%)	1754 (32.4%)	
MFH	5 (0.9%)	5 (1.3%)	96 (2.1%)	106 (2.0%)	
MPNST	6 (1.1%)	6 (1.6%)	42 (0.9%)	54 (1.0%)	
Rare/NOS	96 (17.1%)	90 (24.1%)	974 (21.8%)	1160 (21.5%)	
Grade					<0.0001
Missing	97	71	992	1160	
Well differentiated	172 (36.9%)	85 (28.1%)	1256 (36.1%)	1513 (35.6%)	
Mod differentiated	23 (4.9%)	38 (12.6%)	587 (16.9%)	648 (15.3%)	
Poorly differentiated	99 (21.2%)	111 (36.8%)	1019 (29.3%)	1229 (28.9%)	
Undifferentiated	172 (36.9%)	68 (22.5%)	617 (17.7%)	857 (20.2%)	
Tumor size					0.35
Missing	36	17	327	380	
5–10 cm	98 (18.6%)	80 (22.5%)	848 (20.5%)	1026 (20.4%)	
<5 cm	42 (8.0%)	27 (7.6%)	391 (9.4%)	460 (9.2%)	
>10 cm	387 (73.4%)	249 (69.9%)	2905 (70.1%)	3541 (70.4%)	
AJCC stage group					<0.0001
Stage I	180 (32.0%)	90 (24.1%)	1322 (29.6%)	1592 (29.4%)	
Stage II	49 (8.7%)	39 (10.5%)	560 (12.5%)	648 (12.0%)	
Stage III	204 (36.2%)	140 (37.5%)	1278 (28.6%)	1622 (30.0%)	
Stage IV	38 (6.7%)	20 (5.4%)	314 (7.0%)	372 (6.9%)	
AJCC staging not applicable	22 (3.9%)	27 (7.2%)	275 (6.2%)	324 (6.0%)	
AJCC stage group unknown	70 (12.4%)	57 (15.3%)	722 (16.1%)	849 (15.7%)	
Surgery					<0.0001
No	53 (9.4%)	73 (19.6%)	1198 (26.8%)	1324 (24.5%)	
Yes	510 (90.6%)	300 (80.4%)	3273 (73.2%)	4083 (75.5%)	
Radiation					<0.0001
Missing	0	1	79	80	
No	453 (80.5%)	293 (78.8%)	3196 (72.8%)	3942 (74.0%)	
Yes	110 (19.5%)	79 (21.2%)	1196 (27.2%)	1385 (26.0%)	
Chemotherapy					0.0001
Missing	6	11	188	205	
No	469 (84.2%)	270 (74.6%)	3569 (83.3%)	4308 (82.8%)	
Yes	88 (15.8%)	92 (25.4%)	714 (16.7%)	894 (17.2%)	
Last contact or death, months from Dx					0.68
Mean (SD)	41.7 (27.4)	42.3 (31.6)	43.8 (32.2)	43.5 (31.7)	
Median	37.6	35.8	37.2	37.1	
Q1, Q3	20.0, 58.0	16.8, 61.0	17.9, 64.8	18.1, 63.5	
Range	(0.6–133.1)	(1.2–132.5)	(0.0–142.6)	(0.0–142.6)	
Vital status					<0.0001
Dead	177 (31.4%)	151 (40.5%)	1954 (43.7%)	2282 (42.2%)	
Alive	386 (68.6%)	222 (59.5%)	2517 (56.3%)	3125 (57.8%)	
Hospital volume					<0.0001
Mean (SD)	153.7 (46.5)	62.6 (5.0)	14.4 (12.5)	32.2 (47.1)	
Median	134.0	64.0	10.0	13.0	
Q1, Q3	114.0, 212.0	62.0, 65.0	5.0, 22.0	6.0, 35.0	
Range	(103.0–212.0)	(51.0–68.0)	(1.0–47.0)	(1.0–212.0)	

Tables 1 and 2 also provide descriptive data stratified by annual volume (<5 cases, 5–10 cases, and >10 cases). The number of high-volume centers in the United States performing >10 primary surgical resections on average annually was only 3/678 (0.4%), while the overwhelming majority were low volume 671/678 (99%). Using the same volume cutoffs for all cases of primary RPS treated increased the high-volume centers to four. Correspondingly, low volume centers treated 83% of all patients and also performed 83% of all curative intent surgery, while the same proportion was 10% and 11% for high-volume centers. Overall, high-volume centers were all academic/research centers,

TABLE 2: Patient characteristics: all surgical cases.

	High volume (N = 401)	Medium volume (N = 235)	Low volume (N = 3167)	Total (N = 3803)	p value
Age at diagnosis					0.0045
Mean (SD)	59.6 (13.7)	58.7 (14.5)	61.2 (13.9)	60.9 (14.0)	
Median	60.0	60.0	62.0	62.0	
Q1, Q3	51.0, 69.0	50.0, 69.0	52.0, 71.0	52.0, 71.0	
Range	(20.0–90.0)	(19.0–87.0)	(18.0–90.0)	(18.0–90.0)	
Sex					0.0002
Male	216 (53.9%)	130 (55.3%)	1438 (45.4%)	1784 (46.9%)	
Female	185 (46.1%)	105 (44.7%)	1729 (54.6%)	2019 (53.1%)	
Race					0.0010
Black	21 (5.2%)	15 (6.4%)	350 (11.1%)	386 (10.1%)	
Other	22 (5.5%)	18 (7.7%)	184 (5.8%)	224 (5.9%)	
White	358 (89.3%)	202 (86.0%)	2633 (83.1%)	3193 (84.0%)	
Charlson–Deyo score					0.0061
0	336 (83.8%)	195 (83.0%)	2444 (77.2%)	2975 (78.2%)	
1	55 (13.7%)	34 (14.5%)	565 (17.8%)	654 (17.2%)	
2	10 (2.5%)	6 (2.6%)	158 (5.0%)	174 (4.6%)	
Year of diagnosis					0.20
2004	30 (7.5%)	12 (5.1%)	253 (8.0%)	295 (7.8%)	
2005	31 (7.7%)	19 (8.1%)	259 (8.2%)	309 (8.1%)	
2006	40 (10.0%)	18 (7.7%)	271 (8.6%)	329 (8.7%)	
2007	43 (10.7%)	18 (7.7%)	310 (9.8%)	371 (9.8%)	
2008	51 (12.7%)	22 (9.4%)	306 (9.7%)	379 (10.0%)	
2009	44 (11.0%)	22 (9.4%)	314 (9.9%)	380 (10.0%)	
2010	36 (9.0%)	22 (9.4%)	350 (11.1%)	408 (10.7%)	
2011	38 (9.5%)	42 (17.9%)	389 (12.3%)	469 (12.3%)	
2012	44 (11.0%)	36 (15.3%)	359 (11.3%)	439 (11.5%)	
2013	44 (11.0%)	24 (10.2%)	356 (11.2%)	424 (11.1%)	
Facility type					<0.0001
Missing	31	23	230	284	
Community cancer program	0 (0.0%)	0 (0.0%)	121 (4.1%)	121 (3.4%)	
Comprehensive community cancer program	0 (0.0%)	0 (0.0%)	913 (31.1%)	913 (25.9%)	
Academic/research program	370 (100.0%)	212 (100.0%)	1579 (53.8%)	2161 (61.4%)	
Integrated network cancer program	0 (0.0%)	0 (0.0%)	324 (11.0%)	324 (9.2%)	
Primary payor					<0.0001
Not insured	2 (0.5%)	9 (3.8%)	116 (3.7%)	127 (3.3%)	
Private insurance	175 (43.6%)	109 (46.4%)	1482 (46.8%)	1766 (46.4%)	
Medicaid	6 (1.5%)	18 (7.7%)	189 (6.0%)	213 (5.6%)	
Medicare	102 (25.4%)	96 (40.9%)	1300 (41.0%)	1498 (39.4%)	
Other government	3 (0.7%)	1 (0.4%)	43 (1.4%)	47 (1.2%)	
Insurance status unknown	113 (28.2%)	2 (0.9%)	37 (1.2%)	152 (4.0%)	
Median income quartiles					0.0002
Missing	24	11	119	154	
<$30,000	25 (6.6%)	14 (6.3%)	387 (12.7%)	426 (11.7%)	
$30,000–$35,999	61 (16.2%)	49 (21.9%)	521 (17.1%)	631 (17.3%)	
$36,000–$45,999	93 (24.7%)	61 (27.2%)	807 (26.5%)	961 (26.3%)	
$46,000+	198 (52.5%)	100 (44.6%)	1333 (43.7%)	1631 (44.7%)	
No high school degree quartiles (%)					0.0001
Missing	24	11	119	154	
≥29%	43 (11.4%)	20 (8.9%)	473 (15.5%)	536 (14.7%)	
20–28.9%	62 (16.4%)	55 (24.6%)	694 (22.8%)	811 (22.2%)	
14–19.9%	85 (22.5%)	61 (27.2%)	701 (23.0%)	847 (23.2%)	
<14%	187 (49.6%)	88 (39.3%)	1180 (38.7%)	1455 (39.9%)	
Distance to treating center (miles)					<0.0001
Mean (SD)	259.0 (433.2)	85.3 (149.5)	42.5 (145.9)	68.0 (208.0)	
Median	80.4	49.5	13.7	17.2	
Q1, Q3	22.9, 306.5	22.3, 100.3	5.4, 38.3	6.2, 50.8	
Range	(1.0–4040.1)	(1.0–1495.6)	(1.0–4710.1)	(1.0–4710.1)	

Table 2: Continued.

	High volume (N = 401)	Medium volume (N = 235)	Low volume (N = 3167)	Total (N = 3803)	p value
Histologic subtype					<0.0001
Dedifferentiated liposarcoma	125 (31.2%)	69 (29.4%)	585 (18.5%)	779 (20.5%)	
Fibrosarcoma	6 (1.5%)	4 (1.7%)	45 (1.4%)	55 (1.4%)	
Leiomyosarcoma	64 (16.0%)	38 (16.2%)	715 (22.6%)	817 (21.5%)	
Liposarcoma	143 (35.7%)	64 (27.2%)	1078 (34.0%)	1285 (33.8%)	
MFH	2 (0.5%)	4 (1.7%)	70 (2.2%)	76 (2.0%)	
MPNST	3 (0.7%)	2 (0.9%)	25 (0.8%)	30 (0.8%)	
Rare/NOS	58 (14.5%)	54 (23.0%)	649 (20.5%)	761 (20.0%)	
Grade					<0.0001
Missing	62	53	617	732	
Well differentiated	133 (39.2%)	53 (29.1%)	919 (36.0%)	1105 (36.0%)	
Mod differentiated	15 (4.4%)	19 (10.4%)	426 (16.7%)	460 (15.0%)	
Poorly differentiated	57 (16.8%)	53 (29.1%)	774 (30.4%)	884 (28.8%)	
Undifferentiated	134 (39.5%)	57 (31.3%)	431 (16.9%)	622 (20.3%)	
Tumor size					0.11
Missing	29	6	206	241	
5–10 cm	56 (15.1%)	55 (24.0%)	556 (18.8%)	667 (18.7%)	
<5 cm	29 (7.8%)	17 (7.4%)	236 (8.0%)	282 (7.9%)	
>10 cm	287 (77.2%)	157 (68.6%)	2169 (73.3%)	2613 (73.4%)	
AJCC stage group					0.016
Stage I	128 (31.9%)	63 (26.8%)	989 (31.2%)	1180 (31.0%)	
Stage II	38 (9.5%)	29 (12.3%)	409 (12.9%)	476 (12.5%)	
Stage III	158 (39.4%)	96 (40.9%)	1044 (33.0%)	1298 (34.1%)	
AJCC staging not applicable	17 (4.2%)	18 (7.7%)	196 (6.2%)	231 (6.1%)	
AJCC stage group unknown	60 (15.0%)	29 (12.3%)	529 (16.7%)	618 (16.3%)	
Margins					0.0001
Missing	153	43	810	1006	
Grossly positive (R2)	6 (2.4%)	6 (3.1%)	128 (5.4%)	140 (5.0%)	
Microscopically positive (R1)	40 (16.1%)	61 (31.8%)	621 (26.3%)	722 (25.8%)	
Negative (R0)	202 (81.5%)	125 (65.1%)	1608 (68.2%)	1935 (69.2%)	
30-day mortality					0.027
Patient alive or died more than 30 days after surgery performed	399 (99.5%)	232 (98.7%)	3090 (97.6%)	3721 (97.8%)	
Patient died 30 or fewer days after surgery performed	2 (0.5%)	3 (1.3%)	77 (2.4%)	82 (2.2%)	
90-day mortality					0.0012
Patient alive or died more than 90 days after surgery performed	396 (98.8%)	220 (93.6%)	3000 (94.7%)	3616 (95.1%)	
Patient died 90 or fewer days after surgery performed	5 (1.2%)	15 (6.4%)	167 (5.3%)	187 (4.9%)	
Hospital volume					<0.0001
Mean (SD)	143.5 (38.4)	60.9 (12.1)	12.8 (11.2)	29.5 (44.0)	
Median	108.0	53.0	8.0	11.0	
Q1, Q3	108.0, 185.0	53.0, 78.0	4.0, 18.0	5.0, 32.0	
Range	(108.0–185.0)	(51.0–78.0)	(1.0–45.0)	(1.0–185.0)	

whereas approximately 24% of low-volume centers met that CoC designation. High-volume centers were more likely to provide care to males, Caucasians, those with lower Charlson–Deyo scores, and those who lived in high educational attainment zip codes. The median distance travelled for treatment at a high-volume hospital was 76 miles, compared to 12 miles for a low-volume hospital. High-volume centers were more likely to treat patients whose tumors were larger (17.5 cm versus 15 cm) and of higher grade (58% versus 47%) than low-volume centers. It is important to note that, since the NCDB does not report recurrence, these data only reflect the management of primary RPS and do not provide insight into the management of recurrent RPS.

3.2. Short-Term Outcomes (Surgery-Only Cohort). A total of 82 patients (2.2%) died within 30 days after surgery was performed. The absolute 30-day mortality rates were 0.5%, 1.3%, and 2.4% at high, medium, and low volume centers, respectively. Following adjustment (Table 3), patients undergoing RPS surgery at a low-volume hospital had a greater

TABLE 3: Logistic regression analysis of 30-day postoperative mortality.

Variable	Odds ratio	95% Wald Confidence limits		p value
Age	1.06	1.04	1.09	<0.0001
Female (reference = male)	0.92	0.61	1.40	0.71
Race (reference = white)				
Black	1.16	0.56	2.39	0.69
Other	0.74	0.23	2.37	0.61
Charlson–Deyo (reference = 2)				
0	1.13	0.65	1.95	0.66
1	1.67	0.79	3.50	0.18
Hospital volume (reference = high)				
Medium	2.73	0.65	11.51	0.17
Low	4.66	2.26	9.63	<0.0001

TABLE 4: Logistic regression analysis of *R*0 margin status.

Variable	Odds ratio	95% Wald Confidence limits		p value
Age	0.98	0.98	0.99	<0.0001
Female (reference = male)	1.11	0.94	1.31	0.215
Race (reference = white)				
Black	1.20	0.90	1.60	0.21
Other	0.98	0.69	1.40	0.93
Charlson–Deyo (reference = 2)				
0	0.86	0.69	1.07	0.19
1	0.76	0.51	1.13	0.17
Hospital volume (reference = high)				
Medium	0.38	0.21	0.70	0.0019
Low	0.46	0.31	0.70	0.0003

than fourfold increase in the risk of dying within 30 days of surgery compared to patients undergoing surgery at a high-volume hospital (OR = 4.66, 95% CI 2.26–9.63; $p < 0.001$). On sensitivity analyses, 90-day mortality rates followed a similar trend for absolute and adjusted risk of post-operative mortality.

The overall *R*0 margin rate was 69%. The *R*0 rate was 82%, 65%, and 68% for high-, medium-, and low-volume centers, respectively. Table 4 displays the multivariable analysis for *R*0 margin rate; low-volume centers were less likely to achieve *R*0 margin status compared to high-volume centers (OR = 0.46, 95% CI 0.31–0.70; $P = 0.0003$).

3.3. Long-Term Outcomes (All Cases). The median follow-up to last contact or death is 37 months. There were 2,282 deaths (42%) from all causes over the duration of the study. For all RPS patients, the 5-year overall survival was 57.1% (95% CI 55.6–58.7%). When stratified by the hospital volume, the 5-year overall survival for high-, medium-, and low-volume centers was 66%, 57%, and 56% ($p < 0.001$; Figure 1(a)). For RPS patients who underwent surgical resection for curative intent, the 5-year overall survival rate was 58.6% (95% CI 56.8–60.5). When stratified by the hospital volume, the 5-year overall survival rates for patients undergoing curative intent surgery in high-, medium-, and low-volume centers was 69%, 56%, and 57%, respectively ($p < 0.001$; Figure 1(b)).

Table 5 displays the multivariable analysis for overall survival. After controlling for patient and tumor variables, patients who were treated at a low-volume hospital had a 52% greater risk of all-cause long-term mortality compared to those treated at a high-volume hospital (HR 1.56, 95% CI 1.16–2.11; $p = 0.0032$).

4. Discussion

In this study of patients diagnosed with primary RPS, we show that patients treated at high-volume centers were four times less likely to die within 30 days of the procedure, 54% more likely to have an *R*0 margin status, and 52% more likely to be alive by the end of follow-up when compared to patients in low-volume centers. These results are consistent with a strong volume-outcome association for RPS for both short- and long-term outcomes.

Hospital surgical volume has been suggested to be a proxy for superior outcomes for multiple complex surgical oncologic procedures. Although surgical volume in itself impacts outcomes, it is likely that case volume is also associated with the quality of other processes at the institution. Optimal outcomes in this disease require team-based multidisciplinary care including medical oncology, radiation oncology, radiology, and pathology. The rarity of RPS means that tumor boards, compliance to NCCN guidelines, and coordination of survivorship care are all likely to contribute to better oncologic outcomes. For patients who did undergo surgery, the complexity of the surgical procedure requires processes designed to optimize perioperative care and manage complications such as subspecialty trained surgical oncologists, urologists, vascular surgeons, tertiary anesthesiologists, interventional radiologists, and critical care teams to optimize short-term outcomes. It is likely that increased surgical volume allows for a gain in proficiency both within the operating room as well as at the institutional level, which translates into better perioperative outcomes.

Although an argument could be made that our choice of cutoff to define what constitutes a high-volume institution is somewhat arbitrary, and this is consistent with another large study on the subject. The Transatlantic Retroperitoneal Sarcoma Working Group (TARPSWG) has published on 1,007 primary RPS patients treated in eight North American and European sarcoma centers from 2002 to 2011 [8, 9]. These centers are considered high volume and as a group averaged approximately 12 cases/year, similar to the threshold in this study. When we compare high-volume centers identified in the current study to the TARPSWG, we note other similarities in the outcomes measured. The group investigated the safety of resection of primary RPS and

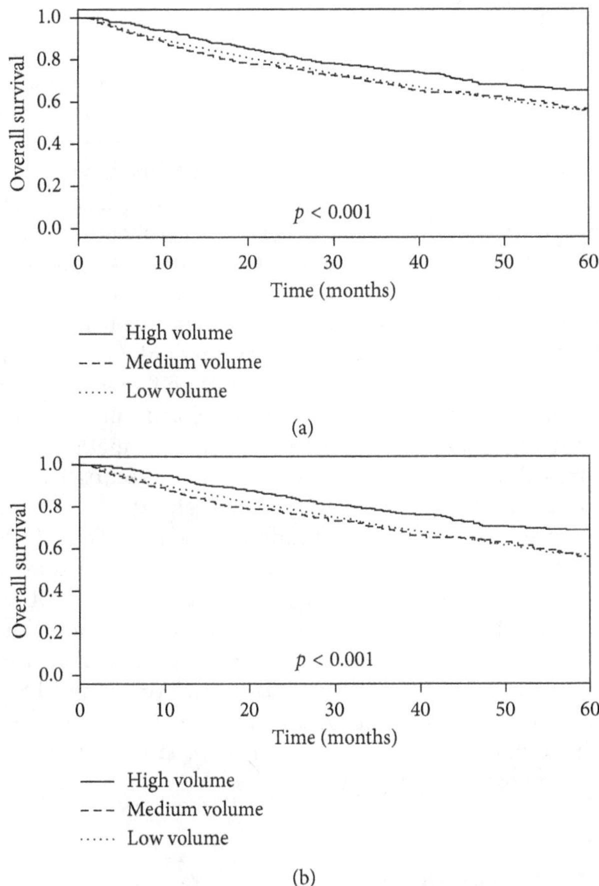

FIGURE 1: Overall survival stratified by hospital volume. (a) All cases. (b) Surgical cases.

TABLE 5: Cox regression model for overall survival: all patients.

Variable	Odds ratio	95% Wald Confidence limits		p value
Age	1.02	1.02	1.03	<0.0001
Female (reference = male)	0.79	0.72	0.87	<0.0001
Race (reference = white)				
Black	0.81	0.69	0.96	0.015
Other	0.88	0.71	1.09	0.23
Insurance (reference = private)				
Medicaid	1.38	1.11	1.70	0.0034
Medicare	1.14	1.00	1.30	0.056
No insured	1.38	1.07	1.79	0.014
Other government	1.18	0.75	1.86	0.47
Unknown	1.23	0.85	1.78	0.28
No high school degree (reference ≥ 29%)				
<14%	0.77	0.67	0.90	0.0007
14–19.9%	0.86	0.73	1.00	0.055
20–28.9%	0.92	0.79	1.08	0.30
Charlson-Deyo (reference = 2)				
0	0.72	0.58	0.88	0.0011
1	0.81	0.65	1.01	0.055
Tumor size (reference = <5 cm)				
5–10 cm	1.02	0.83	1.25	0.85
>10 cm	1.43	1.19	1.73	0.0001
Grade (reference = grade 3)				
Grade 1	0.34	0.28	0.40	<0.0001
Grade 2	0.52	0.44	0.61	<0.0001
Unknown	0.64	0.56	0.73	<0.0001
Margins (reference = $R0$)				
$R1$	1.31	1.15	1.49	<0.0001
$R2$	2.18	1.73	2.75	<0.0001
Unknown	1.61	1.44	1.80	<0.0001
Surgery (reference = yes)				
No	0.93	0.83	1.04	0.21
Radiation (reference = yes)				
No	0.80	0.72	0.90	<0.0001
Chemotherapy (reference = yes)				
No	1.26	1.11	1.42	0.0004
Hospital volume (reference = high)				
Medium	1.44	0.98	2.10	0.064
Low	1.57	1.16	2.11	0.0032

reported that Clavien–Dindo ≥3 events occurred in 16% of patients and that the 30-day mortality was 1.8%. In the current study, high-volume centers had a 30-day mortality of 0.5%, suggesting that the cutoff used in the current study may be appropriate to optimize 30-day mortality.

The TARPSWG also studied oncologic outcomes on the same patients and reported an $R0/R1$ resection rate of 95%. In the current study, high-volume centers had a comparable $R0/R1$ resection rate of 98%; when the negative margin was defined by assessment of microscopic disease; high-volume centers were significantly more likely to achieve $R0$ resection than low-volume centers. However, it should be noted that, since microscopic assessment of the entire tumor surface is not feasible, not all institutions routinely report microscopic margin status. Indeed, approximately 26% of all surgical cases had missing margin data, and therefore, extraction of margin information from pathology reports and subsequent reporting to the NCDB for RPS will need to be improved. Finally, TARPSWG reported a 5-year overall survival rate of 67%, which compares with the 69% seen in our study for high-volume centers. Overall, the comparison with the TARPSWG data suggests that high-volume centers both within and outside of the United States have comparable outcomes.

A review of soft tissue sarcomas identified in the Florida Cancer Data System (FCDS) suggested that high-volume centers—defined as ≥ 5 surgical cases/year—had superior 30-day mortality and 5-year overall survival [10]. Subset analysis of truncal/retroperitoneal sarcomas ($n = 1.745$) showed improved 5-year overall survival for high-volume centers (low volume, 32% versus high volume, 36%). Margin status was not available for analysis. When compared to the 5-year overall survival observed at high-volume centers in the current study and in the TARPSWG study (67% and 69%, resp.), the FCDS study reported a lower 5-year overall survival at high-volume centers (36%). This large difference in overall survival highlights the importance of establishing a cutoff (10 versus 5 cases in this instance) that offers better outcomes for RPS patients.

The association between institutional volume and improved outcomes has been used to advocate regionalization of complex procedures to high-volume centers. Even in the absence of health care policy change, this phenomenon had been observed for a variety of cancer types requiring complex surgery [11, 12]. Finks et al. used Medicare data to examine trends in hospital volume and the proportion of patients undergoing surgical resection in high-volume centers. The authors reported that regionalization of complex cancer resections appears to have occurred in the decade following reports that there is an inverse relationship between hospital volume and outcomes [11]. In the context of regionalization, it is important to note that, in our study, only 3 hospitals met the threshold for high volume (>10 surgical cases/year on average) out of a hospital cohort of 678. However, it is also important to note that the data presented in this study refer to treatment of primary RPS and not recurrent disease. Multiple reports from large volume centers suggest that resection of recurrent RPS constitutes approximately 32–44% of their RPS patient population [13–15]. Since the NCDB does not record recurrence and surgery for recurrence, the number of high-volume centers managing and resecting RPS is certainly underestimated by the current data. Nevertheless, the number of high-volume centers appears to be low, and further research will be needed, likely using qualitative or mixed methods, to investigate why significant regionalization has not occurred with regard to RPS. One clue may be the proximity of patients to a high-volume center. The median distance travelled for treatment at a high-volume center was 76 miles compared to 12 miles for a low-volume center. Whether this was due to referral networks, patient education/income insurance contracts, or other factors is unknown.

In this study, only 3 hospitals qualified as high-volume centers. All commission on cancer-approved hospitals are required to report to the NCDB, and these cancer diagnoses account for 70% of new cancers diagnosed in the United States. Since the cancer programs that report to the NCDB include 19 of 20 National Comprehensive Cancer Network (NCCN) hospitals, 33 or 37 NCI-designated cancer centers, and 69 of 121 major inpatient VA hospitals, it is likely that our study captures most of the major sarcoma centers in the US. One likely explanation for only identifying 3 high-volume hospitals is that the current study only reports treatment for primary RPS and not recurrent RPS. Multiple retrospective studies from large sarcoma centers report that treatment of locally recurrent RPS accounts for 24–35% of all RPS cases [13, 14, 16]. It is highly likely that the inclusion of recurrent RPS would increase the number of high-volume centers and that the current analysis underestimates the number of high-volume centers.

A limitation of this study is that it does not provide surgeon-specific volume data. There is evidence that a surgeon's volume is what drives good outcomes, and that when a surgeon relocates, those good outcomes also relocate to the new institution. Whether this is true for rare malignancy such as RPS is not entirely clear. Another limitation is that the NCDB does not contain ECOG performance status, American Society of Anesthesiologists physical status level, and other indicators of functional status. It does contain components of the Charlson Comorbidity Index which allows for a certain degree of adjustment for functional status. The NCDB also does not report the number of organs resected, the number of intestinal anastomoses, and postoperative complications, and therefore, we cannot comment on complexity of the surgery performed at the institutions. Many of the RPS histologic subtypes were unknown. Recent data suggest that RPS histologic subtype influences pattern of failure and death [8]. Whether histologic subtype influenced the results for high-volume centers cannot be determined. The NCDB also does not report on recurrence and disease-specific mortality. RPS has a high rate of local recurrence, and whether institutional volume affects local recurrence and disease-specific death cannot be ascertained. Moreover, the number of patients undergoing treatment for recurrent RPS cannot be determined, and therefore, the actual patient volume per institution is underestimated in this analysis. Finally, since re-resection for recurrent RPS is not captured in this study, and there may be a separate volume-outcome association that may be stronger than the one we observe for primary tumors.

5. Conclusions

Despite superior short- and long-term outcomes for high-volume institutions treating RPS, the overwhelming majority of patients continue to be seen at low-volume institutions. While it may be impractical to regionalize all RPS care to the few existing high-volume institutions, there is certainly room for consolidation. Other efforts to disseminate expertise, such as remote tumor boards, centralizing pathology review such as seen in Europe, visits by expert surgeons, and telemedicine may need to be explored.

References

[1] C. B. Begg, L. D. Cramer, W. J. Hoskins, and M. F. Brennan, "Impact of hospital volume on operative mortality for major cancer surgery," *JAMA*, vol. 280, no. 20, pp. 1747–1751, 1998.

[2] P. B. Bach, L. D. Cramer, D. Schrag, R. J. Downey, S. E. Gelfand, and C. B. Begg, "The influence of hospital volume on survival after resection for lung cancer," *New England Journal of Medicine*, vol. 345, no. 3, pp. 181–188, 2001.

[3] J. D. Birkmeyer, A. E. Siewers, E. V. Finlayson et al., "Hospital volume and surgical mortality in the United States," *New England Journal of Medicine*, vol. 346, no. 15, pp. 1128–1137, 2002.

[4] B. E. Hillner, T. J. Smith, and C. E. Desch, "Hospital and physician volume or specialization and outcomes in cancer treatment: importance in quality of cancer care," *Journal of Clinical Oncology*, vol. 18, no. 11, pp. 2327–2340, 2000.

[5] Y. Fong, M. Gonen, D. Rubin, M. Radzyner, and M. F. Brennan, "Long-term survival is superior after resection for cancer in high-volume centers," *Annals of Surgery*, vol. 242, no. 4, pp. 544–547, 2005.

[6] D. Schrag, L. D. Cramer, P. B. Bach, A. M. Cohen, J. L. Warren, and C. B. Begg, "Influence of hospital procedure volume on outcomes following surgery for colon cancer," *JAMA*, vol. 284, no. 23, pp. 3028–3035, 2000.

[7] M. Sun, M. Bianchi, Q. D. Trinh et al., "Hospital volume is a determinant of postoperative complications, blood transfusion and length of stay after radical or partial nephrectomy," *Journal of Urology*, vol. 187, no. 2, pp. 405–410, 2012.

[8] A. Gronchi, D. C. Strauss, R. Miceli et al., "Variability in patterns of recurrence after resection of primary retroperitoneal sarcoma (RPS): a report on 1007 patients from the multi-institutional collaborative RPS working group," *Annals of Surgery*, vol. 263, no. 5, pp. 1002–1009, 2016.

[9] A. J. MacNeill, A. Gronchi, R. Miceli et al., "Postoperative morbidity after radical resection of primary retroperitoneal sarcoma: a report from the transatlantic RPS working group," *Annals of Surgery*, vol. 267, no. 5, p. 1, 2017.

[10] J. C. Gutierrez, E. A. Perez, F. L. Moffat, A. S. Livingstone, D. Franceschi, and L. G. Koniaris, "Should soft tissue sarcomas be treated at high-volume centers? an analysis of 4205 patients," *Annals of Surgery*, vol. 245, no. 6, pp. 952–958, 2007.

[11] J. F. Finks, N. H. Osborne, and J. D. Birkmeyer, "Trends in hospital volume and operative mortality for high-risk surgery," *New England Journal of Medicine*, vol. 364, no. 22, pp. 2128–2137, 2011.

[12] P. A. Learn and P. B. Bach, "A decade of mortality reductions in major oncologic surgery the impact of centralization and quality improvement," *Medical Care*, vol. 48, no. 12, pp. 1041–1049, 2010.

[13] J. J. Lewis, D. Leung, J. M. Woodruff, and M. F. Brennan, "Retroperitoneal soft-tissue sarcoma: analysis of 500 patients treated and followed at a single institution," *Annals of Surgery*, vol. 228, no. 3, pp. 355–365, 1998.

[14] T. Lehnert, S. Cardona, U. Hinz et al., "Primary and locally recurrent retroperitoneal soft-tissue sarcoma: local control and survival," *European Journal of Surgical Oncology (EJSO)*, vol. 35, no. 9, pp. 986–993, 2009.

[15] D. A. Anaya, G. Lahat, J. Liu et al., "Multifocality in retroperitoneal sarcoma: a prognostic factor critical to surgical decision-making," *Annals of Surgery*, vol. 249, no. 1, pp. 137–142, 2009.

[16] A. Gronchi, R. Miceli, C. Colombo et al., "Frontline extended surgery is associated with improved survival in retroperitoneal low- to intermediate-grade soft tissue sarcomas," *Annals of Oncology*, vol. 23, no. 4, pp. 1067–1073, 2012.

23

Multimodal Approach of Pulmonary Artery Intimal Sarcoma

S. Secondino,[1] V. Grazioli,[2] F. Valentino,[1] M. Pin,[2] A. Pagani,[1] A. Sciortino,[2] C. Klersy,[3] M. G. Callegari,[4] P. Morbini,[5] R. Dore,[6] M. Paulli,[5] P. Pedrazzoli,[1] and A. M. D'armini[2]

[1]*Division of Medical Oncology, Fondazione IRCCS Policlinico San Matteo, Pavia, Italy*
[2]*Cardiothoracic Surgery Department, Fondazione IRCCS Policlinico San Matteo and Pavia University School of Medicine, Pavia, Italy*
[3]*Service of Biometry & Statistics, Fondazione IRCCS Policlinico San Matteo, Pavia, Italy*
[4]*Unit of Pulmonary Rehabilitation, ICS Maugeri Istituto Scientifico di Montescano, Pavia, Italy*
[5]*Unit of Pathology, Fondazione IRCCS Policlinico San Matteo and Pavia University School of Medicine, Pavia, Italy*
[6]*Division of Radiology, Fondazione IRCCS Policlinico San Matteo, Pavia, Italy*

Correspondence should be addressed to S. Secondino; s.secondino@smatteo.pv.it

Academic Editor: Akira Kawai

Introduction. Pulmonary artery sarcoma (PAS) is a rare tumor, whose therapeutic approach is mainly based on surgery, either pneumonectomy or pulmonary endarterectomy (PEA). The prognosis reported in published series is very poor, with survival of 1.5 months without any kind of treatment. *Patients and Methods*. From January 2010 to January 2016, 1027 patients were referred to our hospital for symptoms of acute or chronic pulmonary thromboembolic disease. Twelve patients having a confirmed diagnosis of PAS underwent PEA. Median age was 64.5 years. Most patients had a long history of symptoms, having a median time of 7.5 months from onset of symptoms to surgery. *Results*. Following PEA and cardiopulmonary rehabilitation, 10 patients received conventional chemotherapy with doxorubicin and ifosfamide, starting at a median of 42 days from surgery. Four patients also received radiotherapy. Four patients have died due to disease progression, while 7 are still alive, with 5 being disease-free at 4–55+ months from diagnosis. *Conclusions*. In patients with PAS, a multimodal approach including PEA, CT, and RT is feasible but it should be evaluated individually, according to the tumor extension and the patient's clinical condition. Apart from improving quality of life mainly by reducing or delaying symptoms due to PH, it may improve life expectancy.

1. Introduction

Pulmonary artery sarcoma (PAS) was first described in 1923 [1]. Since that time, about 300 PAS have been reported in the English-language literature, as case reports or small series. Primary PAS is the most frequent sarcoma of the great arteries [2], in most cases arising in the area derived from the embryologic bulbus cordis, which leads to PAS predominantly occurring in the main pulmonary artery [3] which is involved in 80% of cases: the left pulmonary artery in 58%, the right pulmonary artery in 57%, both arteries in 37%, the pulmonary valve in 29%, and the right ventricle in 8%.

Primary PAS are classified by location as either luminal or mural in origin and then further subclassified histologically. Luminal PAS are thought to derive from pluripotential mesenchymal cells of the intima, while mural sarcomas, less frequent than luminal sarcomas, can be difficult to distinguish from sarcomas of the lung parenchyma due to their growing; they are more likely to appear as mass-like lesions [4]. PAS typically affect middle-aged people, favoring women slightly. Common symptoms at time of presentation often mirror those of pulmonary embolism, including progressive dyspnea, cough, and chest pain [3]. However, symptoms onset is usually more gradual with PAS than pulmonary embolism.

Given the rarity of PAS, only case reports and small series have been published, with the majority focusing on histopathological features and surgical management of the disease [4–7]. Surgery remains the mainstay of management

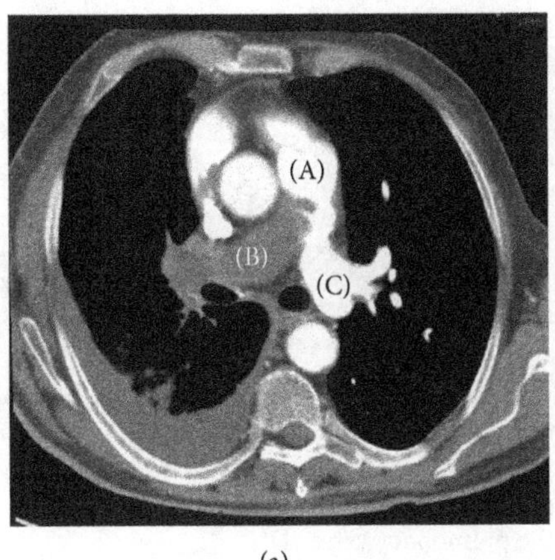

(a)

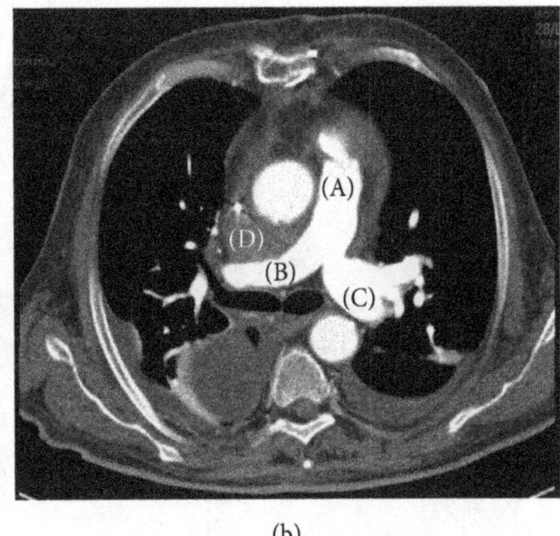

(b)

FIGURE 1: *CT scan of patient number 10*. (a) Presurgical CT scan: right pulmonary artery completely occluded by soft tissue mass (B); proximal aspect of the mass in the pulmonary trunk (A); left pulmonary artery appears preserved (C). (b) Postsurgical CT scan (same level): the intra-arterial mass has been completely removed. Small mediastinal haematoma (D) between ascending aorta and right pulmonary artery.

of patients with PAS and can include pulmonary endarterectomy (PEA), lobectomy, or pneumonectomy, based on the extension of the disease and patient clinical conditions [5, 7, 8]. The prognosis reported in published study is extremely poor, with survival of 1.5 months without surgical resection and 17 months in case of surgery [7–10]. The role of additional chemotherapy (CT) and radiotherapy (RT) after surgical resections remains largely unproven.

In this study, we report our single-institution experience concerning the management of 12 consecutive patients with PAS who were referred to our institution over a period of 6 years period and have been treated with PEA and subsequent CT and RT. A recently published survey has included 20 patients diagnosed over a 14-year period [8], with 14 being treated with PEA.

2. Patients and Methods

Among 1027 patients referred to our Cardiac Surgery Unit for suspected chronic pulmonary hypertension (PH) potentially requiring PEA from January 2010 to January 2016, 574 had a confirmed PH and 448 underwent TEAP. Twenty-two patients had a radiological diagnosis of suspected tumor growing in the pulmonary artery by high-resolution CT scan of the thorax, which is performed within a conventional work-up for chronic thromboembolic PI. CT scan revealed soft tissue masses (Figure 1) occluding the artery; it demonstrated high- or low-attenuation areas consistent with hemorrhage or necrosis, soft tissue density, and variable contrast enhancement, thus suggesting a tumor mass over thrombus [3]. Two patients (numbers 3 and 11) underwent also FDG-PET, resulting in a significant FDG uptake.

All these patients had symptoms of acute or chronic thromboembolic disease. Among 22 patients with radiological diagnosis of tumor, 20 were eligible for surgery: eight patients had metastatic involvement of the pulmonary artery, arising in other sites not yet diagnosed. Twelve patients had PAS at pathology evaluation.

Two patients were referred for chemotherapy due to the presence of nonresectable tumor mass.

The median age of patients undergoing PEA for PAS was 64.5 years (range: 32–84); 9 patients were female. 9 patients had a bilateral disease and 3 had a metastatic disease involving the lung. In most cases (8 patients), the disease involved the main pulmonary artery. Nine patients had pulmonary hypertension (PH), with two with severe hemodynamic instability requiring emergency surgical treatment. Most patients had a long history of symptoms due to pulmonary hypertension, with the median time between onset of symptoms and surgery being 7.5 months (range: 2–33). Relevant patient characteristics are summarized in Table 1. All patients had given their written informed consent to use their data, as approved by the Institutional Ethical Board.

2.1. Surgery. All patients underwent PEA, using a technique identical to that adopted for chronic thromboembolic pulmonary hypertension. As previously described [11], the surgical approach is a median sternotomy and PEA is performed using cardiopulmonary bypass (CPB) and moderate hypothermic ventricular fibrillation. The main pulmonary arteries are sectioned longitudinally, and the dissection plane is accurately identified. Our surgical technique has been the same as that reported in published studies, with some technical changes (e.g., the aorta is left unclamped to reduce the potential risk of embolization of aortic atherosclerotic plaques and myocardial protection relies on hypothermia, left ventricular venting, and frequent reperfusion sections) [12]. The cerebral protection strategy has changed over time mainly to reduce the burden of hypothermic circulatory arrest and currently consists of short periods (7–10 minutes) of moderate hypothermic circulatory arrest followed by short periods (≥5 minutes) of reperfusion, with monitoring using cerebral near-infrared spectroscopy to determine the length of each reperfusion period. At the end of PEA, the left ventricular vent is clamped, and bronchoscopy is performed to verify the absence of airway bleeding. After weaning from

TABLE 1: Patient characteristics ($N = 12$).

Variables	Number of patients (%)
Gender	
(i) Female	9 (75%)
(ii) Male	3 (25%)
Median age	64,5 (range: 32–84)
(i) Male	77 (range: 32–84)
(ii) Female	64 (range: 37–77)
Symptoms	
(i) Dyspnea	10 (83.3%)
(ii) Chest pain	7 (58.3%)
(iii) Cough	2 (16.6%)
(iv) Hemoptysis	2 (16.6%)
(v) Fever	2 (16.6%)
(vi) Cardiovascular event	2 (16.6%)
Dyspnea WHO classification	
(i) II	7 (58.3%)
(ii) III	2 (16.6%)
(iii) IV	3 (25%)
Pulmonary hypertension	
(i) Mild (25–40 mmH)	0
(ii) Moderate (41–55 mmH)	4 (33.3%)
(iii) Severe (>56 mmH)	6 (50%)
Disease stage	
(i) Local disease	9 (75%)
(ii) Metastatic disease	3 (25%)
Histology grading	
(i) G1	0
(ii) G2	5 (41.6%)
(iii) G3	7 (58.3%)
Hospital stay (days)*	
(i) ≤7	0
(ii) >7<15	8 (72.7%)
(iii) ≥15	3 (27.2%)

*Excluding the patient who died after PEA due to cardiovascular event.

CPB, the pericardium is closed to reduce the formation of adhesions and improve postoperative right ventricular function [12].

Pathology evaluation revealed intimal sarcoma of pulmonary artery, being undifferentiated in 7 cases (Table 2). Three patients had pulmonary valve involvement requiring pulmonary valve replacement in two cases and peeling with curettage in one case (Figure 2). One patient (number 12) died after surgery due to cardiovascular complications. After PEA, all patients had a short course of cardiopulmonary rehabilitation.

One patient (number 6) underwent surgical resection of single-lung metastasis 30 days after PEA.

2.2. Chemotherapy and Radiotherapy. Following surgery and cardiologic workup, eligible patients received conventional

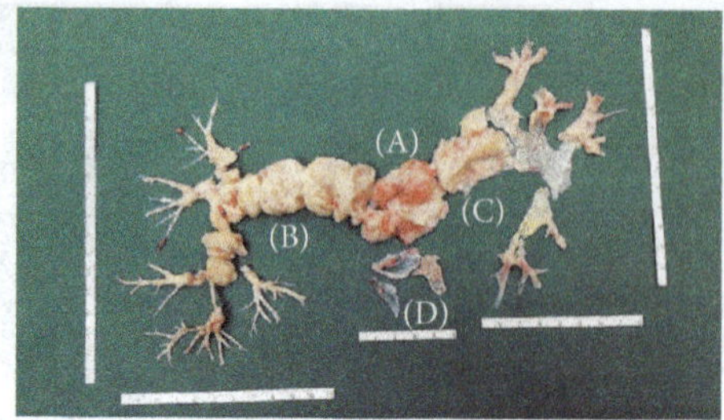

FIGURE 2: Pathological specimen after pulmonary endarterectomy of patient number 10. There is evidence of the tumor growth into the pulmonary artery, particularly the pulmonary trunk (A), the right pulmonary artery (B), and the left pulmonary artery (C); peeling of the pulmonary valve (D).

CT with doxorubicin (20 mg/mq a day, for three consecutive days) and ifosfamide (3000 mg/mq a day, for three consecutive days) for up to six cycles as adjuvant treatment of both local disease and metastatic cancer.

From 2014 onwards, the protocol was modified based on published evidence [7] and patients with local disease were given 4 cycles of the same CT regimen followed by intensity modulated RT (IMRT) at a radical dose of 60 Gy in 30 fractions to surgical bed.

Follow-up after completion of the multimodal approach consisted of high-resolution CT scan of the thorax and CT scan of the abdomen every 4 months during the first year and every 6 months thereafter.

2.3. Statistics. Data were described with median and range if they were continuous and counts and % if they were categorical. The Kaplan-Meier cumulative survival was computed and plotted; median survival was reported. Median follow-up (25th–75th percentiles) was computed with the inverse Kaplan-Meier method. Stata 14 (College Station, TX, USA) was used for computation.

3. Results

The median length of hospital stay for surgery was 13 days (range: 10–22). One patient (number 1) developed neurological defects due to cerebral anoxia requiring long-lasting neurological rehabilitation with partial recovery (lasting memory defects). Atrial fibrillation and anemia requiring blood transfusion were observed in two patients (numbers 5 and 10): one also having haemothorax (patient number 10) and one with mild renal failure (number 5).

Notwithstanding the cardiac surgery, no patient had cardiac dysfunction contraindicating the administration of anthracycline-containing CT.

Ten patients received CT with doxorubicin and ifosfamide starting at a median of 42 days (range: 22–69) after surgery. Nine have completed the planned schedule of CT, receiving a median of 5 cycles (range: 4–6); one patient received only 2 cycles due to early evidence of disease progression. One patient (number 1) did not receive postsurgery CT due to neurologic complications occurring in

TABLE 2: Main characteristics and outcomes of the patients.

Patients (*N*)	Sex Age	Symptoms duration (months)	Symptoms	Date of diagnoses	Histologic type (differentiation)/grading	Site(s) of disease	IP (PAPS) mmHg	Treatment after surgery	Time from surgery to CT (days)	*N* cycles of CT	Disease status	Overall survival (months)
1	F 45	9	Dyspnea Right cardiac failure	2010	IS (fibrosarcoma) G2	Local M+ (lung, kidney, nodes)	85	CT*	10 months*	NA	PD	26†
2	F 65	2	Pain Cough	2011	IS (osteocondroid diff) G2	Local (bilateral)	45	CT	50	6	NED	55
3	M 32	9	Fever Pain Dyspnea	2012	IS (undiff) G3	Local (unilateral)	65	CT	22	6	PD	6†
4	F 74	8	Dyspnea Pain	2012	IS (fibrous histiocytoma diff) G3	Local (unilateral)	—	CT	48	6	PD	8†
5	F 77	7	Dyspnea Pain Cough Hemoptysis	2012	IS (mixofibrous diff) G2	Local M+ (lung)	>60	CT	69	2	PD	6†
6	F 49	33	Dyspnea	2013	IS (leiomuscolar diff) G2	Local M+ (lung)	90	CT	42	5	NED	28
7	F 64	15	Dyspnea Pain Dysesthesia	2014	IS (undiff) G3	Local (bilateral)	45	CT/RT	30	4	NED	21
8	M 77	2	Dyspnea Pain	2015	IS (undiff) G3	Local (bilateral)	100	CT/RT	25	4	PR	11
9	F 49	2	Heart failure	2015	IS (undiff) G3	Local (bilateral)	45	CT/RT	36	4	NED	10
10	M 84	4	Dyspnea Pain	2015	IS (undiff) G2	Local (bilateral)	70	CT	44	4	PD	8
11	F 37	6	Dyspnea Hemoptysis	2016	IS (osteosarcoma diff) G3	Local (bilateral)	—	CT	30	4	NED	4

IS: intimal sarcoma; M+: metastatic disease; CT: chemotherapy (adriamycin and ifosfamide); RT: radiotherapy; NA: not applicable; PD: progressive disease; NED: not evidence of disease; PR: partial response.
†Patient died. *CT was given at disease progression. The patient who died perioperatively was excluded.

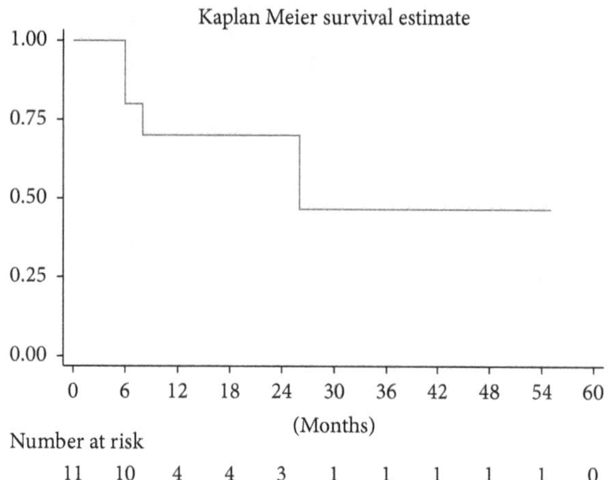

FIGURE 3: *Overall survival of patients with pulmonary artery sarcoma.* Kaplan-Meier survival estimate for patients in the series ($n = 11$), except one who died after surgery.

the rehabilitation phase and was treated at disease recurrence 10 months after PEA.

Overall CT was well tolerated; grade III/IV neutropenia (prophylactic G-CSF was administered in all patients) was observed in 2 patients and grade II mucositis in 1 patient. One patient (number 7) required hospital admission for reversible encephalopathy due to ifosfamide. Four patients underwent IMRT at the end of the CT program, starting at a median of 49 days (range: 49–63) from the end of chemotherapy. With a median follow-up of 21 months, no cardiac complications have been observed.

The median follow-up after surgery was 21 months (25th–75th percentiles, 10–28 months). Four patients have died due to disease progression at 6, 6, 8, and 24 months from surgery, while 7 patients are still alive, with 5 being disease-free at 4, 10, 21, 28, and 55 months from diagnosis. The median survival time was 26 months (Figure 3).

4. Discussion

PAS is a rare disease mimicking acute or chronic thromboembolic disease often causing delay in diagnosis and thus surgical and medical treatment [5, 7, 13–15]. Some specific characteristics can lead to correct differential diagnosis, including the absence of clinical status improvement or mass size reduction after anticoagulant therapy, the absence of thrombophilic risk factors, and the bulky central angiographic presentation [5, 9, 14–16]. However, in our experience, including the present series, patients have been diagnosed with PAS in most cases after being referred for long-lasting PH thought to be of thrombotic origin and therefore potentially requiring PEA. All radiological diagnoses of PAS by high-resolution CT scan of the thorax were confirmed at surgery and pathological examination. We previously reported [5] that PH is a sign of bilateral disease, even in case of a unilateral CT pattern. This is confirmed by the present series as ten out of twelve patients had PH (median: 65 mmHg; range: 45–100 mmHg) and all of them had confirmed bilateral disease at surgery.

Two patients investigated by FDG-PET had significant FDG uptake. Several authors have reported that FDG-PET has been useful in diagnostic workup for differentiating among or staging malignant diseases and monitoring the response to treatment [17, 18]. Among unusual findings, other authors reported case reports of patients with PAS with a lack of uptake of FDG in PET [19, 20]. Therefore, the role of this procedure in the diagnostic workup of PAS remains controversial and requires further investigation.

The prognosis of patients with PAS is generally poor. Surgery, either PEA or lobectomy/pneumonectomy, increases survival and ameliorates symptoms associated with pulmonary artery occlusion, thus allowing patients to receive additional forms of systemic or local therapies [7, 8, 21]. PEA, when feasible, should be considered the treatment of choice. In our series, it provided complete macroscopic tumor removal in most cases and was also effective with palliative intent; eleven out of twelve patients, after rapid recovery of symptoms and heart function improvement, were eligible to receive conventional anthracycline-containing CT with limited side effects. Radiotherapy was also administered after completion of CT in selected patients.

As PAS remains a rare disease, limited data are available on the role of postsurgery treatment. Among 31 patients receiving any surgical procedure [7], 4 died in the postsurgery phase and 15, 2, and 1 underwent CT, RT, or both, respectively. In a more recently published series of 14 patients undergoing PEA [8], there were three perioperative deaths, five patients received postsurgical CT, and, after completion, four also had RT: one of them in adjuvant setting and three for metastatic disease. The CT regimen was different: 3 patients received anthracycline, 1 ifosfamide alone, and 1 the combination of both. Overall, the two studies indicate a trend towards better survival for patients who received postoperative chemotherapy and/or RT compared to those who had surgery alone.

Because of the shorter follow-up and the limited number of patients in our series and although this is one of the largest single-center experiences of PAS treated with a defined multidisciplinary approach, we cannot definitively prove that the addition of CT and RT considerably extend life expectancy over surgery alone. However, survival curves appear to match favorably with previous reports of PAS patients undergoing surgery alone [7, 8, 10, 14].

In summary, while early diagnosis is an essential prerequisite to allow for optimal management of PAS, it is of pivotal importance that patients with suspected diagnosis of PAS be promptly referred to expert centers for PEA where a multidisciplinary team is available. As shown in our study, PEA represents a more effective and the safest surgical procedure. It should be preferred also because it represents a rapid multidisciplinary pathway of care, along with CT and RT. Further clinical research is mandatory to improve the outcome of patients and for a better understanding of the role of systemic anticancer therapy and RT.

Disclosure

An earlier version of this work was presented as an abstract at Annals of Oncology published on 26 September 2015.

Authors' Contributions

P. Pedrazzoli and A. M. D'armini contributed equally to this work.

Acknowledgments

This work was supported by the Fondazione IRCCS Policlinico San Matteo, Pavia (Hospital Research Grant no. 08067611 to P. Pedrazzoli). The authors thank Alice Rossi for data management.

References

[1] M. Mandelstamm, "Über primäre Neubildungen des Herzens," *Virchows Archiv für Pathologische Anatomie und Physiologie und für Klinische Medizin*, vol. 245, no. 1, pp. 43–54, 1923.

[2] E. R. Ferguson, "Sarcomas of the heart and the great vessels," in *Soft tissue sarcomas*, R. Pollock, Ed., pp. 155–171, BC Decker Inc, Lewiston, Me, USA, 2002.

[3] E. C. Bendel, J. J. Maleszewski, and P. A. Araoz, "Imaging sarcomas of the great vessels and heart," *Seminars in Ultrasound, CT and MRI*, vol. 32, no. 5, pp. 377–404, 2011.

[4] Burke A and R. Virmani, *Tumors of the Heart and Great Vessels*, Armed Forced Institute of Pathology, Washington, wash, USA, 1996.

[5] V. Grazioli, N. Vistarini, M. Morsolini et al., "Surgical treatment of primary pulmonary artery sarcoma," *Journal of Thoracic and Cardiovascular Surgery*, vol. 148, no. 1, pp. 113–118, 2014.

[6] A. Neuville, F. Collin, P. Bruneval et al., "Intimal sarcoma is the most frequent primary cardiac sarcoma: clinicopathologic and molecular retrospective analysis of 100 primary cardiac sarcomas," *The American Journal of Surgical Pathology*, vol. 38, no. 4, pp. 461–469, 2014.

[7] S. Mussot, M.-R. Ghigna, and O. Mercier, "Retrospective institutional study of 31 patients treated for pulmonary artery sarcoma," *European Journal of Cardio-Thoracic Surgery*, vol. 43, no. 4, pp. 787–793, 2013.

[8] H. Wong, I. Gounaris, A. McCormack et al., "Presentation and management of pulmonary artery sarcoma," *Clinical Sarcoma Research*, vol. 5, no. 1, pp. 3–8, 2015.

[9] S. W. Jamieson, "Editorial Comment: Pulmonary artery sarcoma," *European Journal of Cardio-Thoracic Surgery*, vol. 43, no. 4, pp. 793-794, 2013.

[10] H. K. Kim, Y. S. Choi, K. Kim et al., "Surgical treatment for pulmonary artery sarcoma," *European Journal of Cardio-thoracic Surgery*, vol. 33, no. 4, pp. 712–716, 2008.

[11] A. M. D'Armini, G. Zanotti, S. Ghio et al., "Reverse right ventricular remodeling after pulmonary endarterectomy," *Journal of Thoracic and Cardiovascular Surgery*, vol. 133, no. 1, pp. 162–168, 2007.

[12] M. Morsolini, S. Nicolardi, E. Milanesi et al., "Evolving surgical techniques for pulmonary endarterectomy according to the changing features of chronic thromboembolic pulmonary hypertension patients during 17-year single-center experience," *Journal of Thoracic and Cardiovascular Surgery*, vol. 144, no. 1, pp. 100–107, 2012.

[13] S. H. Blackmon and M. J. Reardon, "Pulmonary artery sarcoma," in *Methodist Debakey Cardiovasc J*, vol. 6, pp. 38–43, 2010.

[14] S. Lu, T. Hong, and C. Wang, "Clinical treatment for pulmonary artery sarcoma," *European Journal of Cardio-Thoracic Surgery*, vol. 38, no. 1, pp. 115-116, 2010.

[15] M. B. Anderson, J. M. Kriett, D. P. Kapelanski, R. Tarazi, and S. W. Jamieson, "Primary pulmonary artery sarcoma: A report of six cases," *The Annals of Thoracic Surgery*, vol. 59, no. 6, pp. 1487–1490, 1995.

[16] A. J. Peacock and L. J. Rubin, "Hodden Arnold Pubblication," in *Pulmonary Circulation: Diseases and their Treatment*, A. J. Peacock and L. J. Rubin, Eds., pp. 440–457, CRC Press, London, UK, 2nd edition, 2004.

[17] E. L. P. Ote, N. Oriuchi, G. Miyashita et al., "Pulmonary artery intimal sarcoma: The role of 18F- fluorodeoxyglucose positron emission tomography in monitoring response to treatment," *Japanese Journal of Radiology*, vol. 29, no. 4, pp. 279–282, 2011.

[18] K. Strobel, B. Bode, D. Lardinois, and U. Exner, "PET-positive fibrous dysplasia - A potentially misleading incidental finding in a patient with intimal sarcoma of the pulmonary artery," *Skeletal Radiology*, vol. 36, no. 1, pp. 24–28, 2007.

[19] M. Hoiczyk, K. Iliodromitis, S. Bauer et al., "Intimal sarcoma of the pulmonary artery with unusual findings: A case report," *Clinical Research in Cardiology*, vol. 101, no. 5, pp. 397–401, 2012.

[20] D.-H. Lee, T.-E. Jung, J.-H. Lee, D.-G. Shin, W.-J. Park, and J.-H. Choi, "Pulmonary artery intimal sarcoma: Poor 18F-fluorodeoxyglucose uptake in positron emission computed tomography," *Journal of Cardiothoracic Surgery*, vol. 8, no. 1, article no. 40, 2013.

[21] I. Kruger, A. Borowski, M. Horst, E. R. De Vivie, P. Theissen, and W. Gross-Fengels, "Symptoms, diagnosis, and therapy of primary sarcomas of the pulmonary artery," *Thoracic and Cardiovascular Surgeon*, vol. 38, no. 2, pp. 91–95, 1990.

Trial of Angiotensin-(1-7) for the Treatment of Patients with Metastatic Sarcoma

Paul D. Savage,[1,2] James Lovato,[2,3] K. Bridget Brosnihan,[4] Antonius A. Miller,[1,2] and W. Jeffrey Petty[1,2,5]

[1]*Department of Medicine, Section of Hematology and Oncology, Wake Forest School of Medicine, Winston-Salem, NC, USA*
[2]*Comprehensive Cancer Center of Wake Forest University, Wake Forest School of Medicine, Winston-Salem, NC, USA*
[3]*Department of Biostatistical Sciences, Wake Forest School of Medicine, Winston-Salem, NC, USA*
[4]*Department of Surgical Sciences, Center for Hypertension and Vascular Research, Wake Forest School of Medicine, Winston-Salem, NC, USA*
[5]*Department of Cancer Biology, Wake Forest School of Medicine, Winston-Salem, NC, USA*

Correspondence should be addressed to Paul D. Savage; psavage@wakehealth.edu

Academic Editor: Shreyaskumar Patel

Background. Angiotensin-(1-7) [Ang-(1-7)] is an endogenous antiangiogenic hormone with anticancer activity. In a phase I study of Ang-(1-7), two of three patients with metastatic sarcoma experienced disease stabilization. This phase II study examined clinical and biomarker outcomes for patients with metastatic sarcoma. *Methods.* Ang-(1-7) was administered by subcutaneous injection at a dose of 20 mg daily. If excessive toxicities occurred in the first cohort, a dose deescalation cohort was allowed. Blood samples were obtained to measure changes in biomarkers. *Results.* Treatment was well-tolerated and the dose deescalation cohort was not required. Plasma PlGF concentrations following treatment were not statistically significantly changed. A significant increase in plasma Ang-(1-7) was observed at 4 hours after injection. The median progression-free survival was 2.7 months (95% CI; 1.4 to 4.1 months), and the median overall survival was 10.2 months (95% CI; 5.3 to 18.3 months). Two patients with vascular sarcomas demonstrated prolonged disease stabilization of 10 months (hemangiopericytoma) and 19 months (epithelioid hemangioendothelioma). *Conclusions.* Ang-(1-7) at a dose of 20 mg daily was well-tolerated. This prospective phase II study failed to confirm the PlGF biomarker effect identified in the prior phase I study. Prolonged disease stabilization in hemangiopericytoma and epithelioid hemangioendothelioma may warrant further investigation.

1. Introduction

Sarcomas are a diverse group of malignant tumors that arise from mesenchymal tissues including bone and soft tissues. While a few subtypes of sarcomas have specific effective regimens, the majority of patients with advanced sarcomas receive regimens largely based on whether the tumor is of bone or soft tissue origin. For the majority of sarcoma patients, first-line treatments have involved anthracycline-based combination chemotherapy [1]. The doublet of gemcitabine and docetaxel has been studied and also has activity in the front-line setting [2, 3]. As key molecular pathways are elucidated, a number of targeted agents including antiangiogenic therapies are being tested in phase II clinical trials [4, 5]. To date only one such targeted agent, pazopanib, has FDA-approval for treatment of patients with metastatic sarcoma that has progressed after initial treatment [6].

Angiotensin-(1-7) [Ang-(1-7)] is a naturally occurring peptide with antiangiogenic properties [7–11]. Recently, Ang-(1-7) has shown anticancer activity *in vitro* and *in vivo* [12–14]. The effects *in vitro* are linked to the antiproliferative properties of this drug in vascular endothelial cells and reduced secretion of proangiogenic peptides from cancer cells [8–10, 13–15]. Reduced production of angiogenic hormones is triggered by reduced HIF-1α transcription *in vitro* [15].

A phase I trial using subcutaneous administration of Ang-(1-7) for the treatment of patients with advanced solid tumors was previously reported [16]. This study evaluated the maximum tolerated dose (MTD), toxicities, and pharmacokinetics of Ang-(1-7) when given subcutaneously once daily for five consecutive days on a 21-day cycle. This study identified 400 mcg/kg as the MTD for this schedule. Serious adverse events that were at least possibly related to Ang-(1-7) included deep vein thrombosis (400 mcg/kg dose level), stroke (700 mcg/kg dose level), and cranial neuropathy (700 mcg/kg dose level). The observed half-life at the MTD was very short (36 minutes) with considerable intra- and interpatient variability.

Clinical benefit, defined as disease stabilization for more than three months, was observed in two of the three patients with metastatic sarcoma treated in the phase I study. This included one patient with pleomorphic liposarcoma who had a 19% reduction in tumor measurements. Clinical benefit was associated with reduction in plasma levels of the proangiogenic hormone, placental growth factor (PlGF). This effect was statistically significant at several time points following Ang-(1-7) administration, with the greatest reduction observed 4 hours after treatment [15, 16].

The current phase II study sought to confirm and extend the findings from the phase I study by prospectively evaluating radiographic responses by RECIST and changes in PlGF following treatment in a larger cohort of patients with sarcoma. A continuous daily dosing schedule was selected based on the short half-life of the drug and the time course of biomarker changes observed during the phase I study.

2. Materials and Methods

2.1. Patient Eligibility. Patients were required to have a histologically or cytologically confirmed bone or soft tissue sarcoma that was metastatic or unresectable, with measurable disease. Patients had to have disease progression despite 1 or 2 prior treatment regimens with chemotherapy or targeted anticancer agents. Patients were required to be over 18 years of age and have an Eastern Cooperative Oncology Group (ECOG) performance status of 0–2. Patients could not be taking ACE inhibitors or angiotensin II receptor blockers at the time of enrollment. Prior use of these drugs was allowed. Required laboratory criteria at study entry included an absolute neutrophil count $\geq$ 1,500/μL, platelet count $\geq$ 100,000/μL, estimated creatinine clearance > 30 mL/min, total bilirubin < 2 mg/dL, and AST and ALT < 3 times the upper limit of normal.

Prior therapies (including chemotherapy, surgery, and radiation) had to be completed at least 4 weeks before enrollment. Patients were not eligible if they were pregnant or nursing. Women of child-bearing potential and men were required to agree to use adequate contraception (hormonal, double-barrier method of birth control, or abstinence) prior to study entry and for the duration of study participation.

2.2. Study Design. Ang-(1-7) was supplied by Bachem AG (Bubendorf, Switzerland) under good manufacturing protocol (GMP) conditions. Ang-(1-7) was dissolved in bacteriostatic water, filtered, and aliquoted into glass vials. Vials were stored frozen, and after thawing, vials were maintained at refrigerated temperatures for no more than two weeks.

Ang-(1-7) was administered by subcutaneous injection once daily continuously. One cycle was defined as a 21-day period. Toxicities were assessed weekly during the first cycle and on the first day of each subsequent cycle. In the absence of unacceptable treatment-related toxicity, patients continued treatment until disease progression.

This study was approved by the Institutional Review Board of Wake Forest University. It was registered in the National Cancer Institute PDQ Database and ClinicalTrials.gov as NCT00974545 and NCT01553539. Duplicate ClinicalTrials.gov listings were identified and subsequently linked. All patients were required to provide written informed consent.

2.3. Dose Cohorts. Two dose cohorts were planned. In the first cohort, twenty patients were treated at a dose of 20 mg daily which is similar to the weight-based dose of 400 mcg/kg identified as the MTD in the phase I study. Unlike the phase I study, this study utilized continuous daily dosing rather than five days every three weeks. A planned interim safety evaluation was performed after the enrollment of 10 patients in the first cohort. A second cohort of twenty patients was planned as a dose deescalation cohort in the event that excess toxicities were observed in the first cohort. Patients in this cohort would have received Ang-(1-7) at a dose of 10 mg daily if excessive toxicities had been observed in the 20 mg cohort. Safety events that would trigger dose deescalation included 3 strokes in any cohort or other evidence of excessive toxicity.

2.4. Patient Assessment. Tumor measurements were performed using RECIST version 1.1 prior to initiation of treatment and then every two cycles until disease progression or unacceptable toxicity. Toxicities were graded using the Common Terminology Criteria for Adverse Events, version 3.0. Dose limiting toxicities (DLT) were defined as grade 3 or greater toxicities that were felt to be at least possibly related to Ang-(1-7) treatment. In the event of a DLT, the dose of Ang-(1-7) was reduced to 10 mg daily.

2.5. Measurement of Drug and Angiogenic Hormone Levels. In the phase I trial, statistically significant changes in PlGF concentrations were identified 4 hours after the first Ang-(1-7) injection. To prospectively evaluate this biomarker, PlGF levels as well as VEGF, Ang-(1-7), Ang II, and Ang I were measured prior to the first dose, 4 hours after the first dose, and after 21 days of treatment in the phase II trial. Blood samples were immediately placed on ice and processed within 30 minutes of collection. For the angiotensin peptides, blood was taken in an EDTA containing tube with a cocktail of inhibitors to prevent *in vitro* generation or degradation of peptides, as previously described [17]. Plasma samples were stored at −80°C. Concentrations of Ang-(1-7) (developed by laboratory), Ang II (Alpco, Windham, NH), and Ang I (Peninsula, San Carlos, CA) were measured by the Hypertension Core Facility of Wake Forest University using three established radioimmunoassay methods [14]. Aliquots of plasma from the same time points were assayed by Aushon Biosystems (Billerica, MA) using Searchlight ELISA technology to quantify circulating vascular endothelial growth factor

(VEGF) and placental growth factor (PlGF). Samples were blinded prior to shipping.

2.6. Statistical Methods. The study was designed with 87% power to detect a response rate by RECIST criteria of 10% in the study population. Frequency and severity of treatment-related toxicities were examined by cohort. Levels of biomarker expression over time were evaluated using nonparametric, Wilcoxon signed rank tests. All analyses were two-sided, and a P value < 0.05 was considered statistically significant. Analyses were performed using SAS v9.1.3 (SAS Institute, Cary, NC) and Stata v10.1 (StataCorp, College Station, TX) and were performed by the Core Biostatistics Facility of the Comprehensive Cancer Center of Wake Forest University.

3. Results

3.1. Patients. Twenty patients were enrolled between December 2009 and December 2011. Patient demographics are displayed in Table 1. Multiple subtypes of sarcoma were treated on the study, with the most common subtype of sarcoma being uterine leiomyosarcoma.

3.2. Adverse Events. Treatment on the current phase II study was generally well-tolerated. The adverse events are listed in Table 2. Two patients with preexisting headache disorders reported an increase in headaches which was felt to be possibly related to treatment. No strokes or other neurologic toxicities occurred. Only one DLT attributed as at least possibly due to treatment occurred. This was a grade 3 uncomplicated deep vein thrombosis (DVT) which was treated with anticoagulation.

Three deaths occurred, either on study or within 30 days of completing treatment. All three of these deaths were attributed to progressive cancer and were felt to be unrelated to the Ang-(1-7) treatment. Attribution for each of these was independently reviewed by an institutional clinical research oversight committee. Of the three patients who died during this trial, two patients developed respiratory failure from progressive lung metastases and one patient developed biliary obstruction with sepsis attributed to malignant obstruction of the common bile duct.

3.3. Pregnancy. One patient became pregnant while receiving Ang-(1-7) on this study, for which her use of the study drug was immediately suspended; at the time of discontinuation she had taken Ang-(1-7) for more than 1 year. After having an unremarkable fetal ultrasound, she delivered a healthy child, and her child is developing normally. She was felt to have likely benefited from treatment with prolonged stabilization of disease prior to becoming pregnant, and her disease demonstrated minimal change without requiring additional treatment for more than 2 years after discontinuing Ang-(1-7).

3.4. Clinical Outcomes. The study failed to achieve the primary endpoint of a 10% response rate. No partial or complete responses by RECIST were observed; however stabilization of disease for more than 3 months was observed in 9 of 20 (45%) patients. The median overall survival on this study

TABLE 1: Patient characteristics.

Parameter	N (%) or mean ± SD (min–max)
Age (years)	55 (22–78)
Gender	
Male	11 (55)
Female	9 (45)
Race	
Caucasian	19 (95)
African American	1 (5)
Ethnicity	
Hispanic	2 (10)
Non-Hispanic	18 (90)
Sarcoma diagnosis	
Angiosarcoma	1 (5)
Chondrosarcoma	2 (10)
Epithelioid hemangioendothelioma	1 (5)
Hemangiopericytoma	1 (5)
Leiomyosarcoma	4 (20)
Malignant phyllodes	1 (5)
Mesothelioma	1 (5)
Osteosarcoma	3 (15)
Pleomorphic sarcoma (MFH/UPS)	4 (20)
Sclerosing epithelioid fibrosarcoma	1 (5)
Synovial sarcoma	1 (5)
Prior treatment	
Surgery	18 (90)
Radiation therapy	8 (40)
Chemotherapy	20 (100)

TABLE 2: Adverse events at least possibly related to treatment.

Toxicity	Grade			
	1/2	3	4	Total
Headaches	2	0	0	2
Fatigue	2	0	0	2
Muscle pain	1	0	0	1
Injection site reaction	6	0	0	6
Induration	1	0	0	1
Flushing	1	0	0	1
Flu-like symptoms	1	0	0	1
Pruritus	1	0	0	1
Deep vein thrombosis	0	1	0	1
Hyperbilirubinemia	1	0	0	1
Elevated alkaline phosphatase	1	0	0	1
Proteinuria	1	0	0	1
Total	18	1	0	19

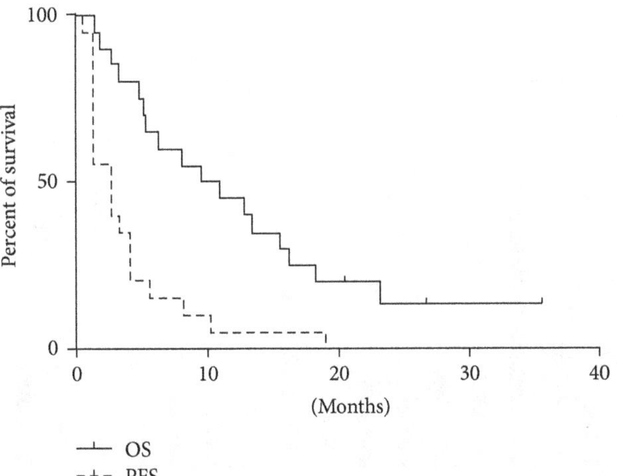

FIGURE 1: Kaplan-Meier graph is shown with progression-free survival (PFS) and overall survival (OS) for all patients enrolled in the study.

was 10.2 months (95% CI; 5.3 to 18.3 months). The median progression-free survival on this study was 2.7 months (95% CI; 1.4 to 4.1 months). The progression-free and overall survival curves are shown in Figure 1.

Two patients with vascular sarcomas experienced prolonged periods of disease stabilization; both patients were demonstrating evidence of disease progression prior to study enrollment. One patient with epithelioid hemangioendothelioma exhibited an 18% increase in the size of lesions measured by the radiologist during a 5-month period of time prior to being enrolled in the study. This patient also developed a new liver lesion five months prior to enrollment. After starting treatment on study, the patient demonstrated stable disease by RECIST for 19 months. One patient with hemangiopericytoma demonstrated 2 new liver lesions as well as 22% increase size in lesions during a 3-month interval prior to enrollment. After starting treatment on study, the patient demonstrated stable disease by RECIST for 10 months. In the opinion of the treating physician, both patients showed evidence of clinical benefit due to a reduction in the pace of disease.

3.5. Biomarker Activity. Concentrations of angiotensin system peptides and angiogenic hormones were measured prior to treatment and at two time points after treatment. The baseline concentrations of angiogenic peptides in plasma samples varied among the patients, as shown in Figure 2. Pretreatment VEGF concentrations were highest in a patient with angiosarcoma while PlGF concentrations demonstrated less variability across histologic subtypes.

Following treatment with Ang-(1-7), plasma Ang-(1-7) concentrations increased at the 4-hour and day 22 time points as shown in Figure 3. There were no changes in the levels of Ang I and Ang II following treatment. Significant changes were not observed in concentrations of VEGF or PlGF peptides although there was a nonsignificant trend to decreasing concentrations of both of these peptides on day 22. PlGF plasma concentrations for pretreatment, 4-hour, and day 22 time points were 4.3, 4.6, and 3 pg/mL. Changes in PlGF plasma concentrations were not statistically significant at these time points ($P = 0.7$ and $P = 0.3$).

4. Conclusions

Sarcomas are considered rare diseases for the purposes of drug development. In clinical practice, however, sarcomas are not a single rare disease but are instead a collection of extremely rare diseases with distinct cells of origin and differing sensitivities to treatment [1–3]. This presents a major challenge for drug development. Functional biomarkers that quantitatively measure biological effects are needed for facilitating clinical drug development decisions in rare and very rare diseases.

The clinical activity manifested by prolonged disease stabilization in our cases of hemangiopericytoma and epithelioid hemangioendothelioma may warrant further investigation in these two subtypes of vascular sarcoma. Other antiangiogenic compounds have been tested and have demonstrated some activity for these histologies [18–23]. The PFS for these two patients on our study of 10 months and 19 months compare favorably to the median PFS achieved with chemotherapy of 4.2 months [22].

Research regarding the anticancer properties of Ang-(1-7) is ongoing. Preclinical studies have shown compelling evidence of antiangiogenic effects using *in vitro*, murine wound healing [8] and murine xenograft models [13]. Our phase I study suggested a mechanistic role for PlGF in mediating its antiangiogenic effects. Although a trend towards decreasing PlGF and VEGF levels was observed on day 22 in the current study, these changes were not statistically significant.

A key pharmacologic barrier to the use of Ang-(1-7) is the short half-life. Stabilizing chemical modifications to the drug may be useful for overcoming this barrier. Alternatively, improved drug exposure could be accomplished by coadministration of an ACE inhibitor which has been demonstrated to inhibit the Ang-(1-7) degradation [24]. Similar chemical modifications and pharmacologic approaches have been explored to enhance the cardioprotective effects of Ang-(1-7)

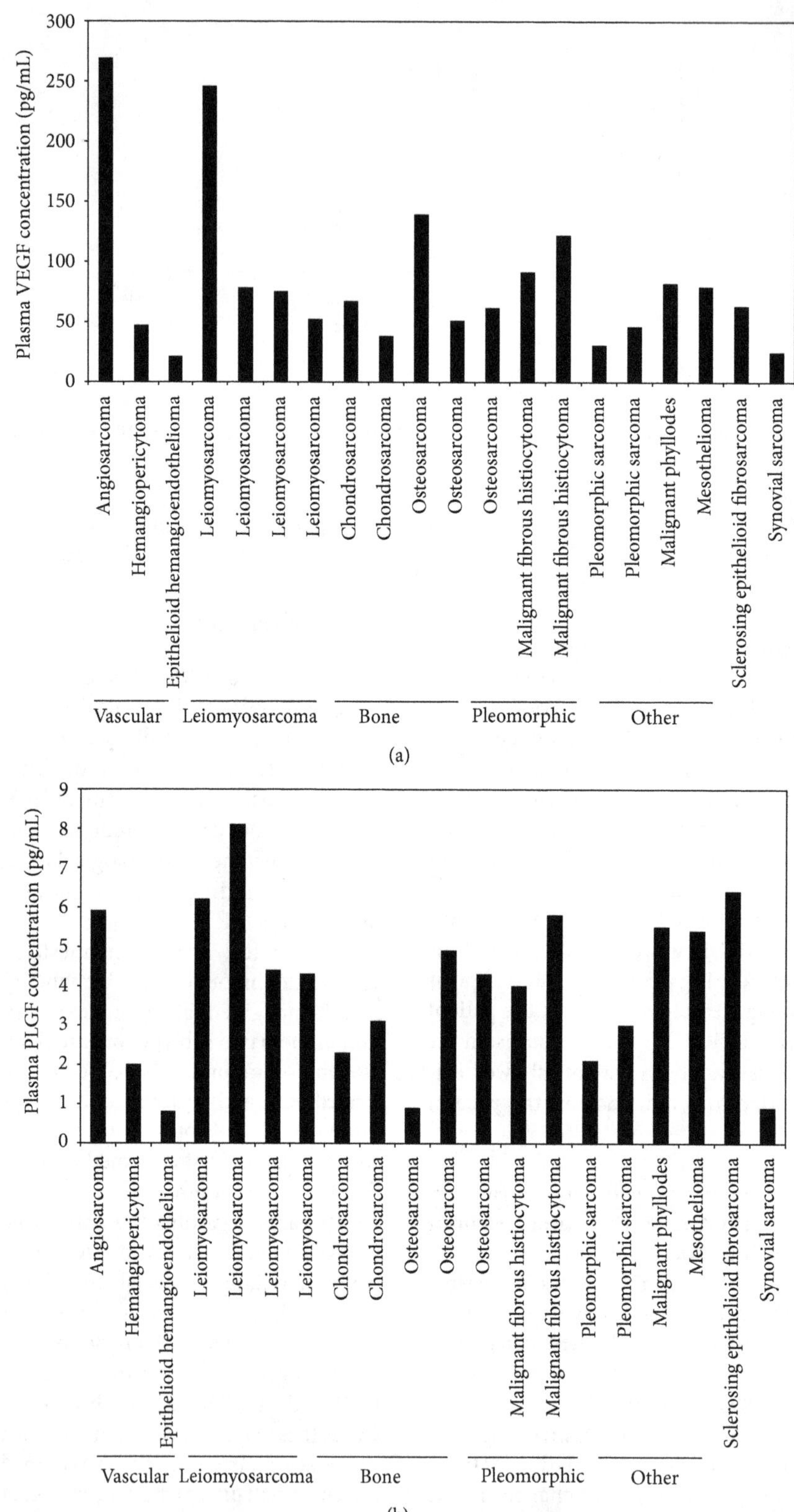

FIGURE 2: Pretreatment plasma concentrations of VEGF (a) and PlGF (b) are shown according to sarcoma subtype. Pretreatment VEGF concentrations were highest in the patient with angiosarcoma.

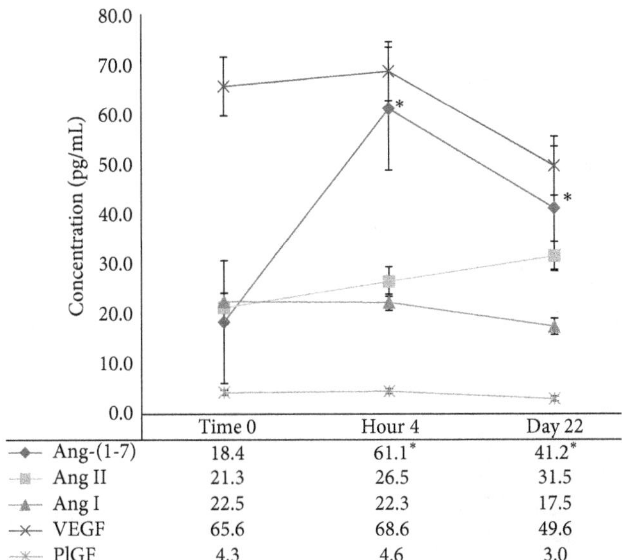

	Time 0	Hour 4	Day 22
Ang-(1-7)	18.4	61.1*	41.2*
Ang II	21.3	26.5	31.5
Ang I	22.5	22.3	17.5
VEGF	65.6	68.6	49.6
PlGF	4.3	4.6	3.0

FIGURE 3: Plasma concentrations of angiotensin system peptides and angiogenic hormones over time are shown. The data points represent median values for the pretreatment (Time 0) and posttreatment blood draws. The 4-hour and day 22 posttreatment Ang-(1-7) levels were increased over baseline ($P < 0.05$). Standard error bars are shown.

treatment [25–28]. The short half-life observed in the current study supports the exploration of these approaches for improving drug exposure and maximizing the anticancer activity of Ang-(1-7).

Competing Interests

W. Jeffrey Petty has a potential financial interest in the development and use of the peptide studied in this project and his interest is being managed in accordance with Wake Forest School of Medicine policies.

Authors' Contributions

Paul D. Savage participated in the design of the study, treated and evaluated all participating patients, and reviewed all clinical outcomes and data analyses. James Lovato participated in the design of the study and conducted data analyses. K. Bridget Brosnihan supervised the conduct of peptide measurements and provided interpretation of the biomarker analyses. Antonius A. Miller participated in the design of the study and reviewed clinical outcomes and data analyses. W. Jeffrey Petty conceived the study, reviewed all clinical outcomes and data analyses, and helped to draft the manuscript. All authors read and approved the final manuscript.

Acknowledgments

This work was supported by the Comprehensive Cancer Center of Wake Forest University (NCI-P30-CA012197) and the Food and Drug Administration, Office of Orphan Products Development (R01-FD003936).

References

[1] B. Bui-Nguyen, J. E. Butrynski, N. Penel et al., "A phase IIb multicentre study comparing the efficacy of trabectedin to doxorubicin in patients with advanced or metastatic untreated soft tissue sarcoma: the TRUSTS trial," *European Journal of Cancer*, vol. 51, no. 10, pp. 1312–1320, 2015.

[2] R. G. Maki, J. K. Wathen, S. R. Patel et al., "Randomized phase II study of gemcitabine and docetaxel compared with gemcitabine alone in patients with metastatic soft tissue sarcomas: results of sarcoma alliance for research through collaboration study 002," *Journal of Clinical Oncology*, vol. 25, no. 19, pp. 2755–2763, 2007.

[3] M. L. Hensley, R. Maki, E. Venkatraman et al., "Gemcitabine and docetaxel in patients with unresectable leiomyosarcoma: results of a phase II trial," *Journal of Clinical Oncology*, vol. 20, no. 12, pp. 2824–2831, 2002.

[4] M. Agulnik, J. L. Yarber, S. H. Okuno et al., "An open-label, multicenter, phase II study of bevacizumab for the treatment of angiosarcoma and epithelioid hemangioendotheliomas," *Annals of Oncology*, vol. 24, no. 1, pp. 257–263, 2013.

[5] J. Lewin, K. K. Khamly, R. J. Young et al., "A phase Ib/II translational study of sunitinib with neoadjuvant radiotherapy in soft-tissue sarcoma," *British Journal of Cancer*, vol. 111, no. 12, pp. 2254–2261, 2014.

[6] W. T. A. van der Graaf, J.-Y. Blay, S. P. Chawla et al., "Pazopanib for metastatic soft-tissue sarcoma (PALETTE): a randomised, double-blind, placebo-controlled phase 3 trial," *The Lancet*, vol. 379, no. 9829, pp. 1879–1886, 2012.

[7] E. A. Tallant, D. I. Diz, and C. M. Ferrario, "Antiproliferative actions of angiotensin-(1–7) in vascular smooth muscle," *Hypertension*, vol. 34, no. 4, pp. 950–957, 1999.

[8] R. D. Machado, R. A. Santos, and S. P. Andrade, "Opposing actions of angiotensins on angiogenesis," *Life Sciences*, vol. 66, no. 1, pp. 67–76, 1999.

[9] E. A. Tallant and M. A. Clark, "Molecular mechanisms of inhibition of vascular growth by angiotensin-(1-7)," *Hypertension*, vol. 42, no. 4, pp. 574–579, 2003.

[10] L. Anton, D. C. Merrill, L. A. A. Neves, and K. B. Brosnihan, "Angiotensin-(1–7) inhibits in vitro endothelial cell tube formation in human umbilical vein endothelial cells through the AT_{1-7} receptor," *Endocrine*, vol. 32, no. 2, pp. 212–218, 2007.

[11] E. J. Freeman, G. M. Chisolm, C. M. Ferrario, and E. A. Tallant, "Angiotensin-(1–7) inhibits vascular smooth muscle cell growth," *Hypertension*, vol. 28, no. 1, pp. 104–108, 1996.

[12] J. Menon, D. R. Soto-Pantoja, M. F. Callahan et al., "Angiotensin-(1-7) inhibits growth of human lung adenocarcinoma xenografts in nude mice through a reduction in cyclooxygenase-2," *Cancer Research*, vol. 67, no. 6, pp. 2809–2815, 2007.

[13] D. R. Soto-Pantoja, J. Menon, P. E. Gallagher, and E. A. Tallant, "Angiotensin-(1–7) inhibits tumor angiogenesis in human lung cancer xenografts with a reduction in vascular endothelial growth factor," *Molecular Cancer Therapeutics*, vol. 8, no. 6, pp. 1676–1683, 2009.

[14] D. R. Soto-Pantoja, W. J. Petty, P. E. Gallagher, and E. A. Tallant, "Angiotensin-(1-7) inhibits triple negative tumor growth through the inhibition of angiogenesis and a reduction in placental growth factor PlGF," *Cancer Research*, vol. 69, no. 2, supplement, abstract 901, 2009.

[15] W. J. Petty, M. Aklilu, V. A. Varela, J. Lovato, P. D. Savage, and A. A. Miller, "Reverse translation of phase I biomarker findings links the activity of angiotensin-(1–7) to repression of hypoxia inducible factor-1α in vascular sarcomas," *BMC Cancer*, vol. 12, article 404, 2012.

[16] W. J. Petty, A. A. Miller, T. P. McCoy, P. E. Gallagher, E. A. Tallant, and F. M. Torti, "Phase I and pharmacokinetic study of angiotensin-(1–7), an endogenous antiangiogenic hormone," *Clinical Cancer Research*, vol. 15, no. 23, pp. 7398–7404, 2009.

[17] K. Kohara, Y. Tabuchi, P. Senanayake, K. B. Brosnihan, and C. M. Ferrario, "Reassessment of plasma angiotensins measurement: effects of protease inhibitors and sample handling procedures," *Peptides*, vol. 12, no. 5, pp. 1135–1141, 1991.

[18] J. Domont, C. Massard, N. Lassau, J.-P. Armand, A. Le Cesne, and J.-C. Soria, "Hemangiopericytoma and antiangiogenic therapy: clinical benefit of antiangiogenic therapy (sorafenib and sunitinib) in relapsed Malignant Haemangioperyctoma /Solitary Fibrous Tumour," *Investigational New Drugs*, vol. 28, no. 2, pp. 199–202, 2010.

[19] S. Stacchiotti, T. Negri, M. Libertini et al., "Sunitinib malate in solitary fibrous tumor (SFT)," *Annals of Oncology*, vol. 23, no. 12, Article ID mds143, pp. 3171–3179, 2012.

[20] M. S. Park, S. R. Patel, J. A. Ludwig et al., "Activity of temozolomide and bevacizumab in the treatment of locally advanced, recurrent, and metastatic hemangiopericytoma and malignant solitary fibrous tumor," *Cancer*, vol. 117, no. 21, pp. 4939–4947, 2011.

[21] T. Valentin, C. Fournier, N. Penel et al., "Sorafenib in patients with progressive malignant solitary fibrous tumors: a subgroup analysis from a phase II study of the French Sarcoma Group (GSF/GETO)," *Investigational New Drugs*, vol. 31, no. 6, pp. 1626–1627, 2013.

[22] A. Constantinidou, R. L. Jones, D. Olmos et al., "Conventional anthracycline-based chemotherapy has limited efficacy in solitary fibrous tumour," *Acta Oncologica*, vol. 51, no. 4, pp. 550–554, 2012.

[23] A. Levard, O. Derbel, P. Méeus et al., "Outcome of patients with advanced solitary fibrous tumors: The Centre Léon Bérard Experience," *BMC Cancer*, vol. 13, article 109, 2013.

[24] M. C. Chappell, N. T. Pirro, A. Sykes, and C. M. Ferrario, "Metabolism of angiotensin-(1–7) by angiotensin-converting enzyme," *Hypertension*, vol. 31, no. 1, pp. 362–367, 1998.

[25] B. S. Pessoa, P. M. Becher, R. Van Veghel et al., "Effect of a stable angiotensin-(1–7) analogue on progenitor cell recruitment and cardiovascular function post myocardial infarction," *Journal of the American Heart Association*, vol. 4, article e001510, 2015.

[26] M. Durik, R. van Veghel, A. Kuipers et al., "The effect of the thioether-bridged, stabilized angiotensin-(1–7) analogue cyclic Ang-(1–7) on cardiac remodeling and endothelial function in rats with myocardial infarction," *International Journal of Hypertension*, vol. 2012, Article ID 536426, 8 pages, 2012.

[27] A. J. Ferreira, T. M. Murça, R. A. Fraga-Silva, C. H. Castro, M. K. Raizada, and R. A. Santos, "New cardiovascular and pulmonary therapeutic strategies based on the angiotensin-converting enzyme 2/angiotensin-(1–7)/mas receptor axis," *International Journal of Hypertension*, vol. 2012, Article ID 147825, 13 pages, 2012.

[28] L. D. Kluskens, S. A. Nelemans, R. Rink et al., "Angiotensin-(1-7) with thioether bridge: an angiotensin-converting enzyme-resistant, potent angiotensin-(1-7) analog," *Journal of Pharmacology and Experimental Therapeutics*, vol. 328, no. 3, pp. 849–854, 2009.

25

Myxoid Liposarcoma: Treatment Outcomes from Chemotherapy and Radiation Therapy

Varun Chowdhry,[1] Saveli Goldberg,[2] Thomas F. DeLaney,[2] Gregory M. Cote,[3] Ivan Chebib,[4] Jason Kim,[5] Santiago A. Lozano-Calderón,[5] and Karen De Amorim Bernstein[2]

[1]*Department of Radiation Medicine, Roswell Park Comprehensive Cancer Center, Buffalo, NY, USA*
[2]*Department of Radiation Oncology, Massachusetts General Hospital, Boston, MA 02114, USA*
[3]*Division of Hematology/Oncology, Massachusetts General Hospital, Boston, MA 02114, USA*
[4]*Department of Pathology, Massachusetts General Hospital, Boston, MA 02114, USA*
[5]*Department of Orthopedic Oncology, Massachusetts General Hospital, Boston, MA 02114, USA*

Correspondence should be addressed to Varun Chowdhry; varun.chowdhry@roswellpark.org

Academic Editor: C. Verhoef

Introduction. Myxoid liposarcoma (MLS) is a subtype of liposarcoma characterized morphologically by lipomatous differentiation with a myxoid stroma. The purpose of this study was to review clinical and pathological information for patients treated for MLS at our institution to better understand neoadjuvant and adjuvant therapy. *Materials and Methods.* An institutional database of sarcomas was queried for patients who were treated for MLS at our institution between 1992 and 2013. Survival curves were constructed using Kaplan–Meier analysis, and univariate and multivariate statistics were performed using the Cox-proportional hazards model and using linear regression. *Results.* A total of 85 patients with myxoid liposarcoma were identified. The mean and median histologic response rate to treatment for patients who received preoperative radiation therapy was 77.6%. Five-year disease-free survival, distant metastasis-free survival, local recurrence-free survival, and overall survival were 78.6% (95% CI: 67.8–86.1), 84.7% (95% CI: 74.5–91.0), 95.6% (95% CI: 86.9–98.6), and 87.5% (95% CI: 77.2–93.3) respectively. On univariate analysis, there was a trend towards higher necrosis or treatment response rates in patients who received concurrent chemotherapy, 84.7% (95% CI: 75.9–93.4) and 69.5% (95% CI: 55.1–83.8), $p = 0.061$. Tumor size was associated with inferior disease-free and overall survival. Hazard ratio for disease-free survival is 1.08 (per cm) (95% CI: 1.01–1.16), $p = 0.019$. *Conclusions.* Myxoid liposarcoma exhibits histological response to chemotherapy and radiation therapy. Tumor size appears to be greatest predictor of long-term disease control and overall survival. We were not able to show that chemotherapy provides a clinical benefit with regard to local control, disease-free survival, or overall survival. However, it is important to note that the selected usage of chemotherapy in the highest risk patients confounds this analysis. Further investigation is needed to help better determine the optimal use of chemotherapy in this group of patients.

1. Introduction

Myxoid liposarcoma (MLS) is a subtype of liposarcoma that represents a distinct pathological entity characterized morphologically by tumor cells within a myxoid stroma with a rich, branching thin-walled vasculature, and focal lipomatous differentiation. The MLS subtype represents approximately 1/3 of all liposarcomas and 10% of adult soft tissue sarcomas [1]. MLS is associated with chromosomal translocations consisting of the FUS and DDIT3 (CHOP) genes t(12; 16)(q13; p11) or the EWS and DDIT3 (CHOP) genes t(12; 22)(q13; q12) [2]. There is evidence to suggest that MLS is both radioresponsive and radiosensitive [3]. Marked reduction of tumor volume has been noted during treatment, with one series showing a median reduction in tumor volume from the start to end of treatment of 59% [4].

Comparative analysis of MLS versus other sarcoma subtypes suggests greater response rates in MLS with the addition of anthracycline-based chemotherapy [5]. In one series, there is a suggestion that doxorubicin and ifosfamide can result in favorable long-term outcomes [6]. However, there is relatively limited information on factors that predict for overall outcome in MLS, particularly with regard to the benefits of combined trimodality therapy. The purpose of this single institution MLS series is to evaluate clinical variables that may predict for improved outcomes and thereby help guide management or future clinical trials.

2. Materials and Methods

After IRB approval, our oncology registry database was queried for patients who were treated for MLS at our institution between 1992 and 2013. Only patients with no evidence of metastatic disease treated with definitive limb-salvage therapy were included in this series. All patients had pathological confirmation by a sarcoma-specialized pathologist either through secondary review of slides from another institution or through direct pathological sampling obtained at our institution. All patients were evaluated in a multidisciplinary care setting for indications and suitability to receive preoperative chemotherapy and radiation therapy. Patients treated with definitive therapy for their disease were included in this analysis. Sixty-nine out of 85 patients (81%) had the initial biopsy performed at our institution, and seventy-nine patients (93%) had definitive surgical resection performed at our institution. Patients diagnosed with MLS, including high-grade MLS (formerly myxoid/round cell liposarcoma), were included in this analysis. Demographic, clinical, radiographic, pathologic, and treatment outcomes were captured. Statistical analysis using both univariate and multivariate models were conducted using SAS software (SAS version 9.4; 100 SAS Campus Drive, Cary, NC 27513). Survival curves were constructed using Kaplan–Meier analysis, and univariate and multivariate statistics were performed using the Cox-proportional hazards model and using linear regression.

3. Results

Demographic information for patients in this series is listed in Table 1. Seventy-three of 85 patients had sarcomas of the lower extremity (85.9%), with complete breakdown by location shown in Table 1. The median follow-up for patients in this series was 85.2 months (range, 4–250 months). Sixty-seven (78.8%) patients were treated with preoperative radiotherapy, and 15 (17.6%) patients were treated with postoperative radiation therapy, generally due to close or positive postoperative margins. Ten patients (11.8%) in this series did not receive any radiotherapy. Seven patients (8.2%) were treated with both pre- and postoperative radiation therapy. Patients were treated with either 2D radiotherapy prior to 2000, 3D conformal radiation therapy (3D-CRT), or intensity-modulated radiotherapy (IMRT). Thirty-nine (45.9%) patients were treated with preoperative chemotherapy, and 22 (25.9%) of these patients received at least one cycle of postoperative chemotherapy. The chemotherapy regimens were almost entirely anthracycline-based, including

Table 1: Demographic information.

Total number of patients	85
Male	48
Female	37
Median age (years)	42 (range, 18–88 years)
Patients treated with preoperative radiation therapy	67 (78.8%)
Patients treated with postoperative radiation therapy	15 (17.6%)
Patients treated with pre- and postoperative radiation therapy	7 (8.2%)
Patients treated with postoperative radiation therapy only	8 (9.4%)
Patients not treated with radiation therapy	10 (11.8%)
Number of patients treated with chemotherapy	39
Location of tumor	
Right thigh	30 (35.3%)
Left thigh	28 (32.9%)
Right lower leg	6 (7.1%)
Left lower leg	4 (4.7%)
Right knee	3 (3.5%)
Buttock	3 (3.5%)
Left knee	2 (2.4%)
Abdomen	2 (2.4%)
Paraspinal	1 (1.2%)
Chest wall	1 (1.2%)
Left shoulder	1 (1.2%)
Back	1 (1.2%)
Vulva	1 (1.2%)
Head and neck	1 (1.2%)
Tumor size	
Mean (cm)	12.0
Median (cm)	10.0
Range (cm)	1.3–35
Median preoperative radiation dose (cGy)	5000 (range, 2000–7100)
Median postoperative radiation dose (cGy)	1600 (range, 1000–7020)
Median postoperative dose in patients receiving preoperative radiation therapy (cGy)	1600 (range, 1000–2200)
Median postoperative dose in patients not receiving preoperative radiation therapy (cGy)	6150 (range, 5940–7020)
Margin status (number of patients)	
Gross positive	2 (2.4%)
Microscopically positive	12 (14.1%)
Close (<1 mm)	50 (58.8%)
Negative	19 (22.3%)
Margin status not reported	2 (2.4%)
Local failures	4/85 (4.7%)
Local failures (patients treated with preoperative radiation therapy)	2/67 (3.0%)
Local failures (patients not treated with preoperative therapy)	2/18 (11%)

mesna, doxorubicin, ifosfamide, and dacarbazine (MAID) or doxorubicin, ifosfamide, and mesna (AIM) chemotherapy, with the exception of one patient who received bevacizumab alone on a clinical trial.

Five-year disease-free survival, distant metastasis-free survival, local control, and overall survival were 78.6% (95% CI: 67.8–86.1), 84.7% (95% CI: 74.5–91.0), 95.6% (95% CI: 86.9–98.6), and 87.5% (95% CI: 77.2–93.3), respectively (Figures 1–4). Four out of 85 (4.7%) patients experienced a local recurrence. Of these four patients, two had received preoperative radiotherapy. One patient received a preoperative dose of 4400 cGy, while the other patient received a preoperative dose of 3000 cGy. Out of these, 1 patient (25%) had received postoperative radiotherapy. This patient had not received preoperative radiotherapy.

Radiotherapy with or without chemotherapy was associated with a high degree of tumor response. The median percent necrosis for patients who received preoperative radiation therapy was 95% (range, 0–100%), with a mean necrosis rate of 77.6% (Table 2). Percent necrosis is a direct indicator of pathological response and was inversely associated with histologically intact residual tumor (e.g., 100% necrosis indicates that no histological tumor was left behind). Ten out of 85 patients had a pathological complete response (11.7%). On univariate analysis, there was a trend towards higher necrosis rates in patients who received concurrent chemotherapy, 84.7% (95% CI: 75.9–93.4) and 69.5% (95% CI: 55.1–83.8), $p = 0.061$, compared with patients who did not receive concurrent chemotherapy. On multivariate analysis, the use of chemotherapy was significantly associated with increased rates of necrosis (Table 3). However, the addition of chemotherapy did not appear to be associated with improvements in disease-free or overall survival. In patients with tumor size ≥5 cm who had chemotherapy, OS: HR (hazard ratio) is 1.69 (95% CI: 0.54–5.25), $p = 0.367$ and DFS: HR is 1.85 (95% CI: 0.81–4.19), $p = 0.143$. Tumor size of <5 cm, 5–10 cm, and >10 cm has been associated with prognosis in sarcoma subtypes [7].

The use of radiation therapy with or without chemotherapy preoperatively resulted in overall very low rates of local recurrence (4.7% in all patients with 2/4 failures occurring in patients with negative margins and 2/4 failures occurring in patients with close (<1 mm) or positive margins).

With regard to pretreatment variables that could predict outcome, large tumor size, as analyzed by a continuous variable, was associated with inferior disease-free survival and local control. Large tumor size and Grade ≥ 2 were associated with inferior overall survival (Tables 4–7).

Short- and long-term toxicity was scored based on retrospective chart review and the RTOG acute and late toxicity scale [8]. Acute toxicity data were available for a total of eighty-three patients. Seventeen out of 83 patients (20%) experienced an RTOG acute skin toxicity Grade 3 or higher. Of these 17 patients, 9 had received chemotherapy (52.9%), while 8 patients did not receive chemotherapy (47.1%). These differences were not statistically significant ($p = 0.771$). Late toxicity data were available for a total of 83 patients. Nine patients (10.8%) experienced an RTOG Grade 3 or higher late skin toxicity.

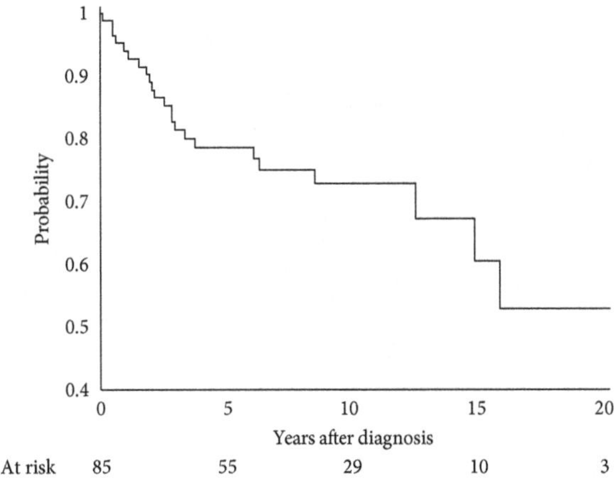

FIGURE 1: Disease-free survival at 5 years, 78.6% (95% CI: 67.8–86.1).

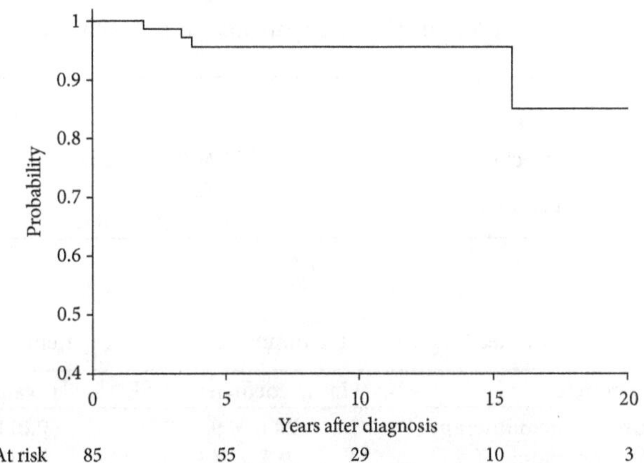

FIGURE 2: Local control at 5 years, 95.6% (86.9–98.6).

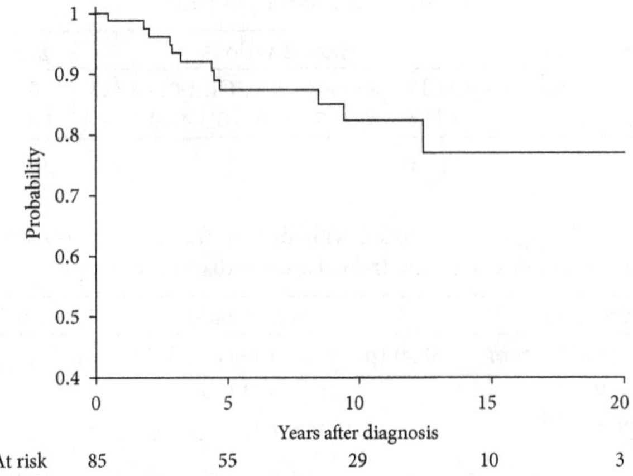

FIGURE 3: Overall survival at 5 years, 87.5% (77.2–93.3).

4. Discussion

In this series of 85 patients, we found a mean necrosis rate of over 77% in patients treated with preoperative radiation therapy. These data support the findings from other published series and clinical experience that suggest that MLS is

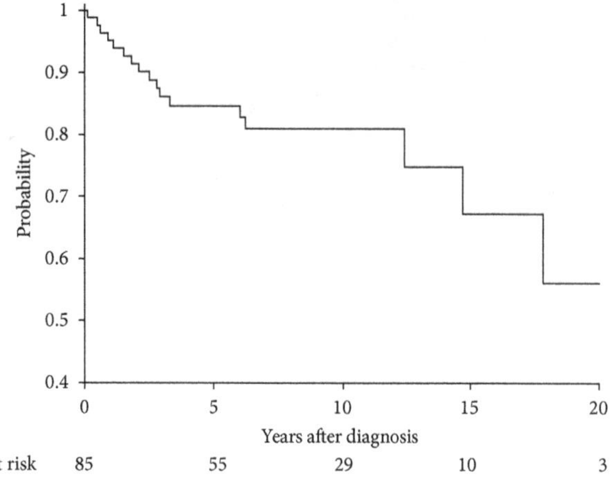

FIGURE 4: Distant metastases-free survival at 5 years, 84.7 (74.5–91.0).

TABLE 2: Mean tumor response (patients treated with radiation therapy).

Pre-op RT	77.6%
No pre-op RT	0%
Concurrent chemotherapy	84.7% (95% CI: 75.9–93.4)
No concurrent chemotherapy	69.5%(95% CI: 55.1–83.8) $p = 0.061$

TABLE 3: Linear regression for tumor response (all patients).

Parameter	Linear coefficient ± SE	p value
Use of chemotherapy	24.6 ± 9.4	0.011
Margin status	9.5 ± 9.3	0.311
Tumor size	0.9 ± 0.7	0.209

TABLE 4: Local control (all patients).

Parameter	Hazard ratio	p value
Tumor size	HR 1.17 (per cm) (95% CI: 1.02–1.33)	0.022
Margin	HR 0.32 (95% CI: 0.02–4.49)	0.396

TABLE 5: Factors associated with disease-free survival on multivariate analysis (patients treated with radiation therapy).

Parameter	Hazard ratio	p value
Necrosis/tumor response	0.90 (per 10% of necrosis) (95% CI: 0.75–1.07)	0.222
High-grade disease	5.97 (95% CI: 0.72–49.67)	0.172
Tumor size	1.08 (per cm) (95% CI: 1.01–1.16)	0.019

a radiosensitive malignancy, as reflected by histological response. While it is not certain how histological response correlates with treatment outcomes, there is a suggestion from some published series that high levels of necrosis may correlate with improved outcomes [9, 10]. Additionally, the results of our series show a trend that the addition of concurrent chemotherapy increased necrosis to a mean of 82.3% as compared with 58.8% patients who were not treated with chemotherapy. Our study findings are also consistent with other sarcoma studies in which large tumor size is associated with inferior disease-free survival [11].

TABLE 6: Factors associated with disease-free survival on multivariate analysis.

Parameter	Hazard ratio	p value
Use of radiation therapy	HR 0.45 (95% CI: 0.13–1.60)	0.218
Size > 10 cm + grade ≥ 2	HR 3.11 (95% CI: 1.17–8.27)	0.023

TABLE 7: Factors associated with overall survival multivariate analysis.

Parameter	Hazard ratio	p value
Any radiation	HR 0.28 (95% CI: 0.06–1.47)	0.133
Size > 10 cm + grade ≥ 2	HR 6.56 (95% CI: 1.32–32.76)	0.022

The high degree of response supports the use of preoperative therapy of these MLS patients.

While it is our practice to consider additional postoperative boost radiation therapy in patients with positive margins after preoperative radiation, the low rates of local failures make it difficult to perform more detailed analysis of related factors that may impact local control and survival. One of the local failures occurred in a patient who had a grossly positive margin and still had a local failure after postoperative radiation therapy.

The results of our series are concordant with other published series in MLS suggesting chemotherapy sensitivity [12]. Furthermore, our series is hypothesis generating in which chemotherapy may enhance the effect of radiotherapy. In our study, chemoradiotherapy was associated with histological response; we did not see a benefit of chemotherapy with disease-free or overall survival.

While patients in this retrospective series received different chemotherapeutic agents, a large randomized study did not show a benefit to histologically tailored chemotherapy, over a standard regimen [13]. Given the low rate of local failures overall, the number of events make statistical analysis about factors that either enhance locoregional control difficult. From the literature, there is uncertainty whether high necrosis rates correlate with improved outcome. Some reports [14, 15] have shown no overall clinical benefit with high tumor necrosis rates, while another has suggested that pathological necrosis does correlate with clinical outcome [16]. Although our series did not demonstrate a definite correlation of the degree of necrosis with disease-free survival or overall survival, it is important to recognize that selection bias likely led to larger, higher risk tumors receiving chemotherapy (which was then associated with greater pathologic necrosis), thus confounding these data. Furthermore, it is possible that mechanisms behind tumor necrosis could vary and that patients with tumor necrosis as a result of a rapidly dividing tumor outgrowing its blood supply could have a different outcome compared with a patient who develops a necrotic tumor due to a significant response. The rarity of this tumor, however, would make a randomized clinical trial designed to address the effectiveness of adjuvant chemotherapy specifically for MLS difficult to complete.

The findings of our study support the importance of multidisciplinary care in the management of patients with MLS. In addition to radiotherapy, chemotherapy also appears to enhance the histological response rates to treatment.

Due to the low numbers of local failures, more definitive conclusions on the impact of chemotherapy on local control in MLS cannot be made. The use of concurrent, neoadjuvant chemotherapy, with the potential to reduce the incidence of metastatic disease has a theoretical appeal because of the poor prognosis of patients who ultimately develop metastatic disease [17].

There are some limitations of study that warrant further discussion. First, as a single institution study, there is inherent selection and management bias. The retrospective nature of our series also limits our ability to draw conclusions regarding specific therapies.

Our series did not find any differences in toxicity in patients who received chemotherapy, although it is likely that chemotherapy adds at least some degree of toxicity in patients who are treated with radiation therapy that may not have been captured in a retrospective analysis. It is possible that chemotherapy may have resulted in higher rates of acute Grade 2 or higher skin toxicity; these may not have been captured due to the retrospective nature of our series. Another limitation of this series was that the patients reviewed performed where largely the population of patients was surveilled using CT imaging to detect distant recurrence. There is a recent report that whole-body MRI may be more sensitive at detecting a pulmonary metastases compared with CT, and it is possible that this is more sensitive with regard to the detection of metastatic disease [18]. Furthermore, it is possible that at least some of the patients in this series could have been found to have metastatic disease even prior to the initiation of definitive therapy.

While the addition of chemotherapy provides for a means of treatment intensification in patients with a high risk of local and distant recurrences, the results of our series also present an opportunity to evaluate the role of treatment deintensification. The high rates of local control with a median preoperative radiotherapy dose of 50 Gy suggest that it may be reasonable to de-escalate therapy in selected patients, which is the subject of an ongoing international clinical trial [19]. However, more investigation is required to better understand in which patients such treatment deintensification is safe.

5. Conclusions

The results of our study support the notion that myxoid liposarcoma has a high rate of histological response with combined chemotherapy and radiotherapy, with low rates of local failure with trimodality therapy. The high pathological response rates to chemotherapy are hypothesis generating. While some reports [16] have suggested that high necrosis rates may correlate with improved clinical outcomes, our study, while not specifically designed to address this issue, did not demonstrate a correlation between necrosis and clinical outcome. We were not able to show that chemotherapy provides a significant clinical benefit with regard to local control, disease-free survival, or overall survival, although the likely selected usage of chemotherapy in the highest risk patients confounds this analysis. We agree with the National Comprehensive Cancer Network (NCCN) guidelines that chemotherapy should be considered in patients with large, high-grade sarcomas [20]. Further research is required to understand which patients benefit the most from chemotherapy, and which patients may benefit from treatment deintensification.

Disclosure

Drs. De Amorim Bernstein and Lozano-Calderón are co-senior authors on this project. This work has been presented as an abstract at the EMSOS 2018, Amsterdam. This work has not been previously published in a peer-reviewed journal.

References

[1] C. Antonescu and M. Ladanyi, "Myxoid liposarcoma," in *World Health Organization Classification of Tumors, Pathology and Genetics of Tumors of Soft Tissue and Bone*, C. D. M. Fletcher, K. K. Unni, and F. Mertens, Eds., pp. 40–43, IARC Press, Lyon, France, 2002.

[2] S. E. ten Heuvel, H. J. Hoekstra, R. J. van Ginkel, E. Bastiaannet, and A. J. H. Suurmeijer, "Clinicopathologic prognostic factors in myxoid liposarcoma: a retrospective study of 49 patients with long-term follow-up," *Annals of Surgical Oncology*, vol. 14, no. 1, pp. 222–229, 2007.

[3] R. S. A. de Vreeze, D. de Jong, R. L. Haas, F. Stewart, and F. van Coevorden, "Effectiveness of radiotherapy in myxoid sarcomas is associated with a dense vascular pattern," *International Journal of Radiation Oncology, Biology, Physics*, vol. 72, no. 5, pp. 1480–1487, 2008.

[4] G. Pitson, P. Robinson, D. Wilke et al., "Radiation response: an additional unique signature of myxoid liposarcoma," *International Journal of Radiation Oncology, Biology, Physics*, vol. 60, no. 2, pp. 522–526, 2004.

[5] R. L. Jones, C. Fisher, O. Al-Muderis, and I. R. Judson, "Differential sensitivity of liposarcoma subtypes to chemotherapy," *European Journal of Cancer*, vol. 41, no. 18, pp. 2853–2860, 2005.

[6] D. Katz, P. Boonsirikamchai, H. Choi et al., "Efficacy of first-line doxorubicin and ifosfamide in myxoid liposarcoma," *Clinical Sarcoma Research*, vol. 2, no. 1, p. 2, 2012.

[7] S. Singer, E. H. Baldini, G. D. Demetri, J. A. Fletcher, and J. M. Corson, "Synovial sarcoma: prognostic significance of tumor size, margin of resection, and mitotic activity for survival," *Journal of Clinical Oncology*, vol. 14, no. 4, pp. 1201–1208, 1996.

[8] J. D. Cox, J. Stetz, and T. F. Pajak, "Toxicity criteria of the radiation therapy oncology group (RTOG) and the European organization for research and treatment of cancer (EORTC)," *International Journal of Radiation Oncology, Biology, Physics*, vol. 31, no. 5, pp. 1341–1346, 1995.

[9] P. W. M. Chung, B. M. Deheshi, P. C. Ferguson et al., "Radiosensitivity translates into excellent local control in extremity myxoid liposarcoma: a comparison with other soft tissue sarcomas," *Cancer*, vol. 115, no. 14, pp. 3254–3261, 2009.

[10] B. A. Guadagnolo, G. K. Zagars, M. T. Ballo et al., "Excellent local control rates and distinctive patterns of failure in myxoid liposarcoma treated with conservation surgery and radiotherapy," *International Journal of Radiation Oncology, Biology, Physics*, vol. 70, no. 3, pp. 760–765, 2008.

[11] P. W. Pisters, D. H. Leung, J. Woodruff, W. Shi, and M. F. Brennan, "Analysis of prognostic factors in 1,041 patients with localized soft tissue sarcomas of the extremities," *Journal of Clinical Oncology*, vol. 14, no. 5, pp. 1679–1689, 1996.

[12] S. R. Patel, M. A. Burgess, C. Plager, N. E. Papadopoulos, K. A. Linke, and R. S. Benjamin, "Myxoid liposarcoma. Experience with chemotherapy," *Cancer*, vol. 74, no. 4, pp. 1265–1269, 1994.

[13] A. Gronchi, S. Ferrari, V. Quagliuolo et al., "Histotype-tailored neoadjuvant chemotherapy versus standard chemotherapy in patients with high-risk soft-tissue sarcomas (ISG-STS 1001): an international, open-label, randomised, controlled, phase 3, multicentre trial," *The Lancet Oncology*, vol. 18, no. 6, pp. 812–822, 2017.

[14] D. R. Lucas, M. P. Kshirsagar, J. S. Biermann et al., "Histologic alterations from neoadjuvant chemotherapy in high-grade extremity soft tissue sarcoma: clinicopathological correlation," *The Oncologist*, vol. 13, no. 4, pp. 451–458, 2008.

[15] J. T. Mullen, F. J. Hornicek, D. C. Harmon et al., "Prognostic significance of treatment-induced pathologic necrosis in extremity and truncal soft tissue sarcoma after neoadjuvant chemoradiotherapy," *Cancer*, vol. 120, no. 23, pp. 3676–3682, 2014.

[16] F. C. Eilber, G. Rosen, J. Eckardt et al., "Treatment-induced pathologic necrosis: a predictor of local recurrence and survival in patients receiving neoadjuvant therapy for high-grade extremity soft tissue sarcomas," *Journal of Clinical Oncology*, vol. 19, no. 13, pp. 3203–3209, 2001.

[17] A. J. Spillane, C. Fisher, and J. M. Thomas, "Myxoid liposarcoma—the frequency and the natural history of nonpulmonary soft tissue metastases," *Annals of Surgical Oncology*, vol. 6, no. 4, pp. 389–394, 1999.

[18] N. Gorelik, S. M. V. Reddy, R. E. Turcotte et al., "Early detection of metastases using whole-body MRI for initial staging and routine follow-up of myxoid liposarcoma," *Skeletal Radiology*, vol. 47, no. 3, pp. 369–379, 2018.

[19] The Netherlands Cancer Institute, "Dose reduction of preoperative radiotherapy in myxoid liposarcomas (DOREMY)," 2014, https://clinicaltrials.gov/ct2/show/NCT02106312.

[20] NCCN, "NCCN clinical practice guidelines in oncology. Soft tissue sarcoma. NCCN evidence blocks. Version 2," 2017, https://www.nccn.org/professionals/physician_gls/pdf/sarcoma_blocks.pdf.

A Systematic Literature Review of Adverse Events Associated with Systemic Treatments used in Advanced Soft Tissue Sarcoma

Ann Colosia,[1] Shahnaz Khan,[1] Michelle D. Hackshaw,[2] Alan Oglesby,[2] James A. Kaye,[3] and Jeffrey M. Skolnik[4]

[1] *Market Access and Outcomes Strategy, RTI Health Solutions, 200 Park Offices Drive, Research Triangle Park, Durham, NC 27709, USA*
[2] *US Health Outcomes, Oncology, GlaxoSmithKline, 5 Crescent Drive, Philadelphia, PA 19112, USA*
[3] *Epidemiology, RTI Health Solutions, 1440 Main Street, Suite 310, Waltham, MA 02451, USA*
[4] *US Medical Affairs, Oncology, GlaxoSmithKline, 5 Crescent Drive, Philadelphia, PA 19112, USA*

Correspondence should be addressed to Ann Colosia; acolosia@rti.org

Academic Editor: Antoine Italiano

This systematic literature review describes adverse events (AEs) among patients with soft tissue sarcoma (STS) who received second-line or later anticancer therapies. Searches were conducted in PubMed, EMBASE, and Cochrane Central Register of Controlled Trials for studies of adults with advanced or metastatic STS who received systemic anticancer therapy before enrollment in a randomized-controlled trial of pazopanib, another targeted cancer agent, or cytotoxic chemotherapy. Of 204 publications identified, seven articles representing six unique studies met inclusion criteria. Additional safety results for pazopanib were identified on ClinicalTrials.gov. Hematologic toxicities were common with all therapies evaluated (pazopanib, trabectedin, dacarbazine ± gemcitabine, gemcitabine ± docetaxel, cyclophosphamide, and ifosfamide). Studies differed in AE type, timing of assessment, and outcomes reported, although patient populations and AE assessment timing were relatively similar for pazopanib and trabectedin. AEs that were more common with trabectedin than pazopanib were anemia, neutropenia, nausea/vomiting, and elevations in aspartate aminotransferase and alanine aminotransferase. An AE that was more common with pazopanib than trabectedin was anorexia. Only the pazopanib study reported AE frequencies versus placebo. A planned meta-analysis was not feasible, as there was no common comparator. More well-designed studies that include common comparators are needed for comparison of safety effects among treatments for STS.

1. Introduction

Soft tissue sarcomas (STS) are malignant tumors that begin in any of the mesodermal tissues of the extremities, trunk, retroperitoneum, or head and neck [1] and include more than 50 histologic subtypes [2]. In 2014, it was estimated that there would be 12,020 new cases of STS and 4740 deaths from STS in the United States (US) [3]. The overall estimated 5-year survival rate is 65.3% in the US, and the 5-year survival is 18.4% in patients with sarcomas with distant spread [3].

Treatment options for STS include surgery, radiotherapy, and systemic anticancer therapy (cytotoxic chemotherapy or targeted cancer agents). Surgery and radiotherapy are the standard initial treatment options for patients with primary resectable STS; however, up to 50% of patients experience recurrence [4]. For patients with advanced, unresectable, or metastatic STS, chemotherapy is the mainstay of treatment. Widely used cytotoxic chemotherapy regimens include dacarbazine, doxorubicin, epirubicin, and ifosfamide as single agents and anthracycline-based combinations (e.g., doxorubicin or epirubicin with ifosfamide, with or without dacarbazine). The National Comprehensive Cancer Network [5] and the European Society of Medical Oncologists [6] recommend an anthracycline (alone or in combination with other agents) as first-line treatment for metastatic STS in most cases, although first-line treatment recommendations may vary by histologic subtype and previous treatment. Other cytotoxic chemotherapy agents that have shown activity in clinical trials are gemcitabine, docetaxel, vinorelbine, pegylated liposomal doxorubicin, temozolomide [5], and trabectedin [6]. All of these agents can be associated with significant adverse events (AEs), including pancytopenia, febrile neutropenia, nausea, alopecia, and fatigue. Some long-term AEs may occur, including cardiomyopathy with doxorubicin and other anthracyclines [4].

Recently, a number of targeted cancer agents, including imatinib, sunitinib, and pazopanib, have demonstrated activity in particular STS histologic subtypes [5]. Imatinib is a tyrosine kinase inhibitor approved for treating gastrointestinal stromal tumors, but it failed to show activity in other histologic subtypes of STS [7]. Sunitinib, a multityrosine kinase inhibitor of vascular endothelial growth factor receptor- (VEGFR-) 2, platelet-derived growth factor receptor- (PDGFR-) β, and c-Kit, showed activity in patients with locally advanced or metastatic STS in a nonrandomized phase II trial [8]. Pazopanib is a multityrosine kinase inhibitor of VEGFR-1, VEGFR-2, VEGFR-3, PDGFR-α, PDGFR-β, and c-Kit. Pazopanib and trabectedin are the only therapies approved in the US for use as monotherapy for the treatment of patients with advanced STS who have received prior chemotherapy [9] (although trabectedin was not approved in the US at the time of the systematic literature review described in this article). Outside the US, trabectedin is approved for treatment in advanced STS after failure of anthracycline and ifosfamide or in patients with advanced STS for whom these agents are not suitable [10]. In the US, it is indicated for patients with advanced liposarcoma or leiomyosarcoma after an anthracycline-containing regimen.

In general, symptom palliation is the goal of treatment with cytotoxic chemotherapy and targeted cancer agents in patients with metastatic disease. There is a paucity of published data from randomized controlled trials (RCTs) evaluating these therapies compared with best supportive care, and no studies of targeted agents have demonstrated a survival advantage in metastatic STS to date [4]. Given the palliative nature of the therapy, lower toxicity regimens are desirable in this population.

There is no single data source that addresses the broad range of AEs associated with systemic anticancer therapy, that is, cytotoxic chemotherapy (classic chemotherapy agents such as doxorubicin and ifosfamide) or targeted cancer agents (drugs developed to target a specific protein in cancer cells such as pazopanib) in STS. To address this gap and to better understand the safety profile of these agents in this disease, we conducted a systematic literature review to review the tolerability and associated toxicities of pazopanib and other targeted cancer agents and cytotoxic chemotherapies used in the treatment of advanced or metastatic STS. A subsequent meta-analysis, if feasible, was planned to compare information on reported AEs associated with pazopanib and other therapies in the management and treatment of STS.

2. Materials and Methods

A systematic literature review was conducted on April 9, 2014, in accordance with the Preferred Reporting Items for Systematic Reviews and Meta-Analyses (PRISMA) guidelines [19]. PubMed, EMBASE, and the Cochrane Central Register of Controlled Trials (CENTRAL) were searched in order to qualitatively assess the frequencies of specific AEs occurring in adult patients with a diagnosis of advanced or metastatic STS other than gastrointestinal stromal tumors (since they are biologically distinct from other STS subtypes regarding their targeted treatment) who received prior systemic anticancer therapy from RCTs, as well as to assess the feasibility of conducting a meta-analysis of identified placebo-controlled trials. There were no date limits, but only publications in English were included. The study (ID: 201358) and protocol can be found at http://www.gsk-clinicalstudyregister.com/study/201358#ps. An example of the search strategies employed is presented in Additional file 1: Table S1 in Supplementary Material available online at http://dx.doi.org/10.1155/2016/3597609.

Bibliographies of included articles were reviewed for additional relevant studies not identified in the electronic database search. Included studies were RCTs in adults (aged ≥18 years) with a diagnosis of advanced/metastatic STS who had received at least one line of systemic anticancer therapy before enrollment in an RCT of pazopanib or another targeted cancer agent or cytotoxic chemotherapy. The original protocol for this systematic literature review included only studies that were blinded, even if only single-blinded. The goal of this inclusion criterion was to reduce bias on the part of patients and/or investigators in the reporting of AEs. After completing level 2 screening (see Section 2.2), we determined that only one study met all of the inclusion criteria (a study of pazopanib by van der Graaf et al. [11]). Because several other studies violated the inclusion criteria only by being open-label, the protocol was amended to include open-label studies to allow a qualitative review of the literature. Other inclusion criteria were that at least one arm of the studies had to evaluate a drug of interest and report an AE of interest.

A list of AEs of interest (Additional file 2: Table S2) was initially developed before conducting the literature review by reviewing product labels, and we further modified this list based on desktop research and clinical expertise. The primary endpoint included any frequency of any grade of the AEs, including separate reporting of grade 3 and/or 4 frequencies. If a meta-analysis had been feasible, the secondary endpoints were to be the same AEs. Studies in which all or most of the patients had gastrointestinal stromal tumor, childhood sarcomas, and other sarcomas or related tumors with unique treatment approaches were excluded.

2.1. Data Extraction. Data extracted from the eligible studies included trial characteristics, treatment information (dosing regimen), patient demographics, descriptions of the AEs captured (e.g., on-treatment only or a specified period beyond treatment, AEs for the intent-to-treat population or only for patients who actually received treatment, most common AE, and AEs occurring in $\geq X\%$ of patients), and data for

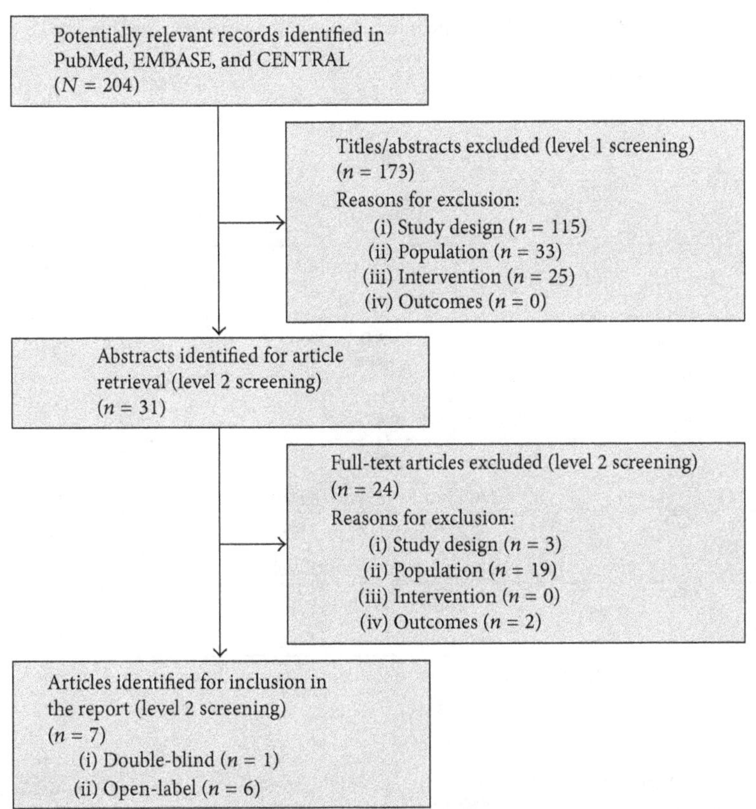

FIGURE 1: PRISMA flow diagram, Amendment 1. CENTRAL: Cochrane Central Register of Controlled Trials; PRISMA: Preferred Reporting Items for Systematic Reviews and Meta-Analyses.

the selected endpoints wherever available. Additionally, the number of patients experiencing any grade of an AE and the total number of patients in the safety population for that treatment arm were captured. Data were extracted by one reviewer, and the accuracy was checked by a second reviewer.

2.2. Quality Control and Assessment. Quality control procedures for inclusion and exclusion of articles included level 1 (titles/abstracts) and level 2 (full-text) screening for eligibility according to the inclusion and exclusion criteria, which were performed independently by two researchers. Articles for which there was any uncertainty about inclusion were discussed with a third researcher. Data were extracted from full-text versions of articles. Resources obtained via the Internet, such as results pages from ClinicalTrials.gov and the Food and Drug Administration Oncologic Drugs Advisory Committee Briefing Document, were saved as PDF files to maintain a record of information in case the electronic source was changed or removed. Quality control procedures for the data extraction included verification by a second researcher of all extracted data with original sources. The quality assessment of evidence from RCTs was based on guidance in the National Institute for Health and Care Excellence single technology appraisal *Specification for Manufacturer/Sponsor Submission of Evidence* [20] and adapted from the Centre for Reviews and Dissemination's guidance for undertaking reviews in health care [21].

2.3. Qualitative Data Synthesis. The qualitative assessment of RCTs identified in the systematic literature review did not involve statistical methods. Results are described qualitatively with more detailed results presented in supporting tables.

3. Results and Discussion

3.1. Search Results. Figure 1 shows the PRISMA flow diagram [22], which documents the number of articles excluded after title/abstract review and full-text review and the number of articles ultimately meeting the inclusion criteria after protocol amendment.

Searches of PubMed, EMBASE, and CENTRAL identified 204 studies after removal of duplicates. The original protocol called for inclusion of RCTs that were single-, double-, or triple-blinded. However, only the pazopanib study by van der Graaf et al. [11] met all of the inclusion criteria. With only one placebo-controlled study, a meta-analysis was not feasible.

The qualitative review was not restricted to placebo-controlled studies and RCTs with active comparators could be included. During level 2 review, five articles representing four open-label RCTs with active comparator arms were identified that met all inclusion criteria for the qualitative review except for blinding (Table 1; Additional file 3: Table S3) [12–14, 16, 17]. Pautier et al. [17] included two multicenter, open-label, phase II studies; patients were stratified by uterine and nonuterine sites of origin of leiomyosarcoma into two

TABLE 1: Characteristics of included studies after protocol amendment.

Reference	Phase	Randomized, n	Treatment	Patient group for safety	n	Median number of cycles (range)
van der Graaf et al., 2012 [11]	III	369	Pazopanib	Treated	239	Median treatment duration, 16.4 weeks (0–79 weeks)
			Placebo		123	Median treatment duration, 8.1 weeks (1–52 weeks)
Bramwell et al., 1986, 1987, 1993 [12–14]	II	171	Cyclophosphamide	Treated	29	2.5 (1–13)
			Ifosfamide		28	3 (1–15)
Demetri et al., 2009 [15]	II	270	Trabectedin 24 h IV every 3 weeks	Treated	130	5 (1–37)
			Trabectedin 3 h IV weekly for 3 of 4 weeks		130	2 (1–21)
García-Del-Muro et al., 2011 [16]	II	113	Dacarbazine	Treated and assessable	52	2 (1–10)
			Gemcitabine + dacarbazine		57	6 (2–12)
Pautier et al., 2012 [17]* Study 1: leiomyosarcoma	II	46	Gemcitabine	Treated	22	5
			Gemcitabine + docetaxel		24	
Study 2: nonuterine leiomyosarcoma	II	44	Gemcitabine	Treated	22	4
			Gemcitabine + docetaxel		22	

*The article by Pautier et al. [17] presents the results of two independent phase II studies: one study in patients with uterine leiomyosarcoma and one in patients with nonuterine leiomyosarcoma. IV, intravenous.

distinct phase II studies conducted in one trial. Based on the protocol amendment, these four studies could be included in the qualitative safety analysis.

The protocol amendment required revisiting the open-label studies excluded at level 1 review. Four open-label studies were identified [15, 23–25]. The full-text articles for these studies were reviewed to determine their eligibility based on the amended protocol, and only one was eligible for inclusion in the qualitative review (a study by Demetri and colleagues [15]).

3.2. Included Studies. A total of six studies from the 7 publications (Bramwell et al. 1986, 1987, and 1993 represented 1 study and Pautier et al. represented 2 studies) were included in this review: one double-blind placebo-controlled study [11] and five open-label RCTs [12–17]. All six studies were multicenter (Table 1; Additional file 3: Table S3): three studies were multinational [11, 12, 15] and three were conducted in only one country [16, 17]. There was one phase III study [11], and the remaining studies were all phase II [12, 15–17]. The treatment arm sizes ranged from 22 to 239. The studies with the largest patient populations were those evaluating pazopanib (n = 369) [11] and trabectedin (n = 270) [15].

The drugs assessed in the trials included pazopanib versus placebo [11]; cyclophosphamide versus ifosfamide (one study in three reports) [12–14]; two different dosing schedules of trabectedin [15]; dacarbazine ± gemcitabine [16]; and gemcitabine ± docetaxel (two studies in one report) [17].

Predictably, the main source of risk of bias was lack of blinding in all included studies except the pazopanib study, which was double-blinded (Additional files 4–9: Tables S4–S9) [11]. The appropriateness of the method of randomization was insufficiently described in four of the studies (in five reports) [12–14, 16, 17].

3.3. Cross Over. The studies differed in whether they allowed patients to cross over to the other study treatment after disease progression occurred on the initially assigned regimen. Patients were allowed to cross over to the other study drug in Bramwell et al. [12–14], which evaluated cyclophosphamide versus ifosfamide and in Demetri et al. [15], which evaluated different dosing schedules of trabectedin. In the study of pazopanib versus placebo by van der Graaf et al. [11], patients were not allowed to cross over when the disease progressed, but postprogression therapy included trabectedin, gemcitabine, taxanes, ifosfamide, dacarbazine, and antiangiogenic agents [26]. There was no discussion of crossover in the García-Del-Muro et al. study of dacarbazine ± gemcitabine [16] or the two studies of gemcitabine ± dacarbazine [17]. It was not explicitly stated that reported AEs were limited to the period prior to crossover, but we made this assumption when reporting the results. The main effect of crossover in clinical trials is to confound overall survival comparisons between randomized treatment groups, but overall survival was not the focus of this review.

3.4. Patient Populations. Most patients in all of the studies had metastatic rather than unresectable locally advanced disease (Additional file 10: Table S10). Although the Bramwell et al. study of cyclophosphamide versus ifosfamide allowed chemotherapy-naïve patients into the study, it presented a separate AE outcome (leukopenia) stratified by whether or not the patient had received previous chemotherapy [12–14].

The performance status of the populations in all of the studies did not differ widely. Although some studies allowed patients with a performance status of 2 to enroll [16, 17], most patients in all of the studies had a performance status of 0 or 1 (Additional file 10: Table S10). The median ages were similar in most of the studies (about 50–54 years) except for the nonuterine leiomyosarcoma group in the study by Pautier et al. [17], in which the median ages were 62 to 64 years for the gemcitabine ± docetaxel groups.

The predominant histology in all of the studies was leiomyosarcoma, representing 100% of the patients in the study of gemcitabine ± docetaxel by Pautier et al. [17] and 27% to 66% of the patients in the other studies. Patients with adipocyte/liposarcoma were excluded from the study of pazopanib [11], but they represented 3% to 34% of the patients in the studies of cyclophosphamide versus ifosfamide [13], dacarbazine ± gemcitabine [16], and trabectedin [15]. Except for the two studies including only patients with leiomyosarcoma (uterine and nonuterine) [17], 10% to 16% of patients had synovial sarcoma.

With the exception of the Pautier et al. study of uterine leiomyosarcoma [17], both sexes were well represented in the studies. Most or all of the patients in the reviewed studies had metastatic disease (versus unresectable locally advanced STS). The median ages were 40 to 64 years (Additional file 10: Table S10).

3.5. Previous Treatment. As a requirement for inclusion in this review, all studies presented data on patients who had received previous chemotherapy. Most or all of the patients were receiving the study drug as second-line therapy.

Only the Bramwell et al. [12] study evaluating cyclophosphamide versus ifosfamide enrolled patients with no previous chemotherapy, and separate AE data were presented for 42% of patients who had received previous chemotherapy. Of these 56 patients (42% of the total study population), 67% had received only one previous drug, which was typically an anthracycline, and 12.5% had received ≥3 drugs. However, the article did not report whether any of the ≥3 drugs were given in combination, which would result in fewer lines of therapy. It was also unclear whether the one drug (usually an anthracycline) was given as neoadjuvant, adjuvant, or first-line therapy for advanced disease. In the pazopanib study [11], 93% of patients had received previous systemic anticancer therapy for advanced disease and 56% had received ≥2 lines of treatment for advanced disease. Similarly, the trabectedin study required that patients had received previous anthracycline and ifosfamide (combined or sequentially) therapy, but it did not restrict this treatment to the advanced-disease setting, so some patients received the study drug as first-line therapy for advanced disease [15]. The median number of previous regimens for advanced disease was one, so at least one-half of the patients in this study received trabectedin as second- or later-line therapy, with some receiving it as up to seventh-line therapy. Also, approximately one-third of the patients had received agents not approved by a regulatory agency for advanced STS, including gemcitabine, docetaxel, and other investigational agents.

In the pazopanib study, 93% of patients had received previous systemic therapy for advanced STS, and 56% of patients received pazopanib as third- or later-line therapy [11]. Compared with the other studies, it appears that patients in the pazopanib study were more heavily pretreated, based on the number of previous systemic anticancer lines administered.

In the study of dacarbazine ± gemcitabine [16], all patients had received previous treatment with an anthracycline, ifosfamide, or both. The authors described the population as "heavily pretreated," which seems to be variably defined with regard to cancer patients. For 77% of the patients in this study, disease progression occurred within 1 year of the prior therapy.

In the two studies of gemcitabine ± docetaxel [17], eligible patients had to receive only one prior doxorubicin-containing regimen. Most patients either received the doxorubicin-containing regimen as first-line therapy or, at disease progression within 1 year of adjuvant therapy, were considered to have received first-line doxorubicin. Few patients had an interval of >1 year after adjuvant therapy with anthracycline.

3.6. Methods of AE Reporting. The methods used for assessing safety in the trials varied (Additional file 11: Table S11). Three studies used the AE definitions from the National Cancer Institute (NCI) Common Terminology Criteria (CTC) [11, 16, 17] and one study used the *Medical Dictionary for Regulatory Activities* definitions with grading of severity by NCI CTC [15]. Another study used World Health Organization grade toxicity [12–14], which was the only study that was clear about the time frame of safety assessment ("after the first course and throughout treatment").

The pazopanib study reported treatment-emergent AEs [11, 27], whereas the other studies did not specify whether all AEs or only treatment-emergent AEs were being reported. The study of dacarbazine ± gemcitabine presented only "clinically relevant toxicities" [16]. Leukopenia was the only AE reported separately for patients with previous chemotherapy experience in the study of cyclophosphamide versus ifosfamide in Bramwell et al. [12–14].

Only the Pautier et al. study of gemcitabine ± docetaxel did not report safety outcomes as the number and percentage of patients experiencing the AE [17]. Instead, this study reported the "percentage of cycles for which patients experienced toxicity." The trabectedin study presented both types of outcomes [15].

This report uses "frequency" to mean the percentage of patients experiencing a particular AE as the worst grade occurrence or the percentage of patients experiencing AEs per cycle. "Rate" is not appropriate for comparisons among studies as the time frame for AE assessment presumably varied because patients were treated for differing amounts of time, as deduced from the median number of cycles administered (Additional file 11: Table S11).

3.7. Adverse Events. As previously mentioned, leukopenia was the only AE reported for patients with previous chemotherapy in the study of cyclophosphamide versus ifosfamide [12–14]. Only two other studies reported leukopenia [11, 16, 18], so this AE is summarized separately from the remaining AEs. In the pazopanib trial, grade 3 leukopenia occurred in three patients (1%) receiving pazopanib and no patients (0%) receiving placebo [11]. Grade 3 and 4 leukopenia occurred in higher percentages of patients treated with cyclophosphamide than with ifosfamide [12–14]. The

TABLE 2: Patients experiencing selected liver-related AEs.

Study	van der Graaf et al., 2012 [11, 18]		Demetri et al., 2009 [15]		García-Del-Muro et al., 2011 [16]	
Patient group	Treated		ITT (independent review)		Treated and analyzed	
Treatment group	Placebo (n = 123)	Pazopanib (n = 239)	Trabectedin q3wk 24 h IV (n = 130)	Trabectedin weekly 3 h IV (n = 130)	Dacarbazine (n = 52)	Gemcitabine + dacarbazine (n = 57)
Liver-related AEs, n (%)						
AST elevation						
All grades	27 (22)*	122 (51)*	122 (94)	85 (65)	—	—
Grade 3	2 (2)*	13 (5)*	41 (32)	4 (3)	—	—
Grade 4	0 (0)*	6 (3)*	0 (0)	0 (0)	—	—
ALT elevation						
All grades	22 (18)*	110 (46)*	126 (97)	100 (77)	—	—
Grade 3	3 (2)*	18 (8)*	59 (45)	12 (9)	—	—
Grade 4	1 (1)*	5 (2)*	3 (2)	0 (0)	—	—
Bilirubin elevation						
All grades	9 (7)*,†	68 (28)*,†	28 (22)	15 (12)	—	—
Grade 3	2 (2)*,†	3 (1)*,†	1 (<1)	1 (<1)	—	—
Grade 4	0 (0)*,†	0 (0)*,†	0 (0)	0 (0)	—	—

*These data were reported on ClinicalTrials.gov: NCT00753688.

†The number of patients with grade 3/4 bilirubin elevation differed slightly for the pazopanib group reporting in the article by van der Graaf et al. [11] and on ClinicalTrials.gov [18]. Because ClinicalTrials.gov had more information (all grades), this table shows the data from ClinicalTrials.gov.

AE: adverse event; ALT: alanine aminotransferase; AST: aspartate aminotransferase; ITT: intention to treat; IV: intravenous; q3wk: every 3 weeks.

Bramwell et al. study also included chemotherapy-naïve patients, and leukopenia was worse in patients with previous chemotherapy. The occurrence of serious infections was similar (~7%) in both treatment groups for all patients (both with and without previous chemotherapy). Leukopenia occurred in more patients receiving gemcitabine + dacarbazine than with dacarbazine alone, but grade 4 leukopenia was observed only in patients receiving dacarbazine alone [16].

An AE comparison of the studies reporting the percentage of patients experiencing AEs of interest [11, 15, 16, 18] is shown in Tables 2–5. In the pazopanib study, AEs that occurred at a higher frequency with pazopanib than placebo were neutropenia, thrombocytopenia, aspartate aminotransferase (AST) elevation, alanine aminotransferase (ALT) elevation, bilirubin elevation, anorexia, weight loss, diarrhea, nausea/vomiting, dysgeusia, mucositis, fatigue, and hypertension [11, 18]. Venous thromboembolic events occurred in a small proportion of patients in both the pazopanib and placebo groups, with a higher frequency in the pazopanib group.

Between the two trabectedin schedules, most on-treatment laboratory abnormalities occurred at a higher frequency with the every 3-week 24-hour infusion schedule than with the weekly 3-hour infusion schedule [15]. These AEs included the nonhematologic AEs elevations in AST, ALT, and bilirubin as well as the hematologic AEs neutropenia and thrombocytopenia. Drug-related nonlaboratory AEs were generally similar between the two treatment groups, except that nausea/vomiting was more common with the every 3-week 24-hour infusion schedule, and dyspnea occurred more often with the less-efficacious weekly 3-hour schedule (28%) and occurred in 17% of patients receiving the recommended every 3-week 24-hour schedule.

In the García-Del-Muro et al. study assessing gemcitabine ± dacarbazine, only the hematologic AE thrombocytopenia occurred more frequently among the AEs reported as clinically relevant in the group receiving dacarbazine alone [16]. All other reported AEs were more common in the dacarbazine + gemcitabine arm, including the hematologic AEs anemia, febrile neutropenia, neutropenia, the nonhematologic AEs diarrhea, and nausea/vomiting.

When AE frequencies were reported by the percentage of cycles during which the AE occurred, the trabectedin every 3-week 24-hour infusion schedule continued to have higher frequencies than the weekly 3-hour infusion schedule [15]. However, bilirubin elevation was equal between the two groups, and constipation occurred at a higher frequency with the every 3-week 24-hour infusion schedule.

Alopecia, asthenia, and fluid retention all occurred in a higher percentage of cycles in patients receiving gemcitabine + docetaxel than in patients receiving gemcitabine monotherapy [17]. Except for few occurrences of grade 3/4 asthenia, these three AEs were grade 1/2 in severity. Fever/infections occurred in a similar percentage of cycles between the two treatment groups, and most of these occurrences were grade 1/2 in severity.

3.8. Liver-Related AEs. More patients in the pazopanib group experienced elevations in AST, ALT, and bilirubin than in the placebo group (Table 2) [11, 18]. The percentage of patients experiencing grade 3 and 4 AST, ALT, and bilirubin elevations was ≤10%, with clinical assessments of safety, including laboratory assessments, done at baseline, weeks 4, 8, and 12,

TABLE 3: Patients experiencing selected gastrointestinal and/or eating-related AEs.

Study	van der Graaf et al., 2012 [11, 18]		Demetri et al., 2009 [15]		García-Del-Muro et al., 2011 [16]	
Patient group	Treated		ITT (independent review)		Treated and analyzed	
Treatment group	Placebo ($n = 123$)	Pazopanib ($n = 239$)	Trabectedin q3wk 24 h IV ($n = 130$)	Trabectedin weekly 3 h IV ($n = 130$)	Dacarbazine ($n = 52$)	Gemcitabine + dacarbazine ($n = 57$)
Gastrointestinal and/or eating-related AEs, n (%)						
Anorexia/decreased appetite						
All grades	24 (20)	95 (40)	29 (22)	21 (16)	—	—
Grade 3	0 (0)	14 (6)	—	—	—	—
Grade 4	0 (0)	0 (0)	—	—	—	—
Grade 3/4	0 (0)	14 (6)	1 (<1)	0 (0)	—	—
Constipation						
Grade 1/2	—	—	45 (35)	42 (32)	—	—
Grade 3/4	—	—	0 (0)	2 (2)	—	—
Decreased weight or weight loss						
All grades	25 (20)	115 (48)	—	—	—	—
Grade 3	0 (0)	0 (0)	—	—	—	—
Grade 4	0 (0)	0 (0)	—	—	—	—
Diarrhea						
All grades	20 (16)	138 (58)	31 (24)	28 (22)	3 (6)	10 (18)
Grade 3/4	1 (1)	11 (5)	1 (<1)	0 (0)	0 (0)	0 (0)
Nausea and/or vomiting						
All grades	34 (28)	129 (54)	97 (75)	67 (52)	8 (15)	23 (40)
Grade 3	2 (2)	8 (3)	—	—	1 (2)	1 (2)
Grade 4	0 (0)	0 (0)	—	—	—	—
Grade 3/4	2 (2)	8 (3)	7 (5)	3 (2)	—	—
Mouth or taste						
Dysgeusia						
All grades	5 (4)	64 (27)	—	—	—	—
Grade 3	0 (0)	0 (0)	—	—	—	—
Grade 4	0 (0)	0 (0)	—	—	—	—
Mucositis						
All grades	4 (3)	29 (12)	—	—	—	—
Grade 3	0 (0)	3 (1)	—	—	—	—
Grade 4	0 (0)	0 (0)	—	—	—	—

AE: adverse event; ITT: intention to treat; IV: intravenous; q3wk: every 3 weeks.

and at 8-week intervals thereafter, and dose modifications possible for AEs.

Nearly all patients receiving trabectedin in the every 3-week 24-hour infusion schedule arm experienced AST or ALT elevations, and ≥32% had grade 3 elevations [15]. Grade 3 and 4 elevations in AST and ALT were noncumulative and transient with a median duration of elevation of 7 to 8 days. Grade 3 increases in AST or ALT were much higher in the 3-week 24-hour infusion schedule arm than in the weekly 3-hour infusion schedule (Table 2). Only one patient in each trabectedin arm had grade 3 bilirubin elevation, and no patients experienced grade 4 bilirubin elevation.

Liver enzyme and bilirubin elevations were not reported in the study of dacarbazine ± gemcitabine [16].

3.9. Gastrointestinal and Eating-Related AEs. Anorexia, weight loss, diarrhea, and nausea/vomiting were all common with pazopanib, occurring in 40%, 48%, 58%, and 54% of patients, respectively (Table 3) [11]. Anorexia was also common in patients receiving trabectedin administered via the every 3-week 24-hour infusion schedule (22%), as were diarrhea (24%) and nausea/vomiting (75%) [15]. In both the pazopanib and trabectedin trials, grade 3/4 events occurred at relatively low frequencies (≤6%). There were no occurrences of grade 3/4 weight loss with pazopanib [11].

TABLE 4: Patients experiencing selected other AEs.

Study	van der Graaf et al., 2012 [11, 18]		Demetri et al., 2009 [15]		García-Del-Muro et al., 2011 [16]	
Patient group	Treated		ITT (independent review)		Treated and analyzed	
Treatment group	Placebo (n = 123)	Pazopanib (n = 239)	Trabectedin q3wk 24 h IV (n = 130)	Trabectedin weekly 3 h IV (n = 130)	Dacarbazine (n = 52)	Gemcitabine + dacarbazine (n = 57)
Other AEs, n (%)						
Alopecia						
Grade 1/2	—	—	—	—	1 (2)*	4 (7)*
Asthenia						
All grades	—	—	—	—	26 (50)	43 (76)
Grade 3	—	—	—	—	5 (10)	4 (7)
Grade 4	—	—	—	—	—	—
Cough						
All grades	—	—	23 (18)	22 (17)	—	—
Grade 3/4	—	—	0 (0)	1 (<1)	—	—
Dyspnea						
All grades	—	—	22 (17)	36 (28)	—	—
Grade 3/4	—	—	5 (4)	8 (6)	—	—
Embolism (including pulmonary and cerebrovascular)						
Venous thromboembolic events						
All grades	3 (2)	13 (5)	—	—	—	—
Fatigue						
All grades	60 (49)	155 (65)	97 (75)	89 (68)	—	—
Grade 3	6 (5)	30 (13)	—	—	—	—
Grade 4	1 (1)	1 (<1)	—	—	—	—
Grade 3/4	7 (6)	31 (13)	10 (8)	9 (7)	—	—
Headache						
All grades	—	—	37 (28)	34 (26)	—	—
Grade 3/4	—	—	1 (<1)	1 (<1)	—	—
Hypertension						
All grades	8 (7)	99 (41)	—	—	—	—
Grade 3	4 (3)	16 (7)	—	—	—	—
Grade 4	0 (0)	0 (0)	—	—	—	—

*All grade 2.
AE: adverse event; ITT: intention to treat; IV: intravenous; q3wk: every 3 weeks.

Adding gemcitabine to dacarbazine increased the frequency of all-grade diarrhea and nausea/vomiting, but there were no grade 3/4 occurrences of diarrhea and similarly low frequencies (2%) of nausea/vomiting in the two treatment groups [16].

3.10. Mouth or Taste. Only the pazopanib study reported on dysgeusia (taste disorder) and mucositis (Table 3). Both were higher in the pazopanib group than in the placebo group. There were no grade 3/4 occurrences of dysgeusia and only three occurrences of grade 3 mucositis in the pazopanib group [11].

3.11. Other AEs. Alopecia was reported in the study of dacarbazine ± gemcitabine; this AE occurred at low frequencies (7% and 2%, resp.), and all occurrences were grade 2 in severity (Table 4) [17]. The frequency of asthenia of any grade increased with the addition of gemcitabine, but grade 3 asthenia frequencies were similar between the two groups [16]. Cough was reported as a drug-related AE in 17% and 18% of patients receiving trabectedin at the weekly 3-hour and the every 3-week 24-hour schedules, respectively [15]. Dyspnea occurred more often with the weekly 3-hour schedule (28%) of trabectedin than with the recommended every 3-week 24-hour schedule (17%).

Embolism of any grade occurred at a low frequency (≤5%) but occurred more often with pazopanib than with placebo [11]. Fatigue was common with either schedule of trabectedin (68%–75%) and was mostly grade 1/2 [15]. Fatigue was also common with pazopanib (65%), but 49%

Study	van der Graaf et al., 2012 [11, 18]		Demetri et al., 2009 [15]		García-Del-Muro et al., 2011 [16]	
Patient group	Treated		ITT (independent review)		Treated and analyzed	
Treatment group	Placebo (n = 123)	Pazopanib (n = 239)	Trabectedin q3wk 24 h IV (n = 130)	Trabectedin weekly 3 h IV (n = 130)	Dacarbazine (n = 52)	Gemcitabine + dacarbazine (n = 57)
Hematologic AEs, n (%)						
Anemia						
All grades	28 (23)*	65 (27)*	126 (97)	117 (90)	34 (65)	47 (82)
Grade 3	1 (1)*	11 (5)*	5 (4)	9 (7)	4 (8)	2 (4)
Grade 4	1 (1)*	4 (2)*	5 (4)	3 (2)	2 (4)	0 (0)
Febrile neutropenia						
All grades	—	—	1 (<1)	1 (<1)	3 (6)	5 (9)
Grade 3	—	—	—	—	2 (4)	4 (7)
Grade 4	—	—	—	—	1 (2)	1 (2)
Neutropenia						
All grades	8 (7)*	79 (33)*	96 (74)	64 (49)	28 (53)	43 (76)
Grade 3	0 (0)*	10 (4)*	34 (26)	15 (12)	7 (13)	18 (32)
Grade 4	0 (0)*	0 (0)*	27 (21)	2 (2)	10 (19)	9 (16)
Grade 3/4	0 (0)*	10 (4)*	61 (47)	17 (13)	17 (32)	27 (48)
Thrombocytopenia						
All grades	7 (6)*	86 (36)*	70 (54)	36 (28)	31 (60)	23 (40)
Grade 3	0 (0)*	7 (3)*	12 (9)	6 (5)	8 (15)	1 (2)
Grade 4	0 (0)*	2 (1)*	3 (2)	1 (<1)	6 (12)	2 (4)

*These data were reported on ClinicalTrials.gov: NCT00753688.
AE: adverse event; ITT: intention to treat; IV: intravenous; q3wk: every 3 weeks.

of patients receiving placebo also reported fatigue [11]. Hypertension, primarily grade 1/2, occurred in 41% of patients receiving pazopanib and 7% of patients receiving placebo.

3.12. Hematologic AEs. For hematologic AEs, patients receiving pazopanib had only a slightly higher frequency of treatment-emergent anemia than patients receiving placebo (Table 5) [18]. The frequencies of all-grade anemia in the pazopanib study were 27% and 23% with pazopanib and placebo, respectively. The frequency of all-grade neutropenia was 33% in patients receiving pazopanib and 7% in patients receiving placebo. The frequency of febrile neutropenia by grade was not reported in the pazopanib study. Thrombocytopenia occurred more frequently in patients receiving pazopanib versus placebo.

For trabectedin, anemia was common with both schedules, but approximately one-half of patients entering the study had preexisting anemia [15]. Neutropenia was the most common grade 3/4 hematologic toxicity and was more common with the every 3-week 24-hour infusion (47%) than with the weekly 3-hour infusion schedule (13%). Grade 4 neutropenia with trabectedin was of short duration, and febrile neutropenia occurred in <1% of patients treated with trabectedin. Thrombocytopenia occurred more frequently in patients receiving trabectedin by the every 3-week 24-hour infusion schedule than by the weekly 3-hour infusion schedule.

Febrile neutropenia occurred in <10% of patients in the dacarbazine ± gemcitabine study [16]. Thrombocytopenia occurred more frequently in patients receiving dacarbazine alone versus dacarbazine + gemcitabine. This finding was true for all grades, grade 3, and grade 4 of thrombocytopenia.

4. Discussion

The goal of this systematic review was to compare a broad array of common AEs that affect patients' health and quality of life based on a list of prespecified AEs, developed by initially reviewing product labels and then modified based on desktop research and clinical expertise. An ideal outcome of this systematic literature review would have been a quantitative comparative assessment of pazopanib with other agents as second or later lines of treatment in previously treated patients with advanced or metastatic STS. However, such a comparison was not possible because there were no common comparators in the studies identified. The only randomized placebo-controlled study was that of pazopanib [11].

Only six RCTs in patients with STS who received previous systemic anticancer therapy met the inclusion criteria for this systematic review (adult patients, randomized design, and previous systemic anticancer therapies for STS), underscoring the paucity of medical evidence available in treating these diseases in the advanced or metastatic setting after first-line therapy. The median overall survival of patients in most arms of these studies was ≤1.5 years [11, 14, 15], with the exception of patients with uterine sarcoma who had a median survival of 20 and 23 months in the gemcitabine and gemcitabine + docetaxel groups, respectively [17]. The short life expectancy of patients in this setting underscores the need for tolerable later-line systemic anticancer therapies.

In addition to the lack of common comparators, comparisons would only be meaningful if the studies had similar patient populations and AE-reporting methods. Although gemcitabine was used in three studies, it was combined with a unique comparator in a study with dacarbazine [16]. The other two studies differed by anatomic location of leiomyosarcoma and were reported together, so the AEs of gemcitabine ± docetaxel were compared within the report [17]. Comparing gemcitabine + dacarbazine with gemcitabine + docetaxel was not possible, because the type of AE reported was not consistent; García-Del-Muro and colleagues reported the percentage of patients with AEs [16], whereas Pautier and colleagues reported the percentage of cycles with AEs [17].

With these limitations in mind, hematologic toxicities were common in the trials of pazopanib, trabectedin, dacarbazine ± gemcitabine, and gemcitabine ± docetaxel. High frequencies of grade 3/4 myelosuppression were observed with trabectedin [15] and dacarbazine + gemcitabine [16]. The toxicity profile of trabectedin and dacarbazine reported here is consistent with those from a phase III trial recently reported by Demetri et al. [28]. For trabectedin versus dacarbazine, rates of neutropenia were 49% versus 29% and rates of thrombocytopenia were 30% versus 36%. In the trabectedin arm, 45% experienced increased ALT levels versus 6% in the dacarbazine arm. In a separate phase III study in the first-line setting, trabectedin plus doxorubicin led to higher rates of grade 3 or 4 thrombocytopenia and liver toxicity, with no improvement in survival compared with doxorubicin alone [29]. Cyclophosphamide produced exceptionally high frequencies of grade 3/4 leukopenia, the only AE reported with higher rates in patients receiving cyclophosphamide, especially those who had prior chemotherapy, in the study by Bramwell et al. [12–14]. In our indirect comparison, grade 4 neutropenia and grade 3 thrombocytopenia were more frequent with trabectedin than pazopanib [11, 15]. Anorexia was more common in the pazopanib trial [11], but both pazopanib and trabectedin were associated with fatigue and elevations in AST and ALT in the two respective trials [11, 15].

Most studies in this review reported AE frequencies as percentages of patients [11–16]. It is unclear whether there is an advantage to reporting the percentage of cycles with a particular AE, and it suggests that the number of patients affected is obscured by the calculation. When AEs are reported by the percentage of patients at risk, the patient is counted once by the worst grade of a particular AE. An additional difficulty is that neither method tells anything about the timing of the AEs (e.g., whether an AE occurred early in treatment and then waned or worsened).

Reporting of the types of AEs was also variable in other ways, impairing comparability. The hematologic AEs in the six studies in this review appear to all to be worst grade while on treatment and therefore would be comparable if the time period of AE assessment and the patient population among studies were similar. Comparison of nonhematologic AEs is made difficult by the variation in the types reported: treatment-emergent (pazopanib) [11], drug-related (trabectedin) [15], and "clinically relevant" (gemcitabine ± dacarbazine) [16]. Besides the type of AE reported, the six studies in this review also differed or appeared to differ in the timing of AE assessments. The ifosfamide versus cyclophosphamide study noted that toxicity was assessed after the first course and throughout treatment but, like the remaining studies, reported only the median number of cycles. Pazopanib was taken orally every day in the clinical trials [11], whereas trabectedin, gemcitabine, dacarbazine, docetaxel, ifosfamide, and cyclophosphamide were all administered intravenously and periodically [12–17]. It is possible that the authors considered reporting the median number of cycles and range as a surrogate for duration of AE assessment. If that is the case, the every 3-week 24-hour infusion schedule in the trabectedin study and both the gemcitabine and gemcitabine + docetaxel arms may have had assessment periods similar to that for pazopanib, with median 3- to 4-week cycles of 5, 5, and 4, respectively [11, 15, 17]. Trabectedin every week, gemcitabine ± dacarbazine, cyclophosphamide, and ifosfamide may have had shorter AE assessment periods [12–16].

Of note, elevations in transaminases and bilirubin were not reported in the studies other than those for pazopanib and trabectedin. However, US labeling for dacarbazine [30] and gemcitabine [31] carry warnings of hepatic toxicity and directives to monitor hepatic function. The dacarbazine label notes that the number of incidences resulting in death is low, and death is mostly observed when dacarbazine is used in combination with other chemotherapy agents. Gemcitabine therapy in other cancers shows high frequencies of all-grade increases in AST and ALT when given as monotherapy, including grade 3/4 frequencies of approximately 10%. Increases in bilirubin were much less common (all grades, 13%) [31].

Cancer type may also have an effect on the frequency of AEs, as may prior therapy. For example, fatigue, nausea, anorexia, weight loss, and dysgeusia appear to occur more frequently in patients receiving pazopanib for STS than for other labeled indications for pazopanib, specifically renal cell carcinoma [11, 32]. In addition, the AEs in patients with nonadipocyte/nonliposarcoma STS receiving pazopanib were primarily grade 1/2 in severity and are AEs commonly managed in clinical practice [11]. Whether prior therapy, disease type, or other factors influence the frequency of reported AEs in clinical trials is unknown.

An earlier systematic literature review on the efficacy and safety of second- or later-line therapy in advanced or metastatic STS summarized grade 3/4, but not all-grade, safety outcomes from RCTs and single-arm studies of patients with advanced STS previously treated with an anthracycline and/or ifosfamide [33]. Of the randomized studies from the Sharma et al. review, five were also identified in this literature review [11, 15–17]. Two of the seven randomized studies in the review by Sharma and colleagues did not meet our inclusion criteria (Pacey et al., 2011: AEs not separated by treatment group; van Oosterom et al., 2002: not powered for comparison of the treatment groups) [34, 35]. We included an additional randomized study [12–14] not included in the Sharma et al. review, possibly because data were not presented separately by histologic subtype. As also found in the review summarized in this report, Sharma and colleagues note the lack of consistency with which AEs were reported among the RCTs [33]. The review by Sharma et al. notes the difference in grade 3/4 AE frequencies in patients treated with pazopanib compared to cytotoxic chemotherapies, the latter being associated with a higher occurrence of grade 3/4 hematologic toxicities [33].

Since our search of the literature, eribulin, a microtubule-dynamics inhibitor, was approved in 2016 for use as a single agent to treat liposarcoma [36]. Although not included in our study, it is worth mentioning that data from phase III trials evaluating eribulin and another agent, ombrabulin, in the relapsed setting have been published [37, 38]. Compared with dacarbazine, eribulin led to lower rates of thrombocytopenia (6% versus 28%) but higher rates of neutropenia (45% versus 24%) and leukopenia (16% versus 10%), and it was associated with peripheral sensory neuropathy (21% versus 4%) [38]. Ombrabulin, a tubulin-depolymerizing tumor vascular-disrupting drug, plus cisplatin was compared with cisplatin plus placebo [37]. Although there was a significant improvement in progression-free survival with ombrabulin, more patients in the ombrabulin group had grade 3 and 4 neutropenia (31% versus 9%) and thrombocytopenia (12% versus 9%).

4.1. Limitations. The major limitation of this review is the small number of randomized trials in previously treated patients with advanced or metastatic STS. Only the study of pazopanib was a phase III study; the remaining studies were phase II trials, a distinction that is perhaps less important in cancer research than the size of a trial. Phase III pazopanib and phase II trabectedin studies were both large (n = 369 and n = 270, resp.) [11, 15]. The population of the phase II study of cyclophosphamide versus ifosfamide was also considerable (n = 171) [12–14], but only a subset of patients had received previous chemotherapy and was eligible for inclusion in this review. With small treatment arm sizes (range, 22 to 57) in most of the studies in this review, common AEs would be detected, but the true risk of infrequent AEs would not be estimated very accurately, and rare AEs (e.g., those occurring in <1% of patients) might not be observed at all.

The quality of the studies was generally acceptable (Additional files 4–9: Tables S4–S9). The open-label design of all but the pazopanib study created a potential bias in the reporting of AEs. However, for practical reasons, many studies in late-stage cancer are open-label, and the risk of bias is tolerated to allow a qualitative review of salvage therapy for advanced or metastatic STS. Additionally, not all patients in the Pautier et al. study received anthracycline-based chemotherapy for metastatic disease [17]. In the nonuterine leiomyosarcoma group, five patients in the gemcitabine-only arm and four patients in the gemcitabine + docetaxel arm had not received first-line anthracycline-based chemotherapy for metastatic disease. In the uterine group, one patient in the gemcitabine arm and seven patients in the gemcitabine + docetaxel arm had not received anthracycline-based chemotherapy for metastatic disease [17].

Other limitations were noted above: the limited amount of safety information reported, including types of AEs; time period of assessment; and the variation in presentation of AEs (percentage of patients versus percentage of cycles). Finally, and very importantly, the limitations inherent in comparing across studies, across years that were a priori not prospectively designed to compare reported AEs by methodology, imply that any comparison of these studies should be made cautiously. However, given the limitations above for an exercise such as this, it is likely that, outside of an RCT, this is the best approach to assessing the frequency and severity of AEs in patients with STS who progress following first-line therapy.

5. Conclusions

Differences in the extent of previous systemic anticancer therapy and the types and timing of AEs reported precluded qualitative comparison of pazopanib with most of the interventions in the six studies in this review. Only the study of trabectedin was reasonably similar in these aspects [15]. A meta-analysis of safety endpoints was not feasible as there was no common comparator allowing for indirect analysis. The AEs that were more common with trabectedin on an every 3-week 24-hour infusion schedule than with pazopanib were all-grade and grade 3/4 anemia and neutropenia, all-grade nausea/vomiting, and all-grade and grade 3 elevations in AST and ALT. The AEs that were more common with pazopanib than with trabectedin were all-grade and grade 3/4 anorexia. More well-designed studies that include one or more comparators in common with the trials identified here are needed to provide additional medical evidence for the best treatment for STS in the advanced and/or metastatic setting.

Abbreviations

AE: Adverse event
ALT: Alanine aminotransferase
AST: Aspartate aminotransferase
CENTRAL: Cochrane Central Register of Controlled Trials
CTC: Common Terminology Criteria
CTCAE: Common Terminology Criteria for Adverse Events
ECOG: Eastern Cooperative Oncology Group
EORTC: European Organisation for Research and Treatment of Cancer
G-CSF: Granulocyte-specific colony-stimulating factor
ITT: Intent to treat
IV: Intravenous
MedDRA: Medical Dictionary for Regulatory Activities
MeSH: Medical subject headings
NA: Not applicable
NCI: National Cancer Institute
NR: Not reported
OS: Overall survival
PDGFR: Platelet-derived growth factor receptor
PFS: Progression-free survival

PRISMA: Preferred Reporting Items for Systematic Reviews and Meta-Analyses
PS: Performance status
q3wk: Every 3 weeks
RCTs: Randomized controlled trials
STS: Soft tissue sarcoma
TTP: Time to progression
VEGFR: Vascular endothelial growth factor receptor
WHO: World Health Organization.

Competing Interests

Ann Colosia, Shahnaz Khan, and James A. Kaye are employees of RTI Health Solutions, which has received funding from GlaxoSmithKline (GSK) for activities related to this study. RTI Health Solutions also received consulting fees and research funding from GSK for activities unrelated to this study. Michelle D. Hackshaw and Jeffrey M. Skolnik were employees of GSK at the time of the study and held stock in GSK. Alan Oglesby is an employee of GSK and holds stock options in GSK.

Authors' Contributions

All authors contributed to the writing of the paper. Ann Colosia contributed to the concept and design of the study, acquisition of data, data analysis, and interpretation of the study. Shahnaz Khan contributed to the concept and design of the study, acquisition of data, data analysis and interpretation. Michelle D. Hackshaw contributed to the concept and design of the study. Alan Oglesby contributed to the data analysis and interpretation of the study. James A. Kaye contributed to the concept and design of the study, data analysis, and interpretation. Jeffrey M. Skolnik contributed to the concept and design, data analysis, and interpretation of the study. All authors had access to the data and contributed to the writing of the paper through critical review, comments, and approval of early drafts of the paper and all authors approved of the final draft for publication.

Acknowledgments

Funding for this study was provided to RTI Health Solutions by GlaxoSmithKline (GSK). All listed authors meet the criteria for authorship set forth by the International Committee for Medical Journal Editors. Editorial support (assembling tables and figures, collating author comments, copyediting, fact checking, and referencing) and graphic services were provided by William R. Pearlman, Ph.D., CMPP, and Nancy Price, Ph.D., of AOI Communications, L.P., and were funded by GSK. GSK employees (listed as authors) contributed to the study design, analysis, and interpretation of the data as well as the writing of the paper.

References

[1] National Cancer Institute, *Adult Soft Tissue Sarcoma Treatment (PDQ®)—Health Professional Version*, National Cancer Institute, Bethesda, Md, USA, 2016, http://www.cancer.gov/types/soft-tissue-sarcoma/hp/adult-soft-tissue-treatment-pdq.

[2] C. Fletcher, J. A. Bridge, P. Hogendoorn et al., *World Health Organization Classification of Tumors. Pathology and Genetics of Tumors of Soft Tissue and Bone*, IARC Press, Lyon, France, 2013.

[3] National Cancer Institute, Surveillance, Epidemiology, and End Results Program, *SEER Stat Fact Sheets: Soft Tissue Including Heart Cancer*, 2016, http://seer.cancer.gov/statfacts/html/soft.html.

[4] R. Wesolowski and G. T. Budd, "Use of chemotherapy for patients with bone and soft-tissue sarcomas," *Cleveland Clinic Journal of Medicine*, vol. 77, supplement 1, pp. S23–S26, 2010.

[5] National Comprehensive Cancer Network, "NCCN clinical practice guidelines in oncology (NCCN Guidelines®): soft tissue sarcoma," Version 2, http://www.nccn.org/professionals/physician_gls/pdf/sarcoma.pdf.

[6] ESMO/European Sarcoma Network Working Group, "Soft tissue and visceral sarcomas: ESMO Clinical Practice Guidelines for diagnosis, treatment and follow-up," *Annals of Oncology*, vol. 23, supplement 7, pp. vii92–vii99, 2012.

[7] R. Chugh, J. K. Wathen, R. G. Maki et al., "Phase II multicenter trial of imatinib in 10 histologic subtypes of sarcoma using a bayesian hierarchical statistical model," *Journal of Clinical Oncology*, vol. 27, no. 19, pp. 3148–3153, 2009.

[8] S. George, P. Merriam, R. G. Maki et al., "Multicenter phase II trial of sunitinib in the treatment of nongastrointestinal stromal tumor sarcomas," *Journal of Clinical Oncology*, vol. 27, no. 19, pp. 3154–3160, 2009.

[9] Votrient [package insert], GlaxoSmithKline (now Novartis), 2016, https://www.pharma.us.novartis.com/sites/www.pharma.us.novartis.com/files/votrient.pdf.

[10] European Medicines Agency, *Yondelis European Public Assessment Report*, 2015, http://www.ema.europa.eu/ema/index.jsp?curl=pages/medicines/human/medicines/000773/human_med_001165.jsp&mid=WC0b01ac058001d124.

[11] W. T. A. van der Graaf, J.-Y. Blay, S. P. Chawla et al., "Pazopanib for metastatic soft-tissue sarcoma (PALETTE): a randomised, double-blind, placebo-controlled phase 3 trial," *The Lancet*, vol. 379, no. 9829, pp. 1879–1886, 2012.

[12] V. H. C. Bramwell, H. T. Mouridsen, A. Santoro et al., "Cyclophosphamide versus ifosfamide: preliminary report of a randomized phase II trial in adult soft tissue sarcomas," *Cancer Chemotherapy and Pharmacology*, vol. 18, supplement 2, pp. S13–S16, 1986.

[13] V. H. C. Bramwell, H. T. Mouridsen, A. Santoro et al., "Cyclophosphamide versus ifosfamide: final report of a randomized phase II trial in adult soft tissue sarcomas," *European Journal of Cancer and Clinical Oncology*, vol. 23, no. 3, pp. 311–321, 1987.

[14] V. H. C. Bramwell, H. T. Mouridsen, A. Santoro et al., "Cyclophosphamide versus ifosfamide: a randomized phase II trial in adult soft-tissue sarcomas. The European Organization for Research and Treatment of Cancer [EORTC], Soft Tissue and Bone Sarcoma Group," *Cancer Chemotherapy and Pharmacology*, vol. 31, supplement 2, pp. S180–S184, 1993.

[15] G. D. Demetri, S. P. Chawla, M. von Mehren et al., "Efficacy and safety of trabectedin in patients with advanced or metastatic liposarcoma or leiomyosarcoma after failure of prior anthracyclines and ifosfamide: results of a randomized phase II study of two different schedules," *Journal of Clinical Oncology*, vol. 27, no. 25, pp. 4188–4196, 2009.

[16] X. García-Del-Muro, A. López-Pousa, J. Maurel et al., "Randomized phase II study comparing gemcitabine plus dacarbazine versus dacarbazine alone in patients with previously treated soft tissue sarcoma: a Spanish Group for Research on Sarcomas study," *Journal of Clinical Oncology*, vol. 29, no. 18, pp. 2528–2533, 2011.

[17] P. Pautier, A. Floquet, N. Penel et al., "Randomized multicenter and stratified phase II study of gemcitabine alone versus gemcitabine and docetaxel in patients with metastatic or relapsed leiomyosarcomas: a fédération nationale des centres de lutte contre le cancer (FNCLCC) french sarcoma group study (TAXOGEM study)," *Oncologist*, vol. 17, no. 9, pp. 1213–1220, 2012.

[18] ClinicalTrials.gov, NCT00753688, Pazopanib versus placebo in patients with soft tissue sarcoma whose disease has progressed during or following prior therapy (PALETTE), 2013, http://clinicaltrials.gov/ct2/show/NCT00753688?term=00753688&rank=1.

[19] A. Liberati, D. G. Altman, J. Tetzlaff et al., "The PRISMA statement for reporting systematic reviews and meta-analyses of studies that evaluate healthcare interventions: explanation and elaboration," *BMJ*, vol. 339, Article ID b2700, 2009.

[20] National Institute for Health and Care Excellence, *Guide to the Single Technology Appraisal Process*, 2009, https://www.nice.org.uk/Media/Default/About/what-we-do/NICE-guidance/NICE-technology-appraisals/Guide-to-the-single-technology-appraisal-process.pdf.

[21] Centre for Reviews and Dissemination, *Systematic Reviews: CRD's Guidance for Undertaking Reviews in Health Care*, 2008, http://www.york.ac.uk/media/crd/Systematic_Reviews.pdf.

[22] D. Moher, A. Liberati, J. Tetzlaff, and D. G. Altman, "Preferred reporting items for systematic reviews and meta-analyses: the PRISMA statement," *The British Medical Journal*, vol. 339, no. 7716, Article ID b2535, pp. 332–336, 2009.

[23] B. Bui-nguyen, I. Ray-coquard, C. Chevreau et al., "High-dose chemotherapy consolidation for chemosensitive advanced soft tissue sarcoma patients: an open-label, randomized controlled trial," *Annals of Oncology*, vol. 23, no. 3, pp. 777–784, 2012.

[24] R. G. Maki, J. K. Wathen, S. R. Patel et al., "Randomized phase II study of gemcitabine and docetaxel compared with gemcitabine alone in patients with metastatic soft tissue sarcomas: results of sarcoma alliance for research through collaboration study 002," *Journal of Clinical Oncology*, vol. 25, no. 19, pp. 2755–2763, 2007.

[25] L. Paz-Ares, A. López-Pousa, A. Poveda et al., "Trabectedin in pre-treated patients with advanced or metastatic soft tissue sarcoma: a phase II study evaluating co-treatment with dexamethasone," *Investigational New Drugs*, vol. 30, no. 2, pp. 729–740, 2012.

[26] FDA Oncologic Drugs Advisory Committee, "Votrient® (pazopanib) tablets for treatment of patients with soft tissue sarcoma," Briefing Document NDA 22-465, 2012, http://www.fda.gov/downloads/AdvisoryCommittees/CommitteesMeetingMaterials/Drugs/OncologicDrugsAdvisoryCommittee/UCM296303.pdf.

[27] GlaxoSmithKline, *VEG110727. A Randomized Double Blind Phase III Trial of Pazopanib Versus Placebo in Patients With Soft Tissue Sarcoma Whose Disease Has Progressed During or Following Prior Therapy. Results Summary*, GlaxoSmithKline, Brentford, UK, 2014, http://www.gsk-clinicalstudyregister.com/study/VEG110727#rs.

[28] G. D. Demetri, M. von Mehren, R. L. Jones et al., "Efficacy and safety of trabectedin or dacarbazine for metastatic liposarcoma or leiomyosarcoma after failure of conventional chemotherapy: results of a phase III randomized multicenter clinical trial," *Journal of Clinical Oncology*, vol. 34, no. 8, pp. 786–793, 2016.

[29] J. Martin-Broto, A. L. Pousa, R. de Las Penas et al., "Randomized phase II study of trabectedin and doxorubicin compared with doxorubicin alone as first-line treatment in patients with advanced soft tissue sarcomas: a Spanish Group for Research on Sarcoma study," *Journal of Clinical Oncology*, vol. 34, no. 19, pp. 2294–2302, 2016.

[30] *Dacarbazine*, Teva Pharmaceuticals, North Wales, Pa, USA, 2014, http://dailymed.nlm.nih.gov/dailymed/lookup.cfm?setid=26e91082-7698-4680-beab-07c47802f0f9.

[31] *Gemzar*, Eli Lilly and Company, Indianapolis, Ind, USA, 2014, http://pi.lilly.com/us/gemzar.pdf.

[32] C. N. Sternberg, I. D. Davis, J. Mardiak et al., "Pazopanib in locally advanced or metastatic renal cell carcinoma: results of a randomized phase III trial," *Journal of Clinical Oncology*, vol. 28, no. 6, pp. 1061–1068, 2010.

[33] S. Sharma, S. Takyar, S. C. Manson, S. Powell, and N. Penel, "Efficacy and safety of pharmacological interventions in second- or later-line treatment of patients with advanced soft tissue sarcoma: a systematic review," *BMC Cancer*, vol. 13, article 385, 2013.

[34] S. Pacey, M. J. Ratain, K. T. Flaherty et al., "Efficacy and safety of sorafenib in a subset of patients with advanced soft tissue sarcoma from a phase II randomized discontinuation trial," *Investigational New Drugs*, vol. 29, no. 3, pp. 481–488, 2011.

[35] A. T. van Oosterom, H. T. Mouridsen, O. S. Nielsen et al., "Results of randomised studies of the EORTC Soft Tissue and Bone Sarcoma Group (STBSG) with two different ifosfamide regimens in first- and second-line chemotherapy in advanced soft tissue sarcoma patients," *European Journal of Cancer*, vol. 38, no. 18, pp. 2397–2406, 2002.

[36] U. S. Food and Drug Administration News Release, *FDA Approves First Drug to Show Survival Benefit in Liposarcoma*, 2016, http://www.fda.gov/NewsEvents/Newsroom/PressAnnouncements/ucm483714.htm.

[37] J.-Y. Blay, Z. Pápai, A. W. Tolcher et al., "Ombrabulin plus cisplatin versus placebo plus cisplatin in patients with advanced soft-tissue sarcomas after failure of anthracycline and ifosfamide chemotherapy: a randomised, double-blind, placebo-controlled, phase 3 trial," *The Lancet Oncology*, vol. 16, no. 5, pp. 531–540, 2015.

[38] P. Schöffski, S. Chawla, R. G. Maki et al., "Eribulin versus dacarbazine in previously treated patients with advanced liposarcoma or leiomyosarcoma: a randomised, open-label, multicentre, phase 3 trial," *The Lancet*, vol. 387, no. 10028, pp. 1629–1637, 2016.

Single-Centre Experience of Systemic Treatment with Vincristine, Ifosfamide, and Doxorubicin Alternating with Etoposide, Ifosfamide, and Cisplatin in Adult Patients with Ewing Sarcoma

Annelies Requilé,[1] Paul M. Clement,[1] Oliver E. Bechter,[1] Herlinde Dumez,[1] Annelies Verbiest,[1] Raf Sciot,[2] Daphne Hompes,[3] Friedl Sinnaeve,[3] Erik Van Limbergen,[4] and Patrick Schöffski[1]

[1]*Department of General Medical Oncology, Leuven Cancer Institute, University Hospitals Leuven, Herestraat 49, 3000 Leuven, Belgium*
[2]*Department of Pathology, University Hospitals Leuven, Leuven, Belgium*
[3]*Department of Oncology, KU Leuven and University Hospitals Leuven, Leuven, Belgium*
[4]*Department of Radiation Oncology, University Hospitals Leuven, Leuven, Belgium*

Correspondence should be addressed to Annelies Requilé; anneliesrequile@gmail.com

Academic Editor: U. Dirksen

The treatment of Ewing sarcoma (ES) in adult patients requires a multidisciplinary approach. Systemic therapy remains an important component of clinical management of this disease. ES is extremely rare in adult patients. Due to the rarity of the disease, no standard of care in terms of chemotherapy for the adult population exists, and the level of evidence for individual agents or some multidrug combinations is limited. Most regimens that are used in both adults and children include anthracyclines, etoposide, vincristine, cyclophosphamide, and ifosfamide. In this report, we describe our experience with the alternating use of triple combination therapies based on vincristine, ifosfamide, and doxorubicin (VIA) and an etoposide, ifosfamide, and cisplatin combination (VIP). We retrospectively evaluated the response rates, outcome, and tolerance of adult patients ($n = 64$) treated with VIA/VIP between 1990 and 2014. The patients included were treated with perioperative chemotherapy (53.1% neoadjuvant therapy and 17.2% adjuvant therapy) or had synchronous metastases at diagnosis (29.7%). Five-year overall survival rate was 52.2% for all patients, 72.2% for patients with localized disease, and 5.3% in patients with synchronous metastases. Overall response rate (ORR) was 37% after 2 cycles of VIA and 2 cycles of VIP. There were no patients with progressive disease (PD).

1. Introduction

The Ewing sarcoma family of tumors (ESFTs) formerly consisted of classical Ewing sarcoma (ES), Askin tumor, and primitive neuroectodermal tumor (PNET) [1] but is now referred to as Ewing sarcoma (ES). The term "PNET" is no longer used as a synonym for ES [2]. ES accounts for 5% of all childhood and adolescent cancers and is the second most common primary bone tumor (after osteosarcoma) in this age group. ES can also occur in soft tissues in about 15 to 30% of cases (extraosseous Ewing sarcoma, EES) [3]. In adult patients (>16 years), ES is very rare and is diagnosed in 8% of patients with a primary bone tumor [4].

ES is a chemotherapy-sensitive disease, as demonstrated by various trials in the last decades evaluating VACA (vincristine, dactinomycin, cyclophosphamide, and doxorubicin), VAC/IE (vincristine, doxorubicin, and cyclophosphamide alternating with ifosfamide-etoposide), VAIA (vincristine, dactinomycin, ifosfamide, and doxorubicin), EVAIA (adding etoposide to VAIA), and VIDE (omitting dactinomycin from EVAIA) [5–10].

The use of chemotherapy in combination with local treatment in patients with localized ES is associated with improved survival outcomes. Five-year overall survival (OS) in patients (all age groups) with nonmetastatic disease at initial presentation is ranging from 65 to 75% in published

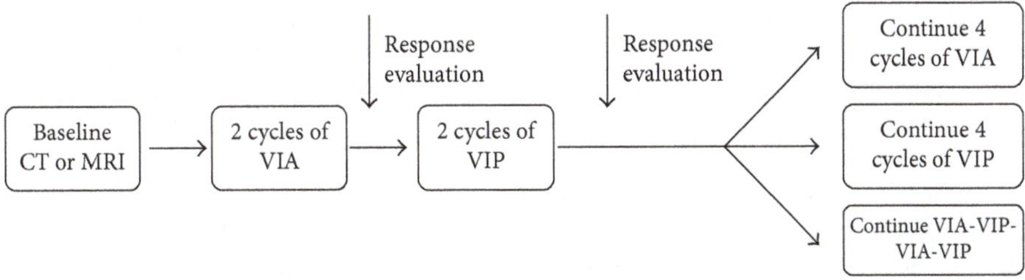

FIGURE 1: Outline of the chemotherapeutic regimen.

series [11]. The treatment of patients with primary metastatic disease, and of patients with ES failing initial multimodal treatment, is an unmet medical need with very unsatisfactory outcome. Of note, 25% of patients have metastatic spread at initial diagnosis [12]. The most common sites of metastases are the lungs (50%), bone (25%), and bone marrow (20%) [13].

Patient outcome has improved over the past decades because of more insight into combination chemotherapies, dose intensification, and better locoregional treatment modalities. The improvement in outcome is especially seen in younger patients (age < 15 years) [4]. Patients older than 16 years have a worse outcome, and in the adult patients, older age is a negative prognostic factor [14–16].

Several other prognostic factors are known. Disease extent (metastatic versus localized disease) is an important risk factor [17], as well as primary tumor site and size in case of localized disease. Axial bone localization is worse than peripheral localization [18, 19]. Higher tumor volume correlates with worse outcome [20].

In our centre, adolescent and adult ES patients (age > 16 years) with localized and metastatic disease have been treated between 1990 and 2014 with two alternating chemotherapy regimens: VIA (vincristine, ifosfamide, and doxorubicin) and VIP (etoposide, ifosfamide, and cisplatin). After completing 2 cycles of VIA followed by an initial response assessment, the alternative protocol VIP is given for 2 further cycles, again followed by radiological assessment. The rationale for applying this alternating treatment scheme was to assess the sensitivity of the individual tumor to both the anthracycline- and the platinum-containing regimens. The treatment used after cycle 4 is based on the initial response assessment. If both regimens were found to be active, they were continued in an alternating schedule (Figure 1).

Between September 1990 and December 2014, a total of 64 patients were treated with this approach. We retrospectively evaluated the response rates to VIA/VIP in all these patients and report patient outcome in terms of overall survival. In patients receiving neoadjuvant treatment, pathological response rates were assessed in terms of percentage of necrosis. Adherence to the planned schedule and the total number of completed cycles and dose modifications are also reported.

2. Patients and Methods

2.1. Patient Selection. All patients diagnosed with ES received a reference number at our pathology department. We reviewed the medical records of all patients diagnosed

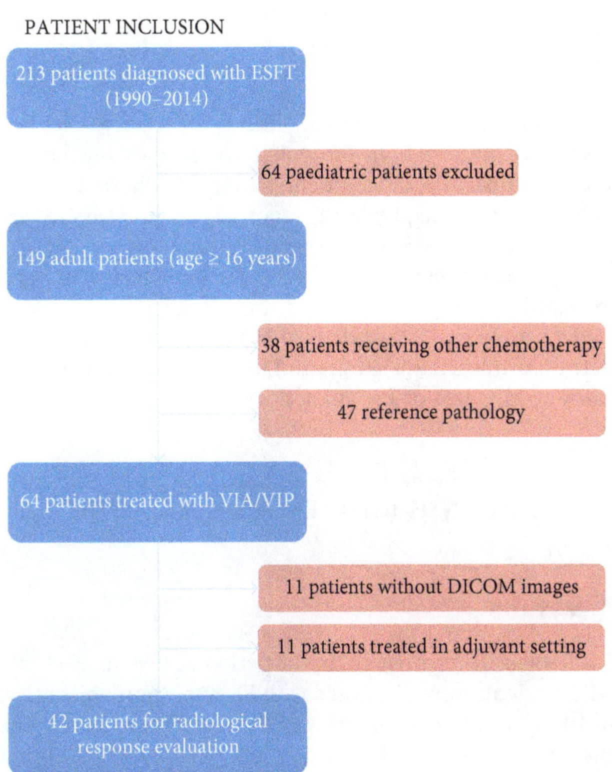

FIGURE 2: Inclusion of patients with diagnosis of ESFT treated in our hospital, aged 16 years and older, and treated with VIA/VIP. Further selection of radiological response evaluation was based on available DICOM images. ESFTs: Ewing's sarcoma family of Tumors; VIA: vincristine, ifosfamide, and doxorubicin; VIP: etoposide, ifosfamide, and cisplatin; DICOM: Digital Imaging and Communications in Medicine.

between 1990 and 2014 and selected patients aged 16 years and older with diagnosis of ES who were treated with VIA/VIP ($n = 64$) (Figure 2). Patients with localized and metastatic disease were included. Patient demographics, disease localization, tumor characteristics, response to treatment, need for dose reduction or schedule modifications, and outcome in terms of response rate and survival were assessed.

We received approval of the ethics committee to perform this retrospective study.

2.2. Radiologic Evaluation. From patients with measurable disease according to the Response Evaluation Criteria in Solid Tumors (RECIST) version 1.1 ($n = 42$), all radiological images were reviewed, and disease evolution was assessed applying the very same criteria. All computed tomography (CT) or magnetic resonance imaging (MRI) scans were reviewed; target and nontarget lesion(s) were assigned and followed over time. Response evaluation was made after two initial cycles of VIA, after two cycles of VIP, and after completion of the chemotherapy. Bone lesions are per definition nonmeasurable according to RECIST, except when there is a measurable soft tissue component. We assessed radiological responses in bone-only disease, taking indirect signs of response into account such as remission of bone oedema on MRI, development of necrosis, and reduction of FDG-activity when PET-CT was performed.

2.3. Statistical Considerations. This is a monocentric, retrospective investigation. The main purpose of this evaluation was to compare the outcome and treatment adherence of our patient cohort with previously reported data in the literature, and results are given in a descriptive fashion.

Five-year overall survival (OS) for both metastatic and localized disease were assessed and displayed as Kaplan-Meier estimates. OS was defined as the interval between the date of histological diagnosis and the date of death from any cause or the date of the last follow-up.

2.4. Review of Literature. We searched http://www.pubmed.com for the MeSH terms "Ewing sarcoma," "ESFT," and adult patients.

3. Results

3.1. Patient Demographics. In the period of 1990 to 2014, 102 adult patients were diagnosed with ES at our hospital, and 64 of those received treatment with VIA/VIP (Figure 2). The main reason for choosing an alternative protocol in the other cases was comorbidity. Median age at diagnosis was 26 years (range of 16 to 67 years). In 51/64 patients (79.7%), the conventional pathological diagnosis was complemented by cytogenetic analysis looking for Ewing sarcoma (EWSR1) gene rearrangement by fluorescent in situ hybridization (FISH). FISH was found positive in tumor material originating from 45/64 patients (70.3%).

The main primary disease localizations were bone (central localization such as vertebral, sacral disease in 37.5% and peripheral localization in 21.9% of patients) and soft tissue (29.7%). Six out of 64 patients (9.4%) had an Askin tumor, defined as a primitive neuroectodermal tumor of the thoracopulmonary region [21]. A total of 29.7% of our cases had synchronous metastatic disease. Patient demographics are shown in Table 1.

Table 1: Patient demographics.

Characteristic	No. of patients (total 64)	—	%
Age at diagnosis			
Median	—	26	—
Range	—	16–67	—
Sex			
M/F	38/26	—	59/41
Localization of primary tumor			
Bone, central	24	—	37.5
Bone, peripheral	14	—	21.9
Soft tissue, abdominal	9	—	14.1
Soft tissue, mediastinal	3	—	4.7
Soft tissue, subcutaneous	2	—	3.1
Soft tissue, other	5	—	7.8
Askin	6	—	9.4
Unknown	1	—	1.6
Metastatic disease at diagnosis	19	—	29.7
Adjuvant therapy	11	—	17.2
Neoadjuvant therapy	34	—	53.1

3.2. Chemotherapy Application. All patients treated with the alternating VIA/VIP schedule started with 2 cycles of VIA (vincristine 1.2 mg/m^2 on days 1, 8, and 15; ifosfamide 3000 mg/m^2 on days 1–3; and doxorubicin 20 mg/m^2 on days 1–3 in a three-weekly schedule). After interim response assessment, cycles 3 and 4 consisted of VIP (etoposide 100 mg/m^2, ifosfamide 2000 mg/m^2, and cisplatin 30 mg/m^2 on days 1–3 also in a three-weekly cycle). The same dose was given to patients in the (neo)adjuvant or metastatic setting. To prevent chemical cystitis, mesna was administered from day 1 to 4 during all cycles. Further supportive care included antiemetic agents, hyperhydration, methylene blue in patients with ifosfamide-induced encephalitis, and haematopoietic growth factors.

After the second cycle of VIP, new imaging was routinely performed, and based on the response assessment, a decision was made to either continue with 4 cycles of VIA or VIP or continue with the alternating schedule with 4 cycles of VIA-VIP until a favourable response was observed with both chemotherapeutic regimens. The criteria taken into account to distinguish between a good or bad response are described below (see Response Evaluation).

In the neoadjuvant setting ($n = 34$), 16 patients underwent local treatment after 4 cycles of chemotherapy, for example, after the sequence VIA-VIA and VIP-VIP. Local therapy consisted of radiotherapy, surgery alone, or surgery plus radiotherapy. The local treatment was based on the advice of a multidisciplinary tumor board. The preference for one or the other option was depending on the localization and size of the tumor, possibility for limb-sparing surgery, and the feasibility of surgery.

After local therapy, adjuvant chemotherapy for 4 cycles was administered (see Response Evaluation). In 18 patients, locoregional therapy was applied after completing the full 8 cycles of chemotherapy due to an insufficient response after 4 cycles. These patients received no further adjuvant chemotherapy.

Fifty-six percentage of patients completed the total of 8 cycles of chemotherapy, and on average, 7 cycles of chemotherapy were given. Most patients (14 patients out of 22) who stopped treatment prematurely had synchronous metastatic disease. In total, 29 patients (45%) needed a dose reduction, on average, after 3 cycles of chemotherapy. Main reasons for early therapy discontinuation or dose reduction were haematological intolerance or poor tolerance. Five patients (7.8%) received an upfront dose reduction either due to comorbidity or due to a cardiac disease localization.

3.3. Pathological Response in Patients Who Received Neoadjuvant Treatment. Among the 34 patients who received neoadjuvant treatment, 17 patients underwent surgery after 4 ($n = 12$) or 8 cycles of chemotherapy ($n = 5$). Sixteen patients underwent radiotherapy only. One patient died during the treatment before initiation of locoregional therapy.

Two patients with metastatic disease underwent surgery after induction chemotherapy: one patient underwent resection of lung metastases and the other patient had only very limited metastatic disease; therefore, based on a multidisciplinary board decision, the primary tumor was operated and the metastatic localizations were irradiated.

In total, we had a group of 19 patients undergoing surgery after chemotherapy with VIA/VIP. Five patients out of these (26%) had a pathological complete response (pCR). In another 6 patients (32%), more than 50% tumor necrosis was seen. In 8 out of 19 cases (42%), viable tumor tissue with necrosis less than 50% was seen.

3.4. Response Evaluation. Among 64 ESFT patients treated with VIA/VIP, 7 (11%) were retreated with the same schedule due to recurrence of the disease. Because the typical dose of doxorubicin in the VIA/VIP schedule is 80 mg/m^2, rechallenge with the same schedule is considered safe taking the cumulative doxorubicin dose into account. For patients diagnosed before 2000, no Digital Imaging and Communications in Medicine (DICOM) images were available ($n = 11$). Another 11 patients were treated in an adjuvant setting, as they had undergone a primary resection and had no postoperatively measurable disease according to RECIST. As a consequence, we were able to review the radiologic images of 42 patients, among whom 1 patient with recurrent disease undergoing rechallenge with VIA/VIP, generating 43 radiological response evaluations (Figure 3).

Among the 43 evaluations were 15 patients with metastatic disease, 27 patients undergoing neoadjuvant treatment, and 1 patient receiving additive VIA-VIP for residual disease after resection which could be followed radiologically.

For response assessment, CT-scan or MRI was used with equal frequency (53.5% versus 46.5%, resp.). In 32 out of 43 radiologically evaluable cases, more than one type of imaging was used to assess response: combination of CT and MRI in 17 cases (39.5%), combination of CT and nuclear imaging (positron emission tomography (PET) and bone scintigraphy) in 4 cases (9.3%), combination of MRI and nuclear imaging in three patients (7%), and combination of 3 or more imaging techniques in 8 patients (18.6%). Bone scintigraphy was used predominantly in patients with skeletal involvement while PET-CT was used in both neoadjuvant and metastatic settings independently of primary tumor localization.

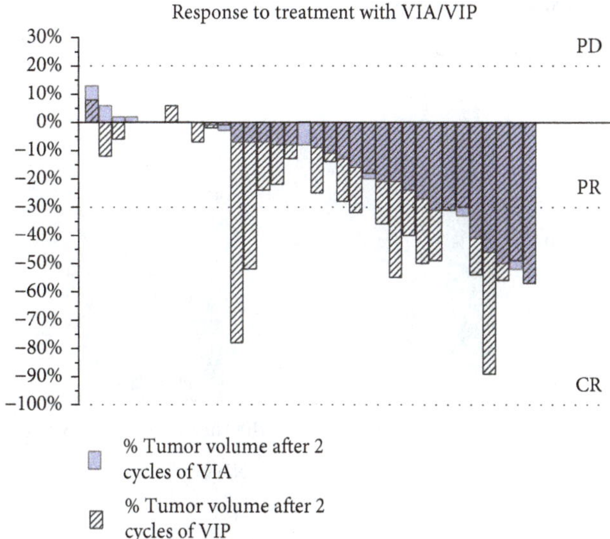

FIGURE 3: Radiologic response to chemotherapy with both VIA and VIP per patient ($n = 34$). Only evaluable patients are shown who had imaging after 2 cycles of VIA and 2 cycles of VIP. VIA: vincristine, ifosfamide, and doxorubicin; VIP: etoposide, ifosfamide, and cisplatin.

After the first 2 cycles of VIA, 11 out of 43 radiologically evaluable patients (26%) had a partial response (PR), 29 patients (67%) had stable disease (SD), none had progressive disease (PD), and 3 patients were not evaluable after the first 2 cycles because they had no imaging at this time point (Figure 4(a)).

Subsequent administration of 2 cycles of VIP led to a further reduction of the disease (PR after initial SD) in 5 patients (11%) and to confirmed SD in 30 patients (70%). Eight patients (19%) were not evaluable due to usage of other imaging techniques rather than baseline, or because they had no imaging at this time point.

The overall response rates after ending treatment with 2 cycles of VIA and 2 cycles of VIP was 37%, and the disease control rate was 84%: SD in 47%, PR in 35%, and complete response (CR) in 2%. Data were insufficient for evaluation in 16% of patients due to the reasons mentioned above (Figure 4(b)).

A total of 36 patients (84%) continued with chemotherapeutic treatment after the first 4 cycles. 28 out of 43 patients (65%) continued with the alternating regimen (i.e., 4 cycles of alternating VIA-VIP). Five patients (12%) continued with 4 cycles of VIA. Three patients (7%) continued with 4 cycles of VIP, the main reason being intolerance to doxorubicin (gastrointestinal intolerance and hepatotoxicity). There was one patient who responded only to the cisplatin-containing regimen. Seven patients (16%) received no further chemotherapy because of side effects.

3.5. Patient Outcome. One patient died prematurely after the first cycle of chemotherapy due to sepsis. There were no other chemotherapy-related deaths.

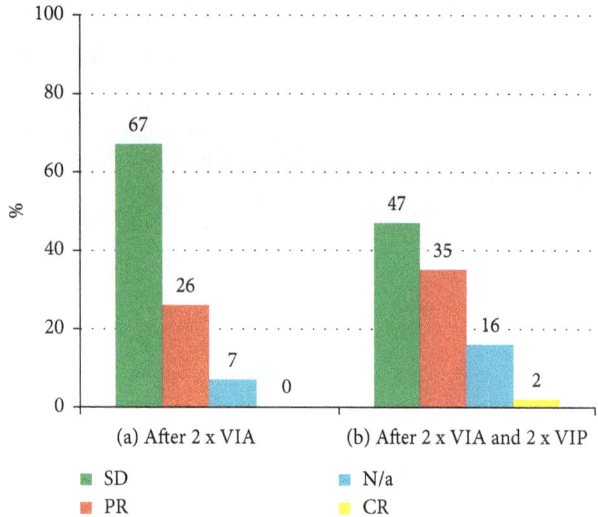

FIGURE 4: (a) Radiological response evaluation after 2 cycles of VIA and (b) radiological response evaluation after 2 cycles of VIA and 2 cycles of VIP according to RECIST 1.1. SD: stable disease; PR: partial response; CR: complete response; N/a: nonevaluable; RECIST: Response Evaluation Criteria in Solid Tumors; VIA: vincristine, ifosfamide, and doxorubicin; VIP: etoposide, ifosfamide, and cisplatin.

The median time of follow-up for all patients ($n = 64$) was 39.6 months. At the time of analysis, 32 out of 64 patients (50%) were alive.

All patients with metastatic disease had died ($n = 19$). The patient with the longest survival lived more than 7 years with metastatic disease at initial diagnosis. Median time between diagnosis and death was 13.3 months (5–88 months), and five-year overall survival was 5.3% in this patient group.

From the 45 patients with localized disease at the start of the treatment, 31 patients (69%) survived with a minimum follow-up period of 27 months. Five-year overall survival in this group of patients was 72.2%. One patient who developed metastases in lymph nodes 3 years after the initial diagnosis was retreated with the VIA/VIP regimen with complete response and received consolidation radiotherapy. He remained disease-free after 9 years of follow-up.

For the group of all patients, five-year overall survival was 52.2% (Figure 5).

4. Discussion

The use of alternating chemotherapeutic regimens is based on the Goldie–Coldman hypothesis that states that the proportion of resistant tumor cells increases over time and that alternating chemotherapy decreases the likelihood of mutations making tumor cells less resistant to a specific drug [22].

This rationale has led to several studies using alternating regimens in different types of cancers. In Burkitt lymphoma, the use of hyperCVAD (cyclophosphamide, vincristine, doxorubicin, and dexamethasone alternating with high-dose methotrexate and cytarabine) is now a standard treatment option [23].

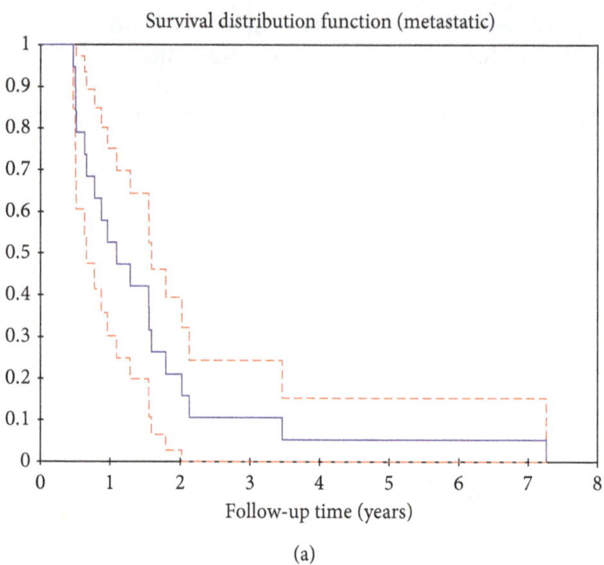

(a)

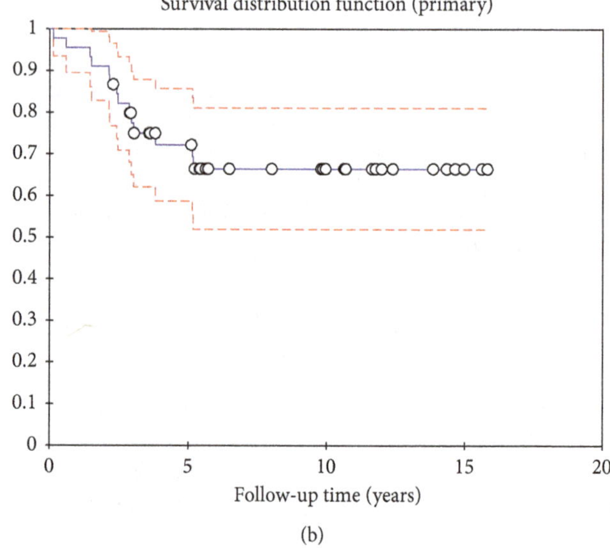

(b)

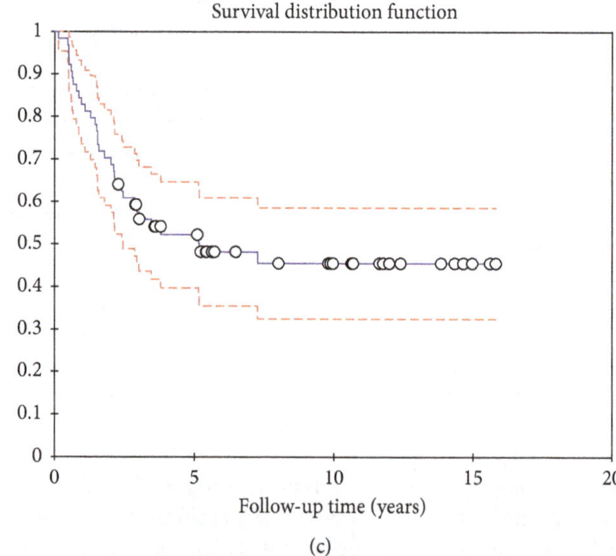

(c)

FIGURE 5: Kaplan–Meier curve survival. OS-curves for (a) patients with synchronous metastatic disease, (b) patients with primary ESFT without metastases, and (c) all patients ($n = 64$).

Treatment with the alternating regimen VAC/IE (vincristine, doxorubicin, and cyclophosphamide alternating with ifosfamide and etoposide) is a standard approach in nonmetastatic ES [8]. Other alternating schedules are not routinely used in the treatment of nonmetastatic or disseminated ES. We have used the alternating triplet combinations VIA and VIP to allow sufficient dosage chemotherapy without obtaining the maximum tolerated dose.

Cisplatin has historically been little used in patients with ES, due to the fact that most of the patients are young, discouraging the use of this chemotherapeutic agent with possible severe late toxicity and morbidity such as renal insufficiency and hearing impairment.

Until today, there is no evidence that supports the use of cisplatin in the first-line treatment of ES. Carboplatin and cisplatin have however been used in recurrent or refractory ES [24–27]. The overall response rate (ORR) to ICE (ifosfamide, carboplatin, and etoposide) in children with recurrent ES was 48% [25]. In one retrospective European study conducted in 106 patients, carboplatin-etoposide was compared to cisplatin-etoposide in patients with refractory ES. Mean age was 20 years (range 2–48) in the carboplatin and 25 years (range 5–46) in the cisplatin group. Five-year overall survival was 24.5% in the carboplatin and 20% in the cisplatin group [26]. VIP as a second-line treatment has been evaluated in adult patients with refractory or recurrent ES in 27 patients [27]. A somewhat different dosing schedule was used compared to our centre (etoposide 75 mg/m^2, ifosfamide 1200 mg/m^2, and cisplatin 20 mg/m^2 on days 1–5 in a three-weekly schedule). Median age was 18 years (range 16–34), and established ORR was 34%, which is good in this setting in an adult patient group.

The results of our analysis reveal that the overall survival for patients with localized disease is comparable to other reports using more common treatment options such as VAC/IE, VIDE, and VAIA, despite the fact that our patient group consisted of a relatively large number of patients with central bone disease (37.5%) which is known to have a negative impact on prognosis.

Cisplatin has given a favourable response to a subgroup of patients, as documented in Figure 3.

Chemotherapeutic adherence to the VIA/VIP schedule was lower in patients with metastatic disease due to worse tolerance, leading to premature discontinuation of the treatment and more dose reductions. This raises the question whether the VIA/VIP schedule might be too intensive in the metastatic setting.

About 50% of the patients were evaluated with MRI, using RECIST and assessing tumor size over time. RECIST could, however, not be applied in bone lesions. In evaluations with MRI, indirect signs of response to treatment such as tumor necrosis and oedema can be assessed. The actual activity of the regimen may therefore be underestimated by RECIST 1.1 response evaluation.

Noteworthy is the high percentage (26%) of pathological complete responses (pCR) in our patient group. Reported pCR rates are approximately 20% depending on the chemotherapeutic regimen that has been used [28]. The high rate of pCR in our series also supports the use of the VIA/VIP regimen in this setting.

5. Conclusion

Treatment of adult patients with ES remains challenging because of the aggressiveness of the disease and lack of standard treatment options.

We treated 64 patients aged 16 years and older with diagnosis of ES with the alternating chemotherapeutic schedule of VIA and VIP. ORR and OS were not inferior compared to reported results using multidrug regimens such as VAC/IE, VIDE, and EVAIA. Using an alternating regimen allows sufficient dosage of antitumor agents with a minimum risk of cumulating toxicity.

The use of cisplatin in first-line needs to be confirmed in a larger, randomized trial, but VIP has proved efficacy in recurrent or refractory disease. Taken into account possible late side effects of cisplatin, caution is warranted using this schedule in younger patients.

Given the fact that, in our analysis, more dose reductions and premature discontinuation of treatment were seen in the metastatic group and that outcome in this group remains very poor, we recommend careful patient selection.

Acknowledgments

A. T. Van Oosterom developed the alternating VIA/VIP regimen in the hospital.

References

[1] J. Miser, T. Kinsella, T. Triche et al., "Treatment of peripheral neuroepithelioma in children and young adults," *Journal of Clinical Oncology*, vol. 5, no. 11, pp. 1752–1758, 1987.

[2] C. D. Fletcher, P. Hogendoorn, F. Mertens, and J. Bridge, *WHO Classification of Tumours of Soft Tissue and Bone*, IARC Press, Lyon, France, 4th edition, 2013.

[3] M. A. Applebaum, J. Worch, K. K. Matthay et al., "Clinical features and outcomes in patients with extraskeletal Ewing sarcoma," *Cancer*, vol. 117, no. 13, pp. 3027–3032, 2011.

[4] K. N. Ganjoo and S. Patel, "The treatment outcome for adult patients with Ewing's sarcoma," *Current Oncology Reports*, vol. 15, no. 4, pp. 372–377, 2013.

[5] N. Jaffe, D. Paed, D. Traggis, S. Salian, and J. R. Cassady, "Improved outlook for Ewing's sarcoma with combination chemotherapy (vincristine, actinomycin D and cyclophosphamide) and radiation therapy," *Cancer*, vol. 38, no. 5, pp. 1925–1930, 1976.

[6] M. E. Nesbit Jr., E. A. Gehan, E. O. Burgert Jr. et al., "Multimodal therapy for the management of primary, nonmetastatic Ewing's sarcoma of bone: a long-term follow-up of the First Intergroup study," *Journal of Clinical Oncology*, vol. 8, no. 10, pp. 1664–1674, 1990.

[7] E. O. Burgert Jr., M. E. Nesbit, L. A. Garnsey et al., "Multimodal therapy for the management of nonpelvic, localized Ewing's sarcoma of bone: intergroup study IESS-II," *Journal of Clinical Oncology*, vol. 8, no. 9, pp. 1514–1524, 1990.

[8] H. E. Grier, M. D. Krailo, N. J. Tarbell et al., "Addition of ifosfamide and etoposide to standard chemotherapy for Ewing's sarcoma and primitive neuroectodermal tumor of bone," *New England Journal of Medicine*, vol. 348, no. 8, pp. 694–701, 2003.

[9] L. Granowetter, R. Womer, M. Devidas et al., "Dose-intensified compared with standard chemotherapy for non-metastatic Ewing sarcoma family of tumors: a Children's Oncology Group Study," *Journal of Clinical Oncology*, vol. 27, no. 15, pp. 2536–2541, 2009.

[10] M. Paulussen, A. W. Craft, I. Lewis et al., "Results of the EICESS-92 study: two randomized trials of Ewing's sarcoma treatment–cyclophosphamide compared with ifosfamide in standard-risk patients and assessment of benefit of etoposide added to standard treatment in high-risk patients," *Journal of Clinical Oncology*, vol. 26, no. 27, pp. 4385–4393, 2008.

[11] N. Gaspar, D. S. Hawkins, U. Dirksen et al., "Ewing sarcoma: current management and future approaches through collaboration," *Journal of Clinical Oncology*, vol. 33, no. 27, pp. 3036–3046, 2015.

[12] M. Paulussen, S. Ahrens, S. Burdach et al., "Primary metastatic (stage IV) Ewing tumor: survival analysis of 171 patients from the EICESS studies. European Intergroup Cooperative Ewing Sarcoma Studies," *Annals of Oncology*, vol. 9, no. 3, pp. 275–281, 1998.

[13] H. E. Grier, "The Ewing family of tumors. Ewing's sarcoma and primitive neuroectodermal tumors," *Pediatric Clinics of North America*, vol. 44, no. 4, pp. 991–1004, 1997.

[14] H. Obata, T. Ueda, A. Kawai et al., "Clinical outcome of patients with Ewing sarcoma family of tumors of bone in Japan: the Japanese Musculoskeletal Oncology Group cooperative study," *Cancer*, vol. 109, no. 4, pp. 767–775, 2007.

[15] G. Bacci, A. Longhi, S. Ferrari, M. Mercuri, M. Versari, and F. Bertoni, "Prognostic factors in non-metastatic Ewing's sarcoma tumor of bone: an analysis of 579 patients treated at a single institution with adjuvant or neoadjuvant chemotherapy between 1972 and 1998," *Acta Oncologica*, vol. 45, no. 4, pp. 469–475, 2006.

[16] E. H. Baldini, G. D. Demetri, C. D. Fletcher, J. Foran, K. C. Marcus, and S. Singer, "Adults with Ewing's sarcoma/primitive neuroectodermal tumor: adverse effect of older age and primary extraosseous disease on outcome," *Annals of Surgery*, vol. 230, no. 1, pp. 79–86, 1999.

[17] S. J. Cotterill, S. Ahrens, M. Paulussen et al., "Prognostic factors in Ewing's tumor of bone: analysis of 975 patients from the European Intergroup Cooperative Ewing's Sarcoma Study Group," *Journal of Clinical Oncology*, vol. 18, no. 17, pp. 3108–3114, 2000.

[18] C. Rodríguez-Galindo, T. Liu, M. J. Krasin et al., "Analysis of prognostic factors in Ewing sarcoma family of tumors: review of St. Jude Children's Research Hospital studies," *Cancer*, vol. 110, no. 2, pp. 375–384, 2007.

[19] K. Fizazi, N. Dohollou, J. Y. Blay et al., "Ewing's family of tumors in adults: multivariate analysis of survival and long-term results of multimodality therapy in 182 patients," *Journal of Clinical Oncology*, vol. 16, no. 12, pp. 3736–3743, 1998.

[20] H. W. Hense, S. Ahrens, M. Paulussen, M. Lehnert, and H. Jürgens, "Factors associated with tumor volume and primary metastases in Ewing tumors: results from the (EI)CESS studies," *Annals of Oncology*, vol. 10, no. 9, pp. 1073–1077, 1999.

[21] F. B. Askin, J. Rosai, R. K. Sibley, L. P. Dehner, and W. H. McAlister, "Malignant small cell tumor of the thoracopulmonary region in childhood: a distinctive clinicopathologic entity of uncertain histogenesis," *Cancer*, vol. 43, no. 6, pp. 2438–2451, 1979.

[22] J. H. Goldie, A. J. Coldman, and G. A. Gudauskas, "Rationale for the use of alternating non-cross-resistant chemotherapy," *Cancer Treatment Reports*, vol. 66, pp. 439–449, 1982.

[23] J. Cortes, D. Thomas, A. Rios et al., "Hyperfractionated cyclophosphamide, vincristine, doxorubicin, and dexamethasone and highly active antiretroviral therapy for patients with acquired immunodeficiency syndrome-related Burkitt lymphoma/leukemia," *Cancer*, vol. 94, no. 5, pp. 1492–1499, 2002.

[24] A. L. Brunetto, L. A. Castillo, A. S. Petrilli et al., "Carboplatin in the treatment of Ewing sarcoma: results of the first Brazilian collaborative study group for Ewing sarcoma family tumors-EWING1," *Pediatric Blood & Cancer*, vol. 62, no. 10, pp. 1747–1753, 2015.

[25] P. Van Winkle, A. Angiolillo, M. Krailo et al., "Ifosfamide, carboplatin, and etoposide (ICE) reinduction chemotherapy in a large cohort of children and adolescents with recurrent/refractory sarcoma: the Children's Cancer Group (CCG) experience," *Pediatric Blood & Cancer*, vol. 44, no. 4, pp. 338–347, 2005.

[26] A. M. van Maldegem, C. Benson, P. Rutkowski et al., "Etoposide and carbo-or cisplatin combination therapy in refractory or relapsed Ewing sarcoma: a large retrospective study," *Pediatric Blood & Cancer*, vol. 62, no. 1, pp. 40–44, 2015.

[27] A. El Weshi, M. Memon, M. Raja et al., "VIP (etoposide, ifosfamide, cisplatin) in adult patients with recurrent or refractory Ewing sarcoma family of tumors," *American Journal of Clinical Oncology*, vol. 27, no. 5, pp. 529–534, 2004.

[28] J. I. Albergo, C. L. Gaston, M. Laitinen et al., "Ewing's sarcoma: only patients with 100% of necrosis after chemotherapy should be classified as having a good response," *Bone & Joint Journal*, vol. 98-B, no. 8, pp. 1138–1144, 2016.

Periosteal Osteosarcoma: A Single-Institutional Study of Factors Related to Oncologic Outcomes

Chung Ming Chan[1] **Adam D. Lindsay**[2] **Andre R. V. Spiguel**[1] **C. Parker Gibbs Jr.**[1] **and Mark T. Scarborough**[1]

[1]*Division of Orthopaedic Oncology, Department of Orthopaedics and Rehabilitation, University of Florida, Gainesville, FL, USA*
[2]*Department of Orthopaedic Surgery, University of Connecticut, Farmington, CT, USA*

Correspondence should be addressed to Chung Ming Chan; chancm@ortho.ufl.edu

Academic Editor: R. Lor Randall

Background. Periosteal osteosarcoma is a rare surface-based variant with a lower propensity to metastasis and better prognosis than conventional osteosarcoma. The literature supporting survival benefit with adjuvant chemotherapy is lacking. Our institutional practice is for chemotherapy to be offered to patients with high-grade disease. *Methods.* We conducted a retrospective cohort study of patients managed for periosteal osteosarcoma from 1970 to 2015 analyzing the survival outcomes and assessing for any relationship of survival to patient- or treatment-related factors. 18 patients were included. The study population presented at a mean of 20.8 years and was followed for a mean of 10.7 years. Factors assessed for an association with survival included age, size of tumor, use of chemotherapy, presence of medullary involvement, presence of high-grade disease, local recurrence, and site of disease. Kaplan–Meier survival analysis and Cox proportional hazard regression were performed to calculate the survival rates and to assess for the effect of any factor on survival. *Results.* 10-year overall survival rate was 77.1%, and 10-year event-free survival rate was 66.4%. No factor was found to have an association with overall or event-free survival. *Conclusion.* These findings add to the available evidence which has failed to find any survival benefit from chemotherapy; patients with this rare disease and their families should be counselled regarding the unclear role of chemotherapy in this rare subtype of osteosarcoma.

1. Introduction

Periosteal osteosarcoma is a rare intermediate-grade malignancy, estimated to represent less than 2% of all osteosarcomas. It is characterized by its histologic appearance of being predominantly chondroblastic with areas of osteoid and its radiographic appearance of a periosteally based lesion with periosteal reaction projecting perpendicularly into the associated soft tissue and has been found to have a lower propensity for metastasis compared to conventional, high-grade medullary osteosarcoma [1–7].

The difference in the natural history of periosteal osteosarcoma as compared to conventional intramedullary osteosarcoma had been observed by the early authors on this topic such as Lichtenstein [6]. This unique and rare subtype of osteosarcoma was further delineated by authors such as Unni et al. [8] and Campanacci and Giunti [4] where the authors made the case for this being recognized as a distinct entity on the grounds of the unique radiographic and histologic features with a clinical behavior distinct from other surface-based osteosarcomas such as parosteal osteosarcoma [9] and high-grade surface osteosarcoma [10]. The importance of making the diagnosis of periosteal osteosarcoma cannot be understated owing to the distinct natural history and that resection alone is a standard treatment for parosteal osteosarcoma [9], while resection and adjuvant chemotherapy are standard treatments for high-grade surface osteosarcoma [10].

While wide resection for local control of this malignancy is accepted as the cornerstone of treatment, strategies differ as to whether adjuvant chemotherapy is administered in patients with this diagnosis. Recent large studies have been inconclusive regarding the utility of adjuvant chemotherapy, with no clear association of the use adjuvant chemotherapy with increased survival [11, 12].

The purpose of this study was to describe our institution's experience of management of patients with this rare malignancy with respect to the characteristics of this patient group and their survival outcomes. We also sought to assess if any patient- or treatment-related factors were associated with improved survival.

2. Materials and Methods

This study is a retrospective case series. The prospectively collected institutional musculoskeletal oncology database was queried to identify patients who had been diagnosed with and managed for periosteal osteosarcoma. We identified 19 patients who had been managed during the period from 1970 to 2015. Of the 19 patients, one had less than one year follow-up and was excluded from statistical analysis. The study population of 18 patients comprised 6 males and 12 females who presented at a mean age of 20.8 years (±9.8) and were followed for a mean of 10.7 years (±7.4).

Data were collected from the patient clinical and pathological charts on demographic characteristics of subjects, tumor-related features, the nature of surgical and medical treatment, and the occurrence of any significant events related to the malignancy (i.e., local recurrence, metastasis, development of a second malignancy, and death). Where patients were histologically graded on the four-point Broder's scale, grades I and II were classified as low grade and grades III and IV were classified as high grade. Patient data regarding certain tumor-related and treatment-related factors were collected for analysis. The factors assessed included the age at diagnosis, size of tumor (as assessed by the maximum dimension measured in centimeters), the presence of high-grade tumor, location of the tumor (axial location versus appendicular), the presence of medullary extension or invasion, and whether chemotherapy was administered. The maximum tumor dimension was recorded for 10 of 18 of our study population. Patients were followed up in the clinic and had radiographic evaluations of the site of disease to monitor for local recurrence as well as of the chest for pulmonary metastasis. Owing to the subjects having been managed from 1970 to 2015, the standard surveillance protocol for pulmonary involvement involved chest radiographs for subjects managed earlier and computed tomography of the lungs for the first 5 years for patients managed more recently. The interval for surveillance was 3 months for the first two years, 4 months for the third-year postsurgery, 6 months for the fourth- and fifth-years postsurgery, and yearly thereafter. Where the death of a study subject could be ascertained, this was included for analysis of overall survival.

Descriptive statistical analysis and Kaplan–Meier survival analysis were performed for the whole study group. Both overall survival and event-free survival were analyzed. Events were defined as local recurrence, metastasis, or mortality. The presence of any association between survival and patient- and tumor-related factors was assessed using the log-rank test and Cox proportional-hazards regression. Patient subgroups were compared and analyzed using a Cox proportional-hazards regression model which was used for analysis to assess for the presence of any association with survival outcome.

Statistical analysis was performed using EZR, a statistical software package based on R (Easy R, Version 2.13.0; Jichi Medical University, Saitama, Japan) [13]. Significance was determined using a 95% confidence level.

3. Results and Discussion

3.1. Results. The commonest site of disease was the femoral diaphysis (5), followed by the tibial diaphysis (3) and the ilium (3) (Figure 1). 12 of 18 patients had tumors that were of high grade, and 11 of these 12 patients received chemotherapy. 17 of 18 patients underwent wide resection of the primary tumor for local control, while the last patient's resection was a marginal resection. The surgery performed was limb sparing in 14 of the 18 patients with an overall 78% limb salvage rate. Medullary involvement was noted in 9 of 18 patients.

One patient (5.3%) developed a local recurrence 9 months after an intralesional excision was performed at the referring institution. This recurrence was not associated with dedifferentiation. Two patients (10.5%) developed metastasis while on follow-up. The first patient developed an isolated lung metastasis at 19 months. This was managed with chemotherapy and pulmonary metastasectomy. There was no evidence of disease for up to 75 months after the diagnosis of the metastasis. The second patient developed a proximal humeral metastasis at 94 months; this was treated with chemotherapy and resection of the proximal humeral metastasis. The patient subsequently developed pulmonary metastases and eventually succumbed to the disease 16 months after the diagnosis of the proximal humeral metastasis.

The 10-year overall survival rate was 77.1% (Figure 2) and 10-year event-free survival rate was 66.4% (Figure 3). No factor was found to have a significant association with survival (Table 1). Notably, no survival benefit was noted with the use of chemotherapy (Figure 4). Multivariate analysis was not performed as no factor was found to have a significant association with survival.

3.2. Discussion. Survival in patients with periosteal osteosarcoma is relatively high compared to other commoner subtypes of osteosarcoma, and the use of adjuvant chemotherapy has not been found in several studies to be associated with increased survival. The 10-year survival rate of 77.1% in this study is comparable to that in the literature [2, 3, 11, 12, 14, 15] (Table 2).

In this study, we did not exclude patients with the presence of medullary involvement. Studies such as by Unni et al. [8] and Rose et al. [2] have excluded patients with medullary involvement from their studies as it is argued that it is not possible to definitively distinguish the tumors in those cases from classic chondroblastic osteosarcoma. Many other contemporary studies [11, 12, 14, 15] have abided by

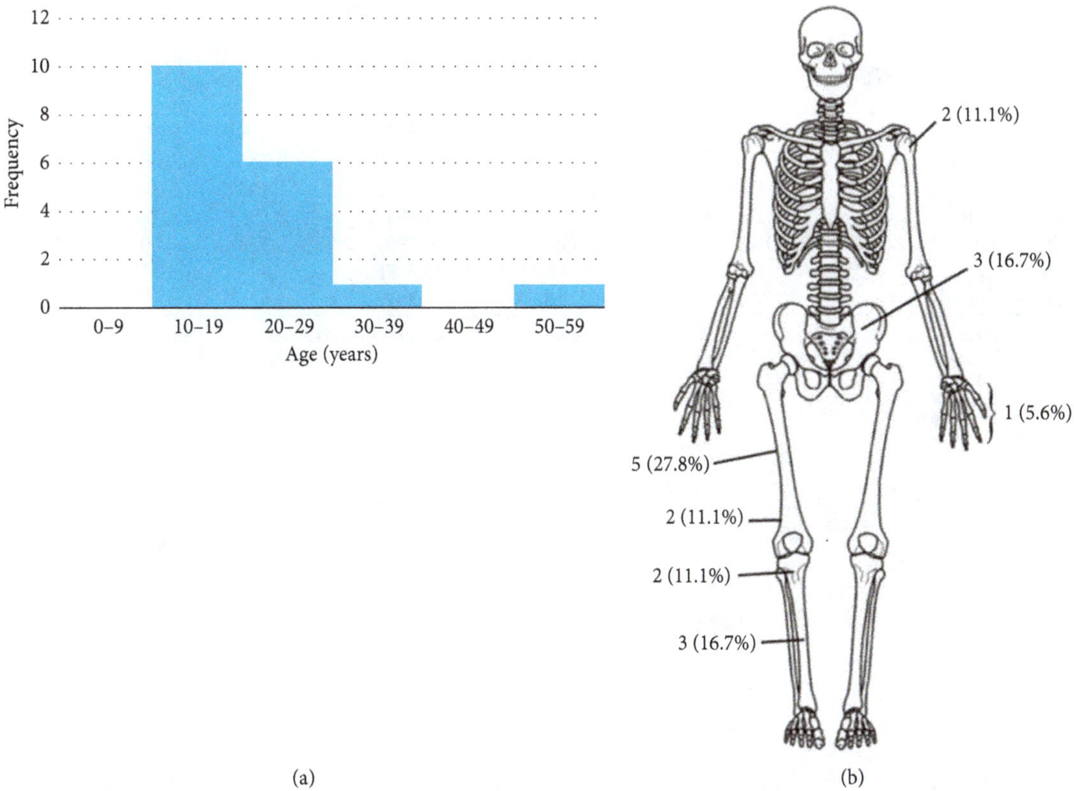

FIGURE 1: Distribution of primary tumors in study population by age and location.

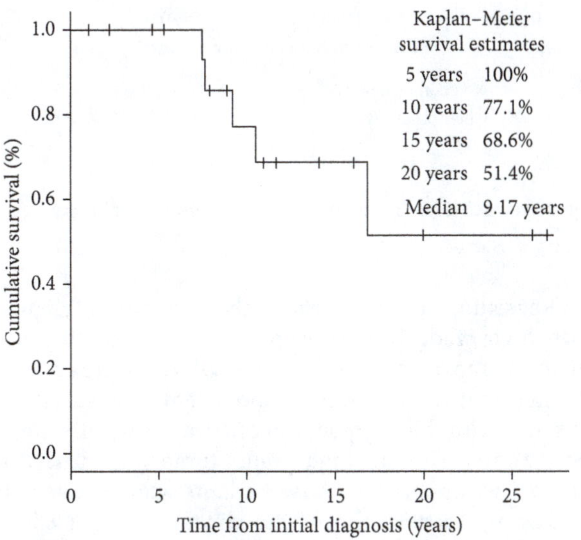

FIGURE 2: Kaplan–Meier curve of overall survival of study population.

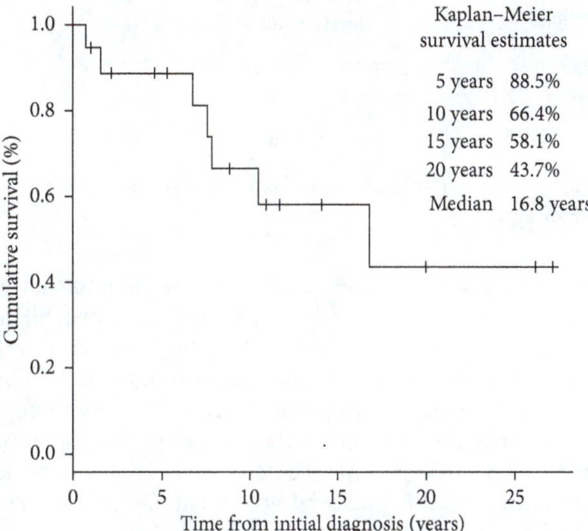

FIGURE 3: Kaplan–Meier curve of event-free survival of study population.

the plea for acceptance of medullary involvement in diagnoses of periosteal osteosarcoma by Hall et al. [16], as this is seen as the natural progression of the disease. This is the practice at our center as well (Table 2).

There is a wide variation in the rates of high-grade tumors in the studies on periosteal osteosarcoma in the literature. In our study, 12 of 18 patients (66%) were classified as having high-grade tumors or tumors with foci of high-grade tumor. Of these 12 patients, 2 were initially graded as low grade on the biopsy specimens and were subsequently reclassified as high grade following complete tumor resection and pathological examination of the entire tumor. In the study by Revell et al. [14], all patients were classified as intermediate or high grade; this was the case as well in the study by Rose et al. [2], with 11 of 29 subjects having

Table 1: Factors assessed for the effect on survival.

	Overall survival			Event-free survival		
	HR	CI	p value	HR	CI	p value
Age (continuous variable)	0.920	0.72–1.175	0.5025	0.9131	0.758–1.10	0.340
Size (continuous variable)	0.864	0.5515–1.354	0.5243	0.738	0.513–1.06	0.103
Use of chemotherapy	2.90	0.3125–26.83	0.3493	1.443	0.275–7.563	0.664
Medullary involvement	1.01	0.1637–6.189	0.9944	2.151	0.411–11.27	0.365
Presence of high-grade disease	1.00×10^9	0–∞	0.9992	2.278	0.272–19.1	0.448
Local recurrence	2.785	0.286–27.13	0.3778	—	—	—
Site (axial versus appendicular)	2.699	0.4407–16.52	0.2826	1.415	0.269–7.44	0.682

Hazard ratios (HRs) with confidence interval (CI) and p values calculated using the Cox proportional-hazards method with each factor being assessed individually.

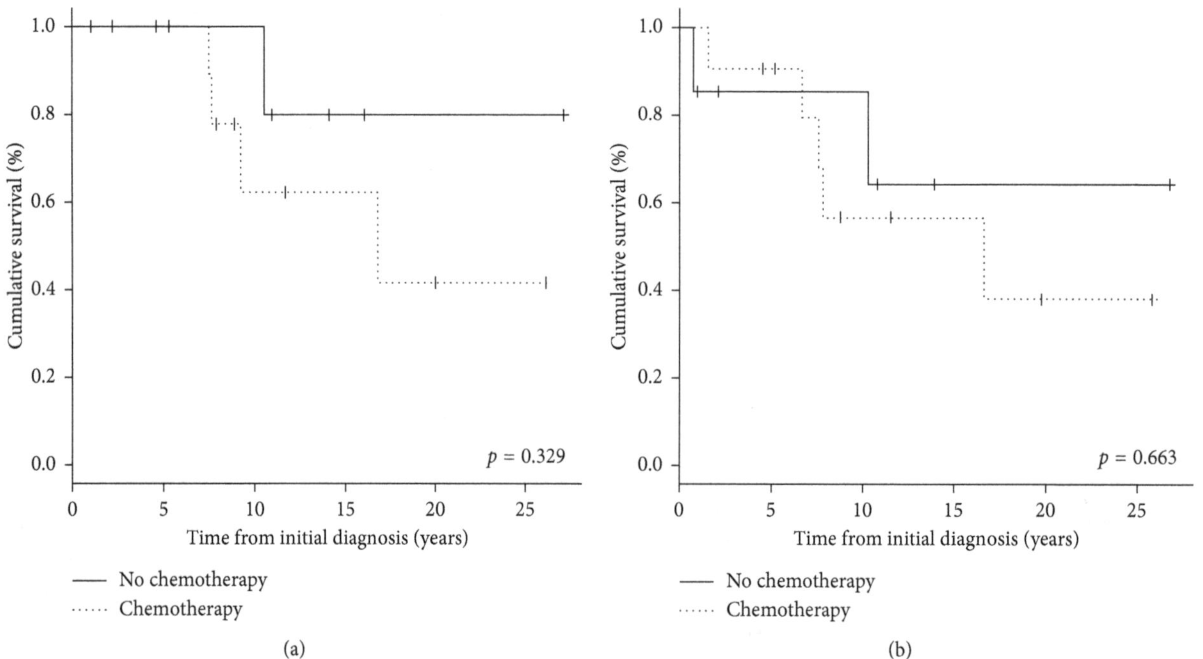

Figure 4: Kaplan–Meier curves comparing overall survival (a) and event-free survival (b) of patients who did and did not receive chemotherapy.

intermediate-grade tumors and 18 of 29 subjects having high-grade tumors. Other studies have significantly higher rates of high-grade tumors. The study by Cesari et al. [11] actually reported a 94% rate of tumors being grade 3/high grade, and in that study, 14 patients received chemotherapy. In that study, the pathology was reviewed specifically for the study and 31 of 33 patients were classified as high grade and it is unclear if this could be accounted for by the areas available for repeat review being areas of higher grade involvement. In the study by Grimer et al. [12], 44 of the 51 patients (86.2%) where the information was available for review had high-grade tumors. In their discussion of the issue of tumor grade, the possibility of a high-grade surface osteosarcomas being misclassified as periosteal osteosarcoma was raised in their discussion owing to the multi-institutional nature of the study and as there was no centralized review of pathology. The importance of correct classification of the tumor grade cannot be overstated as this is often a criterion in deciding on which patients to receive chemotherapy.

Regarding adjuvant chemotherapy, the 12 patients with high-grade tumors were recommended to receive chemotherapy, and all but one of those 12 received chemotherapy. The overall and event-free survival of patients with high-grade tumors was generally poorer than those without high-grade tumor; similarly, the survival was poorer in those patients who received chemotherapy than in those who did not receive chemotherapy. This difference however was not found to be statistically significant on univariate analysis with the log-rank test. Multivariate testing was noted performed owing to the lack of any factor showing statistical significant differences. These findings of there being no significant difference in survival between patients who did and did not receive chemotherapy echo the findings of the multicenter study by Grimer et al. [12] involving 119 subjects and the largest single-institution study by Cesari et al. [11] involving 33 subjects.

Our practice is to recommend neoadjuvant chemotherapy to patients with high-grade tumors on initial biopsy

Table 2: Summary of the contemporary literature regarding periosteal osteosarcoma.

Study	N	Gender ratio (M : F)	Average age of presentation (range) (years)	Mean follow-up (range) (years)	10-year overall survival (%)	Chemotherapy used (%)	Medullary involvement (%)	Local recurrence (%)	Metastasis rate (%)
Bertoni et al. [3]	20	9 : 11	Mean 19.6 (11–53)	7.9 (0.4–39)	85	10	—	40	15
Hall et al. [16]	6	3 : 3	Mean 25.3 (15–40)	2.9 (1.1–5)	—	50	50	0	16.7
Ritts et al. [5]	22	8 : 14	Mean 20.5 (9–47)	10.0 (1.4–29.3)	71.3	9.1	0	13.6	13.6
Revell et al. [14]	17	10 : 7	Median 18 (10–35)	6.8 (0.8–16.7)	88	82	23.5	5.9	0
Grimer et al. [12]	119	54 : 64	Median 18 (8–72)	7.1 (0.5–21)	83	68	—	6.7	14.2
Rose et al. [2]	29	13 : 16	Mean 20.6 (9–47)	15.8 (4–51)*	83	31	0	17.2	17.2
Cesari et al. [11]	33	19 : 14	Median 16 (6–32)	Median 10.1 (0.75–30.5)	84	42	65.2†	21.2	12.1
Gulia et al. [15]	18	12 : 6	Mean 16.3 (5–26)	Median 5.1 (1.5–10.8)	83.3 (5 y OS)	89	44.4	11	22.2
This study	18	6 : 12	Mean 20.8 (10–56)	10.4 (1–27.1)	77.1	61	50	5.6	11.1

*Surviving cohort; †23 of 33 subjects assessed had medullary involvement.

and adjuvant chemotherapy to patients where the resected tumor reveals foci of high-grade disease not found on the initial biopsy. In our study, five of the 12 patients who received chemotherapy received it prior to surgery. The pathology reports for four of these five patients featured estimates of tumor necrosis, and they were <50%, 90%, 92%, and >90%. This may be seen as suggestive that chemotherapy is active against periosteal osteosarcoma. Of particular note, two of these four patients had tumor without evidence of medullary involvement which fits the more restrictive case definition of periosteal osteosarcoma applied in some studies. The tumor necrosis was reported as 90% and >90% in these two patients. These findings are in contrast to those of the study by Rose et al. [2] where tumor necrosis in the two of 29 patients who received neoadjuvant chemotherapy was 10–20%. While the study by Revell et al. [14] did not include a discussion of histologic response to chemotherapy, the 100% 10-year survival rate observed was attributed to the radical tumor resection and the use of chemotherapy.

The survival curves in this study show persistent reduction in the survival estimates with time suggestive of the development of late events with the event-free survival (EFS) dropping from 66% at 10 years to 58% at 15 years and then to 44% at 20 years. This contrasts to the study by Rose et al. [2] where all local and distant recurrences were noted within 36 months and the disease-specific survival curves plateaued, with that data suggesting a low risk of late clinical events. Several explanations could account for these differences: firstly, in our study, events included not only local recurrence and metastasis but also second malignancies and death from all causes. A similar definition for events was used in the series by Cesari et al. [11] where a similar EFS at 10 years of 52% was noted. These events of second malignancy and death from other causes may not be accounted for in some other studies where the disease-specific survival curves plateau. Another significant factor that may account for these differences is the impact of censoring in the calculation of the Kaplan–Meier survival estimates in our small series where at 10 years, 39% of subjects had been censored, while at 15 years, it was 50%. Consider an assumption of censoring in survival analysis is that the subjects censored have a similar prospect of survival as those that continued to be followed. In our study, where patients were found to have died even after their last clinical follow-up, their death was included as an event for survival analysis. If the patients who were lost to follow-up were at a lower chance of events and death, this could have biased the analysis to estimating a poorer rate of survival.

The risk of second malignancy is well known in patients treated for childhood malignancies and in osteosarcoma as well [17]. The benefits of the use of chemotherapy in many childhood cancers outweigh the relatively small risk of a second malignancy, but should be raised as a concern in discussing the use of chemotherapy in patients with periosteal osteosarcoma where its utility has not been well proven. In the study by Ritts et al. [5], of their 22 patients, 3 developed another malignancy, 2 developed acute myelocytic leukemia (AML), and 1 developed liposarcoma, whereas one patient in the study by Revell et al. [14] developed AML as well. In our study, one patient was diagnosed with mesenchymal chondrosarcoma at the same site of her periosteal osteosarcoma 81 months later, and died 8 months after that diagnosis. In the series by Cesari et al. [11], similarly, one patient died from mesenchymal chondrosarcoma at 128 months after the diagnosis of periosteal osteosarcoma, but at a site different from the primary periosteal osteosarcoma. Other second malignancies occurring in that study were breast cancer and acute lymphoblastic leukemia.

Our study has several limitations. It is a small series and it spans 5 decades where some variation in chemotherapy protocols existed. This study also only reports overall survival, as we were not able to ascertain the cause of death on all subjects who died and thus could not report disease-specific survival.

Making strong recommendations regarding the utility of adjuvant chemotherapy of periosteal osteosarcoma is challenging owing to its rarity and the limited and varied data. Owing to the rarity of this disease, it is unlikely that a randomized study will be conducted to answer this question and a large multicenter retrospective study [12] of this rare disease has been unable to provide clear evidence of a survival benefit with the use chemotherapy in this patient group. As in the management of other subtypes of osteosarcoma, wide resection remains the preferred mode of surgical treatment. Similar to other studies on this disease, this study does not conclusively support or refute the use of chemotherapy. The presence of tumor necrosis in four of the six patients in our study who received neoadjuvant chemotherapy could be seen to suggest activity of chemotherapy against periosteal osteosarcoma and lend support to the practice of offering chemotherapy to patients with high-grade disease.

The silence of the literature regarding the efficacy of chemotherapy on periosteal osteosarcoma will lead clinicians to draw on their experience of other subtypes of osteosarcoma, in particular that of high-grade conventional osteosarcoma, to make treatment recommendations. It should be emphasized to patients and their families that little can be said definitively owing to the rarity of the condition, but that current studies have not proven the efficacy of chemotherapy in improving survival outcomes in patients with periosteal osteosarcoma.

References

[1] C. D. M. Fletcher, J. A. Bridge, P. C. W. Hogendoorn, and F. Mertens, *WHO Classification of Tumours of Soft Tissue and Bone*, IARC Press, Lyon, France, 2013.

[2] P. S. Rose, I. D. Dickey, D. E. Wenger, K. K. Unni, and F. H. Sim, "Periosteal osteosarcoma: long-term outcome and risk of late recurrence," *Clinical Orthopaedics and Related Research*, vol. 453, pp. 314-317, 2006.

[3] F. Bertoni, S. Boriani, M. Laus, and M. Campanacci, "Periosteal chondrosarcoma and periosteal osteosarcoma: two distinct entities," *Journal of Bone and Joint Surgery*, vol. 64, no. 3, pp. 370–376, 1982.

[4] M. Campanacci and A. Giunti, "Periosteal osteosarcoma. Review of 41 cases, 22 with long-term follow-up," *Italian Journal of Orthopaedics and Traumatology*, vol. 2, no. 1, pp. 23–35, 1976.

[5] G. D. Ritts, D. J. Pritchard, K. K. Unni, J. W. Beabout, and J. J. Eckardt, "Periosteal osteosarcoma," *Clinical Orthopaedics and Related Research*, vol. 219, pp. 299–307, 1987.

[6] L. Lichtenstein, "Tumors of periosteal origin," *Cancer*, vol. 8, no. 5, pp. 1060–1069, 1955.

[7] M. D. Murphey, J. S Jelinek, H. T. Temple, D. J. Flemming, and F. H. Gannon, "Imaging of periosteal osteosarcoma: radiologic-pathologic comparison," *Radiology*, vol. 233, no. 1, pp. 129–138, 2004.

[8] K. K. Unni, D. C. Dahlin, and J. W. Beabout, "Periosteal osteogenic sarcoma," *Cancer*, vol. 37, no. 5, pp. 2476–2485, 1976.

[9] K. Okada, F. J. Frassica, F. H. Sim, J. W. Beabout, J. R. Bond, and K. K. Unni, "Parosteal osteosarcoma: a clinicopathologic study," *Journal of Bone and Joint Surgery*, vol. 76, no. 3, pp. 366–378, 1994.

[10] K. Okada, K. K. Unni, R. G. Swee, and F. H. Sim, "High-grade surface osteosarcoma: a clinicopathologic study of 46 cases," *Cancer*, vol. 85, no. 5, pp. 1044–1054, 1999.

[11] M. Cesari, M. Alberghini, D. Vanel et al., "Periosteal osteosarcoma: a single-institution experience," *Cancer*, vol. 117, no. 8, pp. 1731–1735, 2011.

[12] R. J. Grimer, S. Bielack, S. Flege et al., "Periosteal osteosarcoma: a European review of outcome," *European Journal of Cancer*, vol. 41, no. 18, pp. 2806–2811, 2005.

[13] Y. Kanda, "Investigation of the freely available easy-to-use software 'EZR' for medical statistics," *Bone Marrow Transplantation*, vol. 48, no. 3, pp. 452–458, 2013.

[14] M. P. Revell, N. Deshmukh, R. J. Grimer, S. R. Carter, and R. M. Tillman, "Periosteal osteosarcoma: a review of 17 cases with mean follow-up of 52 months," *Sarcoma*, vol. 6, no. 4, pp. 123–130, 2002.

[15] A. Gulia, A. Puri, M. Pruthi, and S. Desai, "Oncological and functional outcome of periosteal osteosarcoma," *Indian Journal of Orthopaedics*, vol. 48, no. 3, pp. 279–8, 2014.

[16] R. B. Hall, L. H. Robinson, M. M. Malawar, and W. K. Dunham, "Periosteal osteosarcoma," *Cancer*, vol. 55, no. S9, pp. 165–171, 1985.

[17] L. Aung, R. G. Gorlick, W. Shi et al., "Second malignant neoplasms in long-term survivors of osteosarcoma: Memorial Sloan-Kettering Cancer Center experience," *Cancer*, vol. 95, no. 8, pp. 1728–1734, 2002.

Permissions

All chapters in this book were first published in SARCOMA, by Hindawi Publishing Corporation; hereby published with permission under the Creative Commons Attribution License or equivalent. Every chapter published in this book has been scrutinized by our experts. Their significance has been extensively debated. The topics covered herein carry significant findings which will fuel the growth of the discipline. They may even be implemented as practical applications or may be referred to as a beginning point for another development.

The contributors of this book come from diverse backgrounds, making this book a truly international effort. This book will bring forth new frontiers with its revolutionizing research information and detailed analysis of the nascent developments around the world.

We would like to thank all the contributing authors for lending their expertise to make the book truly unique. They have played a crucial role in the development of this book. Without their invaluable contributions this book wouldn't have been possible. They have made vital efforts to compile up to date information on the varied aspects of this subject to make this book a valuable addition to the collection of many professionals and students.

This book was conceptualized with the vision of imparting up-to-date information and advanced data in this field. To ensure the same, a matchless editorial board was set up. Every individual on the board went through rigorous rounds of assessment to prove their worth. After which they invested a large part of their time researching and compiling the most relevant data for our readers.

The editorial board has been involved in producing this book since its inception. They have spent rigorous hours researching and exploring the diverse topics which have resulted in the successful publishing of this book. They have passed on their knowledge of decades through this book. To expedite this challenging task, the publisher supported the team at every step. A small team of assistant editors was also appointed to further simplify the editing procedure and attain best results for the readers.

Apart from the editorial board, the designing team has also invested a significant amount of their time in understanding the subject and creating the most relevant covers. They scrutinized every image to scout for the most suitable representation of the subject and create an appropriate cover for the book.

The publishing team has been an ardent support to the editorial, designing and production team. Their endless efforts to recruit the best for this project, has resulted in the accomplishment of this book. They are a veteran in the field of academics and their pool of knowledge is as vast as their experience in printing. Their expertise and guidance has proved useful at every step. Their uncompromising quality standards have made this book an exceptional effort. Their encouragement from time to time has been an inspiration for everyone.

The publisher and the editorial board hope that this book will prove to be a valuable piece of knowledge for researchers, students, practitioners and scholars across the globe.

List of Contributors

Alexander L. Lazarides
School of Medicine, Duke University, Durham, NC 27710, USA

William C. Eward, Cindy Green and Brian E. Brigman
Department of Surgery, Division of Orthopedic Surgery, Duke University Medical Center, Durham, NC 27710, USA

Paul J. Speicher, Daniel P. Nussbaum and Dan G. Blazer III
Department of Surgery, Duke University Medical Center, Durham, NC 27710, USA

Chun-Han Hou
Department of Orthopedic Surgery, National Taiwan University Hospital, Taipei 10617, Taiwan

David G. Kirsch
Department of Radiation Oncology, Duke University Medical Center, Durham, NC 27710, USA

Christopher L. Tinkle, Vivian Weinberg, Steve E. Braunstein and Alexander R. Gottschalk
Department of Radiation Oncology, University of California, San Francisco, 1600 Divisadero Street, MZ Building R H1031, San Francisco, CA 94143, USA

Rosanna Wustrack and Richard J. O'Donnell
Department of Orthopaedic Surgery, University of California, San Francisco, San Francisco, CA, USA

Andrew Horvai
Department of Pathology, University of California, San Francisco, San Francisco, CA, USA

Thierry Jahan
Department of Medicine, University of California, San Francisco, San Francisco, CA, USA

M. Matsuda, T. Ichimura, M. Kasai, M. Murakami and T. Sumi
Department of Obstetrics and Gynecology, Osaka City University Graduate School of Medicine, 1-5-7 Asahimachi, Abeno-ku, Osaka 545-8585, Japan

N. Kawamura
Department of Obstetrics and Gynecology, Osaka City General Hospital, Osaka 534-0021, Japan

T. Hayashi
Department of Immunology and Infectious Disease, Shinshu University Graduate School of Medicine, Nagano 390-8621, Japan

Keisuke Ae, Taisuke Tanizawa, Tabu Gokita and Seiichi Matsumoto
Department of Orthopedic Surgery, Cancer Institute Hospital, Ariake 3-8-31, Koutou-ku, Tokyo 135-8550, Japan

Hiroshi Kobayashi
Department of Orthopedic Surgery, Cancer Institute Hospital, Ariake 3-8-31, Koutou-ku, Tokyo 135-8550, Japan
Department of Orthopedic Surgery, The University of Tokyo Hospital, Hongo 7-3-1, Bunkyo-ku, Tokyo 113-8655, Japan

Noriko Motoi
Department of Pathology, Cancer Institute Hospital, Ariake 3-8-31, Koutou-ku, Tokyo 135-8550, Japan

François Gouin and Guillaume Anthony Odri
Clinique Chirurgicale Orthopédique et Traumatologique, CHU Hôtel-Dieu, Place Alexis-Ricordeau 1, 44093 Nantes Cedex 1, France
Laboratoire Physiopathologie de la Résorption Osseuse, Inserm UI957, Faculté de Medecine, Université de Nantes, rue Gaston Veil, 44000 Nantes, France

Laurent Paul and Olivier Cartiaux
Computer Assisted and Robotic Surgery (CARS), Institut de Recherche Expérimentale et Clinique, Université Catholique de Louvain, Avenue Mounier 53, 1200 Brussels, Belgium

Valerie Francescutti, Sartaj S. Sanghera, Joseph J. Skitzki and John M. Kane III
Department of Surgical Oncology, Roswell Park Cancer Institute, Buffalo, NY 14263, USA

Richard T. Cheney
Department of Pathology and Laboratory Medicine, Roswell Park Cancer Institute, Buffalo, NY 14263, USA

Austin Miller
Department of Biostatistics and Bioinformatics, Roswell Park Cancer Institute, Buffalo, NY 14263, USA

Kilian Salerno
Department of Radiation Medicine, Roswell Park Cancer Institute, Buffalo, NY 14263, USA

Rachel Burke
Naval Medical Center Portsmouth, Portsmouth, VA 23708, USA

Kjetil Berner
Department of Oncology, Oslo University Hospital, Norwegian Radium Hospital, 0424 Oslo, Norway
The Norwegian Cancer Registry, 0304 Oslo, Norway

Tom Børge Johannesen
The Norwegian Cancer Registry, 0304 Oslo, Norway

Øyvind S. Bruland
Department of Oncology, Oslo University Hospital, Norwegian Radium Hospital, 0424 Oslo, Norway
Institute of Clinical Medicine, University of Oslo, 0318 Oslo, Norway

Jody E. Hooper
Department of Pathology, Johns Hopkins Medicine, 600 N. Wolfe Street, Pathology B-106, Baltimore, MD 21287, USA

Emma L. Cantor, Macgregor S. Ehlen and Avirup Banerjee
Pediatric Cancer Biology Program, Papé Family Pediatric Research Institute, Oregon Health and Science University, 3181 S.W. Sam Jackson Park Road, Portland, OR 97239, USA
Department of Pediatrics, Oregon Health and Science University, 3181 S.W. Sam Jackson Park Road, Portland, OR 97239, USA

Suman Malempati
Department of Pediatrics, Oregon Health and Science University, 3181 S.W. Sam Jackson Park Road, Portland, OR 97239, USA

Peter Stenzel and Randy L. Woltjer
Department of Pathology, Oregon Health and Science University, 3181 S.W. Sam Jackson Park Road, Portland, OR 97239, USA

Regina Gandour-Edwards
University of California Davis School of Medicine and Cancer Center, Sacramento, CA 95817, USA

Pali Kaur, Carol J. Bult and Susan D. Airhart
The Jackson Laboratory, 1650 Santa Ana Avenue, Sacramento, CA 95838, USA

Neal C. Goodwin
The Jackson Laboratory, 1650 Santa Ana Avenue, Sacramento, CA 95838, USA
Champions Oncology, Hackensack, NJ 07601, USA

Yan Yang
The Jackson Laboratory, 1650 Santa Ana Avenue, Sacramento, CA 95838, USA
Leo Universal, Inc., Torrance, CA 90505, USA

Charles Keller
Pediatric Cancer Biology Program, Papé Family Pediatric Research Institute, Oregon Health and Science University, 3181 S.W. Sam Jackson Park Road, Portland, OR 97239, USA
Department of Pediatrics, Oregon Health and Science University, 3181 S.W. Sam Jackson Park Road, Portland, OR 97239, USA
Children's Cancer Therapy Development Institute, Beaverton, OR 97005, USA

Mei Sheng Duh, Jasmina I. Ivanova, Patrick Lefebvre and Paul Karner
Analysis Group, Inc., 111 Huntington Avenue, Tenth Floor, Boston, MA 02199, USA

Michelle D. Hackshaw and Lesley-Ann N. Miller
GlaxoSmithKline, Philadelphia, PA 19102, USA

Gregory Kruse
University of Pennsylvania, Philadelphia, PA 19104, USA

Bruce Wong
Bruce Wong and Associates, Inc., Wayne, PA 19087, USA

Shailaja Raj, Marilyn M. Bui, Gregory Springett, Xiuhua Zhao, Dungsa Chen, Randy Haysek, Ricardo Gonzalez, G. Douglas Letson, Alberto A. Chiappori and Scott J. Antonia
H. Lee. Moffitt Cancer Center, Tampa, FL 33612, USA

Anthony Conley
MD Anderson Cancer Institute, Houston, TX 77030, USA

Sergio Lavilla-Alonso and Dmitry I. Gabrilovitch
The Wistar Institute, Philadelphia, PA 19104, USA

Steven Eric Finkelstein
21st Century Oncology, Scottsdale, AZ 85251, USA
Christina Kåbjörn Gustafsson, Anders Ståhlberg, Anna Danielsson and Pierre Åman
Sahlgrenska Cancer Center, Department of Pathology, Institute of Biomedicine, University of Gothenburg, 40530 Gothenburg, Sweden

Katarina Engtröm
Department of Oncology, Institute of Medical Sciences, University of Gothenburg, Blå stråket 2, 41345 Gothenburg, Sweden

Ingela Turesson
Department of Oncology, Institute of Medical Sciences, Uppsala University, 75185 Uppsala, Sweden

Ajaz Bulbul
Department of Hematology/Oncology, Kymera Independent Physicians, Carlsbad, NM, USA
Division of Internal Medicine, Department of Hematology/Oncology, Texas Tech University Health Sciences Center School of Medicine, Lubbock, TX, USA

Bridget Noel Fahy
Department of Surgery, University of New Mexico, Albuquerque, NM, USA

Joanne Xiu
Caris Life Sciences, Phoenix, AZ, USA

Sadaf Rashad
All Saints University School of Medicine, Roseau, Dominica

Asrar Mustafa
Acharya Shri Chander College of Medical Sciences and Hospital, Jammu, India

Hatim Husain
Moores Cancer Center, University of California, San Diego, La Jolla, CA, USA

Andrea Hayes-Jordan
Department of Pediatric Surgical Oncology, University of Texas MD Anderson Cancer Center, Houston, TX, USA

Khin Thway, Jayson Wang, Taka Mubako and Cyril Fisher
Sarcoma Unit, Department of Histopathology, The Royal Marsden NHS Foundation Trust, 203 Fulham Road, London SW3 6JJ, UK

Junko Tomikawa, Chiharu Tayama, Kenichiro Hata and Kazuhiko Nakabayashi
Department of Maternal-Fetal Biology, National Research Institute for Child Health and Development, 2-10-1 Okura, Setagaya, Tokyo 157-8535, Japan

Kenzo Sonoda, Norio Wake and Kiyoko Kato
Department of Obstetrics and Gynecology, Graduate School of Medical Sciences, Kyushu University, 3-1-1 Maidashi, Higashi-ku, Fukuoka 812-8582, Japan

Tomoko Miyata
Department of Maternal-Fetal Biology, National Research Institute for Child Health and Development, 2-10-1 Okura, Setagaya, Tokyo 157-8535, Japan
Department of Obstetrics and Gynecology, Graduate School of Medical Sciences, Kyushu University, 3-1-1 Maidashi, Higashi-ku, Fukuoka 812-8582, Japan

Kohji Okamura
Department of Systems Bio Medicine, National Research Institute for Child Health and Development, 2-10-1 Okura, Setagaya, Tokyo 157-8535, Japan

Kayoko Maehara
Department of Maternal-Fetal Biology, National Research Institute for Child Health and Development, 2-10-1 Okura, Setagaya, Tokyo 157-8535, Japan
Department of Health Nutrition, Faculty of Health Science, Kio University, 4-2-4 Umami-naka, Koryo-cho, Kitakatsuragi-gun 635-0832, Japan

Hiroaki Kobayashi
Department of Obstetrics and Gynecology, Graduate School of Medical Sciences, Kyushu University, 3-1-1 Maidashi, Higashi-ku, Fukuoka 812-8582, Japan
Department of Obstetrics and Gynecology, Faculty of Medicine, Kagoshima University, 8-35-1 Sakuragaoka, Kagoshima 890-0075, Japan

D. Nordemar
Department of Radiology, Capio S:t Göran Hospital, S:t Göransplan 1, 112 81 Stockholm, Sweden

J. Öberg
Department of Medical Physics, Karolinska University Hospital, Karolinska Vägen 1, 171 76 Solna, Sweden

O. Brosjö
Department of Orthopaedics, Karolinska University Hospital, Karolinska Vägen 1, 171 76 Solna, Sweden

M. Skorpil
Department of Radiology, Karolinska University Hospital, Karolinska Vägen 1, 171 76 Solna, Sweden
Department of Molecular Medicine and Surgery, Karolinska Institute, Solnavägen 1, 171 77 Solna, Sweden

Sjoerd Kolk
Department of Rehabilitation, Radboud Institute for Health Sciences, Radboud University Medical Center, 6500 HB Nijmegen, The Netherlands

Kevin Cox and Gerjon Hannink
Orthopaedic Research Laboratory, Radboud Institute for Health Sciences, Radboud University Medical Center, 6500 HB Nijmegen, The Netherlands

Vivian Weerdesteyn
Department of Rehabilitation, Radboud Institute for Health Sciences, Radboud University Medical Center, 6500 HB Nijmegen, The Netherlands
Sint Maartenskliniek Research, 6500 GM Nijmegen, The Netherlands

Jos Bramer
Department of Orthopaedic Surgery, Amsterdam University Medical Centre, 1100 DD Amsterdam, The Netherlands

Sander Dijkstra and Michiel van de Sande
Department of Orthopaedic Surgery, Leiden University Medical Centre, 2300 RC Leiden, The Netherlands

Paul Jutte and Joris Ploegmakers
Department of Orthopaedic Surgery, Groningen University Medical Centre, 9700 RB Groningen, The Netherlands

Hendrik Schreuder and Ingrid van der Geest
Department of Orthopaedic Surgery, Radboud Institute for Health Sciences, Radboud University Medical Center, P6500 HB Nijmegen, The Netherlands

Nico Verdonschot
Orthopaedic Research Laboratory, Radboud Institute for Health Sciences, Radboud University Medical Center, 6500 HB Nijmegen, The Netherlands
Laboratory for Biomechanical Engineering, Faculty of Engineering Technology, University of Twente, 7500 AE Enschede, The Netherlands

Zhiwei Qiao and Tadashi Kondo
Division of Rare Cancer Research, National Cancer Center Research Institute, 5-1-1 Tsukiji, Chuo-ku, Tokyo 104-0045, Japan

Daisuke Kubota
Division of Rare Cancer Research, National Cancer Center Research Institute, 5-1-1 Tsukiji, Chuo-ku, Tokyo 104-0045, Japan
Division of Musculoskeletal Oncology, National Cancer Center Hospital, 5-1-1 Tsukiji, Chuo-ku, Tokyo 104-0045, Japan

Nobuyoshi Kosaka, Tomohiro Fujiwara and Takahiro Ochiya
Division of Molecular and Cellular Medicine, National Cancer Center Research Institute, 5-1-1 Tsukiji, Chuo-ku, Tokyo 104-0045, Japan

Akihiko Yoshida
Pathology and Clinical Laboratory Division, National Cancer Center Hospital, 5-1-1 Tsukiji, Chuo-ku, Tokyo 104-0045, Japan

Yasuhito Arai and Akira Kawai
Division of Cancer Genomics, National Cancer Center Research Institute, 5-1-1 Tsukiji, Chuo-ku, Tokyo 104-0045, Japan

Fumitaka Takeshita
Department of Functional Analysis, National Cancer Center Research Institute, 5-1-1 Tsukiji, Chuo-ku, Tokyo 104-0045, Japan

Raymundo A. Quintana, Jose Banchs and Heather Y. Lin
Department of Cardiology, University of Texas MD Anderson Cancer Center, 1515 Holcombe Blvd., Unit 1451, Houston, TX 77030, USA

Ridhi Gupta
Division of Hematology/Oncology, Department of Medicine, Medical University of South Carolina, Charleston, SC 29425, USA

Sean D. Raj, Anthony Conley, Vinod Ravi, Dejka Araujo, Robert S. Benjamin, Shreyaskumar Patel, Saroj Vadhan-Raj and Neeta Somaiah
Department of Sarcoma Medical Oncology, University of Texas MD Anderson Cancer Center, 1515 Holcombe Boulevard, Unit 450, Houston, TX 77030, USA

Magdalena M. Gilg, Christine Wibmer, Marko Bergovec and Andreas Leithner
Department of Orthopaedic Surgery and Traumatology, Medical University of Graz, Graz, Austria

Robert J. Grimer
Royal Orthopaedic Hospital NHS Foundation Trust, Birmingham, UK

Susanna L. Lamers, Rebecca Rose and Andrew E. Barbier
Bioinfoexperts, LLC, 718 Bayou Lane, Thibodaux, LA 70302, USA

David J. Nolan and Marco Salemi
Department of Pathology and Laboratory Medicine, University of Florida, 2055 Mowry Road, Gainesville, FL 32610, USA

Gary B. Fogel
Natural Selection, Inc., 5910 Pacific Center Blvd., 6480Weathers Place, San Diego, CA 92121, USA

Michael S. McGrath
The AIDS and Cancer Specimen Resource, University of California at San Francisco and the Department of Laboratory Medicine, Pathology, and Medicine, University of California at San Francisco, 1001 Poterero Ave, Bldg 3, Rm207, UCSF San Francisco, CA 94110, USA

Drake G. LeBrun
Perelman School of Medicine, University of Pennsylvania, Jordan Medical Education Center, 3400 Civic Center Blvd., Philadelphia, PA 19104, USA

David M. Guttmann, Jacob E. Shabason and William P. Levin
Department of Radiation Oncology, Perelman School of Medicine, University of Pennsylvania, 3400 Civic Center Boulevard, TRC 2West, Philadelphia, PA 19104, USA

Stephen J. Kovach
Department of Plastic Surgery, Perelman School of Medicine, University of Pennsylvania, 3400 Civic Center Boulevard, 7th Floor South Pavilion, Philadelphia, PA 19104, USA

Kristy L. Weber
Department of Orthopaedic Surgery, Perelman School of Medicine, University of Pennsylvania, 3400 Civic Center Boulevard, 10-179 South Pavilion, Philadelphia, PA 19104, USA

Sanjay P. Bagaria and Emmanuel Gabriel
Department of Surgery, Section of Surgical Oncology, Mayo Clinic, Jacksonville, FL, USA

Matthew Neville
Department of Biostatistics, Mayo Clinic, Scottsdale, AZ, USA

Richard J. Gray
Department of Surgery, Section of Surgical Oncology, Mayo Clinic, Phoenix, AZ, USA

Jonathan B. Ashman
Department of Radiation Oncology, Mayo Clinic, Phoenix, AZ, USA

Steven Attia
Division of Hematology/Oncology, Mayo Clinic, Jacksonville, FL, USA

Nabil Wasif
Department of Surgery, Section of Surgical Oncology, Mayo Clinic, Phoenix, AZ, USA
Robert D. and Patricia E. Kern Center for the Science of Health Care Delivery, Surgical Outcomes Division, Mayo Clinic, Phoenix, AZ, USA

S. Secondino, F. Valentino, A. Pagani and P. Pedrazzoli
Division of Medical Oncology, Fondazione IRCCS Policlinico San Matteo, Pavia, Italy

V. Grazioli, M. Pin, A. Sciortino and A. M. D'armini
Cardiothoracic Surgery Department, Fondazione IRCCS Policlinico San Matteo and Pavia University School of Medicine, Pavia, Italy

C. Klersy
Service of Biometry and Statistics, Fondazione IRCCS Policlinico San Matteo, Pavia, Italy

M. G. Callegari
Unit of Pulmonary Rehabilitation, ICS Maugeri Istituto Scientifico di Montescano, Pavia, Italy

P. Morbini and M. Paulli
Unit of Pathology, Fondazione IRCCS Policlinico San Matteo and Pavia University School of Medicine, Pavia, Italy

R. Dore
Division of Radiology, Fondazione IRCCS Policlinico San Matteo, Pavia, Italy

Paul D. Savage and Antonius A. Miller
Department of Medicine, Section of Hematology and Oncology, Wake Forest School of Medicine, Winston-Salem, NC, USA
Comprehensive Cancer Center of Wake Forest University, Wake Forest School of Medicine, Winston-Salem, NC, USA

James Lovato
Comprehensive Cancer Center of Wake Forest University, Wake Forest School of Medicine, Winston-Salem, NC, USA
Department of Biostatistical Sciences, Wake Forest School of Medicine, Winston-Salem, NC, USA

K. Bridget Brosnihan
Department of Surgical Sciences, Center for Hypertension and Vascular Research, Wake Forest School of Medicine, Winston-Salem, NC, USA

W. Jeffrey Petty
Department of Medicine, Section of Hematology and Oncology, Wake Forest School of Medicine, Winston-Salem, NC, USA
Comprehensive Cancer Center of Wake Forest University, Wake Forest School of Medicine, Winston-Salem, NC, USA
Department of Cancer Biology, Wake Forest School of Medicine, Winston-Salem, NC, USA

Varun Chowdhry
Department of Radiation Medicine, Roswell Park Comprehensive Cancer Center, Buffalo, NY, USA

Saveli Goldberg, Thomas F. DeLaney and Karen De Amorim Bernstein
Department of Radiation Oncology, Massachusetts General Hospital, Boston, MA 02114, USA

Gregory M. Cote
Division of Hematology/Oncology, Massachusetts General Hospital, Boston, MA 02114, USA

Ivan Chebib
Department of Pathology, Massachusetts General Hospital, Boston, MA 02114, USA

Jason Kim and Santiago A. Lozano-Calderón
Department of Orthopedic Oncology, Massachusetts General Hospital, Boston, MA 02114, USA

Ann Colosia and Shahnaz Khan
Market Access and Outcomes Strategy, RTI Health Solutions, 200 Park Offices Drive, Research Triangle Park, Durham, NC 27709, USA

Michelle D. Hackshaw and Alan Oglesby
US Health Outcomes, Oncology, GlaxoSmithKline, 5 Crescent Drive, Philadelphia, PA 19112, USA

James A. Kaye
Epidemiology, RTI Health Solutions, 1440 Main Street, Suite 310, Waltham, MA 02451, USA

Jeffrey M. Skolnik
US Medical Affairs, Oncology, GlaxoSmithKline, 5 Crescent Drive, Philadelphia, PA 19112, USA

Annelies Requilé, Paul M. Clement, Oliver E. Bechter, Herlinde Dumez, Annelies Verbiest and Patrick Schöffski
Department of General Medical Oncology, Leuven Cancer Institute, University Hospitals Leuven, Herestraat 49, 3000 Leuven, Belgium

Raf Sciot
Department of Pathology, University Hospitals Leuven, Leuven, Belgium

Daphne Hompes and Friedl Sinnaeve
Department of Oncology, KU Leuven and University Hospitals Leuven, Leuven, Belgium

Erik Van Limbergen
Department of Radiation Oncology, University Hospitals Leuven, Leuven, Belgium

Chung Ming Chan, Andre R. V. Spiguel, C. Parker Gibbs Jr. and Mark T. Scarborough
Division of Orthopaedic Oncology, Department of Orthopaedics and Rehabilitation, University of Florida, Gainesville, FL, USA

Adam D. Lindsay
Department of Orthopaedic Surgery, University of Connecticut, Farmington, CT, USA

Index

www.ingramcontent.com/pod-product-compliance
Lightning Source LLC
Chambersburg PA
CBHW080509200326
41458CB00012B/4142

* 9 7 8 1 6 3 2 4 1 9 0 1 9 *